D0760773

TESTICULAR CANCER

TESTICULAR CANCER

Investigation and management

Second edition

Edited by

Alan Horwich

The Royal Marsden NHS Trust and the Institute of Cancer Research
Academic Unit of Radiotherapy and Oncology
Surrey, UK

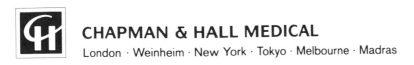

CHAPMAN & HALL MEDICAL

London · Weinheim · New York · Tokyo · Melbourne · Madras

Published by Chapman & Hall,
2–6 Boundary Row, London SE1 8HN, UK

Chapman & Hall, 2–6 Boundary Row, London SE1 8HN, UK

Chapman & Hall GmbH, Pappelallee 3, 69469 Weinheim, Germany

Chapman & Hall USA, 115 Fifth Avenue, New York, NY 10003, USA

Chapman & Hall Japan, ITP-Japan, Kyowa Building, 3F,
2–2–1 Hirakawacho, Chiyoda-ku, Tokyo 102, Japan

Chapman & Hall Australia, 102 Dodds Street, South Melbourne,
Victoria 3205, Australia

Chapman & Hall India, R. Seshadri, 32 Second Main Road, CIT East,
Madras 600 035, India

First edition 1991
Second edition 1996

© 1991, 1996 Chapman & Hall

Typeset in 10/12 Palatino by Photoprint, Torquay, Devon

Printed in Great Britain by The Alden Press, Osney Mead, Oxford

ISBN 0 412 61210 0

A catalogue record for this book is available from the British Library

Library of Congress Catalog Card Number: 96–84537

CONTENTS

CONTRIBUTORS

PROFESSOR A. HORWICH
The Royal Marsden NHS Trust and the
  Institute of Cancer Research,
Academic Unit of Radiotherapy and
  Oncology,
Downs Road, Sutton, Surrey SM2 5PT,
UK

PROFESSOR P.W. ANDREWS
Department of Biomedical Science,
University of Sheffield,
Western Bank, Sheffield S10 2TN,
UK

DR D.F. BAJORIN
Memorial Sloan-Kettering Cancer Center,
1275 York Avenue, New York, NY 10021,
USA

DR C. BOKEMEYER
Department of Internal Medicine II
Hematology, Oncology, Immunology and
  Rheumatology
Eberhard Karls University
Øtfried-Müller Str. 10
D-72076 Tübingen
Germany

DR G.J. BOSL
Head, Division of Solid Tumor Oncology,
Department of Medicine,
Memorial Sloan-Kettering Cancer Centre,
1275 York Avenue, New York, NY 10021,
USA

DR M. BOYER
Head, Department of Medical Oncology,
Royal Prince Alfred Hospital,
Sydney, Australia 2050

DR R.S.K. CHAGANTI
Head, Laboratory of Cancer Genetics,
Memorial Sloan-Kettering Cancer Centre,
1275 York Avenue, New York, NY 10021,
USA

DR M.H. CULLEN
Consultant Medical Oncologist,
Birmingham Oncology Centre,
Queen Elizabeth Hospital,
Edgbaston, Birmingham B15 2TH

DR D.P. DEARNALEY
The Royal Marsden NHS Trust and the
  Institute of Cancer Research,
Academic Unit of Radiotherapy and
  Oncology,
Downs Road, Sutton, Surrey SM2 5PT,
UK

DR L.Y. DIRIX
Department of Oncology,
Universitair Ziekenhuis,
Wilrijkstraat 10, b-2650 Edegem,
Antwerpen, Belgium

DR J.P. DONOHUE
Department of Urology,
Indiana University Cancer Center,
University Hospital,
550 North University Boulevard,
Indianapolis, Indiana 46202–5265,
USA

DR J.-P. DROZ
Centre Régional Léon Bérard,
28 Rue Laennec, 69373 Lyon,
Cedex 08, France

PROFESSOR S.D. FOSSÅ
Department of Medical Oncology and
    Radiotherapy,
The Norwegian Radium Hospital,
Montebello N-0310, Oslo 3,
Norway

MR P. GOLDSTRAW
Consultant Thoracic Surgeon,
Royal Brompton Hospital,
Sydney Street, London SW3 6NP,
UK

MR W.F. HENDRY
Genito-Urinary Surgeon,
149 Harley Street, London W1N 2DE,
UK

DR E.D. HIRSHBERG
Department of Surgical Oncology,
The Princess Margaret Hospital/Ontario
    Cancer Institute,
Toronto, Ontario, Canada

DR J. HUSBAND
Consultant Radiologist,
The Royal Marsden NHS Trust,
Department of Diagnostic Radiology,
Downs Road, Sutton, Surrey SM2 5PT,
UK

DR M.A.S. JEWETT
Professor and Chairman,
Division of Urology,
University of Toronto,
200 Elizabeth Street, EN14–205, Toronto,
Ontario M5G 2C4, Canada

DR P. LOEHRER
Indiana University School of Medicine,
Division of Hematology/Oncology,
University Hospital 1730,
550 North University Boulevard,
Indianapolis, IN 46202–5265,
USA

PROFESSOR DR H. VON DER MAASE
Department of Oncology,
Aarhus University Hospital,
DK-8000 Aarhus C, Denmark

DR M.D. MASON
Velindre Hospital, Velindre NHS Trust,
Whitchurch, Cardiff CF4 7XL,
UK

MS C. MOYNIHAN
The Royal Marsden Hospital NHS Trust,
Downs Road, Sutton, Surrey SM2 5PT,
UK

DR C.R. NICHOLS
Associate Professor of Medicine,
Indiana University School of Medicine,
Division of Hematology/Oncology,
University Hospital 1730,
550 North University Boulevard,
Indianapolis, IN 46202–5265,
USA

PROFESSOR R.T.D. OLIVER
Sir Maxwell Joseph Professor of Medical
    Oncology,
The Medical Schools of the Royal London
    and St Bartholomew's Hospital,
Whitechapel, London E1 1BB,
UK

PROFESSOR J.W. OOSTERHUIS
Scientific Director,
Department of Pathology,
Dr Daniel den Hoed Cancer Center,
Groene Hilledijk 301,
3075 EA Rotterdam, PO Box 5201,
3008 AE Rotterdam, The Netherlands

PROFESSOR A.T. VAN OOSTEROM
Department of Oncology,
Universitair Ziekenhuis,
Wilrijkstraat 10, b-2650 Edegem,
Antwerpen, Belgium

DR G. PIZZOCARO
Instituto Nazionale per lo Studio e La Cura
  dei Tumori,
Divisione de Oncologia Chirurgica Urologica,
20133 Milano, Via Venezian 1,
Italy

DR D. RAGHAVAN
Chief, Departments of Solid Tumor Oncology
  and Investigational Therapeutics,
Division of Medicine,
Roswell Park Cancer Institute,
Elm and Carlton Streets, Buffalo,
NY 14263–0001, USA

PROFESSOR M. RØRTH
Finsen Center,
Department of Oncology 5074,
The National University Hospital
  Rigshospitalet,
9 Belgdamsvej, DK-2100 Copenhagen,
Denmark

DR B.J. ROTH
Indiana University of Medicine,
Division of Hematology/Oncology,
University Hospital 1730,
550 North University Boulevard,
Indianapolis, IN 46202–5265,
USA

DR A. SANDLER
Indiana University School of Medicine,
Division of Hematology/Oncology,
University Hospital 1730,
550 North University Boulevard,
Indianapolis, IN 46202–5265,
USA

PROFESSOR H.-J. SCHMOLL
Department of Hematology/Oncology,
Hannover University Medical School,
Konstanty-Gutschow-Sraße 8,
D-30625 Hannover, Germany

PROFESSOR G. STOTER
Dr Daniel den Hoed Kliniek,
Department of Medical Oncology,
Groene Hilledijk 301, 3075 EA Rotterdam,
PO Box 5201, 3008 AE Rotterdam,
The Netherlands

DR G.M. THOMAS
Toronto–Bayview Regional Cancer Centre,
2075 Bayview Avenue,
Toronto, Ontario M4N 3M5,
Canada

DR J.A. THORNHILL
Department of Urology,
Indiana University Cancer Center,
University Hospital,
550 North University Boulevard,
Indianapolis, Indiana 46202–5265,
USA

DR N.J. VOGELZANG
Department of Medicine,
Section of Hematology/Oncology,
University of Chicago Medical Center,
5841 S. Maryland Ave., MC 2115 Chicago,
Illinois 60637–1470, USA

DR R. DE WIT
Dr Daniel den Hoed Kliniek,
Department of Medical Oncology,
Groene Hilledijk 301, 3075 EA Rotterdam,
PO Box 5201, 3008 AE Rotterdam,
The Netherlands

DR G.K. ZAGARS
MD Anderson Cancer Center,
1515 Holcombe Boulevard,
Houston, Texas 77030,
USA

PREFACE TO THE FIRST EDITION

The radiosensitivity and chemosensitivity of testicular germ cell tumours have given them considerable prominence in oncology despite their rarity. They represent the model of curable cancer, the young age of the patients contributing to the drama of successful treatment but also providing the possibility of prolonged suffering where that treatment is associated with toxicity. Clinicians caring for patients with these diseases bear a great responsibility to ensure appropriate development of surgery, radiotherapy and chemotherapy both to minimize side-effects and also to ensure effective treatment. The very high cure probability for the majority of patients makes all the more tragic those situations where treatment fails.

The pace of clinical investigation of testicular tumours has been rapid and during the last decade there has been extensive investigation of methods of reducing the side-effects of treatment. Topics addressed in this book include the role of nerve-sparing lymphadenectomy, the policy of surveillance postorchidectomy and the reduction of chemotherapy for metastatic disease in terms of both numbers of drugs and number of treatment cycles. It has become clear that success can be achieved via a number of management routes and the challenge which authors in this volume have accepted is to present the advantages and disadvantages of alternative policies so that treatment appropriate to the individual patient can be selected.

The availability of serum tumour markers which reflect accurately the tumour burden has provided a sensitive indicator of response to treatment and a precise endpoint for clinical investigation. A number of basic principles of oncology have been studied in germ cell tumours including dose response of chemotherapy, alternating regimens and treatment intensity. This volume is thus focused on management issues in germ cell tumours. Current practice is discussed in considerable detail and provides the platform from which to consider further advances.

PREFACE

Since it is now five years since the first edition of this monograph was published, the controversies and management recommendations presented then have been informed considerably by results of both laboratory research and clinical investigations. Furthermore, new chapters have been introduced to emphasize the clinical relevance of recent research on the cell and molecular biology of germ cell tumors and to highlight controversies such as in the management of small volume Stage II non-seminoma or entirely new treatment approaches such as the use of adjuvant chemotherapy in Stage I non-seminoma.

Alan Horwich
April 1996

TESTICULAR GERM CELL TUMORS: AN INTRODUCTORY OVERVIEW

A. Horwich

1.1 INTRODUCTION

Testicular germ cell tumors have a particular importance in modern oncology that transcends the emotional prioritization of treating the young patient with a life-threatening disorder. First, the incidence has been rising during this century and has almost doubled over the last 20 years (Fig. 1.1). Secondly, testicular non-seminoma is often associated with the presence within the serum of tumor marker products, namely, alpha-fetoprotein (AFP) and human chorionic gonadotrophin (HCG) as discussed in detail in Chapter 3. When present, these reflect very sensitively any changes in body tumor burden and thus

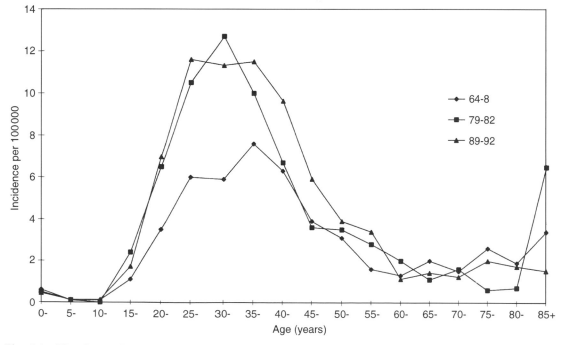

Fig. 1.1 The change in incidence of testicular cancer in the UK comparing the period 1964–8 with 1979–82 and 1989–92. (Data from Thames Cancer Registry.)

Testicular Cancer: Investigation and management. Second edition. Edited by Professor A. Horwich.
Published in 1996 by Chapman & Hall. ISBN 0 412 61210 0.

	Etiology	Diagnosis	Staging	Prognosis	Stage I seminoma	Stage II seminoma	Stage III/IV seminoma	Stage I teratoma	Metastatic teratoma	Response	Follow-up
Management phases	Maldescent CIS Isochromosome 12p Familial risk	Delay Screening	Markers RPLND MRI PET	Histology Stage Markers Age	Surveillance RT Dose and fields	RT Fields Primary chemotherapy	Single agents or Combination chemotherapy	Surveillance RPLND-nerve sparing Adjuvant chemotherapy	Risk-related chemotherapy Salvage chemotherapy Role of high dose	Resection of residual mass	Toxicity Psychosocial effects Fertility 2nd tumor

Controversies

Fig. 1.2 Testicular cancer management overview. MRI, magnetic resonance imaging; PET, positron emission tomography; CIS, carcinoma *in situ*; RPLND, retroperitoneal lymph node dissection; RT, radiotherapy.

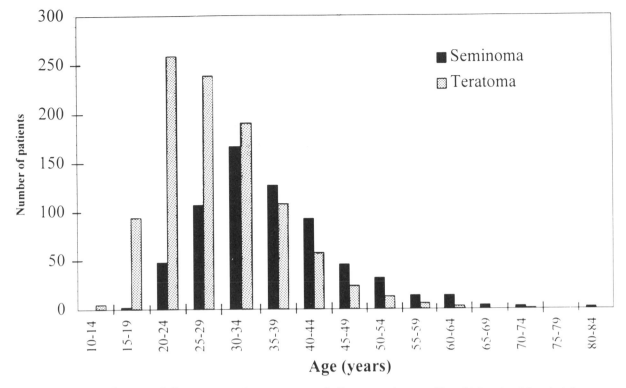

Fig. 1.3 Incidence at different ages of seminoma and all non-seminomas (Royal Marsden Hospital data, 1980–94.)

enable particularly sensitive monitoring of response to treatment. They are used also in diagnosis, prognosis, assessment of relapse and radiolocalization. Thirdly, these tumors are highly sensitive to both chemotherapy and radiotherapy and thus provide a model of a curable neoplasm.

Clinical management of testicular germ cell tumors is optimal in the context of a multi-disciplinary team. Phases of management are simplified in Fig. 1.2, and it is in the over-lap of these phases that the multidisciplin-ary approach most clearly demonstrates its strength. The phases illustrated in Fig. 1.2 will be taken as the structure for presenting an introductory overview to clinical manage-ment of germ cell tumors with reference, where appropriate, to the detailed discussion of controversial issues in subsequent chapters.

1.2 EPIDEMIOLOGY

The peak incidence of testicular cancer is be-tween the ages of 20 and 34 (Fig. 1.3) when it is the most common malignancy in men. A White male has a 1 in 500 chance of develop-ing testicular cancer (Davies, 1981). There is a 10-year age difference between the peak incidence of seminoma (median 37 years) and malignant teratoma (27 years), with com-bined tumors occurring at an intermediate age (Pugh and Cameron, 1976). Germ cell tumors are uncommon over the age of 50 years when most testicular cancers are either malignant lymphoma or spermatocytic sem-inoma. The rise in incidence noted in the UK, USA, Denmark, New Zealand and other developed countries does not affect North American Blacks, in whom there is no early age incidence peak (Schottenfeld and Warshauer, 1982).

The review by Waterhouse *et al.* (1982) *Cancer Incidence in Five Continents* indicates that the highest 5-year incidence rates are in White males from the USA, Scandinavia and western Europe. Low rates are found in Asians, Africans, Puerto Ricans and North American Blacks.

Within Europe there is a particularly low incidence in Spain, with a cumulative risk of less than 1 per 1000 in the 1950 cohort, compared with 3–5 per 1000 in France, Italy or Germany. For both Norway and Denmark there was an intriguing dip in the upward trend in incidence for cohorts born around the time of the Second World War (Coleman *et al.*, 1993).

1.3 ETIOLOGICAL FACTORS

A range of etiological factors have been investigated including cryptorchidism, inguinal hernia, trauma, rural dwelling, marital status, mumps orchitis, religion, occupation and hormonal background. A study of men in the army who developed testicular cancer between 1950 and 1970 reported a relative risk of 8.8 for maldescent and 2.9 for previous hernia operation, although some of these may in fact have been corrections of maldescent. Neither mumps orchitis nor marital status was found to be relevant (Morrison, 1976). A study of US army recruits revealed that 3.6% of those with testicular cancer had maldescent compared with the overall incidence in all recruits of 0.25% (relative risk 14).

Extensive publicity about the use of diethylstilbestrol (DES) in pregnancy led to investigation of this factor. However, this drug was not used in Denmark where testicular cancer incidence has risen at least as rapidly as in the USA and UK. Similarly, time patterns of incidence of testicular cancer do not reflect DES usage in the USA (Schottenfeld, Warshauer and Sherlock, 1980).

Sixty-nine of 724 testicular cancer patients diagnosed at the Royal Marsden Hospital between 1975 and 1984 had a history of undescended testis (Pike, Chilvers and Peckham, 1986). The distribution of age at orchidopexy was not statistically significantly different from the 'expected' distribution (men not developing tumors); however, only four patients had had orchidopexy under the age of 4-years and it is therefore unclear whether early orchidopexy reduces the subsequent risk of developing testicular cancer. Cryptorchidism is found in about 10% of testicular cancer patients and may also increase the risk of bilateral disease, as discussed more fully in Chapter 29.

Cryptorchidism is also increasing in incidence. A study by the John Radcliffe Hospital Cryptorchidism Study Group (1986) revealed a 65% increase between 1960 and 1984. If cryptorchidism and testicular cancer share etiological factors then the rising incidence of cryptorchidism now would suggest that the rise in testicular cancers will continue over the next 20 years.

There is a significant familial risk of testicular cancer. In a case–control comparison of 794 testicular cancer patients, eight patients (1%) had a brother and four patients (0.5%) had a father with a previous diagnosis of testicular cancer at the time of their own diagnosis. Two out of 794 controls (0.3%) had a first degree relative with testicular cancer (Forman *et al.*, 1992). Thus for the brother of a patient with testicular cancer the cumulative risk of developing this tumor by the age of 50 years appeared to be 2.2%, resulting in a relative risk of 9.8 compared with the general population. The Royal Marsden Hospital data base contained 37 families with more than one affected member deriving from a total of 1800 patients on the data base. Most of the families contained only two affected members though there are occasional reports of more. The conclusion would be that a proportion of testis cancer is likely to be due to genetic predisposition. The pattern would best fit a dominant gene with low penetrance,

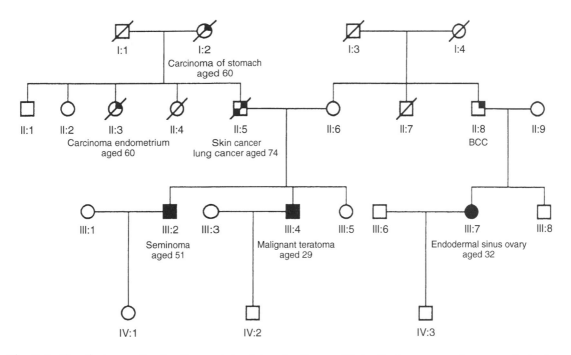

Fig. 1.4 Family tree – the family contained two brothers with testicular cancer whose cousin had an ovarian germ cell tumor. Squares represent males, circles represent females and solid elements indicate incidence of a cancer. (Figure supplied by Dr R. Huddart.)

in which case a significant proportion of sporadic cases could also be related to this gene. Two families were noted also to contain a member with an ovarian germ cell tumor (Fig. 1.4) (Huddart *et al.*, In press).

1.3.1 STUDIES IN PROGRESS

The US collaborative perinatal project provided data for review from pregnancies between 1958 and 1965 and children were examined up to 7 years of age (Depue, 1984). This led to the hypothesis that abnormal levels of free estrogen in the mother led to hypoplastic testes and maldescent; further analyses of this project will provide data on incidence of testicular cancer. Similarly, a prospective analysis of 6000 consecutive male births at the Radcliffe Infirmary in Oxford will also provide information on details of pregnancy, cryptorchidism and orchidopexy.

Carcinoma *in situ* (CIS) is discussed in detail in Chapter 29. A recent interest in CIS as the premalignant phase of testicular germ cell tumors has been stimulated by Danish studies of the contralateral testes of men with testicular cancer. Twenty-seven of 500 patients had CIS and amongst these 27 the risk of progression to invasive tumor was 50% within 5 years (von der Maase, Giwercman and Skakkebæk, 1986). No tumors developed in the contralateral testes of the remaining 473 patients. The lesion was more common in patients with a history of maldescent or with an atrophic contralateral testis, and the diagnosis was worth making since it appears that progression can be prevented by doses of radiotherapy too low to impair hormone production from the testis, although certainly sufficient to cause sterility (von der Maase *et al.*, 1986; Read, 1987).

A current Medical Research Council Testicular Tumour Working Party study suggests routine biopsy of the contralateral testis in those patients with primary germ cell tumors who are at particularly high risk of contralateral CIS, i.e. those with maldescent or an atrophic contralateral testis.

1.4 PATHOLOGY

Two histological classifications of germ cell tumor pathology are in current use, the World Health Organisation (WHO) classification (Mostofi and Sobin, 1977), and the British Testicular Tumour Panel classification (Pugh and Cameron, 1976). These are illustrated in Table 1.1. Both classifications will be used in this book and in general teratoma differentiated will be taken to be synonymous with teratoma mature; malignant teratoma intermediate (MTI) will be taken to be synonymous either with teratoma with malignant transformation, or with embryonal carcinoma with teratoma, malignant teratoma undifferentiated (MTU) will be taken to be synonymous with embryonal carcinoma, and malignant teratoma trophoblastic (MTT) will be taken to be synonymous with choriocarcinoma with or without embryonal carcinoma and/or teratoma.

Of 1750 patients with germ cell tumors presenting to the Royal Marsden Hospital between 1980 and 1994, 659 (38%) were pure seminomas. Occasionally these contain syncytial giant cells and can be associated with elevated serum concentration of HCG, although this is rarely more than a few hundred international units per liter even in the presence of bulky disease. The two major subtypes of seminoma are classical and spermatocytic (about 3%). Some authorities feel that a subgroup of classical seminoma called 'anaplastic seminoma' may be adverse (Maier and Sulak, 1973). Spermatocytic seminoma is not associated with carcinoma *in situ*. It occurs predominantly in elderly men (Talerman, 1980) and metastasis is very rare.

Classical seminoma may be associated with lymphocytic infiltration, although this is not relevant to prognosis. It is characteristically associated with an indolent clinical course. Metastases occur in only 20–30% of patients. First stage nodes are in the para-aortic region unless there has been previous inguinal surgery when the ipsilateral inguinal or femoral regions may be involved; hematogenous spread is rare.

1.4.1   MALIGNANT TERATOMA

The distribution of histological subtypes of non-seminomatous germ cell tumors in 1001 patients presenting to the Royal Marsden Hospital between 1980 and 1994 is shown in Fig. 1.5.

1.4.1.1   Teratoma differentiated

This accounts for approximately 5% of tumors and histologically no malignant tissues can be seen and the cells are morphologically benign. Despite careful examination of the primary

Table 1.1 Histological classifications

British Testicular Tumours Panel *(Pugh and Cameron, 1976)*	World Health Organisation *(Mostofi and Sobin, 1977)*
Seminoma	Seminoma
Teratoma differentiated (TD)	Teratoma Mature Immature
Malignant teratoma intermediate (MTI)	Teratoma with malignant transformation, embryonal carcinoma and teratoma
Malignant teratoma undifferentiated (MTU)	Embryonal carcinoma, polyembryoma
Malignant teratoma trophoblastic (MTT)	Choriocarcinoma with or without embryonal carcinoma and/or teratoma
Yolk sac tumor	Yolk sac tumor

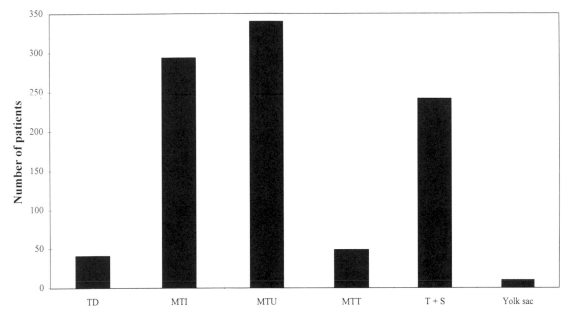

Fig. 1.5 Histological subtypes of primary testicular non-seminomas. TD, teratoma differentiated; MTI, malignant teratoma intermediate; MTU, malignant teratoma undifferentiated; MTT, malignant teratoma trophoblastic; T, teratoma; S, seminoma. (Royal Marsden Hospital data, 1980–94.)

tumor some patients with apparently fully differentiated disease can exhibit metastasis.

1.4.1.2 Malignant teratoma undifferentiated (or embryonal carcinoma)

This form of tumor does not contain differentiated tissue; it is often combined with other germ cell tumor elements and the combination of this tumor with teratoma is designated teratocarcinoma or malignant teratoma intermediate. Malignant teratoma undifferentiated accounts for approximately 37% of patients.

1.4.1.3 Malignant teratoma intermediate

More than 50% of teratoma are of this subtype. It is notable that metastatic disease may be comprised of a range of different morphologies even when the primary appears to be pure embryonal carcinoma (Ray *et al.*, 1974; Donohue, Zachary and Maynard, 1982; Oosterhuis *et al.*, 1983).

1.4.1.4 Malignant teratoma trophoblastic

To diagnose this adverse subgroup of testicular tumors, both syncytiotrophoblast and cytotrophoblast must be present, arranged together in a papillary pattern with syncytial tissue layered over the cytotrophoblast. It is very rarely composed of pure trophoblastic tissue. This variant may pursue a particularly aggressive course, often presenting with widespread metastatic disease throughout the lungs, and also with metastases in the liver or brain (Andreyev, Dearnaley and Horwich, 1993). It is usually associated with a high concentration of serum of HCG. The primary tumor frequently exhibits vascular invasion and the metastatic deposits may be hemorrhagic, causing hemoptysis.

1.4.1.5 Combined tumor

This tumor contains both teratomatous and seminomatous elements and the age incidence is in between that of teratoma and seminoma (Pugh and Cameron, 1976). It forms approximately 14% of testicular tumors and clinically behaves like a non-seminomatous tumor. Combined tumors may metastasize with both or either germ cell tumor elements (Ray *et al.*, 1974).

1.4.2   IMMUNOHISTOCHEMISTRY

As described in Chapter 3, germ cell tumors are associated with relatively specific and sensitive tumor markers including AFP, HCG and placental-like alkaline phosphatase (PLAP). Alpha-fetoprotein is usually associated with evidence of yolk-sac differentiation in germ cell tumors. It can also be produced in hepatocellular carcinomas and some tumors of the gastrointestinal tract. Human chorionic gonadotrophin is associated with trophoblastic elements and it has also been demonstrated in cancers of the liver, pancreas, lung, breast, stomach, uterus, prostate and bladder. Placental-like alkaline phosphatase can be used as an immunohistochemical marker for germ cell tumors. It also stains most of the abnormal cells in carcinoma *in situ* (Jacobsen and Norgaard-Pedersten, 1984).

1.5   CLINICAL PRESENTATION

Approximately 90–95% of men with germ cell tumors present with a testicular primary (Table 1.2), the remainder presenting with metastatic disease with a testicular primary that is either occult or has regressed (Azzopardi, Mostofi and Theiss, 1961; Powell, Hendry and Peckham, 1983). Presentations at extragonadal

Table 1.2 Presentation of germ cell tumors (Royal Marsden Hospital data, 1989–1994)

Tumor	Number
Testicular primary	1623
Occult or retroperitoneal primary	74
Second primary germ cell tumor	18
Mediastinal primary	35

sites are discussed fully in Chapter 28. Some centers regard extragonadal presentation as adverse (Chapter 7); however, this may be because of diagnostic difficulty and delays in diagnosis, such that advanced disease is often extensive at presentation, rather than because the illness is more biologically aggressive (McAleer, Nicholls and Horwich, 1992).

The characteristic findings on examination of a testicular primary are that the tumor is hard and painless. However, about 15% of patients do have pain and this leads to a mistaken diagnosis of epididymo-orchitis and hence delay in diagnosis of tumor. Other differential diagnoses include tuberculosis epididymis, gamma of the testis, torsion, hydrocele or hernia.

Delayed diagnosis is common, but is more often due to delay in seeking medical advice than to delay in the correct diagnosis being made by the physician. It is for this reason that public education campaigns have sought to increase awareness of the illness; there have also been suggestions that health education should include a recommendation to practice regular self-examinations. Self-examination would lead to speedier diagnosis only if the cause of delay was the patient's lack of awareness of an abnormality in the testis rather than a reluctance to bring such abnormality to the attention of the medical profession. In a review of 257 Royal Marsden Hospital patients who had testicular teratoma diagnosed by orchidectomy between 1980 and 1986, the maximum period of delay between symptoms and orchidectomy was 3 years, with a median delay of 2.5 months and mean delay of 3.9 months (Chilvers *et al.*, 1989). Equal numbers of patients fell into three delay categories: 0–49 days, 50–99 days, 100 days or more. Table 1.3 shows the relationship between delay and known prognostic factors. Of those presenting within 100 days of onset of symptoms 55% had Stage I tumors compared with 41% who delayed longer ($p = 0.05$). Of men delaying

Table 1.3 Delay in diagnosis of testicular teratoma and prognostic factors at presentation (Royal Marsden Hospital, 1980–1986)

Prognostic factor	Delay (days)							
	0–49		50–99		100 or more		All	
Stage								
I	45	(54%)	42	(55%)	39	(41%)	126	(49%)
II	17	(20%)	15	(19%)	27	(28%)	56	(23%)
III and IV	22	(26%)	20	(26%)	30	(31%)	72	(28%)
Total	84	(100%)	77	(100%)	96	(100%)	257	(100%)
Markers								
Low*	25	(60%)	22	(61%)	32	(55%)	79	(58%)
High	17	(40%)	14	(39%)	26	(45%)	57	(42%)
Total	42	(100%)	36	(100%)	58	(100%)	136	(100%)
Tumor volume								
Stage I marker-negative	42	(50%)	41	(53%)	38	(40%)	121	(47%)
Small†	29	(35%)	23	(30%)	26	(27%)	38	(30%)
Large†	7	(8%)	8	(10%)	16	(17%)	31	(12%)
Very large†	6	(7%)	5	(6%)	16	(17%)	27	11%)
Total	84	(100%)	77	(100%)	96	(100%)	257	(100%)

See Chilvers *et al.*, 1989.
* AFP <500 IU l^{-1} and HCG <1000 IU l^{-1}.
† MRC classification (MRC 1985).

from 100 days or more 13% had very large tumors with high marker levels (Medical Research Council, 1985), compared with 3% of those with earlier presentation (Chilvers *et al.*, 1989). Some authors have found a relationship between survival and delay in diagnosis (Oliver, 1985; Thornhill, *et al.*, 1987). In Royal Marsden Hospital patients analysis of relapse-free survival after chemotherapy in patients with metastatic disease showed an inverse relationship between delay and survival ($p < 0.5$). However, Fosså, Klepp and Elgjo (1981) found no relationship between survival and delay. The results would not suggest that in the individual patient delay is unimportant, however; the hypothesis would be that rapidly growing tumors may lead to early presentation yet, nevertheless, comprise an adverse subgroup. In the individual, early diagnosis offered the highest chance of finding low stage disease. Raising of public awareness of the tumor and its high curability is an important goal (Jones, 1987).

Diagnosis is confirmed by inguinal orchidectomy. This procedure allows withdrawal of the testis intact and, since the dense membrane of the tunica albuginea tends to limit local spread of tumor, local recurrence is exceptionally rare. In patients where the diagnosis is in doubt or especially when no primary is obvious within a testis, it may be possible to support the diagnosis by assay of tumor markers, testicular ultrasound or needle aspirate or fine needle biopsy of a metastasis. Open surgery for diagnostic purposes is not usually necessary and it appears that extensive initial resection of metastatic disease does not improve the chemotherapy cure rate (Javadpour *et al.*, 1982), possibly because of accelerated repopulation (Lange *et al.*, 1980).

Not all patients who have suffered scrotal interference by needle biopsy or scrotal incision will develop local recurrence and in many cases of germ cell tumor an expectant policy can still be followed (Kennedy, Hendry and

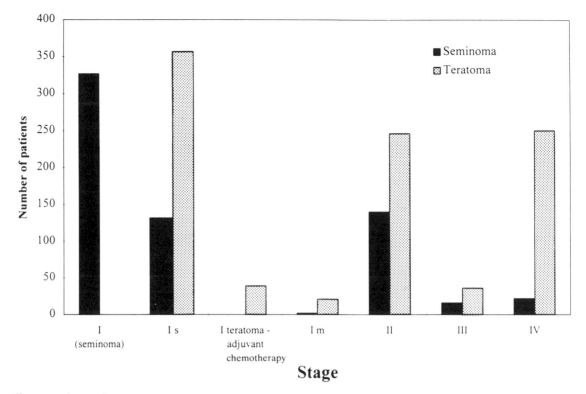

Fig. 1.6 Stage distribution of testicular germ cell tumors staged by CT scan (RMH 1980–94). Stage I is subdivided to indicate those managed by surveillance (Is) by adjuvant radiotherapy (I (seminoma)), by adjuvant chemotherapy or by chemotherapy for metastatic disease identified by rising markers alone (Im).

Peckham, 1986). This is particularly relevant for patients who wish to preserve the fertility of the contralateral testis.

The probability of dissemination is influenced by the local extent of the primary tumor (Pugh and Cameron, 1976). This is most relevant in patients who appear otherwise to have Stage I disease as discussed in Chapter 13.

1.5.1 INVESTIGATIONS

Following histological diagnosis the patient who has had an orchidectomy for germ cell tumor of the testis requires careful assessment, both of his general medical health and of the possibility of metastatic disease. The mainstays of staging are sequential serum tumor marker assays (Chapter 3) and radiological imaging (Chapter 2). Fig. 1.6 shows the stage distribution at presentation of patients with testicular primary tumors presenting to the Royal Marsden Hospital Testicular Tumour Unit between 1980 and 1994, an era when all patients were staged with computer tomography (CT) scanning of the thorax and abdomen and with tumor marker assays. Over the last 5 years, with increasing sophistication of computer tomographic imaging, lymphography has been abandoned as a standard investigation although it is occasionally employed as a supplement for inpatients on surveillance for Stage I disease. It is important to realize that there is some variation in CT scanning techniques between different centers, especially relating to slice thickness and extent of use of intravenous and oral contrast, and that these may lead to a variation in the sensitivity of the investigation. This is discussed more fully in Chapter 2. It is also important to be aware that detailed investigation may discern abnormalities that are unrelated to the diagnosis of germ cell tumor, and noteworthy in the Royal Marsden Hospital experience are six patients with asymptomatic sarcoidosis, one patient with a small hypernephroma, and one patient with a pheochromocytoma arising in the left adrenal gland.

Patients with central nervous system (CNS) symptoms are investigated by either CT or magnetic resonance imaging (MRI), but it is debatable to what extent the CNS should be investigated in patients who do not have relevant symptoms. Our policy is to perform MRI scanning of the brain in patients with more than 20 lung metastases or with serum HCG of more than 20 000 IU l^{-1}.

The assessment of the contralateral testis as it relates to the possible development of a second germ cell tumor is discussed in Chapter 29. However, patients interested in extending their families should also have seminal analysis to determine the possibility of sperm banking. A large proportion of the patients assessed following orchidectomy are either oligospermic or azoospermic (Hendry *et al.*, 1983). However, their fertility may recover spontaneously (Horwich, Nicholls and Hendry, 1988) and many patients with some spermatogenesis prior to either radiotherapy or chemotherapy will recover fertility with time as long as any radiation to the contralateral testis is minimized and as long as their chemotherapy does not contain an alkylating agent (Drury, Hendry and Peckham, 1986; Fosså *et al.*, 1986; Horwich *et al.*, 1991). The probability of recovering fertility has been analyzed in 178 patients treated with cisplatin-based chemotherapy, and was found to be increased in those with high pretreatment count, those aged less than 30

years and in patients receiving more than four chemotherapy cycles (Horwich *et al.*, 1995).

1.6 AN OVERVIEW OF THE MANAGEMENT OF GERM CELL TUMORS

1.6.1 STAGE I SEMINOMA

The conventional management of Stage I seminoma is with adjuvant retroperitoneal irradiation to para-aortic and ipsilateral pelvic nodes Both this policy and the alternative of surveillance alone are discussed in Chapters 8 and 9. The cure rate of this illness is very high and the major issues relating to a treatment decision are the personal circumstances of the patient relating to dependability for surveillance or to plans to start a family.

A second issue is the extent of the radiation field when adjuvant radiotherapy is employed. Some centers include inguinofemoral nodes as well as pelvic and para-aortic nodes. However, the suggestion from surveillance studies (Chapter 9) would be that the initial site of relapse is in the para-aortic nodes and this would be supported by the results of lymphadenectomy for non-seminoma (Chapter 15). The Medical Research Council has therefore carried out a prospective trial comparing a para-aortic field alone with a conventional para-aortic plus ipsilateral pelvic field. Recruitment is complete; the results so far have been presented only in abstract. This indicated that the risk of pelvic recurrence in patients treated only with para-aortic field was of the order of 2% (Fosså *et al.*, 1996).

1.6.2 METASTATIC SEMINOMA

Small volume Stage II seminoma was conventionally treated with radiotherapy; however, the results of treatment worsen as the diameter of the abdominal node enlarges (Gregory and Peckham, 1986). Also, a large para-aortic node mass is difficult to irradiate without renal damage and many centers, therefore, use primary radiotherapy for patients with nodal masses less than 5 cm in diameter. This is extensively discussed in Chapter 10. Recently we have explored the addition of a single cycle of carboplatin to conventional radiotherapy for patients with small volume Stage II seminoma, to reduce the risk of supradiaphragmatic relapse (Yao *et al.*, 1994).

For Stage III and IV seminoma the major modality is combination chemotherapy based on platinum, although there is controversy over how aggressive this chemotherapy need be in view of the results of single agent platinum compounds (Oliver, 1984; Horwich *et al.*, 1989; Horwich and Dearnaley, 1992). There is also controversy over the management of the residual mass. This is a common finding on CT scans, especially when the original mass was bulky and the issue of further treatment was raised since the commonest site of recurrence is also the original involved site. The judgement of seminoma response and assessment and treatment of the residual mass are discussed in Chapter 12. Surgical excision can be difficult since seminoma tends to heal with an infiltrative fibrosis and the major question is whether to employ radiotherapy following chemotherapy. This is easy in Stage II disease, but for more extensive presentations of seminoma radiotherapy would involve very large fields and a subsequent compromise of bone marrow function.

1.6.3   STAGE I NON-SEMINOMA

A number of options exist for management of clinical Stage I non-seminoma, including surveillance and staging lymphadenectomy with chemotherapy either as an adjuvant for node-positive patients or upon relapse. Again the optimal management is likely to depend upon details of the individual patient, including personal preferences and dependability for follow-up. In countries such as England, where follow-up is relatively easy, the policy

of surveillance has been shown to be safe and spares 70% of patients further treatment following their orchidectomy (Chapter 13). The rationale for staging lymphadenectomy and recent innovations in technique designed to avoid the side-effect of dry ejaculation is described in Chapters 15 and 16. A recent innovation has been the investigation of adjuvant chemotherapy following orchidectomy and this is discussed in Chapter 14.

1.6.4   METASTATIC NON-SEMINOMA

The chemotherapy of non-seminoma represents one of the most exciting and successful stories in modern oncology. Results from the Royal Marsden Hospital before 1975 indicate a cure rate in bulky abdominal or more advanced metastatic non-seminoma of less than 10%; this has risen to approximately 90% on current management. The major advances were the development of combinations based on vinblastine and bleomycin (Samuels *et al.*, 1976) and subsequently the incorporation of high dose cisplatin into the platinum/vinblastine/bleomycin (PVB) schedule (Einhorn and Donohue, 1977). The exquisite chemosensitivity of these tumors may relate to their predisposition to undergo apoptosis (Huddart *et al.*, 1995).

Current issues relate to the need for aggressive chemotherapy in patients with good prognosis and, secondly, how to increase efficacy of chemotherapy in the adverse group. Regrettably there is no international uniformity on classification of patients into good and poor prognosis groups and the issues underlying these classifications are discussed in Chapter 7. The Germ Cell Tumour Consensus Conference held in Hull, UK, in 1989 provided a forum for discussion between the European Organisation for Research into Treatment of Cancer (EORTC) Genito-Urinary Group and the Medical Research Council Testicular Tumour Working Party. Some 1400 patients treated with chemotherapy for metastatic non-seminoma were evaluable and consensus was reached on definition of the adverse prognostic subgroup. The Medical Research Council analyzed survival in 795 patients treated with a range of cisplatin-based chemotherapy combinations for metastatic non-seminoma between 1982 and 1986. Prognosis was stable during this era. Median follow-up was 45 months and 96% of the survivors were followed for more than 2 years (Mead *et al.*, 1992). The overall 3-year survival was 85% (95% confidence intervals, range 81–89%). Multivariate analysis revealed that the most significant adverse factors were:

1. liver, bone, or brain involvement;
2. high serum AFP (more than 1000 IU l^{-1}); or high serum HCG (>10 000 IU l^{-1});
3. twenty or more lung metastases;
4. mediastinal mass more than 5 cm in transverse diameter.

The mortality rate was 17% with none of these features, 24% with one feature, 45% with two features and 73% with three features. The adverse prognostic group was thus defined as the patient with at least one of these adverse factors whose 3-year survival probability would therefore be 68%.

As described in Chapter 7, a more recent prognostic factor classification has been agreed between germ cell tumor trial groups on both sides of the Atlantic (Mead, 1995). This identifies three major prognostic groups in metastatic non seminomas; for most patients the classification is based on tumor marker assays, although mediastinal primary site and the presence of liver, bone or brain metastases are retained as important factors. The new classification also includes concentration of lactate dehydrogenase, which is particularly adverse if present in concentration more than ten times the upper limit of normal.

This allows subdivision of patients with metastatic non-seminoma by prognosis. In the adverse group the main challenge is to increase the efficacy of chemotherapy. A number of approaches are outlined in Chapters 21–24, including dose escalation of cisplatin, reduction of intercycle interval (accelerated chemotherapy) and the use of alternating regimens. High dose chemotherapy with autologous bone marrow transplantation has been used predominantly as a salvage chemotherapy, but clearly this technique is likely to be employed earlier in the disease where a particularly adverse prognosis can be recognized (Chapter 25).

Those patients not falling into the adverse subgroup are regarded as having a good prognosis and an important issue is the reduction of treatment-related toxicity. There has now been extensive study of the role of bleomycin in these patients (Chapter 20), a particularly important issue since pneumonitis can be fatal. Other significant advances have been the documentation of the lack of efficacy of maintenance therapy and more recently the demonstration that three rather than four courses of chemotherapy are sufficient in good prognosis patients (Chapter 19). Additionally the use of the less toxic platinum analogues has been investigated and shown to be less effective than cisplatin (Bajorin *et al.*, 1992; Horwich *et al.*, 1994).

Following chemotherapy many patients are left with a residual mass that may contain undifferentiated tumor, fully differentiated teratoma, or merely fibrosis/necrosis (Chapter 26). A standard policy in many centers is to resect this residual mass for both diagnostic and therapeutic purposes, and Chapters 26 and 27 outline these techniques and their results with regard to both thoracic and abdominal metastases. The question remains as to whether this form of surgery is needed in all patients with residual masses, since clearly it would be noncontributory in patients who have only fibrosis or necrosis evident on histology of the resected specimen. An uncertain number of patients with residual differentiated teratoma have suffered late relapse, sometimes of non-germ cell malignancy. Positron emission tomography (PET) of uptake of flurodeoxyglucose may be useful

Table 1.4 Royal Marsden Hospital staging classification

Stage		Definition
I	M	Rising postorchidectomy markers only
II		*Abdominal lymphadenopathy*
	A	<2 cm
	B	2–5 cm
	C	>5 cm
III		*Supradiaphragmatic lymphadenopathy*
	O	No abdominal disease
	ABC	Abdominal node size as in Stage II
IV		*Extralymphatic metastases*
	L1	≤3 lung metastases
	L2	>3 lung metastases all <2 cm diameter
	L3	>3 lung metastases 1 or more >2 cm
	H+	Liver involvement

to determine the presence of residual active disease (Wilson, *et al.*, 1995).

After chemotherapy it is important to maintain close follow-up of patients both to document clearly the long-term success or failure rate and to identify any late toxicity of treatment, which may be relevant to the initial management decision. There is a not insignificant price that the patient pays for successful treatment, in terms of both physical and psychological sequelae. The very success of treatment of this condition with the consequent prolonged and hopefully normal life span of the patient places a great burden of responsibility on the oncologist to take steps to minimize the side-effects of both the illness and its treatment. In this context, the reports of an increased risk of leukemia following etoposide therapy are a cause for concern (Pedersen-Bjergaard *et al.*, 1991; Nichols *et al.*, 1993).

1.7 STAGING

A number of staging systems are in current use (Chapter 7) and will be referred to in individual chapters in this book. Table 1.4 shows the Royal Marsden Hospital staging classification (Peckham, 1971), which is based on CT scans of the thorax and abdomen and on assay of the serum HCG and AFP. The prognoses in Table 1.5 relate to the multi-center prognostic factor analyses performed by the Medical Research Council Working Party on Testicular Tumours (1985) (Mead *et al.*, 1992).

REFERENCES

Andreyev, H.J.N., Dearnaley, D.P. and Horwich, A. (1993) Testicular nonseminoma with high serum human chorionic gonadotrophin: The trophoblastic teratoma syndrome. *Diagn. Oncol.*, **3**, 67–71.

Azzopardi, J.G., Mostofi, F.K. and Theiss, E.A. (1961) Lesions of testes observed in certain patients with widespread choriocarcinoma and related tumors. *Am. J. Pathol.*, **38**, 207–25.

Table 1.5 Medical Research Council prognostic factors analysis

Categories	Stages	Treatment period 1976–1982 Number of patients	Treatment period 1976–1982 3-year survival (%)	Treatment period 1982–1986 Number of patients	Treatment period 1982–1986 3-year survival (%)
Small volume	IM	18	83%	78	95%
	II III AB	106	87%	253	92%
	IV L1 L2 AB	70	75%	200	90%
Large volume	IIC IIIC	104	85%	82	82%
	IV L1 L2 C	43	77%	37	89%
Very large volume	IV L3 H+	117	54%	145	60%

Bajorin, D.F., Sarosdy, M.F., Bosl, G.J. and Mazumdar, M. (1992) Good risk germ cell tumour (GCT): A randomized trial of etoposide + carboplatin (EC) vs etoposide + cisplatin (EP). *Proc. Am. Soc. Clin. Oncol.*, **11**, 203.

Chilvers, C.E.D., Saunders, M., Bliss, J.M., Nicholls, J. and Horwich, A. (1989) Influence of delay in diagnosis on prognosis in testicular teratoma. *Br. J. Cancer*, **59**, 126–8.

Coleman, M.P., Esteve, J., Daniecki, P., Arslan, A. and Renard, H. (1993) Testis cancer, in *Trends in Cancer Incidence and Mortality* (eds WHO), IARC Scientific Publications, Lyon, pp. 521–42.

Davies, J.M. (1981) Testicular cancer in England and Wales: some epidemiological aspects. *Lancet*, **i**, 928–32.

Depue, R.H. (1984) Maternal and gestational factors affecting the risk of cryptorchidism and inguinal hernia. *Int. J. Epidemiol.*, **13**, 311–18.

Donohue, J.P., Zachary, J.M. and Maynard, B.R. (1982) Distribution of nodal metastases in non-seminomatous testis cancer. *Br. J. Urol.*, **128**, 315–20.

Drury, A., Hendry, W.F. and Peckham, M.J. (1986) Recovery of spermatogenesis in patients receiving chemotherapy for advanced testicular cancer, in *Advances in the Biosciences 55 Germ Cell Tumours II* (eds W.G. Jones *et al.*), Pergamon Press, Oxford, pp. 471–3.

Einhorn, L.H. and Donohue, J. (1977) *Cis*-diammine-dichloroplatinum, vinblastine, and bleomycin combination chemotherapy in disseminated testicular cancer. *Ann. Intern. Med.*, **87**, 293–8.

Forman, D., Oliver, R.T.D., Brett, A.R. *et al.* (1992) Familial testicular cancer: a report of the UK family register, estimation of risk and an HLA Class 1 sib-pair analysis. *Br. J. Cancer*, **65**(2), 255–62.

Fosså, S.D., Abyholm, T., Norman, N. and Jetne, V. (1986) Post-treatment fertility in patients with testicular cancer. III Influence of radiotherapy in seminoma patients. *Br. J. Urol.*, **58**, 315–19.

Fosså, S.D., Klepp, O. and Elgjo, R.F. (1981) The effect of patients's delay and doctor's delay in patients with malignant germ cell tumours. *Int. J. Androl.*, **4**, 134.

Fosså, S.D., Horwich, A., Russell, J.M., Roberts, J.P., Jakes, R., Stenning, S. on behalf of MRC Testicular Tumour Working Party, MRC Head Office, London, UK (1996) Optimal field size in adjuvant radiotherapy (XRT) of stage I seminoma – A randomised trial. *Proc. Am. Soc. Clin. Oncol.*, **15**, 239 (Abstract 595).

Gregory, C. and Peckham, M.J. (1986) Results of radiotherapy for stage II testicular seminoma. *Radiother. Oncol.*, **6**, 285–92.

Hendry, W.F., Stedronska, J., Jones, C.R. *et al.* (1983) Semen analysis in testicular cancer and Hodgkin's disease: pre- and post-treatment findings and implications for cryopreservation. *Br. J. Urol.*, **55**, 769–73.

Horwich, A. and Dearnaley, D.P. (1992) Treatment of seminoma. *Semin. Oncol.*, **19**(2), 171–80.

Horwich, A., Dearnaley, D.P., Duchesne, G.M. *et al.* (1989) Simple nontoxic treatment and advanced metastatic seminoma with carboplatin. *J. Clin. Oncol.*, **7**, 1150–6.

Horwich, A., Dearnaley, D.P., Nicholls, J. *et al.* (1991) Effectiveness of carboplatin, etoposide, bleomycin (CEB), combination chemotherapy good prognosis metastatic testicular non seminomatous germ cell tumours. *J. Clin. Oncol.*, **9**(1), 62–9.

Horwich, A., Lampe, H., Norman, A. *et al.* (1995) Fertility after chemotherapy for metastatic germ cell tumours. *Proc. Am. Soc. Clin. Oncol.*, **14**, 236.

Horwich, A., Nicholls, J. and Hendry, W.F. (1988) Seminal analysis post-orchidectomy in stage I teratoma. *Br. J. Urol.*, **62**, 79–81.

Horwich, A., Sleifer, D., Fosså, S. *et al.* (1994) A trial of carboplatin-based combination chemotherapy in good prognosis metastatic testicular non seminoma. *Proc. Am. Soc. Clin. Oncol.*, **13**, 231.

Huddart, R.A., Thompson, C., Nicholls, J., Horwich, A. and Houlston, R. Are ovarian germ cell tumours part of the familial testicular cancer syndrome? *J. Med. Genetic.* (in press).

Huddart, R.A., Titley, J., Robertson, D. *et al.* (1995) Programmed cell death in response to chemotherapeutic agents in human germ cell tumour lines. *Eur. J. Cancer*, **31A**(5), 739–46.

Jacobsen, G.K. and Norgaard-Pedersten, B. (1984) Placental alkaline phosphatase in testicular germ cell tumours and carcinoma *in situ* of the testis. An immunohistochemical study. *Acta Path. Microbiol. Immunol. Scand.*, **92**(A), 323–9.

Javadpour, N., Ozols, R.F., Anderson, T. *et al.* (1982) A randomized trial of cytoreductive surgery followed by chemotherapy versus chemotherapy alone in bulky stage III testicular cancer with poor prognostic features. *Cancer*, **50**, 2004–10.

John Radcliffe Hospital Cryptorchidism Study Group (1986) Cryptorchidism: an apparent substantial increase since 1960. *Br. Med. J.*, **293**, 1401–4.

Jones, W.G. (1987) Testicular cancer. *Br. Med. J.*, **295**, 1488.

Kennedy, C.L., Hendry, W.F. and Peckham, M.J. (1986) The significance of scrotal interference in stage I testicular cancer managed by orchidectomy and surveillance. *Br. J. Urol.*, **58**, 705–8.

Lange, P.H., Hekmut, K., Bosl, G., Kennedy, B.J. and Fraley, E.E. (1980) Accelerated growth of testicular cancer after cytoreductive surgery. *Cancer*, **45**(6), 1498–506.

Maier, J.G. and Sulak, M.H. (1973) Radiation therapy in malignant testis tumors. Part II: Carcinoma. *Cancer*, **32**, 1217–26.

McAleer, J.J.A., Nicholls, J. and Horwich, A. (1992) Does extragonadal presentation impart a worse prognosis to abdominal germ-cell tumors? *Eur. J. Cancer*, **28A**, 825–8.

Mead, G.M. (1995) International consensus prognostic classification for metastatic germ cell tumors treated with platinum-based chemotherapy: final report of the International Germ Cell Cancer Collaborative Group (IGCCCG). *Proc. Am. Soc. Clin. Oncol.*, **14**, 235.

Mead, G.M., Stenning, S.P., Parkinson, M.C. *et al.* (1992) The second Medical Research Council Study of prognostic factors in nonseminomatous germ cell tumours. *J. Clin. Oncol.*, **10**(1), 85–94.

Medical Research Council and Working Party on Testicular Tumours (1985) Prognostic factors in advanced non-seminomatous germ-cell testicular tumours: Results of a multicentre study. *Lancet*, **i**, 8–12.

Morrison, A.S. (1976) Some social and medical characteristics of army men with testicular cancer. *Am. J. Epidemiol.*, **104**, 511–16.

Mostofi, F.K. and Sobin, L.H. (1977) *International Histological Classification of Tumours of Testes*, World Health Organisation, Geneva.

Nichols, C.R., Breeden, E.S., Loehrer, P.J., Williams, S.D. and Einhorn, L.H. (1993) Secondary leukemia associated with a conventional dose of etoposide: review of serial germ cell tumor protocols. *J. Natl. Cancer Inst.*, **85**(1), 36–40.

Oliver, R.T.D. (1984) Surveillance for stage I seminoma and single agent *cis*-platinum for metastatic seminoma. *Proc. Am. Soc. Clin. Oncol.*, **3**, 162.

Oliver, R.T.D. (1985) Factors contributing to delay in diagnosis of testicular tumours. *BMJ*, **290**, 356.

Oosterhuis, J.W., Suurmeyer, A.J.H., Sleyfer, D.T. *et al.* (1983) Effects of multiple-drug chemo-

therapy (*cis*-diammine-dichloroplatinum, bleomycin and vinblastine) on the maturation of retroperitoneal lymph node metastases of non-seminomatous germ cell tumors of the testis. *Cancer*, **51**, 408–16.

Peckham, M.J. (1971) Investigations and staging: general aspects and staging classification, in *The Management of Testicular Tumours* (ed. M.J. Peckham), Edward Arnold, London, pp. 89–101.

Pedersen-Bjergaard, J., Daugaard, G., Hansen, S.W. *et al.* (1991) Increased risk of myelodysplasia and leukaemia after etoposide, cisplatin, and bleomycin for germ-cell tumours. *Lancet*, **338**, 359–63.

Pike, M.C., Chilvers, C. and Peckham, M.J. (1986) Effect of age at orchidopexy on risk of testicular cancer. *Lancet*, **i**, 1246–8.

Powell, S., Hendry, W.F. and Peckham, M.J. (1983) Occult germ-cell testicular tumours. *Br. J. Urol.*, **55**, 440–4.

Pugh, R.C.B. and Cameron, K.M. (1976) Teratoma, in *Pathology of the Testis* (ed. Pugh, R.C.B.), Blackwell Scientific Publications, London, pp. 199–244.

Ray, B., Steven, I., Hajdu, S.I. and Whitemore, W.F., Jr (1976) Distribution of retroperitoneal lymph node metastases in testicular germinal tumors. *Cancer*, **33**, 340–8.

Read, G. (1987) Carcinoma *in situ* of the contralateral testis. *BMJ*, **294**, 121.

Samuels, M.L., Lanzotti, V.J., Holoye, P.Y. *et al.* (1976) Combination chemotherapy in germinal cell tumor. *Cancer Treat. Rev.*, **3**, 185–204.

Schottenfeld, D. and Warshauer, M.E. (1982) Cancer epidemiology and prevention, in *Testis* (eds D. Schottenfeld and J.F. Fraumeni), W.B. Saunders, Philadelphia, pp. 947–57.

Schottenfeld, D., Warshauer, M.E. and Sherlock, S. (1980) The epidemiology of testicular cancer in young adults. *Am. J. Epidemiol.*, **112**, 232–46.

Talerman, A. (1980) Spermatocytic seminoma. Clinicopathological study of 22 cases. *Cancer*, **45**(8), 2169–76.

Thornhill, J.A., Fennelley, J.J., Kelly, D.G., Walsh, A. and Fitzpatrick, J.M. (1987) Patients delay in the presentation of testis cancer in Ireland. *Br. J. Urol.*, **59**, 447.

von der Maase, H., Giwercman, A. and Skakkebæk, N.E. (1986) Radiation treatment of carcinoma *in situ* of testis. *Lancet*, **i**, 624–5.

von der Maase, H., Rørth, M., Walbom-Jorgensen, S. *et al.* (1986) Carcinoma *in situ* of contralateral testis in patients with testicular germ cell cancer: study of 27 cases in 500 patients. *BMJ*, **293**, 1398–401.

Waterhouse, J., Muir, C., Shanmugaratnam, K. and Powell, J. (1982) *Cancer Incidence in Five Continents* (IARC Scientific Publications No. 42), International Agency for Research on Cancer, Lyon.

Wilson, C.B., Young, H.E., Ott, R.J. *et al.* (1995) Imaging metastatic testicular germ cell tumours with 18FDG positron emission tomography: prospects for detection and management. *Eur. J. Nucl. Med.*, **22**, 508–13.

Yao, W.Q., Fosså, S.D., Dearnaley, D.P. and Horwich, A. (1994) Combined single course carboplatin with radiotherapy in treatment of Stage IIA, B seminoma – a preliminary report. *Radiother. Oncol.*, **33**, 88–90.

ADVANCES IN TUMOR IMAGING 2

J. Husband

2.1 INTRODUCTION

During the last 15 years dramatic advances in the treatment of testicular tumors have been paralleled by exciting technological advances in radiology. In 1975 the first whole-body computed tomography (CT) scanners were introduced into clinical practice, and since then the technique has been rigorously researched and developed. Today highly sophisticated fast scanners with superb image quality are readily available and CT scanning has become an integral part of the management of testicular tumors. In addition to CT scanning there have been other important developments in imaging with new approaches to ultrasound and nuclear medicine techniques. Magnetic resonance imaging (MRI), the latest and most complex of all the imaging techniques, is now established as a useful tool in cancer radiology, and in certain situations may provide unique diagnostic information.

The radiological assessment of patients with testicular tumors is of critical importance, both at the time of staging and during follow-up. Following orchidectomy, the most important role of the radiologist is to identify small volume metastases but, even in those patients with obvious large volume disease, precise information about the extent of spread is required. Radiology continues to play a key role during the follow-up of patients with metastatic disease by monitoring treatment response, documenting the presence of resid-ual disease and detecting post-treatment relapse. Regular radiological studies also form an integral part of the surveillance policy in patients considered to be Stage I at the time of diagnosis. The most important radiological investigations currently used are plain chest radiographs, CT scanning and ultrasound. Lymphography, which used to play a key role in lymph node staging of testicular tumors, is now rarely used.

The detection of testicular tumor metastases will be considered according to the sites of disease, and the advantages and limitations of the different techniques discussed.

2.2 DIAGNOSIS

Imaging has a very limited role in the detection of testicular cancer, and careful examination of the swollen testicle remains the best method of diagnosis. However, during recent years ultrasound has become a useful method of imaging the testis, and is particularly valuable in patients who are difficult to examine clinically and those who present with metastases in whom an occult primary tumor of the testis is suspected (Hendry *et al.*, 1984). Ultrasound is also valuable for examining the contralateral testis to identify the small number of patients with bilateral tumors. MRI imaging may also be used to distinguish solid tumors from cysts, but is inaccurate for local staging of the primary tumor (Thurnher *et al.*, 1988).

Testicular Cancer: Investigation and management. Second edition. Edited by Professor A. Horwich. Published in 1996 by Chapman & Hall. ISBN 0 412 61210 0.

2.3 STAGING

2.3.1 LYMPH NODE METASTASES

2.3.1.1 Pattern of tumor spread

Lymphatic spread of testicular tumors occurs along lymphatic channels, which pass from the mediastinum of the testis through the inguinal ring to accompany testicular vessels. After crossing the ureter the lymphatics spread out and enter the retroperitoneal lymph nodes.

Right-sided tumors spread to the interaortic–caval nodes, the precaval nodes and right para-aortic nodes. Left-sided tumors spread to the left para-aortic nodes and the preaortic nodes. The upper para-aortic nodes just below the renal vessels are more commonly involved than the lower para-aortic nodes in left-sided tumors, but in right-sided tumors nodes may be seen anywhere between the renal hilum and the aortic bifurcation (Fig. 2.1a and b). Approximately 20% of patients show crossover with involvement of left-sided nodes in patients with right-sided-node tumors (Ray, Hadju and Whitmore, 1974; Dixon, Ellis and Sikora, 1986). In addition to these sites, spread may occur directly to the so-called 'echelon' node, first described by Rouvière (1938). This node is situated on the right, lateral to the para-aortic node between the level of the first and third lumbar vertebrae. There is also evidence to suggest that an 'echelon' node exists on the left (Macdonald and Paxton, 1976). Occasionally lymph node spread is first to an ipsilateral upper external iliac node or common iliac node. Nodes adjacent to the iliopsoas muscle may also be involved. This site of spread is unusual and is more likely to be observed at the time of relapse than at that of initial staging (Williams, Cook and Duchesne, 1989).

The distribution of involved nodes at lymphography was studied by Wilkinson and Macdonald (1975). In 71% of patients the involved nodes were on the ipsilateral side of the tumor, in 9% involvement of the contra-lateral side was seen and in 20% there was bilateral involvement. Using CT scanning the distribution of involved nodes appears to be different from that demonstrated by lymphography. Dixon and his colleagues (1986) were unable to demonstrate contralateral involvement without ipsilateral disease. They suggest that the difference in their results compared with those of Wilkinson and Macdonald (1975) was due to the demonstration of involved ipsilateral 'echelon' nodes with CT that are not opacified at lymphography.

Lymph nodes above the renal hila are involved by direct spread from lower para-aortic nodes and extension of disease is then to the retrocrural nodes. Supradiaphragmatic spread of testicular tumors occurs via the thoracic duct, which leads to involvement of supraclavicular and superior mediastinal nodes. Direct spread through the diaphragm from the retrocrural space results in posterior mediastinal and subcarinal nodal involvement.

2.3.1.2 Lymphography

Lymphography has now become almost completely replaced by CT, but there are still occasions when the technique is helpful for staging testicular tumor patients, for example, in a patient with an equivocal CT scan in whom percutaneous biopsy of the suspicious node is not possible and serum marker estimations are unhelpful.

Following injection of oily contrast medium into the lymphatic vessels, lymph nodes in the external iliac, common iliac and para-aortic chains are opacified. Metastases appear as filling defects within involved nodes and contrast medium, which opacifies normal lymphoid tissue, is compressed around the deposit. Metastases can, therefore, be identified in nodes that are not significantly enlarged (Fig. 2.2). As a lymph node metastasis grows it compresses the nodal capsule and eventually breaks through it into the surrounding tissues. At this stage the lympho-

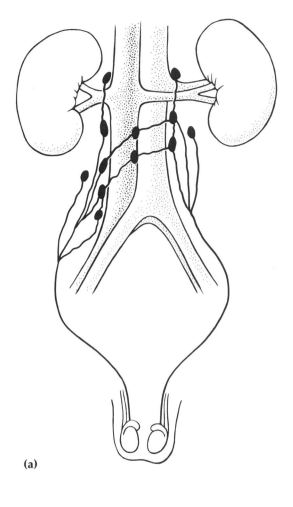

Fig. 2.1 Schematic representation of (a) lymphatic drainage from the testis to the retroperitoneal nodes and (b) the retroperitoneal nodes in cross-section at the level of the second lumbar vertebra. (Published by kind permission of Churchill Livingstone, Edinburgh.)

(a)

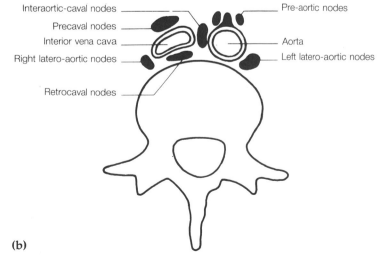

Interaortic-caval nodes

Precaval nodes

Interior vena cava

Right latero-aortic nodes

Retrocaval nodes

Pre-aortic nodes

Aorta

Left latero-aortic nodes

(b)

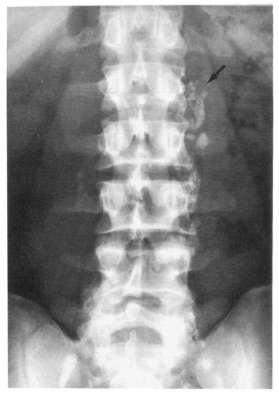

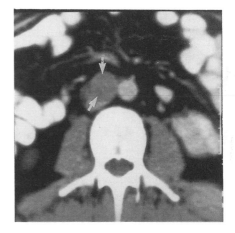

Fig. 2.3 CT scan showing minimally enlarged node (arrows) in the interaorticocaval space in a patient with a right-sided seminomatous germ cell tumor.

Fig. 2.2 Lymphogram showing the lymph node metastases at the level of L1 in the left para-aortic chain. The node is minimally enlarged.

gram demonstrates only that portion of the node that is not replaced by tumor; the precise extent of disease is therefore not shown. Further major limitations of lymphography that have contributed to its replacement by CT are that it is an unpleasant procedure for the patient, it may be technically difficult to perform and it opacifies only lymph nodes up to the level of the first or second lumbar vertebra. Thus, in patients with testicular tumors, high para-aortic node involvement and retrocrural nodal disease are demonstrated.

2.3.1.3   Computed tomography

With CT, normal lymph nodes appear as soft tissue density structures that are usually no more than 5 mm in diameter. Lymph node metastases are diagnosed on the basis of lymph node enlargement because tumor cannot be distinguished from the normal components of the lymph node. Thus metastases in normal-sized nodes cannot be detected.

Lymph node metastases are frequently of soft tissue density (Figs 2.3 and 2.4). Large masses produce displacement of the kidneys and/or hydronephrosis and these features are well shown on CT (Fig. 2.5). In patients with non-seminomatous germ cell tumors, low density 'cystic' lymph node deposits may be seen (Fig. 2.6).

A major advantage of CT over lymphography is the ability to image a tumor directly, thus providing information on tumor volume (Husband, Peckham and MacDonald, 1980). A further asset of CT is the ability to detect nodes high in the retroperitoneal space, in the retrocrural space (Fig. 2.7) and deposits in the 'echelon' nodes lateral to the para-aortic chain.

2.3.1.4   Ultrasound

Although ultrasound techniques have improved enormously during recent years, full

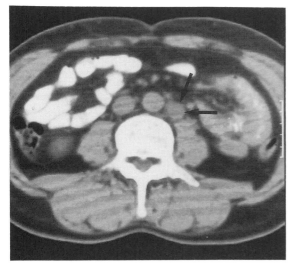

Fig. 2.4 CT scan showing minimally enlarged node (arrows) in the left para-aortic chain in a patient with a left-sided seminoma.

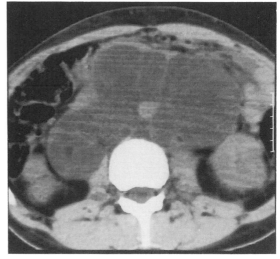

Fig. 2.6 CT scan showing large volume metastatic disease in a patient with a non-seminomatous germ cell tumor. The mass is almost entirely cystic.

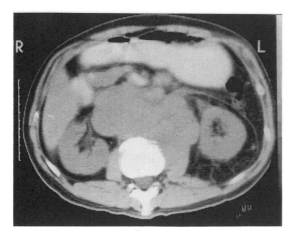

Fig. 2.5 CT scan in a patient with metastatic seminoma. The nodal mass measures 12 cm in diameter. Note displacement of both kidneys.

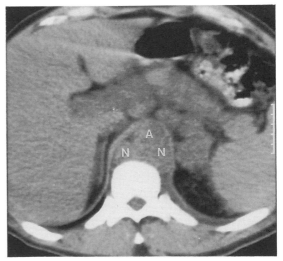

Fig. 2.7 CT scan in a patient with seminoma showing enlarged lymph nodes in the retrocrural space (N). The outline of the aorta (A) is obscured.

evaluation of the retroperitoneum remains difficult owing to the limitations imposed by adipose tissue and excessive bowel gas. In practice this means that precise tumor extent is difficult to assess and minimal degrees of lymph node enlargement may be missed. Failure to visualize the retroperitoneum adequately in patients with testicular tumors

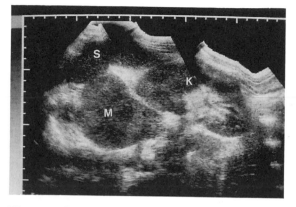

Fig. 2.8 Coronal ultrasound scan showing a large volume retroperitoneal mass (M) in a patient with a non-seminomatous germ cell tumor. K, kidney; S, spleen.

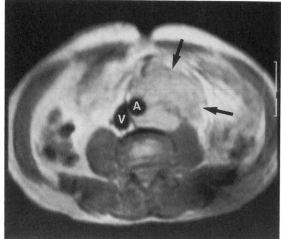

Fig. 2.9 Magnetic resonance imaging scan (T2-weighted sequence) showing a high signal retroperitoneal mass in a patient with a left-sided non-seminomatous germ cell tumor. Note the aorta (A) and inferior vena cava (V) are clearly distinguished from the mass.

ranges from 8 to 17% (Rowland *et al.*, 1982). However, in thin patients with little retroperitoneal fat CT may be difficult to interpret and, on occasion, ultrasound may be superior.

Enlarged nodes from testicular cancer appear as relatively echo-free soft tissue masses and, as with CT, in patients with non-seminomatous germ cell tumors, cystic areas may be seen within the mass (Burney and Klattie, 1979) (Fig. 2.8).

2.3.1.5 Magnetic resonance imaging

Magnetic resonance imaging (MRI) can demonstrate lymph node metastases provided the nodes are enlarged. In the early days of MRI it was hoped that information derived from T1- and T2-weighted images would be useful in distinguishing enlargement due to malignant disease from that due to benign pathology. Unfortunately, however, this has not proved possible and it appears that the limitations of MRI in detecting malignant involvement are similar to those of CT. The potential advantages of MRI over CT in the evaluation of enlarged lymph nodes are the ability to obtain images in multiple planes

and the ability to detect lymph node enlargement without the need for intravenous contrast medium to distinguish vessels from minimal degrees of lymphadenopathy. In patients with extensive tumors, coronal images might be helpful for defining the upper and lower limits of tumor more precisely than conventional CT, and for demonstrating the relationship of the mass to important structures such as the aorta, inferior vena cava and renal vessels prior to resection (Fig. 2.9). Coronal images can now be obtained using spiral (helical) CT. This technique, combined with the use of intravenous contrast medium, provides excellent anatomical detail in the same way as MRI (Brink *et al.*, 1994).

Recent investigation of new contrast agents for MRI has revealed some promising results in the evaluation of lymph node metastases. Initial animal experiments have shown that iron oxide particles are taken up by normal lymphoid tissue and tumor within a lymph node is therefore displayed as an area of **negative** uptake (Hamm *et al.*, 1992).

2.4 ACCURACY AND ROLE OF IMAGING TECHNIQUES

2.4.1 LYMPH NODE INVOLVEMENT: THE ABDOMEN

Data obtained at staging laparotomy have shown that approximately 20–30% of patients considered to be Stage I harbour occult metastases in retroperitoneal nodes that cannot be detected by imaging techniques (Wallace and Jing, 1970; Kademian and Wirtanen, 1977; Thomas, Bernardino and Bracken, 1981). Thus false negative imaging results are inevitable, but in addition false negative examinations result from observer error and limitations of the particular technique used.

With CT, size is the key criterion for diagnosing lymph node deposits, but in nonseminomatous germ cell tumors the density of the suspected node is also significant. In the early days of CT the upper limit of normal for a retroperitoneal node was considered to be 1.5 cm in diameter. This criterion worked reasonably well in practice, but today the superior image quality available, as well as increased expertise in interpreting CT scans, permits a more stringent evaluation of minimally enlarged nodes. Two important studies have addressed the issue of size criterion for diagnosing lymph node involvement in testicular cancer (Lien *et al.*, 1986; Stomper *et al.*, 1987). Lien and colleagues (1986) showed that if the criterion of 5 mm (upper limit of normal) was used the negative predictive value was 76%, the positive predictive value 61%, the sensitivity 71% and specificity 67%. When 15 mm was used as the upper limit of normal the negative predictive value and sensitivity decreased to 68% and 30%, respectively, and the positive predictive value and specificity increased to 93% and 98%, respectively. The results of Stomper and colleagues (1987) were similar and these authors concluded that, in patients with lymph nodes measuring less than 20 mm, histological confirmation of metastatic disease should be obtained by fine needle aspiration unless the serum markers were raised. We regard lymph nodes of 8–10 mm in diameter as suspicious and nodes greater than 10 mm as definitely enlarged. We agree with Stomper and colleagues that other confirmatory evidence should be sought. Earlier studies using a CT nodal diameter of 10–15 mm as the sole criterion of metastatic disease have revealed false negative rates ranging from 29 to 44% (Thomas, Bernardino and Bracken, 1981; Richie, Garnick and Finberg, 1982; Rowland *et al.*, 1982). Although lymphography is now seldom used as a staging investigation, it is interesting to note that, although lymphography can detect metastases in normal-sized nodes, the false negative rates reported are similar to those for CT, ranging from 10 to more than 40% (Thomas, Bernardino and Bracken, 1981; Lien *et al.*, 1983; Tesoro-Tess *et al.*, 1986). In the retrocrural space, lymph nodes greater than 6 mm in diameter are considered enlarged, but care must be taken to distinguish such minimally enlarged nodes from the thoracic duct and azygos vein.

Follow-up studies using CT in patients with clinical Stage I disease entered into a surveillance program have permitted further evaluation of CT in patients not undergoing radical lymphadenectomy. This has provided information on the development of demonstrable disease and its relationship to elevated marker estimations. In a study conducted at the Royal Marsden Hospital in which 147 patients were entered into the surveillance program, 37 patients relapsed. Computed tomography scanning identified relapse in 76% of patients and serum marker estimations in 68% of patients. The majority of relapses not identified by CT were in patients with elevated serum markers only (22%) and one patient in whom the lymphogram was positive and the CT examination was negative.

The accuracy of ultrasonography has been compared with that of CT and lymphography in testicular cancer. Results show that ultrasound is equally accurate to CT for identifying bulky retroperitoneal disease, but the extent of tumor is not so accurately delineated. Furthermore, ultrasound is inferior to CT and lymphography for detecting minimally enlarged nodes (Williams *et al.*, 1980; Rowland *et al.*, 1982; Poskitt, Cooperberg and Sullivan, 1985).

To date there is little information on the accuracy of MRI in the detection of lymph node metastases in the retroperitoneum, but an early report by Ellis *et al.* (1984) did not demonstrate any obvious benefit of MRI over CT for staging testicular tumors. However, the enormous technological advances in MRI, even over the last few years, have now resulted in very fast highly flexible systems with superb image quality. This now opens the way to routine abdominal imaging. Since many patients with testicular tumors require several serial imaging studies, MRI is likely to become the imaging method of choice in the not too distant future, thus avoiding irradiation in patients considered to have an excellent long-term prognosis.

2.4.2 LYMPH NODE INVOLVEMENT: THE CHEST

The most common sites of supradiaphragmatic lymph node involvement are the supraclavicular fossae subcarinal region and posterior mediastinum.

Posterior mediastinal lymphadenopathy appears as a mass that produces a convex outline to the mediastinal contour (Fig. 2.10). This abnormal contour may be appreciated on penetrated conventional chest films, but is more easily seen on CT than with plain radiography. Several authors have demonstrated a significant proportion of patients with positive CT scans and negative chest radiographs (Husband and Grimer, 1985; Williams *et al.*, 1987; Lien *et al.*, 1988). As in the retroperitoneum, lymph nodes of 1 cm in diameter or greater are considered to be definitely abnormal, but in the posterior mediastinum and subcarinal area minimal

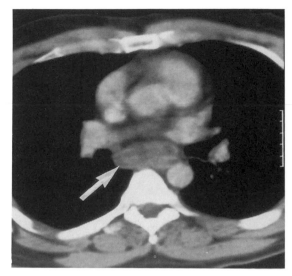

Fig. 2.10 CT scan showing subcarinal lymphadenopathy in a patient with a non-seminomatous germ cell tumor. The mediastinal contour in the region of the axygoesophageal recess is abnormal, indicating a mass (arrow).

degrees of lymphadenopathy may be difficult to identify even with intravenous contrast medium. MRI may be helpful in cases of doubt because the superior contrast resolution of MRI, together with the multiplanar capability, frequently commits lymph nodes to be shown with greater clarity than with CT.

2.4.3 PULMONARY METASTASES

It is widely accepted that CT scanning is the most sensitive radiological technique for identifying pulmonary metastases because nodules can be identified at the lung periphery down to a size of 3–4 mm in diameter (Muhm, Brown and Crowe, 1977; Schaner *et al.*, 1978) (Fig. 2.11). Computed tomography has now completely replaced whole lung tomography, and one study in the early 1980s demonstrated an increased yield of 5% for CT in the detection of pulmonary metastases (Husband, Peckham and MacDonald, 1980).

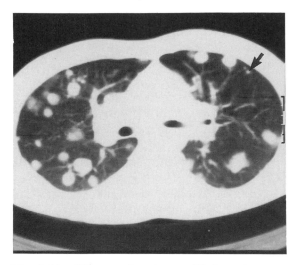

Fig. 2.11 CT scan showing multiple pulmonary metastases in a patient with a non-seminomatous germ cell tumor. Very small metastases are seen at the lung periphery (arrow).

A more recent study using current CT technology has shown that CT was the only positive technique in 20 out of 47 patients with lung metastases from testicular tumors (Lien *et al.*, 1988). A major problem with CT is that the technique is nonspecific and well-circumscribed round lesions may not only represent metastases, but may also represent granulomas, subpleural lymph nodes or areas of inflammation. If multiple nodules are demonstrated then the likelihood of metastases is greater, but if a single lesion is seen it may be necessary to repeat the examination after an interval of 4–6 weeks to see if there has been any change in size before a diagnosis of pulmonary involvement is made. In the UK granulomatous disease is uncommon and problems relating to lack of specificity are therefore not so great as in other countries such as the USA, where granulomatous disease (e.g., histoplasmosis) has a high incidence. Other problems encountered in the diagnosis of pulmonary deposits include: (a) the distinction between major blood vessels and metastases in the region of the hila, and (b) small metastases (<1 cm in diameter),

which may be missed if breath holding is not carried out at the same level of inspiration/expiration for each CT slice. However, the advent of spiral/helical CT promises to eliminate problems of misregistration because the technique allows multiple CT slices to be obtained in a single breath hold.

2.4.4   OTHER SITES OF DISEASE

2.4.4.1   The liver

Liver metastases are seldom seen at the time of initial diagnosis, and even in patients who have relapsed liver involvement is uncommon.

Ultrasound, CT and MRI may all be used to identify liver metastases. Since CT is currently used for staging the retroperitoneum, examination of the liver is automatically included in the upper abdominal scan; it is therefore unnecessary to undertake further investigation of the liver at this time. However, it should be borne in mind that an ultrasound examination may reveal a liver metastasis that is not visible on CT. It may also be helpful for characterizing focal lesion demonstrated on the staging CT scan that may or may not be malignant. MRI may also be useful in occasional patients in whom other information regarding the number of metastases or character of a lesion is required (Whitney *et al.*, 1993).

With ultrasound, as in other primary tumors, liver metastases in testicular cancer appear as low echogeneity lesions compared with normal liver parenchyma (Fig. 2.12a). With CT they appear as areas of diminished density with ill-defined borders. In patients with non-seminomatous germ cell tumors, liver metastases may be cystic (Fig. 2.12b).

The use of MRI in the detection of liver metastases is currently being evaluated and several studies have already been reported in the literature comparing the detectability of liver metastases by CT, MRI and ultrasound in different tumor types. With MRI the liver

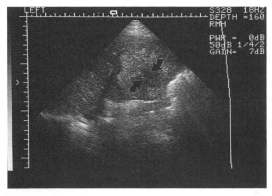

(a)

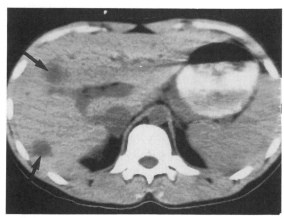

(b)

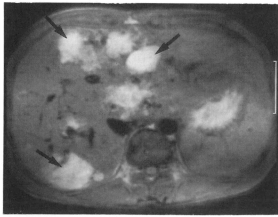

(c)

Fig. 2.12 Liver metastases in a patient with a non-seminomatous germ cell tumor. (a) Ultrasound showing low echogeneity metastases (arrows). (b) CT scan showing low density metastases (arrows). (c) Magnetic resonance imaging scan (T2-weighted sequence) showing multiple metastases (arrows).

metastasis appears as a bright lesion on a T2-weighted sequence (high intensity) and as a dark lesion (low intensity) on a T1-weighted sequence (Fig. 2.12c) (Ferrucci, 1986; Semelka *et al.*, 1992). Although there is considerable variation between the results, overall there is probably little difference between the accuracies of contrast-enhanced dynamic CT and MRI at the present time. The introduction of specific contrast agents for liver imaging with MRI may, however, change the situation by increasing the sensitivity of MRI (Reinig *et al.*, 1987; Bernardino *et al.*, 1991).

2.4.4.2   Bone

Bone metastases are rare and seldom seen at presentation. Symptoms usually indicate the site of involvement, and conventional radiology, radionuclide scanning, CT and even MRI may all be helpful in revealing the nature and extent of disease.

2.4.4.3   Central nervous system

Brain metastases may be seen at presentation in patients with aggressive disseminated disease and are more common in patients with trophoblastic teratomas than any other histological type on either MRI or CT (Fig. 2.13a)

MRI has also been shown to be the method of choice for detecting meningeal involvement for both the brain and spinal canal. Contrast-enhanced T1-weighted sequences elegantly display the presence and extent of involvement (Fig. 2.13b)

2.4.4.4   Unusual sites of metastases

The widespread use of CT has revealed disease in many different sites not previously recognized. A retrospective analysis of 600 patients from the Royal Marsden Hospital demonstrated unusual thoracoabdominal metastases in 22 patients. These sites included the kidneys, adrenal glands, striated muscle,

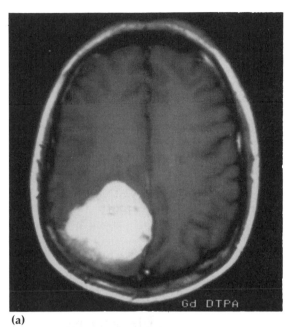

(a)

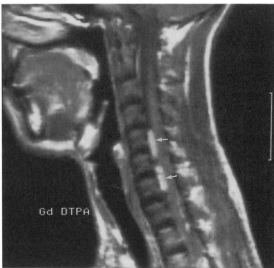

(b)

Fig. 2.13 (a) MRI scan of the brain in a patient with a non-seminomatous germ cell tumor of the testis. T1-weighted image following injection of intravenous contrast medium (gadolinium–DTPA) shows a 4 cm enhancing mass in the right posterior parital representing a solidary metastasis. (b) MRI scan of the cervical spinal canal in a patient with a non-seminomatous germ cell tumor of the testis. This sagitall post-contrast T1-weighted image shows deposits of enhancing meningeal metastatic tumor (arrows).

the spleen, stomach, seminal vesicles, prostate and pericardium (Husband and Bellamy, 1985).

2.5 MONITORING TREATMENT RESPONSE

Radiology is equally as important during patient follow-up as at the time of initial staging. Timing and frequency of follow-up investigations should be designed according to treatment protocols, and clearly vary in different centers. In general, patients are re-evaluated fully following initial treatment, and continued radiological assessment is then dependent on the initial stage of disease, measured treatment response and future management strategy.

2.5.1 THE ABDOMEN

Before the days of ultrasound and CT, post-lymphangiogram films were the only method of assessing regression or regrowth of retro-peritoneal tumors. However, CT has now replaced lymphography, not only at the time of staging but also for follow-up purposes, because accurate measurements of tumor volume change in relation to therapy can be made (Husband, Peckham and MacDonald, 1980). In addition to changes in tumor volume, changes in tumor composition may also be identified (Husband, Hawkes and Peckham, 1982). In patients undergoing post-chemotherapy lymphadenectomy, CT is a highly accurate technique for localizing the site of residual disease, the size of the mass and its relationship to major vessels (Kennedy *et al.*, 1985). This information is useful for surgical planning because residual masses above the renal hilar require a thoraco-abdominal incision, whereas disease confined below the renal vessels may be approached using a midline abdominal incision.

Seminoma nodal metastases show marked regression in response to treatment, but in the majority of patients a soft tissue residuum is seen in the retroperitoneum (Figs. 2.14a

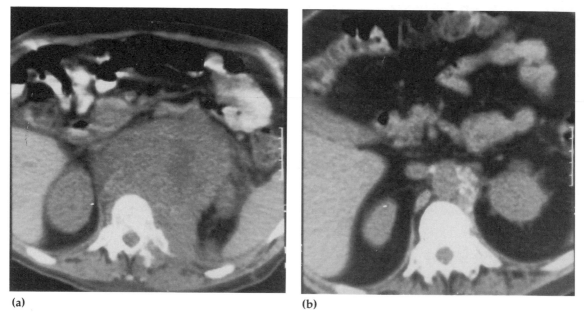

(a)   (b)

Fig. 2.14   (a) Axial CT scan showing large mass of metastatic seminoma in the upper para-aortic region extending around the vertebral body; (b) the same patient following chemotherapy; the mass has regressed considerably but a residuum is present adjacent to the aorta and has calcified.

and b) (Stomper *et al.*, 1985; Williams *et al.*, 1987). These masses usually persist and may show further minimal regression for up to 2 years following treatment (Williams *et al.*, 1987). On CT these residua appear as irregular masses closely applied to the aorta and/or inferior vena cava and are of soft tissue density. Occasionally calcification is seen.

Non-seminomatous germ cell tumor masses show different patterns of response. For example, a large soft tissue density metastasis may respond in a similar way to a seminomatous mass, leaving a small residuum after treatment, or may completely disappear. Masses that contain cystic elements at the time of diagnosis may remain cystic and become larger on treatment (Figs 2.15a and b). Even masses of soft tissue density at the time of diagnosis may become cystic during treatment (Husband, Hawkes and Peckham, 1982). Over recent years there has become considerable interest in the possibility of detecting persistent active malignancy in resid-

ual teratomatous masses demonstrated on imaging following chemotherapy. We correlated the mean attenuation values of residual teratomatous masses with histology in 26 patients. The results showed that masses of low attenuation (<30 Hounsfield units) represented cysts and there was good correlation between these low attenuation values and the presence of mature differentiated teratoma, with no evidence of active malignancy. Studies were also carried out by Stomper *et al.* (1985) and Scatarige *et al.* (1983). The work by Stomper and coauthors agreed with our data and suggests that residual masses with uniform low attenuation values are not associated with persistent malignancy, but the study by Scatarige and colleagues reported two patients with low attenuation masses in which active residual disease was found. As yet insufficient information is available to determine whether MRI may be useful in distinguishing differentiating teratoma from active malignancy, but

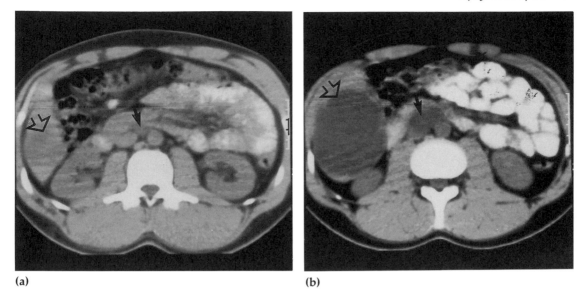

(a)   **(b)**

Fig. 2.15 CT scans in a patient with a non-seminomatous germ cell tumor. (a) Before treatment. There is a 1 cm interaorticocaval soft tissue density nodal deposit (solid arrow). Note liver metastases (open arrow). (b) Following chemotherapy. The small nodal deposit (solid arrow) has become larger and 'cystic' following chemotherapy. Note the large 'cystic' deposit in the liver (open arrow), which was not so clearly identified on the previous scan.

early work at the Royal Marsden Hospital suggests that MRI, like CT, is not wholly reliable. Clearly, at the present time, imaging methods cannot obviate the need for post-chemotherapy lymphadenectomy in patients with demonstrable residual disease.

2.5.2 THE CHEST

Chest radiographs are the mainstay of monitoring tumor regression of pulmonary metastases, provided they can be clearly identified on standard films. As in the abdomen, surgery may be indicated following chemotherapy to remove residual lung and mediastinal disease (Goldstraw, 1986). Immediately prior to resection, CT is useful for depicting the number and position of obvious metastases and may also identify deposits not readily visible on plain radiographs.

The small pulmonary metastases only initially identified on CT usually disappear completely after treatment, and it is only the larger deposits that remain as residual irregular lesions. Occasionally, treated metastases cavitate, leaving an air-containing space with a thin rim of soft tissue density around the edge (Charig and Williams, 1990).

Regression of mediastinal lymph node disease is well shown on CT and residual nodes are often present when the chest radiograph appearance is normal. Occasionally, a teratomatous lymph node deposit enlarges and becomes cystic in the mediastinum, just as in the abdomen. In this situation a plain chest radiograph may suggest progressive disease, whereas CT reveals the underlying cystic change.

2.6 BIOPSY TECHNIQUES

Occasionally biopsy of a retroperitoneal mass is required. This may be to confirm metastatic disease in patients with negative serum markers at the time of presentation or to determine the nature of the mass at the time of suspected relapse. Retroperitoneal masses may be successfully biopsied percutaneously

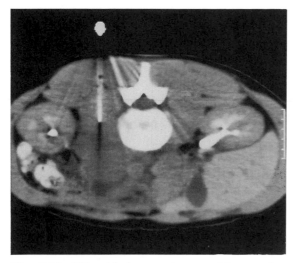

Fig. 2.16 CT-guided percutaneous biopsy of a retroperitoneal mass in a patient with relapsed seminoma.

under ultrasound or CT guidance (Fig. 2.16). However, CT guidance is the preferred technique for fine needle aspiration of small volume metastases because visualization of the retroperitoneum with CT is superior to ultrasound.

2.7   EFFECT OF TREATMENT ON NORMAL TISSUE

During recent years the treatment of testicular cancer has become so refined that the common complications previously demonstrated on CT, such as radiation fibrosis of the lungs and bleomycin-induced lung damage, are seldom seen. Today radiotherapy is not usually given to the mediastinum and the doses of bleomycin used have been reduced. However, it is important to recognize that bleomycin damage does cause characteristic appearances on plain chest radiographs in patients with moderate or severe damage and early changes that are invisible on plain chest films may be seen on CT (Bellamy *et al.*, 1985). Recognition of such damage is important because it may otherwise be confused with developing metastases or areas of infect-

ive consolidation. Typical features of bleomycin injury include diffuse bilateral pleural and pulmonary infiltrates, which may be linear, nodular or reticulonodular and which appear 6 weeks to 3 months after treatment has commenced. Changes are confined to the lung bases in a third of patients and are solely peripheral in about 25% (Mills and Husband, 1990).

True thymic hyperplasia is an important side-effect of chemotherapy that is thought to represent thymic rebound following a period of stress-induced atrophy. We found an incidence of obvious thymic growth in 11.6% of patients treated with chemotherapy of the testis (Kissin *et al.*, 1987). The recognition of this phenomenon as a cause of an enlarging anterior mediastinal mass in a patient who has recently undergone chemotherapy may avoid the erroneous diagnosis of mediastinal relapse.

2.8   CONCLUSIONS

A strategy for the use of imaging in testicular tumors should be agreed by close liaison between clinicians and radiologists, with CT playing the most important role of all imaging investigations. However, there are certain occasions when other imaging methods may be appropriate; for example, an enlarged retroperitoneal node shown on CT may not necessarily contain tumor, and in the absence of raised serum markers or positive cytology a lymphogram may be helpful. In a similar way ultrasound, MRI and nuclear medicine techniques may be helpful for resolving specific problems in symptomatic patients. The role of MRI in the management of testicular tumors appears to be limited currently, but in centers where the technique is available it is already the method of choice for the detection of intracerebral metastases and meningeal involvement. In the next few years as technology advances, MRI is likely to become increasingly used in other areas such as in the evaluation of retroperitoneal and mediastinal disease, and even in the diagnosis of lung involvement.

ACKNOWLEDGEMENTS

I am most grateful to the Cancer Research Campaign for supporting the work of this department. I would also like to thank Paula Ursell for her secretarial assistance and Janet MacDonald for helping to prepare the illustrations. Finally I would like to thank Dr D.O. Cosgrove for providing the ultrasound illustrations (Figs 2.8 and 2.12a). Figs 2.1a and b are published by kind permission of Churchill Livingstone, Edinburgh.

REFERENCES

Bellamy, E.A., Husband, J.E., Blaquiere, R.M. *et al.* (1985) Bleomycin-related lung damage: CT evidence. *Radiology*, **156**, 155–8.

Bernardino, M.E., Young, S.W., Lee, J.K.T. *et al.* (1991) Contrast-enhanced magnetic resonance imaging of the liver with Mn-DPDP for known or suspected focal hepatic disease. *Radiology*, **26**, S148.

Brink, J.A., Heiken, J.P., Wang, G. *et al.* (1994) Helical CT: principles and technical considerations. *RadioGraphics*, **14**, 887–93.

Burney, B.T. and Klattie, E.C. (1979) Ultrasound and computed tomography of the abdomen in the staging and management of testicular carcinoma. *Radiology*, **132**, 415–19.

Charig, M.J. and Williams, M.P. (1990) Pulmonary lucanae: sequelae of metastases following chemotherapy. *Clin. Radiol.*, **42**, 93–6.

Dixon, A.K., Ellis, M. and Sikora, K. (1986) Computed tomography of testicular tumours: Distribution of abdominal lymphadenopathy. *Clin. Radiol.*, **37**, 519–23.

Ellis, J.H., Blies, J.R., Kopecky, K.K. *et al.* (1984) Comparison of NMR and CT imaging in the evaluation of metastatic retroperitoneal lymphadenopathy from testicular carcinoma. *J. Comput. Assist. Tomogr.*, **8**, 709–19.

Ferrucci, J.T. (1986) MR imaging of the liver. *Am. J. Roentgenol.*, **147**, 1103–16.

Goldstraw, P. (1986) Thoracic surgery for germ cell tumours, in *Germ Cell Tumours II, Advances in the Biosciences*, Volume 55 (eds W.G. Jones, A.M. Ward and C.K. Anderson), Pergamon Press, Oxford, pp. 419–21.

Hamm, B., Taupitz, M., Hussmann, P. *et al.*, (1992) MR lymphography with iron oxide particles: dose–response studies and pulse sequence optimization in rabbits. *Am. J. Roentgenol.*, **158**, 183.

Hendry, W.F., Garvie, W.H.H., Ah-See, A.K. *et al.* (1984) Ultrasonic detection of occult testicular neoplasms in patients with gynaecomastia. *Br. J. Radiol.*, **57**, 571–2.

Husband, J.E. and Bellamy, E.A. (1985) Unusual thoracoabdominal sites of metastases in testicular tumors. *Am. J. Roentgenol.*, **145**, 1165–71.

Husband, J.E. and Grimer, D.P. (1985) Staging testicular tumours: the role of CT scanning. *J. Royl Soc. Med.*, **58**, 429–36.

Husband, J.E., Hawkes, D.J. and Peckham, M.J. (1982) CT estimations of mean attenuation values and tumour volume in testicular tumours: a comparison with operative findings and histology. *Radiology*, **144**, 553–8.

Husband, J.E., Peckham, M.J. and MacDonald, J.S. (1980) The role of abdominal computed tomography in the management of testicular tumours. *Comput. Tomogr.*, **4**, 1–6.

Kademian, M. and Wirtanen, G. (1977) Accuracy of bipedal lymphography in testicular tumours. *Urology*, **9**, 218–20.

Kennedy, C.L., Husband, J.E., Bellamy, E.A. *et al.* (1985) The accuracy of CT scanning prior to para-aortic lymphadenectomy in patients with bulky metastases from testicular teratoma. *Br. J. Urol.*, **57**, 755–8.

Kissin, C.M., Husband, J.E., Nicholas, D. *et al.* (1987) Benign thymic enlargement in adults after chemotherapy: CT demonstration. *Radiology*, **163**, 67–70.

Lien, H.H., Fosså, S.D., Ous, S. *et al.* (1983) Lymphography in retroperitoneal metastases in non-seminoma testicular tumour patients with a normal CT scan. *Acta Radiol.*, **24**, 319–22.

Lien, H.H., Lindskold, L., Fosså, S.E. *et al.* (1988) Computed tomography and conventional radiography in intrathoracic metastases from non-seminomatous testicular tumor. *Acta Radiol.*, **29**, 547–9.

Lien, H.H., Stenwig, A.E., Ous, S. *et al.* (1986) Influence of different criteria for abnormal lymph node size on reliability of computed tomography in patients with nonseminomatous testicular tumour. *Acta Radiol.*, **27**, 199–203.

Macdonald, J.S. and Paxton, R.M. (1976) Lymphography, in *Scientific Foundations of Urology*, Volume II (eds D.I. Williams and G.D. Chisholm), Heinemann Medical, Oxford, p. 226.

Mills, P. and Husband, J.E. (1990) Computed tomography of pulmonary bleomycin toxicity. *Seminars in Ultrasound, CT and MR.*, **11**, 417–22.

Muhm, J.R., Brown, L.R. and Crowe, J.K. (1977) Detection of pulmonary nodules by computed tomography. *Am. J. Roentgenol.*, **128**, 267–70.

Poskitt, K.J., Cooperberg, P.L. and Sullivan, L.D. (1985) Sonography and CT in staging nonseminomatous testicular tumors. *Am. J. Roentgenol.*, **144**, 939–44.

Ray, B., Hadju, S.I. and Whitmore, W.F. (1974) Distribution of retroperitoneal lymph node metastases in testicular germinal tumours. *Cancer*, **33**, 340–8.

Reinig, J.W., Dwyer, A.J., Miller, D.L. *et al.*, (1987) Liver metastasis detection: comparative sensitivities of MR imaging and CT scanning. *Radiology*, **162**, 43–7.

Richie, J.P., Garnick, M.H. and Finberg, H. (1982) Computerized tomography: how accurate for abdominal staging of testis tumors? *J. Urol.*, **27**, 715–17.

Rouvière, H. (1938) *Anatomy of the Human Lymphatic System* (translation edited by M.J. Tobias), Edwards Brothers, Ann Arbor, pp. 216–26.

Rowland, R.G., Weisman, D., Williams, S.D. *et al.* (1982) Accuracy of preoperative staging in stages A and B non-seminomatous germ cell testis tumors, *J. Urol.*, **127**, 718–20.

Scatarige, J.C., Fisherman, E.K., Kuhajda, F.P. *et al.*, (1983) Low attenuation nodal metastases in testicular carcinoma. *J. Comput. Assist. Tomogr.*, **7**, 682–7.

Schaner, E.G., Chang, A.E., Doppman, J.L. *et al.*, (1978) Comparison of computed and conventional whole lung tomography in detecting pulmonary nodules: a prospective radiologic–pathologic study. *Am. J. Roentgenol.*, **131**, 51–4.

Semelka, R.C., Shoenut, J.P., Kroeker, R.M. *et al.* (1992) Focal liver disease: Comparison of dynamic contrast-enhanced CT and T2-weighted fat-suppressed, FLASH, and dynamic gadolinium-enhanced MR imaging at 1.5T. *Radiology*, **184**, 687.

Stomper, P.C., Fung, C.Y., Socinski, M.A. *et al.* (1987) Detection of retroperitoneal metastases in early-stage nonseminomatous testicular cancer: Analysis of different CT criteria. *Am. J. Roentgenol.*, **149**, 1187–90.

Stomper, P.C., Jochelson, M.S., Garnick, M.B. *et al.* (1985) Residual abdominal masses after chemotherapy for nonseminomatous testicular cancer: correlation of CT and histology. *Am. J. Roentgenol.*, **145**, 743.

Tesoro–Tess, J.D., Pizzocaro, G., Zanoni, F. *et al.* (1986) Lymphangiography and computerized tomography in testicular carcinoma: how accurate in early stage disease? *J. Urol.*, **133**, 967–70.

Thomas, J.L., Bernardino, M.E. and Bracken, R.B. (1981) Staging of testicular carcinoma: comparison of CT and lymphangiography. *Am. J. Roentgenol.*, **137**, 991–6.

Thurnher, S., Hricak, H., Carrol, P.R. *et al.*, (1988) Imaging the testis: comparison between MR imaging and US. *Radiology*, **167**, 631–6.

Wallace, S. and Jing, B.S. (1970) Lymphangiography: Diagnosis of nodal metastases from testicular malignancies. *JAMA*, **213**, 94–6.

Whitney, W.S., Herfkens, R.J., Jeffrey, R.B. *et al.* (1993) Dynamic breath-hold multiplanar spoiled gradient-recalled MR imaging with gadolinium enhancement for differentiating hepatic hemangiomas from malignancies at 1.5T. *Radiology*, **189**, 863.

Wilkinson, D.J. and Macdonald, J.S. (1975) A review of the role of lymphography in the management of testicular tumours. *Clin. Radiol.*, **26**, 89–98.

Williams, M.P., Cook, J.V. and Duchesne, G.M. (1989) Psoas nodes – An overlooked site of metastasis from testicular tumours. *Clin. Radiol.*, **40**, 607–9.

Williams, R.D., Feinberg, S.B., Knight, L.C. *et al.* (1980) Abdominal staging of testicular tumours using ultrasonography and computed tomography. *J. Urol.*, **123**, 872–5.

Williams, M.P., Naik, G., Heron, C.W. *et al.*, (1987) Computed tomography of the abdomen in advanced seminoma: response to treatment. *Clin. Radiol.*, **38**, 629–33.

TUMOR MARKERS

3

M.D. Mason

3.1 INTRODUCTION

No tumor marker is ideal. For many years it has been known that human germ cell tumors secrete human chorionic gonadotrophin (HCG) and alpha-fetoprotein (AFP), which are now the principal testicular tumor markers in widespread clinical use. In the last ten years, the patterns of their secretion in testicular tumors before and during treatment have been extensively described, and some understanding of the underlying biological implications of marker production is being reached. Despite this, AFP and HCG are not ideal, since, among other reasons, at least 20% of patients with testicular teratomas do not produce either of these markers, and no specific marker for testicular seminoma exists. Hence, in recent years much effort has been devoted to the search for new testicular tumor markers.

In the last ten years, the scope of what constitutes a 'marker' has widened, with the use of immunohistochemistry to identify marker production in tissue sections, with new cytogenetic analysis of chromosomal abnormalities in tumor cells, and with attempts to measure molecules of possible biological significance such as oncogene products in serum.

In this chapter, attention will be focused on AFP and HCG. Lactate dehydrogenase (LDH), considered separately, is now regarded as an important marker but its uptake into routine clinical practice has been slow.

3.2 THE CELLULAR ORIGINS OF ALPHA-FETOPROTEIN AND HUMAN CHORIONIC GONADOTROPHIN IN TESTICULAR TUMORS

Testicular non-seminomatous germ cell tumors (NSGCT) consist of a mixture of undifferentiated stem cells and varying amounts of differentiated derivatives. Recent studies of cultured cells from human teratomas have suggested that the stem cells comprise embryonal carcinoma (EC), two distinct yolk sac carcinoma stem cells (Pera, Blasco-Lafite and Mills, 1987) and malignant cytotrophoblastic stem cells (Yamazaki *et al.*, 1987). The cell lineage in germ cell tumors, and the relationship of these stem cells to each other, is only just beginning to be understood, but the resistance of seminoma to growth in tissue culture has hampered our understanding of its relationship to these other cell types.

Human choriocarcinoma mimics normal trophoblastic development with mature postmitotic syncytiotrophoblast arising from malignant cytotrophoblast. Immunohistochemical studies show that, as with normal trophoblast, HCG production is mainly from syncytiotrophoblast cells, and not from the malignant stem cells (Mostofi, 1984). Pure choriocarcinoma is characterized by extremely high serum levels of HCG, but production of HCG is seen in other types of NSGCT and even in seminoma, where its significance will be discussed later. Production of modest

Testicular Cancer: Investigation and management. Second edition. Edited by Professor A. Horwich.
Published in 1996 by Chapman & Hall. ISBN 0 412 61210 0.

amounts of HCG by EC cells in tissue culture has also been seen, but it is not produced by either of the two types of yolk sac stem cell (Pera, Blasco-Lafite and Mills, 1987). It is possible that this represents early differentiation along a trophoblastic lineage.

Alpha-fetoprotein is an embryonic protein produced by the yolk sac, and subsequently by the fetal liver. It is structurally similar to albumin, and probably services a similarly diverse number of functions in the fetus. Serum levels of AFP fall dramatically around birth as AFP production is switched off, and albumin production is switched on.

Alpha-fetoprotein production in NSGCT is usually associated with yolk sac differentiation. Such areas may be identified in histological sections by immunohistochemistry (Mostofi, 1984) and the conventional view is that the presence of such elements, or of an elevated serum AFP level, should always indicate the presence of a non-seminomatous component to a germ cell tumor.

Do seminomas ever produce AFP? The answer to this question must remain that they do not, at least within our current understanding of what constitutes seminoma. However, some reports of AFP-producing seminomas exist. Raghavan and colleagues (1982) described a series of cases treated as seminomas, which exhibited morphology similar to yolk sac and produced AFP, and proposed that seminoma and yolk sac carcinoma were closely related cell types, with a spectrum of differentiation between the two. However, several possible explanations exist for this finding, including histological confusion between seminoma and the solid form of yolk sac carcinoma (Kohn and Raghavan, 1981), a view also expressed by Mostofi (1984), who felt that all of these cases were yolk sac tumors. Indeed, a cell line isolated from one of these so-called seminomas has, *in vitro*, characteristics of yolk sac carcinoma resembling visceral endoderm (Pera, Blasco-Lafite and Mills, 1987). Therefore, for the present it must be assumed that elevation of serum AFP reflects non-seminomatous

elements in a tumor, which must be treated as such. The two types of yolk sac stem cell identified by Pera differ in their capacity to produce AFP. The first, which gives rise to yolk sac tumors resembling rodent visceral endoderm when implanted in nude mice, is characterized by the production of large amounts of AFP. By contrast, the second type gives rise to yolk sac tumors resembling rodent parietal endoderm (endodermal sinus tumors), and among many features distinguishing it from the first type is the production of only very modest amounts of AFP. As with HCG, some degree of AFP production has also been seen in EC cells in tissue culture (Pera, Blasco-Lafite and Mills, 1987), possibly indicating early yolk sac differentiation.

3.3   BASIS AND INTERPRETATION OF MARKER ASSAYS

Early assays for HCG and AFP required either bioassays or gel immunoelectrophoresis, and were crude and insensitive. With the advent of the radioimmunoassay it was possible to use much greater sensitivity and precision (Vaitukaitis, Braunstein and Ross, 1972; Waldmann and McIntire, 1974), and the double antibody techniques used in those early studies still form the basis of the assays currently in use, the principle of which is shown in Fig. 3.1.

Among the newer techniques available are monoclonal antibody enzyme-linked immunosorbent assays (ELISA), and immunoradiometric assays (IRMA), which are shown in Fig. 3.2. Using these assays, normal values of <4 IU l^{-1} for HCG, and <10 kU l^{-1} for AFP are obtained at the regional tumor marker laboratory at Charing Cross Hospital.

Human chorionic gonadotrophin is a polypeptide consisting of two subunits designated alpha and beta. The alpha subunit has homology with a number of other hormones such as luteinizing hormone (LH), while the beta subunit confers the immunological specificity and functional activity. The homology

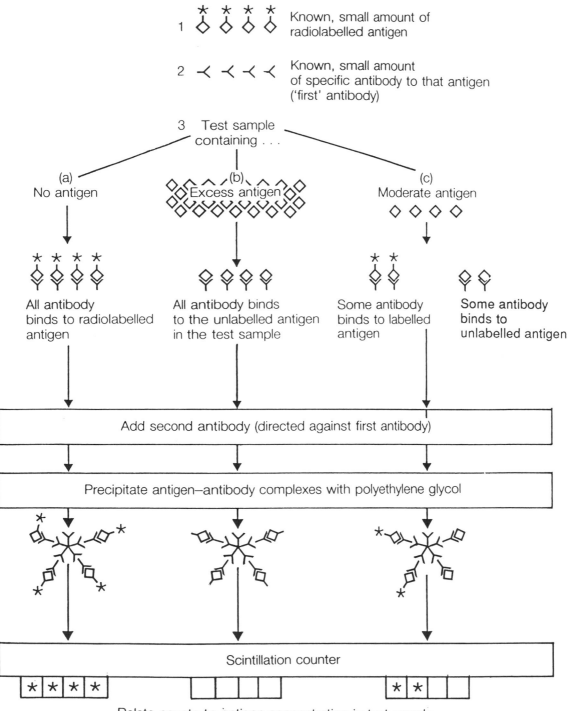

Fig. 3.1 The principle of radioimmunoassay.

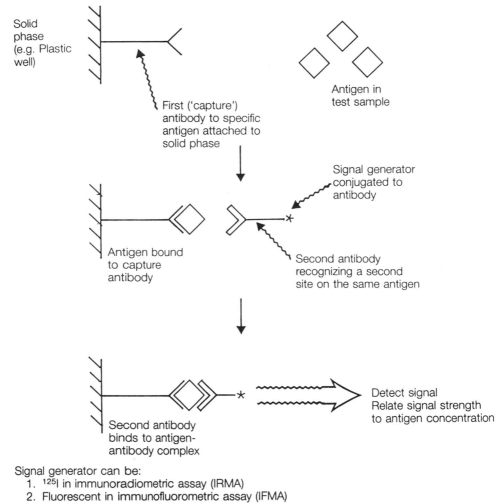

Signal generator can be:
  1. ^{125}I in immunoradiometric assay (IRMA)
  2. Fluorescent in immunofluorometric assay (IFMA)
  3. Peroxidase in enzyme-linked immunosorbent assay (ELISA)
     (signal generated by addition of substrate)

Fig. 3.2 Sandwich techniques.

of alpha-HCG and LH created difficulties with early antibody assays, until a radio-immunoassay using a polyclonal antiserum against beta-HCG was developed (Vaitukaitis, Braunstein and Ross, 1972), and the specificity was further improved by the use of antibodies to the carboxy terminal end of the beta subunit (Javadpour, 1986).

It has recently been shown that some germ cell tumors are characterized by the secretion of the free beta subunit, either alone, or in combination with the alpha subunit and the intact molecule (Mann and Karl, 1983; Paus *et al.*, 1988). It has also been shown that heterogeneity in the degree of glycosylation of the HCG molecule exists, as indicated by its binding characteristics to concanavalin A (Mann and Karl, 1983). This may reflect liberation of HCG by cell lysis as opposed to active secretion, but the significance of all

Table 3.1 Differential diagnosis of elevated serum alpha-fetoprotein (AFP) and human chorionic gonadotrophin (HCG) in adult testicular tumors

	AFP	*HCG*

Gastrointestinal	Liver damage
	    Infective
	    Drug/alcohol induced
	    Metastases (e.g. colon carcinoma)	

Technical	Error	Error
		Cross-reaction (assay not specific
		    enough to distinguish between
		    HCG and LH)

Secretion by non-germ cell tumors	Hepatocellular carcinoma	Carcinomas
		    Pancreas
		    Stomach
		    Colon
		    Bladder
		    Small intestine
		    Bronchus
		    Breast
		Hematological
		    Hodgkin's disease
		    Non-Hodgkin's lymphoma
		    Myeloma
		    Leukemias
		Miscellaneous
		    Retroperitoneal sarcoma
		    Melanoma
		    Insulinoma

Congenital	Ataxiatelangiectasia Hereditary tyrosinemia Hereditary persistence of AFP	

LH, luteinizing hormone.

these findings is as yet unknown. There has also been recent interest in a fragment of HCG, the so-called urinary gonadotrophin peptide (UGP), excreted in the urine of patients with germ cell tumors and a variety of non-germ cell tumors (Kardana *et al.*, 1988), which complicates the notion that estimation of HCG in concentrated urine specimens may be more sensitive than serum measurements (Javadpour, 1986). The demonstration that some normal tissues express the UGP is of great interest, supporting the suggestion that the HCG peptide may be a widespread cell membrane component (Mann and Karl, 1983; Kardana *et al.*, 1988).

Conditions in which AFP or HCG may be detected other than in germ cell tumors are shown in Table 3.1 (Braunstein *et al.*, 1973; Kohn and Raghavan 1981; Coppack *et al.*, 1983; Staples, 1986). Production of AFP other than by germ cell tumors can be a source of much diagnostic difficulty, particularly as it may occur in patients treated for testicular tumors during or after chemotherapy. This is often associated with other parameters suggestive of hepatic dysfunction (which may be an underlying problem), and has been reported with several chemotherapy regimens, including cisplatin/vinblastine/bleomycin (PVB), bleomycin/etoposide/cisplatin (BEP), vinblastine/cyclophosphamide/actinomycin-D/bleomycin/cisplatin (VAB-6) and POMB/ACE (Coppack *et al.*, 1983; Grem and Trump, 1986; Hida *et al.*, 1986; Staples, 1986). It was hoped that differences in glycosylation between AFP of germ cell tumor and other origins, as shown by their pattern of binding to concanavalin A, would allow distinction between the two, but there is still not uniform agreement that this is reliable enough to be used routinely (Coppack *et al.*, 1983; Vessella *et al.*, 1984), and further evaluation of this test is needed. It is apparent that AFP is also produced by certain differentiated teratoma tissues, for example, primitive gut-like epithelium and liver (Krag Jacobsen and Talerman, 1989), and could conceivably add to the diagnostic confusion. Serum AFP levels in these circumstances are modest; AFP levels between 10 and 20 kU l^{-1} may be regarded as abnormal provided the patient is not receiving, or has not recently received, cytotoxic chemotherapy. Plateau levels of between 10 and 30 kU l^{-1} for 12 weeks without any other evidence of active disease are compatible with complete remission (Coppack *et al.*, 1983).

False positive estimations of HCG are extremely uncommon now that antibodies to the carboxy terminal end of the beta subunit are in use (Javadpour, 1986). It has been stated in the past that cannabinoids increase serum HCG levels, but this has been disputed (Hogan *et al.*, 1983).

3.4 THE ROLE OF TUMOR MARKERS IN DIAGNOSIS AND STAGING

The association of serum AFP and HCG with testicular germ cell tumors is so well established that elevation of serum markers may be diagnostic in a young adult with a metastatic tumor, even without a biopsy. Similarly, immunohistochemistry on a tumor specimen using antibodies to AFP and HCG may lead to a tissue diagnosis even when the clinical picture is not typical. Newer tissue markers such as placental-like alkaline phosphatase, membrane monoclonal antibodies and genetic markers such as *i* (12p), *c-kit*, or *hst-1*, may also have an application in this respect, and will be discussed later (Strohmeyer *et al*, 1991; Rajpert-De Meyets and Skakkebæk, 1994).

The incidence of marker positivity based on serum assays is similar in most studies (Table 3.2). What is apparent is the large number of patients who are marker negative in several series. It is still important to monitor serum AFP and HCG in these patients. At the Royal Marsden Hospital 271 patients with marker negative NSGCT were treated between January 1978 and June 1989, of whom 44 relapsed, 16 with marker negative disease and 28 with raised serum markers (seven AFP, nine HCG and 12 both AFP and HCG). Hence, it is important to continue to measure serum AFP and HCG following therapy even in patients who are marker negative.

The principal use of tumor markers in staging is in the distinction between Stage I and metastatic disease; failure of serum markers to normalize with the appropriate half-life in a patient with no macroscopic disease is usually taken to indicate metastatic disease. Attempts to correlate pre- or postoperative serum marker levels with clinical stage in metastatic disease have met with variable success as reported in the literature. It is not surprising that most authors have found that in NSGCT the proportion of marker positive patients rises with advancing clinical stage (Willemse *et al.*, 1981a; Vugrin *et al.*, 1982; Nørgaard-Pedersen *et al.*, 1984), but this does not mean that marker-secreting tumors are more likely to metastasize (Krag Jacobsen, 1983). It can be difficult to define the volume of metastatic disease in NSGCT accurately, but when this has been done a close correlation with marker levels has been

Table 3.2 Incidence of marker positivity in testicular cancer patients

Source	Histology	AFP	HCG	AFP and/or HCG
Bosl *et al.* (1983)	NSGCT	95/201 (47%)	146/245 (60%)	–
Javadpour (1986)	Seminoma	0/160 (0%)	14/160 (9%)	14/160 (9%)
	NSGCT	147/226 (65%)	129/226 (57%)	190/226 (84%)
Nørgaard-Pedersen *et al.* (1984)	Seminoma	3/307* (1%)	21/307 (7%)	24/307 (8%)
	NSGCT	155/296 (52%)	92/296 (31%)	179/296 (60%)
Royal Marsden Hospital Jan. 1978–June 1989	Seminoma	18/403* (4%)	59/403 (15%)	73/403 (18%)
	NSGCT	299/623 (47%)	224/623 (36%)	352/623 (56%)

* See text for discussion of this finding.
AFP, alpha-fetoprotein.
HCG, human chorionic gonadotrophin.

observed (Horwich *et al.*, 1987). With modern imaging techniques, serum marker level estimations have little to contribute to staging in germ cell tumors where metastatic disease is demonstrable, but it remains to be seen whether radioimmunoscintigraphy will complement standard staging investigations.

Serum marker estimations have important roles in surveillance programs for Stage I disease, and this is discussed in Chapters 9 and 13.

3.4.1 ESTIMATION OF MARKERS IN SPERMATIC VEIN BLOOD

Although the currently used assays for HCG and AFP are extremely sensitive, some patients whose tumors produce very small quantities of markers will be incorrectly labelled as 'marker negative' based on peripheral blood tests. Several authors have studied marker levels in the spermatic vein blood taken at the time of orchidectomy in an attempt to overcome this, and there is general agreement that such levels are higher than those in peripheral blood, and that some patients have markers detectable only in spermatic vein blood (Tsukamoto *et al.*, 1986; Light and Tyrrel, 1987). Furthermore, the proportion of seminomas that secrete HCG as determined using spermatic vein blood may be much higher than suggested by peripheral blood estimations, although the numbers of patients reported is small (Tsukamoto *et al.*, 1986). It will be of interest to see whether this method may also detect low levels of AFP production by combined seminoma/teratoma as yet unidentified by current peripheral blood and immunohistochemical techniques.

3.4.2 THE USE OF MARKERS IN DIAGNOSIS OF CENTRAL NERVOUS SYSTEM INVOLVEMENT

Estimation of the levels of AFP and HCG in the cerebrospinal fluid (CSF) has been investigated in several centers as a possible means of diagnosing central nervous system (CNS) involvement in metastatic disease. Kaye *et al.* (1979) found that AFP levels were unhelpful in this context, but that a CSF HCG level more than 1/40th of the simultaneous serum level was strongly suggestive of CNS metastases, although lower levels did not exclude it. Marrink *et al.* (1984) have suggested that the AFP index, defined as the quotient between the CSF/serum AFP level and the CSF/serum albumin level (so taking into account possible damage to the blood–brain barrier) might be similarly used. Patients with CNS metastases would be expected to have indices higher than the mean value of 1.07 found in patients without CNS disease.

Further studies will be required to determine whether these methods add any useful information to that gained by modern imaging techniques.

3.4.3 THE SIGNIFICANCE OF ELEVATED HUMAN CHORIONIC GONADOTROPHIN IN SEMINOMA

The production of HCG by seminomas is a well-recognized phenomenon, but the exact proportion of tumors that do so is unclear (Paus *et al.*, 1988). In a review of previous studies, Nørgaard-Pedersen found a total incidence of 8%, in agreement with the Danish Testicular Carcinoma study, and with data from the National Cancer Institute (Nørgaard-Pedersen *et al.*, 1984; Javadpour, 1986; Table 3.2). Some more recent studies suggest rates of 50% or even higher, and the sensitivity of the individual assays may have a bearing on this (Tsukamoto *et al.*, 1986; Paus *et al.*, 1988). Immunohistochemical studies have been illuminating in developing understanding of this phenomenon, indicating that in many instances HCG-positive cells can be identified that are either typical syncytiotrophoblast cells or individual mononuclear cells (Mostofi, 1984). The latter may also be cells committed to syncytiotrophoblastic differentiation (Mostofi, 1984). In many cases where these cells are not identified, an overt non-seminomatous component in the form of choriocarcinoma or embryonal carcinoma may be identified, although occasionally no HCG-secreting elements are found even after careful sectioning. Seminoma with syncytiotrophoblast cells should be regarded as being distinct from combined teratoma/seminoma, but it is unclear how to distinguish reliably between the two when the histology is unhelpful.

The question of the prognostic significance of HCG production in seminoma is still unresolved, despite some views to the contrary in the literature. Although some recent studies suggest that such patients have a worse prognosis stage for stage (Morgan *et al.*, 1982; Nørgaard-Pedersen *et al.*, 1984; Butcher *et al.*, 1985; Paus *et al.*, 1987), others have not demonstrated this (Kuber *et al.*, 1983; Swartz *et al.*, 1984; Scheiber *et al.*, 1985; Tsukamoto *et al.*, 1986; Mirimanoff *et al.*, 1993). What does seem apparent is that seminoma with syncytiotrophoblast is associated with modest elevations of HCG (Javadpour, 1986), higher levels being suggestive of a non-seminomatous component.

3.5 THE PROGNOSTIC SIGNIFICANCE OF TUMOR MARKER ELEVATION

There is no doubt that serum marker levels at presentation are of prognostic significance. This has been demonstrated in a number of studies of prognostic factors in metastatic NSGCT using multivariate analyses, discussed further in Chapter 5. Inevitably, different studies came to different conclusions regarding the precise details of the cutoff point between 'good' and 'poor' prognostic groups, but a review of studies published up to 1986 indicated that, in terms of serum markers, HCG was the most important prognostic factor (Vaeth *et al.*, 1984; Vogelzang, 1987). It has been elegantly demonstrated that the application of different models to the same group of patients yields different assessments of which patients are in a poor prognostic group (Bosl, Bajorin and Geller, 1987). Several studies indicated that serum LDH was an independent prognostic factor, an important observation for those centers that were not routinely using this marker. Serum markers appear to be of prognostic value with regard to the probability of achieving complete remission on chemotherapy, to relapse after complete remission, and to survival (Vaeth *et al.*, 1984; Vogelzang, 1987; Geller, Bosl and Chan, 1989). The correlation between tumor bulk and marker levels has already been mentioned, and both appear to correlate with prognosis (Horwich *et al.*, 1987).

An important observation from these studies is that serum markers are continuous variables with regard to prognosis, i.e. the prognosis steadily worsens as marker levels increase. The concept of a 'cutoff' between good and bad prognostic groups is, to an extent, artificial in this sense, but is of practical use in assigning an appropriate treatment regimen to an individual patient. The cutoff levels derived from the second MRC prognostic factor analysis (HCG >10 000 IU l^{-1}, AFP >1000 IU l^{-1}), are currently in widespread use in the United Kingdom (Mead *et al.*, 1992).

Much of the confusion generated by the multiplicity of prognostic models should be resolved when the International Germ Cell Cancer Collaborative Group publishes in full its prognostic factor analysis, based on 6000 evaluable patients drawn from a worldwide database of evaluable patients treated with cisplatin-based chemotherapy. The precise details of this extensive analysis are awaited, but certain conclusions can already be drawn from presentations and the conference abstract (Mead and Stenning, 1995).

1. The tumor markers AFP, HCG and LDH are all of independent prognostic significance, and all three should be incorporated into routine clinical management.
2. On the basis of tumor marker levels, plus other factors (presence or absence of a primary mediastinal teratoma, and presence or absence of non-pulmonary visceral metastases), patients will be assigned to one of three prognostic groups: good, intermediate and poor.
3. The stratification marker divisions are as follows: Good Prognosis, HCG <1000 mg/ml

(<5000 IU/L) and AFP <1000 mg/ml and LDH <1.5 × N (N = upper limit of normal range). Poor Prognosis, HCF >10 000 mg/ml (>750 000 IU/L) or AFP >10 000 mg/ml or LDH >10 × N. Intermediate Prognosis markers are between the above levels.

3.6 THE KINETICS OF SERUM ALPHA-FETOPROTEIN AND HUMAN CHORIONIC GONADOTROPHIN

3.6.1 THE MARKER SURGE PHENOMENON

Contrary to the expectation that serum AFP and HCG levels would fall immediately following the onset of chemotherapy for non-seminomas, a transient elevation is often seen. This alarming phenomenon was described for HCG in gestational choriocarcinoma (Bagshawe, 1973), and subsequently by Vogelzang *et al.* (1982), and by Horwich and Peckham (1986) in testicular tumors. It can occur with both AFP and HCG, and tends to occur early; in these studies, the median time to peak marker levels was 5 days, with a range of 1 to 12 days, and markers were below their day 1 levels by 16 days. This may be seen in as many as 70% of patients if frequent marker estimations are performed, and can on occasions be dramatic (up to 400%). Based on relatively small numbers, neither of these studies has demonstrated any clear prognostic significance to this phenomenon, which has been termed the marker 'surge' (Horwich and Peckham, 1986).

Several mechanisms have been proposed to explain the marker surge phenomenon, including continued tumor growth, altered marker metabolism or excretion, tumor cell lysis and differentiation of stem cells to HCG-producing cells, since this phenomenon has been observed with choriocarcinoma cells treated with cytotoxic drugs *in vitro* (Browne and Bagshawe, 1982).

There is no direct evidence as to which, if any, of these mechanisms are important *in vivo*. However, in at least one series describing HCG-secreting seminomas, a transient elevation of HCG level was seen following radiotherapy (Kuber *et al.*, 1983). Furthermore, a new tumor marker, TRA-1–60, a surface molecule on EC cells that disappears during differentiation, is under evaluation (Marrink *et al.*, 1991). Preliminary results suggest that with this marker too a transient rise in serum levels occurs after the onset of chemotherapy. Tumor cell lysis is probably the explanation for these results, and is therefore at least contributory to this phenomenon in some circumstances. The possibility of a false positive rise in AFP should also be borne in mind, related to underlying liver dysfunction or to the induction chemotherapy, as discussed above.

3.6.2 MARKER REGRESSION RATES

The first information about the behavior of AFP and HCG as tumor markers came from the physiological characterization of these molecules in the 1960s. Of particular relevance were the observations on the metabolism of HCG and AFP in normal individuals, in whom plasma levels of each declined in an exponential fashion, with quoted clearance rates from the blood of approximately 5 days for AFP and 30 hours for HCG. Subsequently, it was noted that these figures were also applicable to patients with germ cell tumors following complete surgical removal of all marker-producing tumor (Lange *et al.*, 1982b).

However, in the context of chemotherapy or radiotherapy for a marker-producing tumor the situation is more complex, in that tissue is still present, albeit in microscopic amounts, for a period of some time after the onset of treatment. Although the marker levels should decline in this setting, their rate of decline is determined by a complex interplay between marker production on the one hand, and removal by excretion or metabolism on the other. In these circumstances the rate of

disappearance from the serum is not a true half-life, and the term 'apparent half-life' (AHL) was introduced (Kohn, 1979). In practice, the AHL (which can be calculated in several ways from measured serum marker levels), is similar to the true half-life for AFP, but can be slightly longer for HCG (Kohn, 1979; Willemse *et al.*, 1981b; Vogelzang *et al.*, 1982; Horwich and Peckham, 1984). This naturally prompted the question whether a prolonged AHL in a patient on chemotherapy carried any prognostic significance. It is still unclear whether rates of marker decline on chemotherapy are useful guides to treatment and prognosis, some studies suggesting that they are (Bosl, 1993) and some reaching the opposite conclusion (Stevens *et al.*, 1995). It is of interest that a pattern of initially normal AHL followed by a late increase may be associated with residual mature teratoma (Willemse *et al.*, 1981b; Horwich and Peckham, 1984).

A simple index comprising the ratio of the HCG level at day 22 to that at day 1, and the AFP level at day 43 to that at day 1, has been reported to be an accurate predictor of treatment failure in individuals with indices greater than 0.005 and 0.0025 for AFP and HCG, respectively (Picozzi *et al.*, 1984; Nielsen *et al.*, 1984). It is interesting that this method should succeed where the more sophisticated AHL estimation did not, and it needs to be further evaluated.

3.7 THE USE OF SERUM MARKERS IN ESTIMATING MARKER PRODUCTION

The proportion of the marker-producing subpopulation in a germ cell tumor varies from individual to individual and, as indicated earlier, may not consist entirely of mitotically active cells. The question arises whether estimates of the total burden of marker-producing cells can be informative. To arrive at this estimate it must be assumed that the body burden of these cells per day is related to the amount of marker produced by them per day. Unfortunately marker production and serum levels are not related in a simple way; marker clearance from the body depends on the total amount of marker present (hence its exponential elimination), and not on its rate of production. These considerations led Price and colleagues to develop a mathematical means of calculating marker production (Price *et al.*, 1990). The mathematics are complicated, which has restricted the use of this method, but it requires further evaluation.

3.8 TESTICULAR TUMOR MARKERS IN IMAGING

The first attempts at imaging using radiolabeled antitumor antibodies date from the 1950s. The advent of monoclonal antibody techniques reawakened interest in this field, and several studies examined the use of monoclonal antibodies to AFP, carcinoembryonic antigen (CEA) and HCG in radioimmunolocalization (Javadpour *et al.*, 1981; Van Cangh *et al.*, 1985; Begent, 1986), indicating that circulating antigen did not prevent the uptake of radiolabeled antibody by tumor, and that on occasions it was possible to demonstrate tumor not visible by any other means. However, the scans produced can be difficult to interpret, and improved techniques are required. Progress is likely to be made by advances in scanning, with the use of techniques such as single photon emission computerized tomography (SPECT), or by a better choice of detecting antibody. Attempts have already been made to use newer markers such as placental-like alkaline phosphatase as the basis for monoclonal antibody scanning (Epenetos *et al.*, 1985b). However, it may be that antibodies to surface antigens (therefore not requiring internalization), and those that recognize determinants on malignant stem cells rather than on differentiated derivatives, will be better candidates than anti-AFP or anti-HCG antibodies. Antibodies that meet these criteria have been described (Pera *et al.*, 1988; Marrink *et al.*,

1992; Mason and Pera, 1992), but not as yet employed in this context in humans, though the use of a monoclonal antibody to a mouse EC surface antigen, SSEA-1, has been successful in an animal model (Solter and Knowles, 1986).

In addition to a role in the staging of testicular cancer, these techniques might also find application in the localization of isolated residual or recurrent disease in patients suitable for curative surgery. This approach has already resulted in occasional long-term remission (Begent, 1986).

3.9 OTHER MARKERS OF TESTICULAR CANCER

In the last decade, the search for new markers of testicular cancer has yielded a bewildering array of candidates, which are summarized in Table 3.3. In many instances the potential clinical benefit is unproven, although a few appear promising, and a few, such as CEA, and CA 125 do not (Bosl *et al.*, 1983; Buamah *et al.*, 1987).

Of the placental proteins SP_1, or pregnancy-specific beta-1 glycoprotein, has been the most studied, but it has not yet been shown that it adds any useful information to serum AFP and HCG in NSGCT, and it is not elevated in pure seminoma (de Bruijn *et al.*, 1985; Javadpour, 1986).

The B5 antigen is either undetectable or present in small amounts on the erythrocyte surface in normal people, except in a few who express it strongly, and its density on the cell remains constant in any one individual unless a malignancy develops, including a testicular cancer (Metcalfe and Jones, 1987). It is detectable in the majority of patients with seminoma and NSGCT, and could have a role in monitoring the clinical course of disease.

Of the enzymes being evaluated, placental-like alkaline phosphatase and lactate dehydrogenase deserve special mention and are discussed below. It has recently been

Table 3.3   Other markers of testicular germ cell tumors

Class	Reference
Placental/pregnancy associated	
SP$_1$	Javadpour (1986)
	de Bruijn *et al.* (1985)
Placental proteins 5, 10, 15	Javadpour (1986)
PAPP–A	Bischoff and Mégevand (1986)
EPF	Rolfe *et al.* (1983)
HPL	Javadpour (1986)
Fetal proteins	
Basic fetoprotein	Harada *et al.* (1987)
Erythrocyte associated	
B5	Metcalfe and Jones (1987)
Hemoglobin F	Dainiak and Hoffman (1980)
Enzymes	
Lactate dehydrogenase	Sugawara *et al.* (1986)
	Javadpour (1986)
	von Eyben *et al.* (1988)
Placental alkaline phosphatase	Lange *et al.* (1982a)
	Epenetos *et al.* (1985a)
	Javadpour (1986)
	Hofmann and Millan (1993)
Neuron-specific enolase	Kuzmits, Schernthaner and Krisch (1987)
	Kawata *et al.* (1989)
	Fosså, Klepp and Paus (1992)
Gamma-glutamyl transpeptidase	Javadpour (1986)
Cell-surface antigens	
TRA-1-60	Marrink *et al.* (1991)
GCTM-2	Mason, Pera and Cooper (1991)
Others	
Estradiol	Uysal and Bakkaloglu (1987)
Prolactin	MacLean and Holdaway (1980)
Ferritin	Szymendera *et al.* (1985)
Gene markers	
i(12p)	Atkin and Baker (1982)
hst-1	Strohmeyer *et al.* (1991)
c-kit	Rajpert-de Meyts and Skakkebæk (1994)

shown that germ cell tumors express neuron-specific enolase, particularly in seminoma-dysgerminoma, and in neural elements of malignant teratoma intermediate (MTI), and this, too has potential as a monitor of disease, particularly seminoma, although like B5 its lack of specificity limits its usefulness in diagnosis.

Monoclonal antibody studies have defined cell surface antigens on EC which disappear during *in vitro* differentiation; one of these antibodies, TRA-1–60, has been detected in the sera of 32 out of 42 patients with an EC component to their tumor (Marrink *et al.*, 1991). Preliminary studies on GCTM-2, a monoclonal antibody to an extracellular matrix antigen on EC (Mason, Pera and Cooper, 1991), suggest that it too might be of value, and it is being further evaluated.

The finding of a specific chromosomal change in NSGCT, the isochromosome of the short arm of chromosome 12 (Atkin and Baker, 1982) provides a cellular marker which is being evaluated for its use in diagnosis and prognosis. Other genetic abnormalities associated with germ cell tumors include over-expression of *c-kit* in carcinoma *in situ* and seminomas, and *hst-1*, which is associated with NSGCT (Strohmeyer *et al.*, 1991; Rajpert-de Meyts and Skakkebaek, 1994). These, too, may yield new approaches to markers of diseases.

3.9.1 PLACENTAL-LIKE ALKALINE PHOSPHATASE

It was found some years ago that malignant tumors could produce placental-like alkaline phosphatase (PLAP) substances. The first description was in a patient with bronchogenic carcinoma that produced an isoenzyme, termed the Regan isoenzyme after the patient. A second subtype, termed the Nagao iso-enzyme, was discovered soon afterwards which, as well as being present in trace amounts in testis and thymus, is strongly expressed in germ cell tumors (Hofmann and Millan, 1993), particularly seminoma, where it can be demonstrated using immunohisto-chemistry. Studies from Europe and the USA indicate that serum PLAP levels are elevated in 40–100% of seminoma patients (Lange *et al.*, 1982a; Epenetos *et al.*, 1985a; Javadpour, 1986), and mirror the clinical course of disease. It seems less useful in NSGCT. Its major drawback is its elevation in up to 35% of patients without disease, many of whom smoke, this being the likely reason for many false positives. Its prognostic significance and relation to clinical stage are as yet unclear, and its main application may be in combination with other markers (Munro *et al.*, 1991).

To date it has still not found universal application.

It seems that the isoenzyme 1 is particularly associated with germ cell tumors (Sugawara *et al.*, 1986; von Eyben *et al.*, 1988), and selective measurement of this fraction might overcome some of its disadvantages.

3.10 FUTURE PROSPECTS

A number of new potential tumor markers are available for evaluation; clearly, none is ideal, and should not deter efforts to find others, particularly in seminoma. However, as new markers become available, they should be critically evaluated to assess whether they provide useful information in patients currently designated 'marker negative' for AFP and HCG. It seems likely that any new marker will be more valuable in combination with others than when used singly, but the optimum combinations of existing markers have still not been adequately delineated. Radioimmunoscintigraphy and chromosomal analysis have still not yet revealed their full potential, and need to be further explored.

Major efforts are underway to find useful tumor markers in malignancies other than testicular tumors. If they succeed, we must not be slow to apply the lessons we have learned.

REFERENCES

Atkin, N.B. and Baker, M.C. (1982) Specific chromosome change, *i*(12p), in testicular tumours? *Lancet*, **ii**, 1349.

Bagshawe, K.D. (1973) Recent observations related to the chemotherapy and immunology of gestational choriocarcinoma. *Adv. Cancer Res.*, **18**, 231–63.

Begent, R.H.J. (1986) Radioimmunolocalisation of germ cell tumours, in *Germ Cell Tumours II* (eds W.G. Jones, A. Milford Ward and C.K. Anderson), Pergamon Press, Oxford, pp. 159–62.

Bischof, P. and Mégevand, M. (1986) Pregnancy-associated plasma protein-A concentrations in men with testicular and prostatic tumours. *Arch. Androl.*, **16**, 155–60.

Bosl G.J. (1993) Prognostic factors for metastatic testicular germ cell tumours: the Memorial Sloan-Kettering cancer model. *Eur. Urol*, **23**, 182–7.

Bosl, G.J., Bajorin, D. and Geller, N.L. (1987) An analysis of poor risk assignment in patients with germ cell tumours. *Int. J. Androl.*, **10**, 285–9.

Bosl, G.J., Geller, N.L., Cirrincione, C. *et al.* (1983) Serum tumour markers in patients with metastatic germ cell tumours of the testis – a ten year experience. *Am. J. Med.*, **75**, 29–35.

Braunstein, G.D., Vaitukaitis, J.L., Carbone, P.P. and Ross, G.T. (1973) Ectopic production of human chorionic gonadotrophin by neoplasms. *Ann. Intern. Med.* **78**, 39–45.

Browne, P. and Bagshawe, K.D. (1982) Enhancement of human chorionic gonadotrophin production by antimetabolites. *Br. J. Cancer*, **46**, 22–9.

de Bruijn, H.W.A., Sleijfer, D.Th., Koops, H.S. *et al.* (1985) Significance of human chorionic gonadotrophin, alpha-fetoprotein, and pregnancy-specific beta-1-glycoprotein in the detection of tumour relapse and partial remission in 126 patients with nonseminomatous germ cell tumours. *Cancer*, **55**, 829–35.

Buamah, P.K., Cornell, C., Skillen, A.W. *et al.* (1987) Initial assessment of tumour-associated antigen CA-125 in patients with ovarian, cervical, and testicular tumours. *Clin. Chem.*, **33**, 1124–5.

Butcher, D.N., Gregory, W.M., Gunter, P.A. *et al.* (1985) The biological and clinical significance of HCG-containing cells in seminoma. *Br. J. Cancer*, **51**, 473–8.

Van Cangh, P.J., Ferrant, A., Ninance, J. *et al.* (1985) Radioimmunodetection of primary and secondary germ cell tumours. *Prog. Clin. Biol. Res.*, **203**, 127–38.

Coppack, S., Newlands, E.S., Dent, J. *et al.* (1983) Problems of interpretation of serum concentrations of alpha-fetoprotein (AFP) in patients receiving cytotoxic chemotherapy for malignant germ cell tumours. *Br. J. Cancer*, **48**, 335–40.

Dainiak, N. and Hoffman, R. (1980) Hemoglobin F production in testicular malignancy. *Cancer*, **45**, 2177–80.

Epenetos, A.A., Munro, A.J., Tucker, D.F. *et al.* (1985a) Monoclonal antibody assay of serum placental alkaline phosphatase in the monitoring of testicular tumours. *Br. J. Cancer*, **51**, 641–4.

Epenetos, A.A., Snook, D., Hooker, D. *et al.* (1985b) Indium-111 labelled monoclonal antibody to placental alkaline phosphatase in the detection of neoplasms of testis, ovary, and cervix. *Lancet*, **ii**, 350–3.

von Eyben, F.E., Blaabjerg, O., Petersen, P.H. *et al.* (1988) Serum lactate dehydrogenase isoenzyme I as a marker of testicular germ cell tumour. *J. Urol.*, **140**, 986–90.

Fosså, S.D., Klepp, O. and Paus, E. (1992) Neuron-specific enolase – a serum tumour marker in seminoma? *Br.J.Cancer*, **65**, 297-9.

Geller, N.L., Bosl, G.J. and Chan, E.Y.W. (1989) Prognostic factors for relapse after complete response in patients with metastatic germ cell tumours. *Cancer*, **63**, 440–5.

Grem, J.L. and Trump, D.L. (1986) Reversible increase in serum alpha-fetoprotein content associated with hepatic dysfunction during chemotherapy for seminoma. *J. Clin. Oncol.*, **4**, 41–5.

Harada, K., Morishita, S., Itani, A. *et al.* (1987) Clinical evaluation of basic fetoprotein in testicular cancer. *J. Urol.*, **138**, 1178–80.

Hida, S., Kawakita, M., Oishi, K. *et al.* (1986) False positive elevation of alpha-fetoprotein during the induction chemotherapy of patients with testicular cancer. *Hinyokika Kiyo*, **32**, 1859–66.

Hofmann, M.C. and Millan, J.L. (1993) Developmental expression of a alkaline phosphatase genes; reexpression in germ cell tumours and *in vitro* immortalised germ cells. *Eur. Urol*, **23**, 38–45

Hogan, P., Sharpe, M., Smedley, H. and Sikora, K. (1983) Cannabinoids and HCG levels in patients with testicular cancer. *Lancet*, **ii**, 1144.

Horwich, A., Easton, D., Husband, J. *et al.* (1987) Prognosis following chemotherapy for metastatic malignant teratoma. *Br. J. Urol.*, **59**, 578–83.

Horwich, A. and Peckham, M.J. (1986) Transient tumour marker elevation following chemotherapy for germ cell tumours of the testis. *Cancer Treat. Rep.*, **70**, 1329–31.

Horwich, A. and Peckham, M.J. (1984) Serum tumour marker regression rate following chemotherapy for malignant teratoma. *Eur. J. Cancer Clin. Oncol.*, **20**, 1463–70.

Javadpour, N. (1986) Serum and cellular markers in testicular cancer, in *Principles and Management of Testicular Cancer* (ed. N. Javadpour), Thieme Inc., New York, pp. 155–65.

Javadpour, N., Kim, E.E., DeLand, F.H. *et al.* (1981) The role of radioimmunodetection in the management of testicular cancer. *JAMA*, **246**, 45–9.

Kardana, A., Taylor, M.E., Southall, P.J. *et al.* (1988) Urinary gonadotrophin peptide-isolation and purification, and its immunohistochemical distribution in normal and neoplastic tissues. *Br. J. Cancer*, **58**, 281–6.

Kawata, M., Sekiya, S., Hatakeyama, R. and Takamizawa, H. (1989) Neuron-specific enolase as a serum marker for immature teratoma and dysgerminoma. *Gynecol. Oncol.*, **32**, 191–7.

Kaye, S.B., Bagshawe, K.D., McElwain, T.J. and Peckham, M.J. (1979) Brain metastases in malignant teratoma: a review of four years' experience and an assessment of the role of tumour markers. *Br. J. Cancer*, **39**, 217–23.

Kohn, J. (1979) The value of apparent half-life assay of alpha-1 fetoprotein in the management of testicular teratoma, in *Carcino-Embryonic Proteins*, Volume II (ed. F.G. Lehmann), Elsevier/North Holland Biomedical Press, Amsterdam, pp. 383–6.

Kohn, J. and Raghavan, D. (1981) Tumour markers in malignant germ cell tumours, in *The Management of Testicular Tumours*, (ed. M.J. Peckham), Edward Arnold, London, pp. 59–69.

Krag Jacobsen, G. (1983) Tumour markers in testicular germ cell tumours related to the stage of the disease at the time of diagnosis. *Oncodev. Biol. Med.*, **4**, C39–C44.

Krag Jacobsen, G. and Talerman, A. (1989) *Atlas of Germ Cell Tumours*, Munksgaard, Copenhagen.

Kuber, W., Kratzik, Ch., Schwarz, H.P. *et al.* (1983) Experience with beta-HCG-positive seminoma. *Br. J. Urol.*, **55**, 555–9.

Kuber, W., Kratzik, Ch., Schwarz, H.P. *et al.* (1983) Experience with beta-HCG-positive seminoma. *Br. J. Urol.*, **55**, 555–9.

Kuzmits, R., Schernthaner, G. and Krisch, K. (1987) Serum neuron-specific enolase – a marker for response to therapy in seminoma. *Cancer*, **60**, 1017–21.

Lange, P.H., Millan, J.L., Stigbrand, T. *et al.* (1982a) Placental alkaline phosphatase as a tumour marker for seminoma. *Cancer Res.*, **42**, 3244–7.

Lange, P.H., Vogelzang, N.J., Goldman, A. *et al.* (1982b) Marker half-life analysis as a prognostic tool in testicular cancer. *J. Urol.*, **128**, 708–11.

Light, P.A. and Tyrrell, C.J. (1987) Testicular tumour markers in spermatic vein blood. *Br. J. Urol.*, **59**, 74–5.

MacLean, G.D. and Holdaway, I.M. (1980) The serum prolactin level in testicular tumours – a new tumour marker? *Aust. N.Z. J. Surg.*, **50**, 384–6.

Mann, K. and Karl, H.J. (1983) Molecular heterogeneity of human chorionic gonadotrophin and its subunits in testicular cancer. *Cancer*, **52**, 654–60.

Marrink, J., Andrews, P.W., van Brummen, P.J., de Jong, HJ., Sleijfer, D.T., Schraffordt Koops, H. and Oosterhuis, J.W. (1991) TRA-1-60: a new serum marker in patients with germ cell tumours. *Int. J. Cancer*, **49**, 368–72.

Marrink, J., Sleijfer, D.Th., Kok, A.J. *et al.* (1984) AFP index, a parameter for the detection of brain metastases in non-seminomatous germ cell tumours of the testis. *Eur. J. Cancer Clin. Oncol.*, **20**, 1207–8.

Mason, M.D. and Pera, M.F. (1992) Immunohistochemical and biochemical characterisation of the expression of a human embryonal carcinoma cell proteoglycan antigen in human germ cell tumours and other tissues. *Eur. J. Cancer*, Abstract 28, 1090–8.

Mason, M.D., Pera, M.F. and Cooper, S. (1991) Possible presence of an embryonal carcinoma-associated proteoglycan in the serum of patients with testicular germ cell tumours. *Eur. J. Cancer*, **27**(3), 300.

Mead, G.M. and Stenning, S.P. (1995) International consensus prognostic classification for metastatic germ cell tumours treated with platinum based chemotherapy: final report of the international germ cell cancer collaboration group (IGCCCG). *Proc. Am. Assoc. Clin. Oncol.*, **235**.

Mead, G.M., Stenning, S.P., Parkinson, M.C., Horwich, A., Fosså, S.D., Wilkinson, P.M., Kaye, S.B., Newlands, E.S. and Cook, P.A. (1992) The second MRC study of prognostic factors in non-seminomatous germ cell tumours. *J. Clin. Oncol.* **10**, 85–94.

Metcalfe, S. and Jones, W.G. (1987) Testicular cancer: B5, a new tumour marker? *Urol. Int.*, **42**, 254–9.

Mirimanoff, R.O., Sinzig, M., Kruger, M., Miralbell, R., Thoni, A., Ries, G., Bosset, J.F., Bernier, J., Bolla, M., Nguyen, T.D., Lutolf, U.M., Hunig, R., Kurtz, J., Greiner, R. and Couke, P.A. (1993) Prognosis of human chorionic gonadotrophin-producing seminoma treated by postoperative radiotherapy. *Int. J. Rad. Oncol. Biol. Phys.*, **27**, 17–23.

Morgan, D.A.L., Caillaud, J.M., Bellet, D. and Eschwege, F. (1982) Gonadotrophin-producing seminoma: a distinct category of germ cell neoplasm? *Clin. Radiol.*, **33**, 149–53.

Mostofi, F.K. (1984) Tumor markers and pathology of testicular tumors. *Prog. Clin. Biol. Res.*, **153**, 69–87.

Munro, A.J., Nielsen, O.S. Duncan., W., Stureon, J., Gospodarowicz, M.K., Malkin, A., Thomas, G.M. and Jewett, M.A. (1991) An assessment of combined tumour markers in patients with seminoma: placental alkaline phosphatase (PLAP), lactate dehydrogenase (LD) and β human chorionic gonadotrophin (βHCG). *Br.J. Cancer*, **64**, 537–42.

Nielsen, H., Hansen, S.W., Ernst, P. and Rørth, M. (1984) Prognostic value of changes in tumor marker concentrations during treatment of patients with testicular cancer. *Cancer Treat. Rep.*, **68**, 1422–3.

Nørgaard-Pedersen, B., Schultz, H.P., Arends, J. *et al.* (1984) Tumour markers in testicular germ cell tumours; five year experience from the DATECA Study 1976–1980. *Acta Radiol. Oncol.*, **23**, 287–94.

Paus, E., Fosså, A., Fosså, S.D. and Nustad, K. (1988) High frequency of incomplete human chorionic gonadotrophin in patients with testicular seminoma. *J. Urol.*, **139**, 542–4.

Paus, E., Fosså, S.D., Risberg, T. and Nustad, K. (1987) The diagnostic value of human chorionic gonadotrophin in patients with testicular seminoma. *Br. J. Urol.*, **59**, 572–7.

Pera, M.F., Blasco-Lafite, M.J., Cooper, S. *et al.* (1988) Analysis of cell differentiation lineage in human teratomas using new monoclonal antibodies to cytostructural antigens to embryonal carcinoma cells. *Differentiation*, **39**, 139–49.

Pera, M.F., Blasco-Lafite, M.J. and Mills, J. (1987) Cultured stem cells from human testicular teratomas: the nature of embryonal carcinoma, and its comparison with two types of yolk sac carcinoma. *Int. J. Cancer*, **40**, 334–43.

Picozzi, V.J., Freiha, F.S., Hannigan, J.F. and Torti, F.M. (1984) Prognostic significance of a decline in serum human chorionic gonadotrophin levels after initial chemotherapy for advanced germ cell carcinoma. *Ann. Intern. Med.*, **100**, 183–6.

Price, P., Hogan, S.J., Bliss, J.M. and Horwich, A. (1990) The growth rate of metastatic non-seminomatous germ cell testicular tumours measured by marker production doubling time–II.

Prognostic significance in patients treated by chemotherapy. *Eur. J. Cancer*, **26**, 453–7.

Raghavan, D., Sullivan, A.L., Peckham, M.J. and Munro Neville, A. (1982) Elevated serum alpha-fetoprotein and seminoma. Clinical evidence for a histologic continuum? *Cancer*, **50**, 982–9.

Rajpert-de Meyts, E. and Skakkebaek, N.E. (1994) Expression of the *c-kit* protein product in carcinoma-in-situ and invasive testicular germ cell tumours. *Int. J. Androl.*, **17**, 85–92.

Rolfe, B.E., Morton, H., Cavanagh, A.C. and Gardiner, R.A. (1983) Detection of an early pregnancy factor-like substance in sera of patients with testicular germ cell tumours. *Am. J. Reprod. Immunol.*, **3**, 97–100.

Scheiber, K., Mikuz, G., Frommhold, H. and Bartsch, G. (1985) Human chorionic gonadotrophin-positive seminoma: is this a special type of seminoma with a poor prognosis? *Prog. Clin. Biol. Res.*, **203**, 97–104.

Solter, D. and Knowles, B.B. (1986) Cell surface antigens of germ cells, embryos, and teratocarcinoma cells, in *Principles and Management of Testicular Cancer* (ed. N. Javadpour), Thieme Inc., New York, pp. 88–98.

Staples, J. (1986) Alphafetoprotein, cancer, and benign conditions. *Lancet*, **ii**, 1277.

Stevens, M.J., Norman, A.R., Dearmley, D.P. and Horwich A. (1995) Prognostic significance of early serum tumor marker half-life in metastatic testicular teratoma. *J. Clin. Oncol.*, **13**, 87–92.

Strohmeyer, T., Peter, S., Hartmann, M., Munemitsu, S., Ackermann, R., Ullrich, A. and Slamon, D.J. (1991) Expression of the *hst-1* and *c-kit* protooncogenes in human testicular germ cell tumours. *Cancer Res.*, **51**, 1811–16.

Sugawara, T., Furuhata, T., Ogawa, K. and Hosaka, M. (1986) A clinical study of testicular tumor-usefulness of serum lactate dehydrogenase (LDH). *Nippon Hinyokika Gakkai Zasshi*, **77**, 948–53.

Swartz, D.A., Johnson, D.E. and Hussey, D.H. (1984) Should an elevated human chorionic gonadotrophin titer alter therapy for seminoma? *J. Urol.*, **131**, 63–5.

Szymendera, J.J., Kozlowicz-Gudzinska, I., Madej, G. *et al.* (1985) Clinical usefulness of serum ferritin measurements in patients with testicular germ cell tumours. *Oncology*, **42**, 253–8.

Tsukamoto, T., Kumamoto, Y., Oshmura, K. *et al.* (1986) Clinical studies of testicular tumour I-analysis of 27 patients with seminoma: the clinical significance of HCG-beta determination and of retroperitoneal lymph node dissection for stage I patients. *Hinyokika Kiyo*, 7, 989–97.

Uysal, Z. and Bakkaloglu, M. (1987) Serum estradiol as a tumor marker for non-seminomatous germinal cell tumors (NSGCT) of the testis. *Int. Urol. Nephrol.*, 19, 415–18.

Vaeth, M., Schultz, H.P., von der Maase, H. *et al.* (1984) Prognostic factors in testicular germ cell tumours – experiences from 1058 consecutive cases. *Acta Radiol. Oncol.*, 23, 271–85.

Vaitukaitis, J.L., Braunstein, G.D. and Ross, G.T. (1972) A radioimmunoassay which specifically measures human chorionic gonadotrophin in the presence of human luteinizing hormone. *Am. J. Obstet. Gynecol.*, 113, 751–8.

Vessella, R., Santrach, M.A., Bronson, D. *et al.* (1984) Evaluation of AFP glycosylation heterogeneity in cancer patients with AFP-producing tumors. *Int. J. Cancer*, 34, 309–14.

Vogelzang, N.J. (1987) Prognostic factors in metastatic testicular cancer. *Int. J. Androl.*, 10, 225–37.

Vogelzang, N.J., Lange, P.H., Goldman, A. *et al.* (1982) Acute changes of alpha-fetoprotein and human chorionic gonadotrophin during induction chemotherapy of germ cell tumours. *Cancer Res.*, 42, 4855–61.

Vugrin, D., Whitmore, W.F., Nisselbaum, J. and Watson, R.C. (1982) Correlation of serum tumor markers and lymphangiography with degrees of nodal involvement in surgical stage II testis cancer. *J. Urol.*, 127, 683–4.

Waldman, T. and McIntire, K.R. (1974) The use of a radioimmunoassay for alpha-fetoprotein in the diagnosis of malignancy. *Cancer*, 34, 1510–15.

Willemse, P.H.B., Sleijfer, D.Th., Schraffordt Koops, H. *et al.* (1981a) Tumor markers in patients with non-seminomatous germ cell tumors of the testis. *Oncodev. Biol. Med.*, 2, 117–28.

Willemse, P.H.B., Sleijfer, D.Th., Schraffordt Koops, H. *et al.* (1981b) The value of AFP and HCG half lives in predicting the efficacy of combination chemotherapy in patients with non-seminomatous germ cell tumors of the testis. *Oncodev. Biol. Med.*, 2, 129–34.

Yamazaki, II., Kotera, S., Ishikawa, H. and Machida, T. (1987) Characterisation of a human chorionic gonadotrophin producing testicular choriocarcinoma cell line. *J. Urol.* 137, 548–51.

MOLECULAR BIOLOGY OF MALE GERM CELL TUMORS

4

R.S.K. Chaganti and G.J. Bosl

4.1 INTRODUCTION

Male gonadal tumors capable of differentiation into all germinal lineages have traditionally been thought to arise in primordial germ cells (PGC) because of their implicit totipotentiality. Histologically, male germ cell tumors (GCT) are divided into two major groups: seminomas, which do not display embryonal differentiation, and non-seminomas, which do display embryonal differentiation and exhibit embryonal (embryonal carcinoma), extraembryonal (choriocarcinoma, yolk sac tumor), and somatic (teratoma) patterns of tissue differentiation. Clinically, germ cell tumors (GCT) are highly treatable, with more than 90% of patients with newly diagnosed testicular GCT attaining cure following initial treatment and 70–80% of patients with advanced disease achieving cure with cisplatin-based chemotherapy (Bosl and Chaganti, 1994). Their origin in a totipotential cell, ability to express embryonal differentiation patterns, and exquisite sensitivity to antineoplastic therapy make GCT an ideal system for studies aimed at understanding the molecular basis of transformation, differentiation, and cell death pathways in germ cells.

4.2 PATHOBIOLOGY OF GERM CELL TUMORS

Seminomatous GCT (SGCT) retain the morphology of spermatogonial germ cells and are exquisitely sensitive to treatment by radiation as well as chemotherapy (Bosl and Chaganti, 1994). Non-seminomatous GCT (NSGCT) display embryonal-like differentiation and are sensitive to chemotherapy, although they are relatively less sensitive to radiation treatment compared with SGCTs (Bosl and Chaganti, 1994). Pure forms of SGCT and NSGCT account for approximately 40% of all GCT. NSGCT usually present as mixed tumors, comprising both differentiated and undifferentiated elements. Among tumors with differentiated elements, mature teratomas exhibit the most complete differentiation, often presenting such mature cell types as cartilage, neural tissue and mucinous and nonmucinous glands. These tissue elements, however, develop in an unorganized fashion. On occasion, mature cell types in teratomatous lesions undergo malignant transformation into neoplastic elements which show histological features characteristic of *de novo* tumors affecting multiple cell lineages (e.g. sarcoma, carcinoma or leukemia) (Ulbright *et al.*, 1984; Chaganti *et al.*, 1989).

GCT of all types are frequently associated with carcinoma *in situ* (CIS) and intratubular

4

Testicular Cancer: Investigation and management. Second edition. Edited by Professor A. Horwich.
Published in 1996 by Chapman & Hall. ISBN 0 412 61210 0.

germ cell neoplasia. In nearly all cases, CIS lesions progress to invasive lesions. Notably, both SGCT and NSGCT are suggested to arise from cytologically identical CIS lesions, suggesting a common cell of origin of all GCT. Thus, the totipotentiality of the presumed progenitor cell and its pathways to transformation, and expression of complex patterns of differentiation, invasion, metastasis and response to treatment by radiation and chemotherapy by GCT, make these tumors a model system for the molecular genetic analysis of malignant transformation and regulation of differentiation.

4.3   CHROMOSOMAL CHANGES IN GERM CELL TUMORS

The clonal chromosome abnormalities studied in over 200 GCT represented by all histological subsets showed that chromosomes 1 and 12 are most frequently involved in aberration in these tumors (Rodriguez *et al.*, 1992; Chaganti, Rodriguez and Bosl, 1993). The chromosome 1 abnormalities were in the form of deletions and rearrangements and affected both the short arm (1p) and the long arm (1q). The most common nonrandom chromosome abnormality to be detected in GCT, however, was an isochromosome for the short arm of chromosome 12 [*i*(12p)] (Rodriguez *et al.* 1992; Chaganti, Rodriguez and Bosl, 1993) (Fig. 4.1). A number of studies have now shown that one or more copies of *i*(12p) can be detected in >80% of GCT with clonal chromosome abnormalities in all histologic subsets presenting at gonadal as well as extragonadal sites as primary or metastatic lesions. Notably, the *i*(12p) has been noted in lesions as early as CIS (Voss *et al.*, 1990). This abnormality results in the net increase in the copy number of 12p, either as multiple copies of *i*(12p) or as marker chromosomes with tandemly duplicated 12p segments (Rodriguez *et al.*, 1993) (Fig. 4.1). Recently, a number of groups have developed fluorescence *in situ* hybridization (FISH)

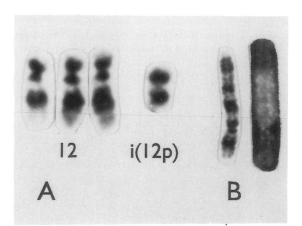

Fig. 4.1   Amplification of 12p in GCT. (a) A partial karyotype of a tumor metaphase showing the *i*(12p) marker. (b) A partial karyotype of a tumor metaphase showing tandem duplication of 12p segments. On the left is a G-banded picture of a marker chromosome with novel tandemly arranged chromosomal segments attached at the end of 12p. On the right is the same marker chromosome hybridized ('painted') with a probe comprising DNA sequences from the entire 12p that recognize the novel segments and establish their derivation from 12p.

methods utilizing chromosome 12-derived probes (centromere, short arm, entire chromosome) to determine the copy number of 12p at interphase (Mukherjee *et al.*, 1991; Suijkerbuijk *et al.*, 1992; Rodriguez *et al.*, 1993). These studies showed that virtually all GCT show multiple copies of 12p. The consistent amplification of 12p in CIS as well as in all histological subsets of GCT indicates an important role for this genetic abnormality in the etiology of this tumor type. Amplified chromosomal regions in tumor cells classically have been indicators of amplification of specific genes associated with origin, progression, or drug resistance of tumors. The second consistent aberration affecting chromosome 12 is deletion in the long arm, which may be seen in as many as 20% of tumors (Murty *et al.*, 1990; Samaniego *et al.*, 1990; Rodriguez *et al.*, 1992). Consistent cytogenetic deletion classically has been the indicator for loss of tumor suppressor genes (TSG), as has been shown in the case of retinoblastoma (*RB* gene), Wilm's tumor (*WT1* gene), and other inherited cancers. Thus, cytogenetic data alone have provided evidence for possible amplification of one or more genes on 12p and possible loss of several TSG on chromosomes 1 and 12 in the development of GCT. The molecular analysis of these and other lesions in GCT identified independently of cytogenetic clues will be discussed below.

4.4 MOLECULAR CHANGES IN GERM CELL TUMORS

A recently developed measure to assess genetic alteration affecting the entire genome of a tumor, termed the 'allelotype', measures loss of heterozygosity (LOH) at multiple polymorphic loci spanning all the chromosomal arms. Allelotype analysis has provided important molecular (loss) correlates of clinical outcome as well as identified sites of novel candidate TSGs in colorectal and other solid tumors (Goddard and Solomon, 1993). A number of studies analyzed LOH and determined the allelotype of GCT. These studies molecularly defined the deletions affecting chromosomes 1 and 12q previously detected by cytogenetic analysis as well as those on 3p and 11p; they also provided new insights into molecular changes affecting GCT (Lothe *et al.*, 1989, 1993; Radice *et al.*, 1989; Murty *et al.*, 1992, 1994a; Mathew *et al.*, 1994).

A recent detailed LOH study of chromosome 1 utilizing 22 polymorphic markers mapped to specific chromosomal bands identified four specific regions of LOH: three on 1p (1p13,1p22,1p31.3–32.2) and one on 1q (1q32) (Mathew *et al.*, 1994). These deletions thus identify sites of many candidate TSGs yet to be isolated and characterized. Chromosome 1 has previously been shown to undergo rearrangement and deletion at the cytogenetic as well as molecular levels in multiple tumor types (hematopoietic as well as solid tumors). A comparison of molecular deletion data between losses on GCT and multiple other

solid tumor types revealed that the deleted sites are common to most tumors, indicating that the loss of the candidate TSG on chromosome 1 may be associated with functions common to the development of most tumors, such as progression (Mathew *et al.*, 1994).

LOH studies of chromosome 12, on the other hand revealed two specific sites of deletion: one at 12q13 and the other at 12q22 (Murty *et al.*, 1992). Although the 12q13 site has been shown to be extremely important in tumorigenesis because of rearrangement or amplification of a number of tumor-associated genes in sarcomas and lymphomas, deletions have previously not been noted in any tumor type other than GCT. Likewise, the 12q22 deletions so far appear to be restricted to GCT. Thus, unlike chromosome 1 deletions, the chromosome 12 deletions appear to be GCT-specific and have the potential to reveal specific genetic mechanisms associated with the development of these tumors (Murty *et al.*, 1992).

A major allelotype analysis of GCT utilizing a panel of 56 tumors and 63 polymorphic probes mapped to each of the chromosomal arms in the genome revealed several novel molecular genetic features of GCT (Murty *et al.*, 1994a). Thus, frequent deletion of several previously recognized TSG (*RB1*, *DCC*, *NME*) and a number of previously described sites of candidate TSG (3p, 9p, 9q, 10q, 11p, 11q and 17p) was noted (Table 4.1). In addition, several novel sites of frequent deletion not previously reported in any other tumor type also were identified (2p, 3q, 5p, 12q, 18p and 20p). Another new finding was that well-differentiated teratomas showed a significantly higher level of allelic loss than did the less differentiated embryonal carcinomas (Murty *et al.*, 1994a). In addition, certain loci and genes exhibited frequent nonrandom deletion in teratomas (D3S32, D3S42, D5S12, D10S25, D11S12, *RB1*, *TP53*, *NME1*, *NME2*, D18S6, and D20S6) and embryonal carcinomas (*IFNB*, D9S27). Among these loci the *NME* genes were notable for a high degree of

Table 4.1   Chromosomal regions that showed high frequency loss of heterozygosity (LOH) in male germ cell tumors (GCT) and their relationship to tumor suppressor genes*

Chromosome region	Polymorphic probe	% LOH	Candidate gene(s)	Gene(s) shown to be deleted in GCTs
1p31.3–32.3	D1S17	33	?	
1p22	D1S16	39	?	
1p13	D1S73	26	?	
1q32	REN	27	?	
2p	D2S44	27	hMSH2	
3p21.33	D3S32	46	VHL, hMLH1	
3q28–29	D3S42	27	?	
5p15.2–15.1	D5S12	42	?	
9p22	IFNB	71	MTS1, MTS2	
9q34	D9S7	49	?	
10q26	D10S25	27	?	
11p15.5	D11S12	30	BWS	
11q13	WNT2	50	MEN1	
12q13.1–q13.3	D12S17	27	?	
12q13.1–q13.3	D12S6	42	?	
12q22	D12S7	42	BTG1	
12q22	D12S12	47	?	
13q14.2	RB1	35	RB1	RB1
13q22	D13S2	29	?	
13q32	D13S3	40	?	
17p13	D17S28	41	TP53, ?	
17q21.3	NME1, NME2	38	NME1, NME2, BRCA1	NME1, NME2
17q23–25.3	D17S4	40	?	
18p11	D18S6	27	?	
18q21.3–ter	D18S5, DCC	46	DCC	DCC
20p12	D20S6	41	?	

* Data from Cullen *et al.*, 1994; Studer *et al.*, 1993;

genetic loss (± 70%) in teratomas (Murty *et al.*, 1994a). These results suggest that non-random loss or inactivation of certain genes may be associated with tumor development and loss or inactivation of other genes may be associated with somatic differentiation. They also provide opportunities for isolation of novel candidate deleted genes and investigation of their role in normal and malignant development and differentiation of germ cells.

Four of the genes whose genomic perturbation (or lack of it) has been indicated by the allelotype analysis have been subjected to further analysis, namely, TP53, NME, RB and DCC (Table 4.1). The TP53 gene encodes a 53 kD (p53) cytoplasmic protein that plays a critical role in several cellular functions.

Thus, it regulates mitotic G_1/S checkpoint through transcriptional control of the 21 kD (p21) cyclin kinase inhibitor (WAF1), and promotes DNA integrity in cycling cells by inducing repair mechanisms and inhibiting entry into S phase of cells with DNA damage (Sherr, 1994). In addition, it acts as a transcriptional regulator of many genes by direct DNA binding. Thus, loss of function of TP53 through deletion, mutation, or both leads to loss of control of the cell cycle leading to neoplastic proliferation (loss of tumor suppression). Indeed, TP53 is the most frequently deleted/mutated gene in a variety of tumor types. Another important function of p53 is to regulate apoptosis (programmed cell death) in cells with DNA damage (strand breaks). In such cells, p53 can initiate cell cycle arrest and enable repair of DNA lesions and restore the normal cell cycle. Alternatively, in the presence of excess DNA damage, p53 can initiate apoptosis. Since most cancer therapy involves DNA damage, treatment response is increasingly thought of in terms of availability of conditions for successful induction of apoptosis, rather than induction of physiological cell death by these agents. Cells harboring p53 mutations will therefore be unable to regulate apoptosis and hence have increased potential for resistance to treatment with DNA-damaging agents. On the other hand, the presence of normal p53 will enable induction of apoptosis in cells with DNA damage, and hence favorable response to treatment. Although a region closely contiguous with the *TP*53 gene shows frequent LOH in GCT, a number of studies of the *TP*53 gene itself have identified no mutations in exons 4–9 (Peng *et al.*, 1993; Murty *et al.*, 1994a), and most tumors express abundant, apparently normal, p53 protein. These findings suggest that the basis for the high degree of responsiveness of GCT to antineoplastic treatment is p53-based apoptosis. Of considerable biological and clinical interest are the ± 10% treatment-resistant tumors. Mechanisms that possibly account for their treatment resistance include as yet unrecognized p53-inactivating mutations or induction of anti-apoptotic genes such as *BCL*2.

The phosphorylation of the retinoblastoma gene (*RB*1) product, a 105–110 kD nuclear phosphoprotein (Rb), is mediated by D-type cyclins and their associated kinases and initiates the G_1/S transition of the mitotic cycle. Loss of *RB* gene function through deletion and/or mutation results in loss of G_1 regulation and suppression of inappropriate cycling. Therefore, the *RB*1 gene has often been called the prototype tumor suppressor gene. Besides retinoblastoma, *RB*1 loss has been noted in a variety of tumors, e.g. breast, bladder and small cell lung carcinomas, and soft tissue sarcomas. In one study of GCT, the level of

*RB*1 mRNA was noted to be decreased 3–15 fold in tumor cells of all histological subsets compared with surrounding epithelial cells (Strohmeyer *et al.*, 1991). In addition, *RB*1 expression by immunohistochemical staining was undetectable in undifferentiated GCT, while it was detectable in nearly all differentiated GCT. In another study, LOH for *RB*1 gene was noted in as many as 40% of tumors belonging to all histological subsets (Murty *et al.*, 1994a). Thus, loss and/or deregulation of the *RB*1 gene seems to be an important genetic event in GCT development; however, its mechanistic basis and significance are yet to be determined.

The *NME*1 and *NME*2 genes encode the A and B subunits, respectively, of the housekeeping enzyme nucleoside diphosphate kinase (NDPK) (Steeg, Cohn and Leone, 1991). The *NME* genes have been suggested to be metastasis suppressor genes because, in some tumors, progression towards a metastatic phenotype was associated with decreased *NME* expression (Steeg, Cohn and Leone, 1991). On the other hand, the level of mRNA expression, as well as enzymatic activity of NDPK, has been found to be increased in certain types of human tumors in comparison with surrounding normal tissues. Mutational disruption of the homologous *awd* gene in *Drosophila* leads to multiple somatic abnormalities during postembryonic development, suggesting that in *Drosophila* the *NME* homologue may be involved in regulation of differentiation. Among male GCT, teratomas exhibit a significantly higher LOH at the *NME* loci and a four to five-fold lower *NME* protein level, compared with embryonal carcinomas. These data suggest a potential role for the *NME* genes in the regulation of somatic differentiation in human male GCT, as in *Drosophila* (Backer *et al.*, 1994).

The product of the *DCC* tumor suppressor gene shares a high degree of homology with neural cell adhesion molecules (NCAM) which are involved in cell–cell and cell–

basement membrane interactions and cell homing. Allelic loss and reduced expression of *DCC* were first identified in colon carcinoma as late events in tumor development. Since then significant deletion and/or decreased expression of the *DCC* gene have been reported in a wide variety of tumors such as breast, pancreatic, gastric and prostate carcinomas, glioblastomas and leukemias (reviewed in Murty *et al.*, 1994b). In GCT, overall *DCC* allelic loss was noted in 45% of tumors, including two cases with homozygous deletion (Murty *et al.*, 1994b). *DCC* mRNA levels were either reduced or absent in a number of tumors. Interestingly, *DCC* perturbations were unrelated to the primary or metastatic state of the tumors and were equally common in all histological subsets, suggesting that *DCC* loss is an early event in germ cell tumorigenesis. This observation is consistent with a possible role for normal *DCC* in regulation of germ cell migration and intratubular cell communications necessary for proper germ cell development (Murty *et al.*, 1994b). One of the requirements for neoplastic growth would be abrogation of such controls.

Genomic instability detected as microsatellite variations, also called the replication error (RER) phenotype, has recently been identified as a novel genetic mechanism associated with the development of many tumor types. Defects in a family of genes responsible for DNA mismatch repair (*hMLH1*, *hMSH2*, *hPMS1*, *hPMS2*) have been implicated in the generation of a high rate of genome-wide somatic instability in hereditary nonpolyposis colon cancer and other types of cancers. In a recent study, RER phenotype localized to the 1q42–43 chromosomal region was reported, with a higher frequency in embryonal carcinomas and yolk sac tumors, compared with teratomas (Murty *et al.*, 1994c). The significance of this instability to GCT development and histological differentiation remains to be determined.

4.5 A GENETIC MODEL FOR GERM CELL TUMOR DEVELOPMENT

The cytogenetic and molecular data on GCT discussed above allowed us to develop a novel, testable hypothesis regarding GCT origin and development. Thus, GCT as a group exhibit heteroploid (triploid–tetraploid) chromosome numbers, express wild-type p53, show high frequency of allelic loss affecting *RB*, *DCC* and *NME* genes and a number of previously identified as well as novel chromosomal sites. Virtually all tumors as well as CIS exhibit multiple copies of 12p segments, suggesting that amplification and overexpression of a gene on this chromosomal arm may be linked to transformation. Two candidate genes mapped to this chromosomal arm are *CCND2* (cyclin D2) and *KRAS2*, although a number of studies have shown that the *KRAS2* gene does not undergo activating mutations in GCT (Dmitrovsky *et al.*, 1990). These data suggest that the target cell for transformation is one with replicated chromosomes that expresses wild-type p53, harbors DNA breaks, and may be prone to apoptosis. The pachytene spermatocyte fulfils these requirements: it contains replicated DNA undergoing recombination; p53 is expressed at this stage presumably to arrest the cell cycle to facilitate recombinational repair. Apoptotic cell death is a feature of normal germ cells. Based on these data we suggest a model of germ cell transformation according to which aberrant recombination at pachytene leads to amplification of 12p and overexpression of a gene on 12p (such as *CCND2*), which may reinitiate the cell cycle and rescue a cell otherwise destined to undergo apoptosis. In such cells, downstream events such as *RB1* loss may lead to neoplastic proliferation.

4.6 A GENETIC MODEL FOR GERM CELL TUMOR DIFFERENTIATION

The ability of highly heteroploid and chromosomally abnormal GCT derived from germ cells prior to completion of meiosis to express embryonal-like differentiation is a paradox. These cells do not contain the appropriately imprinted genomes characteristic of post-fertilization embryos, which are normally programmed to express such differentiation. At the same time, the molecular data described above permit recognition of several possible levels of differentiation control:

1. **Switches in expression of major lineage-associated genes.** Thus *KIT*, which normally is expressed by germ cells through the pachytene stage, is expressed mainly by CIS and SGCT, which retain a germ cell-like phenotype. NSGCT, on the other hand, appear to down-regulate *KIT* and up-regulate *MGF*, which is consistent with their loss of germ cell phenotype and acquisition of somatic fates (Murty *et al.*, 1992).

2. **Loss of dominant regulation of induction of differentiation cascades.** Detailed allelotype analysis of GCT showed that teratomas with somatic differentiation exhibit significantly greater genetic loss compared with undifferentiated embryonal carcinomas, suggesting that loss of certain types of genes may lead to loss of dominant negative control of initiation of differentiation cascades constitutive to proliferating embryonal cells. The role of these genes in differentiation control would be analogous to that of tumor suppressor genes in the control of cell cycle (Murty *et al.*, 1994a). One such gene, as discussed above, may be *NME*, which shows significantly higher LOH and reduced protein levels in teratomas compared with embryonal carcinomas (Backer *et al.*, 1994). Several genes with similar functions may be expected to be identified in future.

3. **Re-imprinting.** Parental imprinting is erased in normal germ cells early (prior to meiosis) in their differentiation and a new set of imprints are laid down during gametogenesis. Therefore, the target cell proposed (pachytene cell at mid prophase) would be imprint erased, which is consistent with recent observation of biallelic expression of *IGF2* and *H*19, which normally show monoallelic expression in post-fertilization somatic tissues (van Gurp *et al.*, 1994). One possible mechanism by which embryonal and extraembryonal lineages may be initiated in imprint-erased transformed germ cells is DNA methylation in critical chromosomal regions.

In this brief review, we have attempted to bring together the rapidly developing genetic view of human male GCT. The new data generated by us and others allow us to construct new and testable hypotheses regarding GCT development and differentiation. Experimental verification of these hypotheses will lead to a fuller understanding of these fascinating and challenging tumors.

REFERENCES

Backer, J.M., Murty, V.V.V.S., Potla, L. *et al.* (1994) Loss of heterozygosity and decreased expression of *NME* genes correlate with teratomatous differentiation in human male germ cell tumors. *Biochem. Biophys. Res. Commn.*, **202**, 1096–103.

Bosl, G.J. and Chaganti, R.S.K. (1994) The use of tumor markers in germ cell malignancies. *Hematol/Oncol. Clin. North Am.*, **8**, 573–87.

Chaganti, R.S.K., Ladanyi, M., Samaniego, F. *et al.* (1989) Malignant hematopoietic differentiation of germ cell tumors. *Genes. Chrom. Cancer.*, **1**, 83–7.

Chaganti, R.S.K., Rodriguez, E. and Bosl, G.J. (1993) Cytogenetics of male germ-cell tumors. *Urol. Clinics North Am.*, **20**, 55–66.

Dmitrovsky, E., Murty, V.V.V.S., Moy, D. *et al.* (1990) Isochromosome 12p in non-seminoma cell lines: karyologic amplification of c-ki-ras$_2$ without point-mutational activation. *Oncogene*, **5**, 543–8.

Goddard, A.D. and Solomon, E. (1993) Genetic aspects of cancer, in *Advances in Human Genetics*, vol.21. eds H. Harris and K. Hirshhorn, Plenum Press, New York, pp. 321–76.

van Gurp, R.J.H.L.M., Oosterhuis, J.W., Kalscheuer, V., Mariman, E.C.M. and Looijenga,

L.H.J. (1994) Biallelic expression of the *H19* and *IGF2* genes in human testicular germ cell tumors. *J. Natl Cancer Inst.*, **86**, 1070–5.

Lothe, R.A., Fosså, S.D., Stenwig, A.E. *et al.* (1989) Loss of 3p or 11p alleles associated with testicular cancer tumors. *Genomics*, **5**, 134–8.

Lothe, R.A., Hastie, N., Heimdal, K., Fosså, S.D., Stenwig, A.E. and Borresen, A.-L. (1993) Frequent loss of 11p13 and 11p15 loci in male germ cell tumors. *Genes Chrom. Cancer*, **7**, 96–101.

Mathew, S., Murty, V.V.V.S., Bosl, G.J. and Chaganti, R.S.K. (1994) Loss of heterozygosity identifies multiple sites of allelic deletions on chromosome 1 in human male germ cell tumors. *Cancer Res.*, **54**, 6265–9.

Mukherjee, A.B., Murty, V.V.V.S., Rodriguez, E., Reuter, V.E., Bosl, G.J. and Chaganti, R.S.K. (1991) Detection and analysis of origin of *i*(12p), a diagnostic marker of human male germ cell tumors, by fluorescence *in situ* hybridization. *Genes Chrom. Cancer*, **3**, 300–7.

Murty, V.V.V.S., Bosl, G.J., Houldsworth, J. *et al.* (1994a) Allelic loss and somatic differentiation in human male germ cell tumors. *Oncogene*, **9**, 2245–51.

Murty, V.V.V.S., Dmitrovsky, E., Bosl, G.J. and Chaganti, R.S.K. (1990) Nonrandom chromosome abnormalities in testicular and ovarian germ cell tumor cell lines. *Cancer Genet. Cytogenet.*, **50**, 67–73.

Murty, V.V.V.S., Houldsworth, J., Baldwin, S. *et al.* (1992) Allelic deletions in the long arm of chromosome 12 identify sites of candidate tumor suppressor genes in male germ cell tumors. *Proc. Natl Acad. Sci. USA*, **89**, 11006–11.

Murty, V.V.V.S., Li, R.-G., Houldsworth, J. *et al.* (1994b) Frequent allelic deletions and loss of expression characterize the *DCC* gene in male germ cell tumors. *Oncogene*, **9**, 3227–31.

Murty, V.V.V.S., Li, R.-G., Mathew, S. *et al.* (1994c) RER-type instability at 1q42–43 in human male germ cell tumors. *Cancer Res.*, **54**, 3983–5.

Peng, H.-Q., Hogg, D., Malkin, D. *et al.* (1993) Mutations of the p53 gene do not occur in testis cancer. *Cancer Res.*, **53**, 3574–8.

Radice, P., Pierotti, M.A., Lacerenza, S. *et al.* (1989) Loss of heterozygosity in human germinal tumors. *Cytogenet. Cell Genet.*, **52**, 72–6.

Rodriguez, E., Houldsworth, J., Reuter, V.E. *et al.* (1993) Molecular cytogenetic analysis of *i*(12p)-negative human male germ cell tumors. *Genes Chrom. Cancer*, **8**, 230–6.

Suijkerbuijk, R.F., Looijenga, L., de Jong, B., Oosterhuis, J.W., Cassiman, J.J., Geurts van Kessel, A. (1992) Verification of isochromosome 12p and identification of other chromosome 12 aberrations in gonadal and extragonadal human germ cell tumors by bicolor double fluorescence *in situ* hybridization. *Cancer Genet. Cytogenet.*, **63**, 8–16.

Rodriguez, E., Mathew, S., Reuter, V., Ilson, D.H., Bosl, G.J. and Chaganti, R.S.K. (1992) Cytogenetic analysis of 124 prospectively ascertained male germ cell tumors. *Cancer Res.*, **52**, 2285–91.

Samaniego, F., Rodriguez, E., Houldsworth, J. *et al.* (1990) Cytogenetic and molecular analysis of human male germ cell tumors: Chromosome 12 abnormalities and gene amplification. *Genes Chrom. Cancer*, **1**, 289–300.

Sherr, C.J. (1994) G1 phase progression. Cycling on cue. *Cell*, **79**, 551–5.

Steeg, P.S., Cohn, K.H. and Leone, A. (1991) Tumor metastasis and nm23: current concepts. *Cancer Cells*, **3**, 257–62.

Strohmeyer, T., Reissmann, P., Cordon-Cardo, C., Hartmann, M., Ackermann, R. and Slamon, D. (1991) Correlation between retinoblastoma gene expression and differentiation in human testicular tumors. *Proc. Natl Acad. Sci. USA*, **88**, 6662–6.

Ulbright, T.M., Loehrer, P.J., Roth, L.M., Einhorn, L.H., Williams, S.D. and Clark S.A. (1984) The development of non-germ cell malignancies within germ cell tumors. A clinicopathologic study of eleven cases. *Cancer*, **54**, 1824–33.

Voss, A.M., Oosterhuis, J.W., de Jong, B., Buist, J. and Koops, H.S. (1990) Cytogenetics of carcinoma *in situ* of the testis. *Cancer Genet. Cytogenet.*, **46**, 75–81.

DIFFERENTIATION IN GERM CELL TUMORS

J.W. Oosterhuis and P.W. Andrews

5.1 INTRODUCTION

Germ cell tumors (GCT) and teratomas form a heterogeneous group of neoplasms occurring in the gonads and extragonadal localizations. The testicular GCT will be discussed in the context of other GCT, teratomas and gestational trophoblastic disease. It appears that GCT and teratomas can be clustered according to patterns of differentiation. The clusters differ with regards to cytogenetic characteristics and pathogenesis. We propose that genomic imprinting is important among the factors determining the developmental potential and therefore the patterns of histological differentiation in GCT and teratomas.

5.2 CLUSTERING ACCORDING TO DEVELOPMENTAL POTENTIAL

The five developmental clusters to be distinguished are summarized in Table 5.1.

5.2.1 CLUSTER I: (IMMATURE) TERATOMA/ YOLK SAC TUMOR

The tumors of cluster I are, with rare exceptions, composed of pure mature or immature teratoma, pure yolk sac tumor, or a combination of the two (Dehner, 1983; Hawkins, 1990). Tumors originally diagnosed as teratoma may recur as yolk sac tumor. This sequence of events is well documented for tumors in the sacrococcygeal region and in the neck, and experimentally in embryo-derived teratomas of the mouse (van Berlo *et al.*, 1990). The most frequent anatomical site of these lesions is the sacrococcygeal region. With an incidence of about one to two per 100 000 live-born infants, it is the most frequent solid tumor in neonates. It is much rarer in the other anatomical sites: testis, ovary and extragonadal localizations along the midline of the body such as the retroperitoneum, mediastinum, head and neck and midline of the brain. The sacrococcygeal tumors have a male to female ratio of 1:3. A yolk sac component endowing the tumor with malignant potential is more frequent in boys than in girls.

Tumors of cluster I occur in neonates and very young children. Only in the ovary do they occur in somewhat older children and adolescents, at a median age of about 12. Extragonadal (immature) teratomas/yolk sac tumors are extremely rare in adults. Recently we described two adult patients with extragonadal immature teratomas, characterized by specific chromosomal translocations involving chromosomes 6 and 11 (van Echten *et al.*, 1995). In contrast to immature teratomas at the pediatric age, the tumors were highly malignant, presenting with blood-borne metastases.

The majority of GCT of cluster I are (pseudo)diploid; some are (near) tetraploid.

Testicular Cancer: Investigation and management. Second edition. Edited by Professor A. Horwich.
Published in 1996 by Chapman & Hall. ISBN 0 412 61210 0.

Table 5.1 Clustering of germ cell tumors, teratomas and complete mole according to developmental potential

Cluster	Histology	Anatomical site(s)	Age	Ploidy	Numerical Abbn.	Structural Abbn.
I	(Immature) teratoma and/or yolk sac tumor	Testis Ovary	1,5 (0–4) >4 (child–adult)	Teratoma: diploid; YST: diploid/aneuploid	+ X;1;3;8;12;14	Deletions of 1p, in part. 1p36, rarely i(12p) and in YST also aberrations of 3p and 6q
		Sacral region	Neonatal			
		Retroperitoneum	Children			
		Mediastinum	Children		− Y;10	
		Head and neck	Neonatal			
		Midline brain	Neonatal			
		Other rare sites				
II	'Adult testicular type' histology	Testis	>15	Hypotriploid	+ X;7;8;12;	i(12p) and other abbr. of 12p, abberr. of 1 i.p. deletions of 1p
		Nonseminoma	Median 25	Hypo- and hypertriploid		
		Combined tumor	Median 30	Hypertriploid		
		Seminoma	Median 35	Peritetraploid		
		Ovary	>4 (child–adult)	Diploid/peritetrapl./aneupl.	− Y;11;13;18;	
		Dysgenetic gonad	Second decade	Diploid/peritetrapl./aneupl.		
		Anterior mediast.	Adolescents	Diploid/peritetrapl./aneupl.		
		Midline brain	Children			
III	Dermoid cyst	Ovary	Child–adult	Diploid	+ X;7;12;15	–
IV	Spermatocytic seminoma	Testis	Older age	Diploid/peritetrapl./aneupl.	too few analyzed	No i(12p)
V	Complete mole	Uterus	Reproductive age	Diploid	–	–

The yolk sac tumors may be aneuploid. Numerical chromosomal aberrations include: overrepresentation of chromosomes 1, 8, 12 and X and underrepresentation of chromosomes 10 and Y. With regard to structural aberrations, deletions of 1p, in particular the region 1p36, are the most frequent. The cells of diploid tumors are genetically identical to the normal host cells (Perlman *et al.*, 1994; Stock *et al.*, 1994).

Murine spontaneous GCT of the testis in 129 strain mice and in the ovary of LT mice as well as embryo-derived tumors resemble the human GCT of cluster I. The spontaneous tumors are present at birth; most are diploid teratomas in which in the course of time, sometimes only after retransplantation, a yolk sac component may develop.

5.2.2 CLUSTER II: ADULT TESTICULAR TYPE

5.2.2.1 Histological differentiation

GCT of cluster II typically occur in the sexually mature, adult testis. Basically there are two histological types: seminoma, composed of the neoplastic counterparts of primordial germ cells (Jørgensen *et al.*, 1993), and non-seminomatous GCT (non-seminomas), which are neoplastic caricatures of early embryonic development. Carcinoma *in situ* (CIS) of the seminiferous tubules is the precursor of both seminoma and non-seminoma (Skakkebæk *et al.*, 1987). The cells of CIS preceding and accompanying seminoma and non-seminoma are at the morphological level similar to each other and to seminoma cells. It appears that CIS cells have two differentiation options when they become invasive. Either they keep their phenotype of neoplastic primordial germ cells to give rise to seminoma, or they are reprogrammed to become non-seminomas composed of the neoplastic counterparts of pluripotent embryonal stem cells: embryonal carcinoma (EC) cells (Oosterhuis and Looijenga, 1993). This process may be similar to the reprogramming of

murine primordial germ cells grown *in vitro* (Matsui, Zsebo and Hogan, 1992). EC cells may develop into embryoid bodies, resembling 10-day-old human embryos, various immature or mature somatic tissues, or extra-embryonic tissues: yolk sac tumor and choriocarinoma. About 40% of the GCT of the adult testis are pure seminomas; 15% have a seminoma and a non-seminoma component. These tumors are termed 'combined tumors' in the British classification but labeled as non-seminomas in the WHO classification. Their clinical behavior is determined by the more aggressive non-seminoma component. The remaining 45% are non-seminomas lacking a seminoma component. Only a minority of the non-seminomas have a pure histology of EC, (immature) teratoma, yolk sac tumor or choriocarcinoma. Indeed, the better these tumors have been studied histologically the higher are the reported figures of mixed histologies (Ulbright, 1993), reflecting the pluripotent nature of the EC stem cells. This is in sharp contrast with tumors of the other developmental clusters, which as a rule have pure histologies. The very close clonal relationship between EC and its differentiated derivatives in mixed non-seminomas is borne out by their usually identical ploidy (Oosterhuis *et al.*, 1989) and close karyotypic resemblance (de Graaff *et al.*, 1992). Cell lines derived from testicular germ tumors, in particular, have allowed the study of differentiation of EC cells *in vitro*. This aspect is discussed in the final paragraph of this chapter. Animal models for GCT of developmental cluster II do not exist.

5.2.2.2 Seminoma: relative or precursor of non-seminoma?

The pathogenetic relationship between seminoma and non-seminoma is not so obvious (Damjanov, 1989). Evidence is growing that non-seminoma may develop through a seminoma stage. All non-seminomas appear to be derived from an *in situ* precursor cell with a seminomatous phenotype. Pure seminomas may give rise to non-seminomatous metastases. Seminomas themselves appear to be phenotypically heterogeneous. In addition to classical seminoma there are intermediate phenotypes with non-seminomatous features. Seminoma with trophoblastic giant cells, about 10% of all seminomas, is a well-known example. More recently, intermediate phenotypes between seminoma and yolk sac tumor have been described (Czaja and Ulbright, 1992). A clonal relationship between seminoma and non-seminoma is further supported by the cytogenetic similarity between the two (see below). The consistently lower ploidy of non-seminomas, compared with seminomas, hypotriploid and hypertriploid respectively (Oosterhuis *et al.*, 1989), suggests that seminoma may progress to become a non-seminoma through a net loss of chromosomes, among them chromosome 15, which has significantly fewer copies in non-seminoma than in seminoma (de Jong *et al.*, 1990), probably already at the CIS level (Looijenga *et al.*, 1993). In addition, cytogenetic data suggest that the two components of combined tumors are usually of monoclonal origin (Gillis *et al.*, 1994). Taken together these data suggest that seminoma is not as separate from non-seminoma as was previously assumed. Experimental demonstration of reprogramming of seminoma cells *in vitro* would prove the validity of the concept. The methods to grow seminoma cells *in vitro* need further development before such experiments can be done (Berends *et al.*, 1991; Olie *et al.*, 1995).

5.2.2.3 Differentiation of metastases

The different components of combined tumors and mixed non-seminomas differ in their metastatic potential (Oosterhuis, 1983). Teratoma and seminoma are the least aggressive types; choriocarcinoma on the other hand is highly metastatic, giving rise to blood-borne metastases. Thus, aggressiveness of a germ cell tumor is determined not only by its stage

of progression, but also by the differentiation lineages it develops.

The histology of metastases can be predicted from the composition of the primary tumors. Accordingly, residual mature teratoma after chemotherapy is associated with primary tumors with a teratoma component (Oosterhuis *et al.*, 1983). A secondary non-germ cell malignancy, observed in metastatic lesions of patients who fail chemotherapy, is usually already present in the primary tumor (Ulbright *et al.*, 1990). Components of low metastatic potential tend to be underrepresented in regional metastases and even more so in distant metastases (de Graaff *et al.*, 1991).

5.2.2.4 Primary sites other than the testis

GCT of the adult testicular type occur, apart from the testis, in the ovary and only two extragonadal localizations: the anterior mediastinum and midline of the brain. They are rare in these anatomical sites, however. In the ovary they may present at a younger age than in the testis. Mediastinal GCT of the adult testicular type occur most often in male adolescents. Klinefelter's syndrome poses a higher risk. Adult testicular type GCT of the brain occur mainly in the pineal gland and in the hypothalamic region in older children, more often in boys than in girls.

The spectrum of histological differentiation is the same as in the adult testis. The counterparts of seminoma are called 'dysgerminoma' in the ovary and 'germinoma' in the brain. Yolk sac tumor seems a more prominent component of mediastinal GCT than in those of the adult testis. Combined tumors occur in the ovary, anterior mediastinum and midline of the brain. Secondary non-germ cell malignancies are also encountered in these sites. Secondary hematopoietic malignancies, not induced by therapy, may originate in perhaps the yolk sac component of mediastinal GCT, and rarely in midline of the brain lesions, but not in testicular or ovarian GCT (Nichols *et al.*, 1990). This is the more striking since hematopoietic activity may be seen in GCT of the adult testis.

5.2.2.5 Ploidy and cytogenetics

GCT of the adult testicular type of all sites are prone to polyploidization. The testicular tumors are virtually always aneuploid: CIS and seminoma are hypertriploid and non-seminoma is hypotriploid. Dysgerminomas of the ovary are peritetraploid. Data on non-seminomas of this site are too scanty to allow generalizations. Mediastinal tumors are pseudo-diploid, peritetraploid or aneuploid (Ooster-huis *et al.*, 1990). Lesions of the midline of the brain have not been studied in sufficient detail. Existing data suggest a similar ploidy pattern to that in mediastinal tumors (Ooster-huis, Castedo and de Jong 1990).

All GCT of the adult testicular type irre-spective of anatomical localization are cyto-genetically characterized by amplification of the short arm of chromosome 12. In about 80% of the non-seminomas and 60% of the seminomas, this occurs by forming iso-chromosomes of 12p, and in the remaining tumors by other rearrangements involving 12p (Suijkerbuijk *et al.*, 1993).

Histology and cytogenetic findings suggest that all GCT of the adult testicular type are derived from premeiotic primordial germ cells that have migrated to the gonadal blastema or to the anterior mediastinum or the midline of the brain. Initiation probably takes place during intrauterine life. Poly-ploidization of the tumor cells is a frequent and early event, followed during tumor progression by amplification of 12p (Geurts van Kessel *et al.*, 1989) and nonrandom losses and gains of certain other chromosomes (de Jong *et al.*, 1990).

5.2.3 CLUSTER III: DERMOID CYST

The dermoid cyst is the most frequent GCT, occurring almost exclusively in the ovary. In children it constitutes 60–70% of all GCT. In patients older than 15 years over 95% of the ovarian GCT are dermoid cysts. They consist of cysts lined by mature skin with append-ages or by glandular epithelium. The lumen is filled with hairs and sebaceous material. A nodular thickening of the wall of the cyst, protruding into the lumen, is composed of mature somatic tissues, most often of neuro-ectodermal derivation.

Dermoid cysts are diploid with a normal female karyotype. Cytogenetic and molecular studies have demonstrated that they are derived from parthenogenetically activated meiotic oöcytes via at least three mechan-isms: failure of first meiosis, failure of second meiosis or duplication of a mature ovum (Surti *et al.*, 1990).

5.2.4 CLUSTER IV: SPERMATOCYTIC SEMINOMA

Spermatocytic seminoma is a rare GCT that occurs only in descended testes of elderly men, and is composed of neoplastic germ cells at a stage of maturation between sper-matogonia and spermatocytes (Eble, 1994, for review). It is not a variant of seminoma and is not associated with GCT of the adult testicu-lar type, including CIS. The intratubular variant is probably the *in situ* precursor of spermatocytic seminoma. Microscopically it is composed of sheets of small, medium and large cells with round nuclei. The chromatin is dense in the small, more open in the medium, and often filamentous in the large nuclei. The overall picture has some super-ficial resemblance to the early stage germ cells of the testis. The tumors have very low metastatic potential. In less than 5%, sar-comas have developed in testes with sper-matocytic seminoma. The DNA content is pseudodiploid or peritetraploid and less often aneuploid. The only karyotyped case did not have isochromosomes 12p (unpublished data), and *in situ* hybridization suggests that chromosome 12 is not overrepresented (unpublished data). The pathogenesis of spermatocytic seminoma and GCT of the adult testicular type is different. The latter originate from transformed primordial germ cells. Spermatocytic seminoma is probably the result of neoplastic transformation of somewhat more mature cells in the spermatogenetic lineage. Seminomas reported in animals, in particular dogs, have more in common with spermatocytic seminoma than seminoma (Looijenga *et al.*, 1994).

5.2.5 CLUSTER V: COMPLETE MOLE AS PROTOTYPE OF GESTATIONAL TROPHOBLASTIC DISEASE

Gestational trophoblastic disease is not normally listed among the GCT and teratomas. In anticipation of the discussion of genomic imprinting and its possible role in determining the developmental potential of GCT, they are mentioned here. Complete moles are discussed in some more detail as a prototype of gestational trophoblastic growths.

The term 'gestational trophoblastic disease' encompasses the following entities: complete mole, partial mole, invasive mole, choriocarcinoma, and placental site trophoblastic tumor. All have in common that they are exclusively composed of trophoblastic tissue: cyto- and syncytiotrophoblast and intermediate trophoblast in varying proportions.

Complete moles are composed of grossly swollen chorionic villi, resembling a bunch of grapes. The villi are lined by proliferating trophoblast. They result from the fertilization of eggs that have lost their chromosomes. There are two variants: the most common form is homozygous 46,XX, resulting from androgenetic activation of an X-bearing sperm, and the less common form is heterozygous 46,XX or 46,XY, caused by dispermic fertilization (Arima *et al.*, 1994).

5.3 DEVELOPMENTAL CLUSTERS BY SITE AND AGE

The broad classification of GCT and teratomas in a small number of developmental clusters enforces the notion that these tumors occur in a limited number of anatomical sites (gonads and midline of the body) and in these sites in the same chronological order (Table 5.2). (Immature) teratoma/yolk sac tumor occurs most often in neonates and infants. In the four sites where GCT of the adult testicular type occur, cluster I tumors may be encountered, but at an earlier age. The karyotypes of the tumors of cluster I and II are different, but there is some overlap (Table 5.1), again suggesting a close relationship between the two.

In the testis the cluster II tumors are followed by spermatocytic seminoma; in the ovary the dermoid cysts occur on average at an older age than the tumors of cluster I and II. These findings suggest that the GCT and teratomas of the different clusters may originate from closely related cells, probably germ cells in different stages of maturation. One of the factors that will probably influence the developmental potential of germ cells and

Table 5.2 Chronological order of developmental clusters by anatomical site

Anatomical site	Chronological order of developmental clusters
Testis	I; II; IV
Ovary	I and II; III
Sacrum	I*
Retroperitoneum	I**
Mediastinum	I; II
Head and neck	I*
Midline brain	I; II
Uterus	V

* (Immature) teratoma may be followed by yolk sac tumor.
** Tumors of adult testicular type are usually metastases from testicular primary tumors.
I = (immature) teratoma/yolk sac tumor; II = GCT of the adult testicular type; III = dermoid cyst; IV = spermatocytic seminoma; V = complete mole.

their primitive precursors is their genomic imprinting status.

5.4 GENOMIC IMPRINTING

During the 1980s a new phenomenon important in early embryonal development was discovered, when expression of certain genes did not appear to obey the normal Mendelian rules of inheritance. Pronuclear transfer experiments in mice indicated that the developmental potential of a manipulated diploid zygote was determined by the parental origin of the haploid sets of chromosomes present. Uniparental embryos always failed early in pregnancy; they rarely survive beyond day ten. Androgenotes, zygotes with an exclusively paternal genome, show a poor development of somatic tissues, but the extraembryonic tissues, in particular the trophoblast, develop relatively well. In contrast, the gynogenotes, zygotes with a completely maternally derived genome, have a relatively normal development of somatic tissues and a very poor growth of the trophoblast. Apparently, for normal embryonic development certain chromosomal regions must be donated by the father and some by the mother. This difference in functionality between homologous chromosomal regions based on their parental origin is defined as genomic imprinting. Somewhere during the development from primitive germ cell to mature gamete, the genomic constitution of paternally and maternally imprinted chromosomes present in the normal zygote has to be changed into either a totally maternal pattern (during oogenesis), or a totally paternal pattern (during spermatogenesis) (Solter, 1988). It is also along this route that GCT are initiated.

5.4.1 GENOMIC IMPRINTING AND GCT

The suspicion that genomic imprinting might play a role in the pathogenesis of GCT is based on the assumption that the dermoid cyst of the ovary is the human counterpart of the mouse gynogenote, which favors somatic differentiation. Indeed the dermoid cyst of the ovary (developmental cluster III) is exclusively composed of somatic tissues, and is the result of parthenogenetic activation of a meiotic ovum, of which the chromosomes most likely have completed erasement and possess only female imprinting. On the other hand, the complete mole (developmental cluster V) is the human counterpart of the mouse androgenote, which favors trophoblastic differentiation. The complete mole consists of trophoblastic tissue only and results from the fertilization of an empty ovum. It has, therefore, an exclusively male imprint.

The role of genomic imprinting in the remaining developmental clusters is more speculative. The truly pluripotent nature of the non-seminomas of developmental cluster II, with somatic differentiation, yolk sac tumor and trophoblast, might require a biparental imprinting. This would imply that the primordial germ cells from which they derive are not yet erased. The seminomas and (dys)germinomas, also in cluster II, are tumors of primordial germ cells not readily reprogrammable to pluripotency. This could be due to the fact that these cells, in the course of specialization towards germ cells, have undergone erasement.

Spermatocytic seminoma (developmental cluster IV), originating from even more specialized germ cells, cannot be activated to pluripotency.

The tumors of cluster I in the gonads are most probably derived from germ cells. They have the same developmental potential as the testicular GCT of the strain 129 mice and the ovarian GCT of LT mice. The extragonadal tumors of developmental cluster I, with their typical localization in the midline of the body, are probably also derived from primitive germ cells with a biparental imprint, prior to erasement. The limited spectrum of differentiation in these tumors as compared with tumors of cluster II might be due to a more primitive phenotype of their cells of origin, resembling embryonal stem cells. This view is supported by the finding that transplanted embryos devoid of germ cells give rise to similar tumors as the spontaneous GCT in the gonads of 129 and LT mice (Solter, 1983). Clearly, these hypotheses need to be tested.

5.5   HUMAN GCT IN CULTURE

Isolation of a large number of cell lines from explants of human GCT, virtually all of them from developmental cluster II, has provided a valuable resource for experimentally investigating the biology of these tumors, the relationships between the various histological subtypes and the characterization of various markers that can be useful in clinical practice, and for testing new approaches to treatment and diagnosis.

5.5.1   EC CELL LINES

Any extensive analysis of GCT biology tends to center upon the EC component of these tumors, ever since early reports suggested that EC cells represent the critical malignant stem cell population of such tumors. Initial studies of human EC cell lines were hampered by the lack of definitive markers for identification and by the lack of differentiation that would have indicated their pluripotent nature. However, many human GCT-derived cell lines resembled cultured murine EC cells in their morphology, growth patterns and expression of high levels of alkaline phosphatase (Andrews *et al.*, 1980; Cotte, Easty and Munro-Neville, 1981). Also, when injected into immunosuppressed mice (typically nude, nu/nu, athymic mice), several such lines produced xenograft tumors that, histologically, closely resembled clinical examples of human EC. Using one such cell line, 2102Ep, which had been derived from a primary testicular non-seminoma GCT, with EC components, several surface antigen markers that

appeared to be typically expressed by human EC cells were defined (Andrews *et al.*, 1982). These antigens included stage specific embryonic antigens-3 and -4 (SSEA-3 and -4), which are carried as globoseries glycolipids that are expressed by cleavage stage mouse embryos, but not by mouse EC cells, and high molecular weight glycoproteins, defined by monoclonal antibodies such as TRA-1–60 and TRA-1–81 (Andrews, 1988). EC cell marker antigens have also been defined by other groups, including additional high molecular weight glycoproteins defined by monoclonal antibodies K4 and K21 (Rettig *et al.*, 1985) and GCTM2 (Pera *et al.*, 1988).

Recently, a large panel of human GCT-derived cell lines was examined for expression of glycolipids (Wenk *et al.*, 1994) and certain surface antigens (Andrews *et al.*, 1996). From that study it was clear that this panel included a distinct subset of cell lines that appeared to correspond to the EC cell component of human GCT and could be defined by its pattern of marker expression. Thus globoseries glycolipids and surface antigens SSEA-3, SSEA-4, TRA-1–60, TRA-1–81, K4, K21 and GCTM2, as well as surface antigens associated with the liver/bone/kidney isoform of alkaline phosphatase, were all typically expressed by the putative EC subset of cell lines, but only sporadically expressed, or not at all, by various other lines corresponding to yolk sac carcinoma, choriocarcinoma or miscellaneous more differentiated cell types derived from GCT.

Accordingly, studies of GCT-derived cell lines have provided clear objective criteria for recognition of EC cell components of GCT, and at least one EC cell marker antigen, TRA-1–60, is shed by the cells and has been proposed as a serum marker for monitoring therapy, supplementing the more traditional serum markers human chorionic gonadotrophin and alpha-fetoprotein (Marrink *et al.*, 1991). It remains to be determined whether expression of these markers might provide new prognostic criteria in a clinical setting.

5.5.2 DIFFERENTIATION OF EC CELLS *IN VITRO*

Most of the human EC cell lines defined in culture show little capacity for differentiation, although some (e.g. 2102Ep cells) do exhibit limited differentiation in mostly undefined directions when culture condition or cell densities are modified (Andrews *et al.*, 1982). This may reflect the prevalence of pure EC components in GCT without associated teratoma components. It can also be rationalized by realizing that EC cell differentiation is often associated with loss, or at least a reduction in malignant potential; one could imagine that mutations or other changes that reduced an EC cell's propensity to differentiate would also provide a selective advantage during tumor evolution and adaptation to conditions *in vitro*. Nevertheless, a full understanding of the biology of GCT must include a study of EC cells that have retained a capacity for differentiation under defined conditions. Several such lines have now been identified and include GCT27, NCCIT and NCR-G3 (Teshima *et al.* 1988; Pera *et al.* 1989; Hata *et al.* 1993). These cells exhibit the same patterns of markers, cell morphology and growth behavior as those EC cells that do not differentiate, and thus serve to underline the notion that pluripotent EC cells do exist in human GCT and are probably the stem cells that can give rise to the various somatic and extraembryonic cell types that characterize the different components of mixed nonseminomas.

Of all the pluripotent EC cell lines, the various clones derived from the TERA2 cell line are probably the best characterized and most widely studied (Andrews *et al.*, 1984; Thompson *et al.*, 1984). This is particularly true for the clonal derivative NTERA2 cl. D1 (abbreviated NT2/D1), which epitomizes the properties of most of these clones. NT2/D1 cells closely resemble other human EC cells when maintained continuously at high cell densities and passaged by scraping rather than by trypsinization. However, when injected into nude mice these cells form well-differentiated tumors that contain neural elements and well developed glandular structures. In culture, they differ from most other human EC cell lines by differentiating extensively when exposed to retinoic acid (Andrews, 1984). This retinoic acid-induced differentiation is almost complete when the cells are exposed to concentrations of 10^{-5} or 10^{-6} mol l^{-1} all-trans retinoic acid for several days, and is characterized by loss of EC cell markers, the appearance of new surface antigens, the appearance of heterogeneous cell morphologies and the activation of various genes, notably those of the *HOX* complexes. In the latter case, the *HOX* genes induced are dependent upon the concentration of retinoic acid used, which may reflect the possible role of retinoic acid as a morphogen during embryonic development (Simeone *et al.*, 1990). Whereas the undifferentiated EC cells can be passaged indefinitely, their differentiation induced by retinoic acid is accompanied by a reduced growth rate and eventual cessation of cell division, although the differentiated cells can subsequently be maintained in culture for several months.

Neurons are especially prominent differentiated cells to appear in NT2/D1 cultures after exposure to retinoic acid (Andrews, 1984) (Fig. 5.1). These neurons express neurofilaments and other neural markers, including receptors and ion channels suggestive of CNS neurons (Lee and Andrews, 1986; Pleasure, Page and Lee, 1992; Rendt, Erulkar and Andrews, 1989). The NT2/D1 cells therefore provide particularly useful tools for investigating the regulation of neurogenesis during human embryonic development. NT2/D1, EC cells possess pluripotent capacities with the ability to differentiate into somatic cell types. Other cell lines have shown yolk sac and trophoblastic differentiation *in vitro*, sometimes in combination with somatic lineages. Seminoma cell lines have not yet been established. Thus human EC cell lines cover the develop-

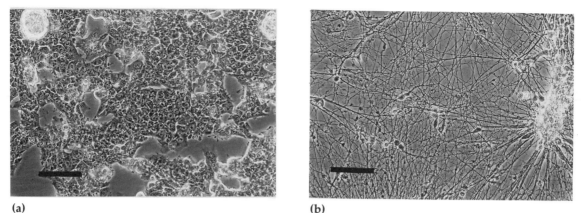

(a)   **(b)**

Fig. 5.1 Cultures of (a) NTERA2 cl.D1 human EC cells and (b) purified neurons derived from them following differentiation. The cells were cultured and induced to differentiate as previously described by exposure to 10^{-5} mol l^{-1} retinoic acid for 3 weeks (Andrews, 1984). Under these conditions, almost all the EC cells disappear and are replaced by various cells with distinct phenotypes; those cells exhibiting a definitive neuronal phenotype constitute only a few per cent of the differentiated cells, but they can be purified by shaking cells off the differentiated cultures and replating on matrigel. Bar = 100 μm.

mental potential of the non-seminomas of the adult testicular type.

5.6 CONCLUSIONS

The differentiation occurring in GCT is clinically relevant for its role in determining their aggressiveness and patterns of metastases. However, from the point of view of tumor biology more generally, the relationships between tumor progression and cell differentiation underline the notion that cancer is often a disease in which the mechanisms that regulate a balance between cell proliferation and cell differentiation are disturbed. Lastly GCT offer models to study fundamental developmental questions concerning the regulation of differentiation in the early embryo and the role of genomic imprinting in the maturation of germ cells.

REFERENCES

Andrews, P.W. (1984) Retinoic acid induces neuronal differentiation of a cloned human embryonal carcinoma cell line in vitro. *Dev. Biol.* **103**, 285–93.

Andrews, P.W. Human teratocarcinoma (1988). *Biochim. Biophys. Acta*, **948**, 17–36.

Andrews, P.W., Bronson, D.L., Benham, F., Strickland, S. and Knowles, B.B. (1980) A comparative study of eight cell lines derived from human testicular teratocarcinoma. *Int. J. Cancer.*, **26**, 269–80.

Andrews, P.W., Casper, J., Damjanov, I., Duggan-Keen, M., Giwercman, A., Hata, J., von Keitz, A., Looijenga, L., Millán, J.L., Oosterhuis, J.W., Pera, M., Saurada, M., Schmoll, H.J., Skakkebæk, N.E., van Putten, W. and Stern, P. (1996) Comparative analysis of cell surface antigens expressed by cell lines derived from human germ cell tumours. *Int. J. Cancer*, **66**, 806–16.

Andrews, P.W., Damjanov I., Simon, D. *et al.* (1984) Pluripotent embryonal carcinoma clones derived from the human teratocarcinoma cell line TERA-2: differentiation in vivo and in vitro. *Lab. Invest.*, **50**, 147–62.

Andrews, P.W., Goodfellow, P.N., Shevinsky, L., Bronson, D.L. and Knowles, B.B. (1982) Cell surface antigens of a clonal human embryonal carcinoma cell line: morphological and antigenic differentiation in culture. *Int. J. Cancer.*, **29**, 523–31.

Arima, T., Imamura, T., Amada, S. *et al.* (1994) Genetic origin of malignant trophoblastic neoplasms. *Cancer Genet. Cytogenet.*, **73**, 95–102.

Berends, J.C., Schutte, S.E., van Dissel-Emiliani, F.M.F. *et al.* (1991) Significant improvement of the survival of seminoma cells *in vitro* by use of a rat Sertoli cell feeder layer and serum-free medium. *J.Natl. Cancer Inst.*, **83**, 1400–3.

Cotte, C.A., Easty, G.C. and Munro-Neville, A. (1981) Establishment and properties of human germ cell tumours in tissue culture. *Cancer Research*, **41**, 1422–7.

Czaja, J.T. and Ulbright, T.M. (1992) Evidence for the transformation of seminoma to yolk sac tumor, with histogenetic considerations. *Am. J. Clin. Pathol.*, **97**, 468–77.

Damjanov, I. (1989) Editorial. Is seminoma a relative or a precursor of embryonal carcinoma? *Lab. Invest.*, **60**, 1–3.

de Graaff, W.E., Oosterhuis, J.W., de Jong, B. *et al.* (1992) Cytogenetic analysis of the mature teratoma and the choriocarcinoma component of a testicular mixed nonseminomatous germ cell tumor. *Cancer Genet. Cytogenet.*, **61**, 67–73.

de Graaff, W.E., Oosterhuis, J.W., van der Linden, S. *et al.* (1991) Residual mature teratoma after chemotherapy for nonseminomatous germ cell tumors of the testis occurs significantly less often in lung than in retroperitoneal lymph node metasases. *J. Urol. Pathol.*, **1**, 75–81.

de Jong, B., Oosterhuis, J.W., Castedo, S.M.M.J. *et al.* (1990) Pathogenesis of adult testicular germ cell tumors. A cytogenetic model. *Cancer Genet. Cytogenet.*, **48**, 143–67.

Dehner, L.P. (1983) Gonadal and extragonadal germ cell neoplasia of childhood. *Hum. Pathol.*, **14**, 493–511.

Eble, J.N. (1994) Spermatocytic seminoma. *Hum. Pathol.*, **25**, 1035–42.

Geurts van Kessel, A., van Drunen, E., de Jong, B. *et al.* (1989) Chromosome 12q heterozygosity is retained in i(12p)-postive testicular germ tumor cells. *Cancer Genet. Cytogenet.*, **40**, 129–34.

Gillis, A.J.M., Looijenga, L.H.J., de Jong, B. *et al.* (1994) Clonality of combined testicular germ cell tumors of adults. *Lab. Invest.*, **71**, 874–8.

Hata, J., Fujimoto, J., Ishii, E. *et al.* (1993) Differentiation of human germ cell tumour cells *in vivo* and *in vitro*. *Acta Histochem. Cytochem.* **25**, 563–7.

Hawkins, E.P. (1990) Pathology of germ cell tumors in children. *Crit. Rev. Oncol./Hemat.*, **10**, 165–79.

Jørgensen, N., Giwercman, A., Müller, J. *et al.* (1993) Immunohistochemical markers of carcinoma in situ of the testis also expressed in normal infantile germ cells. *Histopathol.*, **22**, 373–8.

Lee, V. M.- Y. and Andrews, P.W. (1986) Differentiation of NTERA-2 clonal human embryonal carcinoma cells into neurons involves the induction of all three neurofilament proteins. *J. Neurosci.* **6**, 514–21.

Looijenga, L.H.J., Gillis, A.J.M., van Putten, W.L.J. *et al.* (1993) *In situ* numeric analysis of centromeric regions of chromosomes 1, 12, and 15 of seminomas, nonseminomatous germ cell tumors, and carcinoma *in situ* of human testis. *Lab. Invest.*, **68**, 211–19.

Looijenga, L.H.J., Olie, R.A., van der Gaag, I. *et al.* (1994) Seminomas of the canine testis. Counterpart of spermatocytic seminoma of men? *Lab. Invest.*, **74**, 490–6.

Marrink, J., Andrews, P.W., van Drummen, P.J. *et al.* (1991) TRA-1-60: A new serum marker in patients with germ-cell tumors. *Int. J. Cancer*, **49**, 368–72.

Matsui, Y., Zsebo, K. and Hogan, B.L.M. (1992) Derivation of pluripotent embryonic stem cells from primordial germ cells in culture. *Cell*, **70**, 841–7.

Nichols, C., Roth, B., Heerema, N. *et al.* (1990) Hematologic neoplasia associated with primary mediastinal germ cell tumours – an update. *N. Engl. J. Med.*, **322**, 1425–9.

Olie, R., Looijenga, L.H.J., Dekker, M.C. *et al.* (1995) Heterogeneity in the *in vitro* survival and proliferation of human seminoma cells. *Br. J. Cancer*, **12**, 110–16.

Oosterhuis, J.W. (1983) The metastasis of human teratomas, in *The Human Teratomas, Experimental and Clinical Biology*, (eds I. Damjanov, B.B. Knowles and D. Solter), Humana Press Inc., Clifton, pp. 137–71.

Oosterhuis, J.W., Castedo, S.M.M.J. and de Jong, B. (1990) Cytogenetics, ploidy and differentiation of human testicular, ovarian and extragonadal germ cell tumours. *Cancer Surv.*, **9**, 321–32.

Oosterhuis, J.W., Castedo, S.M.M.J., de Jong, B. *et al.* (1989) Ploidy of primary germ cell tumors of the testis. *Lab. Invest.*, **60**, 14–21.

Oosterhuis, J.W. and Looijenga, L.H.J. (1993) The biology of human germ cell tumours: retrospective speculations and new prospectives. *Eur. Urol.*, **23**, 245–50.

Oosterhuis, J.W., Rammeloo, R.H.H., Cornelisse, C.J. *et al.* (1990) Ploidy of malignant mediastinal germ cell tumors. *Hum. Pathol.*, **21**, 729–32.

Oosterhuis, J.W., Suurmeyer, A.J.H., Sleijfer, D.Th. *et al.* (1983) Effects of multiple-drug chemotherapy (cis-diammine-dichloroplatinum, bleomycin, and vinblastine) on the maturation of retroperitoneal lymph node metastases of nonseminomatous germ cell tumors of the testis. *Cancer*, **51**, 408–16.

Pera, M.F., Blasco-Lafita, M.F., Cooper, S., Mason, M., Mills, J. And Monoghan, P. (1988) Analysis of cell-differentiation lineage in human teratomas using new monoclonal antibodies to cytostructural antigens of embryonal carcinoma cells. *Differentiation*, **39**, 139–49.

Pera, M.F., Cooper, S., Mills, J. and Parrington, J.M. (1989) Isolation and characterization of a multipotent clone of human embryonal carcinoma cells. *Differentiation*, **42**, 10–23.

Perlman, E.J., Cushing, B., Hawkins, E. *et al.* (1994) Cytogenetic analysis of childhood endodermal sinus tumors: A pediatric onology group study. *Pediatr. Pathol.*, **14**, 695–708.

Pleasure, S.J., Page, C. and Lee, V.M.Y. (1992) Pure, post mitotic polarised human neurons derived from NTERA-2 cells provide a system for expressing exogenous proteins in terminally differentiated neurons. *J. Neurosci.*, **12**, 1802–15.

Rendt, J., Frulkar, S. and Andrews, P.W. (1989) Presumptive neurons derived by differentiation of a human embryonal carcinoma cell line exhibit tetrodotoxin-sensitive sodium currents and the capacity for regenerative responses. *Exp. Cell Res.*, **180**, 580–4.

Rettig, W.J., Cordon-Cardo, C., Ng, J.S.C., Oetggen, H.F., Old, L.J. and Lloyd, K.O. (1985) High molecular weight glycoproteins of human teratocarcinoma defined by monoclonal antibodies to carbohydrate determinants. *Cancer Res.*, **45**, 815–21.

Simeone, A., Acampora, D., Arcioni, L., Andrews, P.W., Boncinelli, E. and Mavilio, F. (1990) Sequential activation of *HOX2* homeobox genes by retinoic acid in human embryonal carcinoma cells. *Nature Lond.*, **346**, 763–6.

Skakkebæk, N.E., Berthelsen, J.G., Giwercman, A. *et al.* (1987) Carcinoma-*in-situ* of the testis: possible origin from gonocytes and precursor of all types of germ cell tumors except spermatocytoma. *Int. J. Androl.*, **10**, 19–28.

Solter, D. (1983) Experimental mouse teratocarcinoma, in *The Human Teratomas, Experimental and Clinical Biology* (eds I. Damjanov, B.B. Knowles

and D. Solter), Humana Press Inc., Clifton, pp. 343–56.

Solter, D. (1988) Differential imprinting and expression of maternal and paternal genomes. *Annu. Rev. Genet.*, **22**, 127–46.

Stock, C., Ambros, I.M., Lion, T. *et al.* (1994) Detection of numerical and structural chromosome abnormalities in pediatric germ cell tumors by means of interphase cytogenetics. *Genes Chromosom. Cancer*, **11**, 40–50.

Suijkerbuijk, R.F., Sinke, R.J., Meloni, A.M. *et al.* (1993) Overrepresentation of chromosome 12p sequences and karyotypic evolution in i(12p)-negative testicular germ cell tumors revealed by fluorescence *in situ* hybridization. *Cancer Genet. Cytogenet.*, **70**, 85–93.

Surti, U., Hoffner, L., Chakravarti, A. *et al.* (1990) Genetics and biology of human ovarian teratomas. I. Cytogenetic analysis and mechanism of origin. *Am. J. Hum. Genet.*, **47**, 635–43.

Teshima, S., Shimosato, Y., Hirohashi, S. *et al.* (1988) Four new human germ cell tumor cell lines. *Lab. Invest.*, **59**, 328–36.

Thompson, S., Stern, P.L., Webb, W. *et al.* (1984) Cloned human teratoma cells differentiate into neuron-like cells and other cell types in retinoic acid. *J. Cell Sci.*, **72**, 37–64.

Ulbright, T.M. (1993) Germ cell neoplasms of the testis. *Am. J. Surg. Pathol.*, **17**, 1075–91.

Ulbright, T.M., Loehrer, P.J., Donohue, J.P. *et al.* (1990) Spindle cell tumors resected from male patients with germ cell tumors: a clinicopathologic study of 14 cases. *Cancer*, **15**, 148–56.

van Berlo, R.J., Oosterhuis, J.W., Schrijnemakers, E., Schoots, C.J.F., de Jong, B. and Damjanov, I. (1990) Yolk-sac carcinoma develops spontaneously as a late occurence in slow-growing teratoid tumors produced from transplanted 7-day mouse embryos. *Int. J. Cancer*, **45**, 153–55.

van Echten, J., de Jong, B., Sinke, R.J. *et al.* (1995) Definition of a new entity of malignant extragonadal germ cell tumors. *Genes Chromosom. Cancer*, **12**, 8–15.

Wenk, J., Andrews, P.W., Casper, J. *et al.* (1994) Glycolipids of germ cell tumours: Extended globoseries glycolipids are a hall-mark of human embryonal carcinoma cells. *Int. J. Cancer*, **58**, 108–15.

PROGNOSTIC CLASSIFICATION OF METASTATIC SEMINOMA

6

R.T.D. Oliver

6.1 INTRODUCTION

Since the demonstration by Friedman (Friedman, 1944) that patients with metastatic seminoma had more lasting complete remissions with lower doses of radiation than malignant teratoma or non-seminoma, seminomas have always been regarded as a different clinicial entity and treated differently. With the advent of curative cisplatin-based chemotherapy this has meant that the response of metastatic seminoma to cisplatin-based single agent and combination chemotherapy has been distorted by the continued inclusion of up to 30% of previously irradiated patients in most reports, so making any prognostication overview from literature reports on previously untreated patients difficult. Today the overall cure rate of all germ cell cancer patients, i.e. both seminoma and non-seminoma, exceeds 95% and even for metastatic disease patients the difference in cure between seminoma and good risk non-seminoma is relatively small (Table 6.1). As a consequence the question arises of whether there is any justification for prognostication in patients with seminomas or for treating them any differently to good risk non-seminomas. The principal reason for doing so is the increasing body of evidence that seminoma is more chemosensitive than non-seminoma, with single agent platinum being nearly as good as combination therapy,

Table 6.1 Anglian Germ Cell Tumour Studies (11.5.1983–17.3.1994)

	No. of cases	Relapses (%)	Currently alive and well (%)
Stage I			
Malignant teratoma	205	19	97
Metastatic teratoma	212	24	85
Stage I seminoma	251	2	99
Metastatic seminoma	72	17	95
Total	940	10	95

both for curing metastatic patients (Oliver, Love and Ong, 1990) and for eliminating the risk of relapse after a single course used as adjuvant treatment for those with Stage I disease (Oliver, *et al.*, 1994). It has now been established that use of etoposide, the second most important drug in combination for non-seminoma, is associated with a medium-term (3–5 year) risk of leukemia (Boshoff *et al.*, 1995) and follow-up is too short to exclude a risk of late solid cancers at 15 and 20 years, as has emerged on follow-up of previously irradiated patients (van Leeuwen *et al.*, 1993), so there remains a need to prognosticate in order to identify patients in whom it is safe to minimize use of chemotherapy.

It is the aim of this chapter, after briefly reviewing modern understanding of etiology, pathology and treatment results of these

Testicular Cancer: Investigation and management. Second edition. Edited by Professor A. Horwich.
Published in 1996 by Chapman & Hall. ISBN 0 412 61210 0.

tumors, to focus on the prognostic factors that have emerged and then end with consideration of the priorities for future studies.

6.2 RELEVANCE OF MODERN VIEWS ON PATHOLOGY OF GERM CELL CANCER TO PROGNOSTICATION OF METASTATIC SEMINOMA

It is 15 years since cytogenetic data first suggested that non-seminomas may arise by clonal evolution from seminoma due to chromosomal loss (Oliver, 1990). The discovery of premalignant carcinoma *in situ* (CIS) in men with infertility (Skakkebæk *et al.*, 1993) and the demonstration that these cells were present in the rim of normal testis that remains in all types of germ cell cancer (Jacobsen, Henricksen and von der Maase, 1981), has helped explain the cytogenetics. CIS areas had higher chromosome numbers than non-seminoma with seminomas intermediate. However, only a minority of tumors containing both seminoma and non-seminoma elements had a gradient in DNA content between *in-situ* carcinoma, seminoma and non-seminoma components (Looijenga *et al.*, 1993), suggesting that in some patients chromosomal loss occurred before development of the solid tumor element.

There has been no cytogenetic abnormality predictive of metastasis, whether of seminoma or non-seminoma component, though as Oosterhuis *et al.* (Oosterhuis *et al.*, 1994) have reported that loss of chromosome 15 is associated with progression from seminoma to non-seminoma even at the *in situ* stage and development of non-seminoma is the feature most predictive of metastases for germ cell cancers (Table 6.2), there may be some element involved in the metastatic process regulated by this chromosome. Patients who present with Stage III pure seminoma with glands in the neck amenable to biopsy at the same time as orchidectomy could provide important cytogenetic data to understand the development of the metastatic phenotype in seminoma.

Age is a significant predictor of seminoma metastasis (Table 6.2), also demonstrable in combined seminoma/non-seminoma but not in non-seminoma (Oliver, Leahy and Ong, 1995). Delay in diagnosis may be playing a role in this age difference as the faster growth of non-seminoma does not allow the long delay that can occur in seminoma before metastases develop. That combined seminoma/non-seminoma patients also have a difference between the age of Stage I and metastatic disease patients suggests such patients could have had a longer period of delay during

Table 6.2 Combined tumors as an intermediate prognosis subgroup of testicular germ cell tumors (Oliver, 1995)

	Seminona n = 248	Combined seminoma non-seminoma n = 116	Non-seminoma n = 241
Median age Stage I	36 yrs	31 yrs	29 yrs
Median age metastatic patients	42 yrs	37 yrs	29 yrs
Proportion presenting in Stage I	79%	51%	41%
Relapse Stage I after adjuvant chemotherapy	1%	6%	0%
Relapse Stage I after surveillance only	23%	31%	38%
Primary cure of all metastatic patients	91%	93%	86%
Proportion of metastatic cases with high markers	0%	16%	21%
Cure rate low markers	91%	94%	92%
Cure rate high markers	–	89%	65%

Table 6.3 Impact of cigarette smoking on disease-free survival of germ cell tumors (Oliver *et al.*, 1995)

	Seminoma or combined seminoma/ non-seminoma		Non-seminoma		
	No. of cases	Disease-free survival	No. of cases	Disease-free survival	
>10 per day	37	68%	27	70%	x^2 0.14 p = NS
≤10 per day	82	94%	81	70%	x^2 16.7 p <0.0005
Significance	x^2 13.9 p <0.0005		x^2 0.08 p = NS		

their seminoma phase before rather than after transformation to non-seminoma. The slower growth rate of the pure seminoma and combined seminoma/non-seminoma by allowing longer exposure may also explain why smoking increases their risk of chemotherapy-resistant tumor but not that of non-seminoma (Table 6.3).

One other pathological risk factor for seminoma metastasis is tumor size. Three authors, one studying Stage I seminoma relapses on surveillance (von der Maase *et al.*, 1993) and two comparing Stage I patients and those with *de novo* metastatic disease (Marks *et al.*, 1990; Zagars, 1993), have demonstrated that large tumors have a higher probability of metastasis. The demonstration from one study that there is a correlation between delay and tumor size (Oliver *et al.*, 1995) would explain why large tumors have more metastases.

The data in Table 6.2 demonstrate that, for all parameters, combined seminoma/non-seminoma display characteristics that are intermediate between those of pure seminoma and pure non-seminoma. This gradient of malignant potential and the morphological similarity between seminoma cells and the spermatogonia justify applying the principles used to grade other solid cancers to germ cell cancers. On this basis seminoma would be considered as Grade 1 or well-differentiated germ cell cancer (G1 GCC) with respect to its cell of origin (Oliver, Leahy and Ong, 1994). Pure non-seminoma without cells resembling the differ-

entiated stem cell would be considered as undifferentiated or Grade 3 germ cell cancer (G3 GCC), while combined seminoma/non-seminoma would be considered as Grade 2 or intermediate germ cell cancer (G2 GCC).

Although this explains the relationship between seminoma and the embryonal carcinoma elements, the occurrence of extra-embryonic tissue such as trophoblast, yolk sac or fetal cartilage, glandular or neural elements is not so easily explained. The frequency with which immunocytochemistry identifies these elements in other solid tumors (Oliver *et al.*, 1989) and classifies them as metaplastic components provides a nomenclature that could be combined with grading in germ cell cancer classification. That GCC with these somatic elements have a higher level of loss of heterozygosity than other GCC (Murty *et al.*, 1994) provides a justification for considering the clonal grading evolution and fetal/somatic tissue differentiation as two separate dimensions of the pathological classification relevant to the prognosis of germ cell cancer metastasis.

If this interpretation is correct, it makes the seminoma element in combined tumors of greater consequence than was previously considered in the current WHO/UICC classification and suggests the need for re-examination of the prognostic significance of alpha-fetoprotein and beta-human chorionic gonadotrophin expression in otherwise pure seminomas. The need to reduce exposure to drugs and radiation because of the issue of late non-germ cell cancer (van Leeuwen *et al.*, 1993; Boshoff *et al.*, 1995) is increasing the value of identifying risk factors that make it safe to reduce treatment of metastatic disease patients, though exploring such approaches is only justified in the setting of reliable approaches for salvage treatment of the minority who fail conventional treatment.

6.3 HIV AND PROGNOSIS OF GERM CELL TUMORS

The situation with respect to the survival of HIV-positive germ cell cancer patients is far from clear. Although there have been several publications of small series that have given some early indications (Tables 6.4, 6.5), the small amount of data published makes it difficult to obtain a complete picture. Two groups have demonstrated an increased

incidence of testis cancer in HIV-positive individuals. Lyter *et al.* (1994) reported three in 430 HIV-positive men compared with nil in 769 HIV-negative gay men followed for 5 years, while Moyle *et al.* reported three in 2205 HIV-positives compared with 0.2 expected. Paradoxically, given its better prognosis, there has been a trend for those tumors that do occur to have a slight excess of seminoma, though the disease presents at a more advanced stage. Damstrup *et al.* (1989) demonstrated that with judicious use of chemotherapy it was possible to achieve a similar cure rate to that in normal individuals, despite their patients having a more frequent incidence of metastatic disease. A review of smaller series reported in the literature by Buzelin (Buzelin *et al.*, 1994) also observed an excess of metastatic disease patients. This series and those reported by an Italian group (Vaccher *et al.*, 1994), in which

Table 6.4   Clinical and pathological staging in HIV-positive and -negative germ cell cancer

	Seminoma		*Non-seminoma*	
	No. of cases	*Final stage 1*	*No. of cases*	*Final stage I*
Buzelin *et al.*, 1994	6	2	9	2
Vacher *et al.*, 1994	13	NA	10	2
Damstrup *et al.*, 1989	2	1	2	0
Krain and Dieckmann, 1994	2	0	NA	–
Moyle, Hawkins and Gazzard, 1991	3	3	NA	–
Total	13	46%	21	19%
Control Series (30)	248	61%	357	29%

Table 6.5   Survival of HIV-positive germ cell cancer

	No. of cases	*Tumor progression*	*Dead from AIDS*	*Lost FU or dead other cause*	*Nem after exclusion + AIDS or lost FU (%)*
Buzelin *et al.*, 1994	11	4	2	0	46
Vacher *et al.*, 1994	23	4	9	5	56
Krain and Dieckmann, 1994	2	0	0	0	100
Moyle *et al.*, 1991	3	0	0	0	100
Damstrup *et al.*, 1989	4	0	0	0	100
Timmerman, Northfelt and Small, 1995	14	1	5	0	89
All HIV+	57	9	16	5	78
Control (30)	605		nil		95

intravenous drug abusers predominated, definitely had a poorer survival than conventionally treated patients (Buzelin *et al.*, 1994). These reports would support the view that immunosuppression reduces cure of chemotherapy-curable germ cell cancer. However, because it is such an important question to be absolutely sure, there is a need for an international data base to try and collect more substantive data to clarify this uncertainty. As data from studying lymphomas arising in this situation suggest that they can be cured by *in vitro* expanded specific antitumor T lymphocytes (Papadopoulos *et al.*, 1994), such an approach would offer an extra dimension that could be added to the treatment of germ cell cancers arising in HIV-positive patients.

There are now at least three publications that have confirmed that these tumors have a total lack of HLA class I and II expression (for review see Nouri *et al.*, 1993) and particularly in seminoma. The absence of HLA expression on sperm has long been established, though one of the most important observations from our work has been the demonstration that spermatogonia, the stem cells for these tumors, have reactivity with an antibody, HC10, which identifies determinants on the monomorphic part of the HLA class I heavy chain (Nouri *et al.*, 1993), though this reactivity is lost on malignant germ cells.

As discussed above, seminoma is the germ cell tumor whose morphology most closely resembles the original starting stem cell, the spermatogonium, and can therefore be functionally considered as well differentiated. This tumor has an excessive level of lymphocyte infiltrate, the level of which correlates with prognosis (Dayan and Marshall, 1964) and a high frequency of spontaneous regression (Oliver, 1990). The idea discussed earlier, that germ cell cancers develop in a clonal way (Oliver, 1990) in association with chromosomal loss from near-tetraploid carcinoma *in situ* via seminoma (DNA content 3.6) and combined tumors (mixed content populations) to embryonal carcinoma (DNA content 2.8 N), fits closely to the accepted clonal evolution with increasing escape from immune surveillance from Grade 1 to Grade 3 tumors in other adult cancers. It would also explain why seminoma, like other Grade 1 tumors such as superficial bladder cancer, demonstrates more evidence for the importance of anti-tumor immune response. Equally supportive of this view, given the knowledge that normal germ cells are the most radiosensitive tissue in the body (Ash, 1980), is the fact that radiation and chemosensitivity decrease with evolution from G1 to G3 germ cell cancer.

Further support for this increasing evidence that immune response may be playing a role in the responsiveness of germ cell cancer to chemotherapy comes from a recent *in vitro* study of immune response to renal cell cancer. Gold *et al.* have demonstrated that treatment of the tumor cells *in vitro* with cisplatin increases their susceptibility to cytolytic T cells (Gold *et al.*, 1995). Such changes happening *in vivo* after platinum treatment of seminoma could explain why a single treatment with carboplatin is so effective in eliminating a 20% risk of relapse in Stage I seminoma (Oliver *et al.*, 1994).

6.4 PROGNOSTICATION OF METASTATIC SEMINOMA ON THE BASIS OF RESPONSE TO THERAPY

Because of the relative rarity of patients with metastatic seminoma there have been very few studies reporting more than 50 patients. The setting up of the International Germ Cell Cancer Collaborative Group (IGCCCG) enabled information on more than ten times that number of cases to be studied (Table 6.6). Although the impact of age, era when treated, the presence of lung or visceral non-lung metastases such as liver, bone and brain, as well as a history of previous radiation, had a similar poor prognostic effect to that demonstrated in studies of non-seminoma, tumor

Table 6.6 International germ cell cancer collaborative group prognostic factors for metastatic seminoma (Mead and Stenning, ASCO, 1995)

	No. of cases	5 year progression free (%)
Age		
<30	146	86
30–50	415	81
>50	99	73
Primary site		
Testis	559	80
Mediastinal	41	80
Retroperitoneum	45	88
Other	15	88
Lung mets		
No	543	81
Yes	78	67
Visceral met (nonlung)		
No	508	81
Yes	64	67
HCG IU m/l^{-1}		
<5000	526	79
5000–50 000	9	67
>50 000	6	50
Years treated		
<1985	221	80
1985–89	355	85
>1989	84	91
Radiation before chemotherapy		
Nil	342	83
Yes	103	74
LDH		
<1.5 × n	226	87
1.5–10 × n	213	77
>10 × n	24	83

n = upper limit of normal range

Table 6.7 MRC Testicular Tumour Working Party prognostic factors for metastatic seminoma (Duchesne, Oliver and Stenning, in preparation)

	No. of cases	3 year progression free (%)
Stage 2/3 (no radiation)		
BEP	39	95
Other	85	86
Lung ± nodes (no radiation)		
BEP	3	100
Other	17	71
Liver/bone/brain ± node ± lung (no radiation)		
BEP	3	33
Other	8	75

markers, particularly LDH and HCG, were less impressive risk factors than in non-seminoma, as was the presence of a mediastinal or retroperitoneal primary.

In a subset of this data, i.e. that from the UK MRC collaborating centers, more information was available on chemotherapy regimen (Table 6.7). The apparently better survival of patients treated with bleomycin/etoposide/cisplatin (BEP) could be a factor in the continued improvement since 1990 in the IGCCCG study; though a 96% cure rate of patients with metastatic seminoma with this regimen was reported in 1985 (Peckham, Horwich and Hendry, 1985), it did not become widely used immediately. This was because of studies into the use of regimens without bleomycin.

The high cure rate with BEP leaves very little margin for prognostication. Clearly it would be scientifically unsound to consider the 4% lower (92%) survival in the reports of seminoma patients treated with etoposide and cisplatin (Mencel, Motzer and Mazumdar, 1994) as clinically significantly worse because it is not statistically significant. However, in non-seminoma it is increasingly accepted that it is unsafe to omit bleomycin. Despite early warnings of high relapse rates in good risk patients from phase II studies (Horwich and Peckham, 1985; Oliver *et al.*, 1988) and preliminary reports that use of prolonged infusion bleomycin instead of the rapid IV bolus of the Einhorn regimen was a better way of reducing bleomycin lung deaths (Oliver *et al.*, 1988; Chisholm *et al.*, 1992), it has taken four trials involving 859 patients, all of which had worse survival in the arm without bleomycin with an overall 9% worse survival without bleomycin, before a consensus has been reached that it is perhaps not safe to eliminate bleomycin from combination therapy even in good risk patients.

Although only two of these trials had a statistically significant difference, one of the others compared EP with VAB-6 as a control arm. As this later regimen has, unlike BEP (Williams *et al.*, 1987), not been proven to be any better than BVP, equivalence in this trial could be misleading. In view of this minor difference, given the added safety from use of bleomycin by infusion, it would seem prudent to continue using bleomycin for patients with both metastatic seminoma and non-seminoma. To reduce risk of lethal lung toxicity, treatment should be by infusion rather than bolus, the total dose kept below 270 mg and the use of bleomycin drastically reduced if there is any fall-off in renal function while on treatment (Dalgleish *et al.*, 1984).

Despite the excellent results with BEP, there is a need to resolve the issue of whether histology should play any role in discrimination of treatment or, as is currently the case for non-seminoma, whether prognostication should be totally based on tumor marker levels and volume/site of metastases. The strongest advocates of this have been the Memorial Group. Given that there are differences between seminoma and non-seminoma, as demonstrated for some of the prognostic factors presented in Table 6.6, there is a need for more data on this issue comparing seminoma, combined and pure non-seminoma patients who have been treated with BEP without any previous chemotherapy or radiation before the issue can be resolved. The opportunity to do this is presented by the current MRC/EORTC good risk protocol, which compares a 3- versus 5-day regimen of BEP chemotherapy and three versus four courses of treatment.

6.5 PROGNOSTIC FACTORS AND SINGLE AGENT PLATINUM FOR LYMPH NODE METASTATIC STAGE II AND III SEMINOMA

One of the most important issues of prognostication for metastatic seminoma patients that needs resolving relates to whether it is possible to identify a subgroup in whom single agent platinum therapy is justified (Oliver, Love and Ong, 1990). Cisplatin, vinblastine and bleomycin (PVB) combination chemotherapy became the regimen for metastatic seminoma after only two patients (one a long-term survivor) had been treated with single agent cisplatin in the initial Phase II study, which consisted primarily of patients with metastatic non-seminoma (Higby *et al.*, 1974). In 1980 Samuels reported on five patients treated with weekly cisplatin 100 mg m^{-2} and then changed to cisplatin plus cyclophosphamide (Logothetis, Samuels and Ogden, 1987). Our own unit explored conventional cisplatin dosage of 100 mg m^{-2} every 3 weeks and then changed to carboplatin when that drug became available (Oliver, Hope-Stone and Blandy, 1984; Oliver 1987). Table 6.8 summarizes the admittedly far too small series treated by either cisplatin alone or carboplatin alone. After cisplatin 100% of Stage IIC/III patients ($n = 12$) achieved durable progression-free survival, while after carboplatin it has been only 73% ($n = 85$). There were two factors that possibly explain the poor performance of carboplatin. Firstly, in two of the studies

Table 6.8 Single agent platinum studies for metastatic seminoma

		Progression free Stage 2 and 3	Stage 4	Overall primary cure (%)	Current NEM (%)
Oliver, Hope-Stone and Blandy, 1984	Cisplatin q21	12/12	1/4	82	88
Oliver *et al.*, 1990	Carboplatin q21	15/18			
Schmoll *et al.*, 1993	Carboplatin q28	27/36	3/6	71	95
Horwich *et al.*, 1992	Carboplatin q28	20/31	7/10	68	94

(Horwich *et al.*, 1992; Schmoll *et al.*, 1993) most of the patients received their treatment every 4 weeks. Only 70% of these patients achieved durable primary progression-free survival compared with 83% in the smaller series treated with a similar dose every 21 days.

A second factor may be the method used for calculating the dosage of carboplatin, which is based on a formula developed by Calvert, Newell and Gumbrell (1989) studying females with ovarian cancer who were on average 30 years older. This aimed to correct dosage based on area under the curve formula. Because most carboplatin is excreted via the kidneys, dosage was calculated by the formula: dose = AUC (area under the curve) × (GFR + 25). There was no correction for surface area. Although this may have been unnecessary for the small females in the ovarian studies, analysis of the cases treated in our studies showed that most of the failures were in larger-than-average males, and when progression-free survival was recalculated with a correction for surface area those receiving adequate carboplatin dosage achieved 89% progression free survival (Oliver, in preparation).

Clearly the numbers are too small to know if this correction is justified. Even so the level of cisplatin response in Stages IIC/D/III (100%) is close to that achieved with BEP (Table 6.8, in similar cases, while that after corrected carboplatin dosage (89%) is closer to the 92% achieved with EP (Mencel, Motzer and Mazumdar, 1994). Horwich *et al.* (1992) salvaged 12 out of 14 of carboplatin failures using weekly bleomycin, oncovin and cisplatin, Schmoll *et al.* (1993) salvaged ten of 12 carboplatin failures using PEI (platinum/etoposide/ifosfamide) and our group salvaged two of three carboplatin failures using BEP, giving an overall survival of single agent treated patients of 95%. This would seem to justify further exploration of single agent carboplatin as an alternative to BEP even if one ignores the fact that this approach reduces the cost of treatment by at least two-thirds, to say nothing of the reduced toxicity.

The debate revolves around whether the level of quality of life gain for the 75–90% who avoid the extra toxicity of immediate combination treatment exceeds the extra toxicity for the 10–25% extra who have to have more intensive treatment of relapse.

The MRC trial TE12, which compared carboplatin with etoposide/cisplatin, was set up to investigate this issue. It was terminated in November 1993 when there was a non-significant excess of relapses in the carboplatin arm. This was because the Working Party and the trial data monitoring committee, worried by the results from a large trial in non-seminoma where there had been a significantly worse progression-free survival in the carboplatin combination arm compared with those receiving cisplatin combination (Horwich and Sleijfer, 1993), felt it inappropriate to allow the trial to proceed until more information was available. The trial data is currently in the process of maturing and will be analyzed in 1 year's time when all patients will have been followed for 2 years. In the mean time given the phase II data presented in Table 6.8 further exploration of single agent studies in Stage II/III, i.e. N+, M0 seminoma is undoubtedly justified. As there is such poor survival of M+ seminoma cases, whether lung or other visceral sites (see Tables 6.6 and 6.7), it would be prudent to treat these cases like good risk non-seminoma to establish if there is any difference in responsiveness between pure seminoma, combined tumors and pure non-seminoma, by including them in the European good risk trial comparing three versus four courses of BEP and 2 versus 5 days of cisplatin treatment.

6.6 RELEVANCE OF PROGNOSTIC CLASSIFICATION OF GERM CELL CANCER TO FUTURE TRIALS IN METASTATIC SEMINOMA

As the recent distressing experience of trials using carboplatin in combination instead of cisplatin in non-seminoma patients has demonstrated, there is little doubt that risking less treatment for patients with good prognosis is far harder to do than give ever increasingly toxic treatment to poor risk patients (Oliver *et al.*, 1988). Today bleomycin, etoposide and cisplatin remains the gold standard of treatment for all metastatic germ cell cancer including seminoma. For the immediate future the European trial of three versus four courses and two versus five fractions of cisplatin will dominate recruitment to trials. As discussed in Section 6.5 the increasing recognition that the prognosis of seminoma patients that are M0 is so good may justify excluding them from these studies to pilot other approaches. The toxicity profile of carboplatin, in terms of less nephrotoxicity, ototoxicity and neurotoxicity, is clearly better than cisplatin. In terms of health economics something that can be given over 2 hours without hospitalization compares favorably with the 5-day inpatient regimen currently standard in Europe. Clearly there is a need for further attempts to get the dosage of carboplatin right. Additional evidence to justify such a view comes from the reports that high dose carboplatin in association with stem cell transplants salvages a substantial number of patients failing conventional treatment (Motzer and Bosl, 1992). Equally relevant is the very steep dose–response curve in the Phase I data on incorporating carboplatin into combination therapy for patients with non-seminoma (Childs, Nicholls and Horwich, 1992) and the evidence from a study of elderly ovarian cancer patients (Jodrell, Egorin and Canetta, 1992), demonstrating that they can tolerate more than double the dosage used in the current testis trials without getting serious marrow toxicity complications. Preliminary studies in six patients with problems that precluded use of conventional dosage cisplatin in our unit has demonstrated that dosage of carboplatin of AUC 8 may be safe to give in combination with conventional dose etoposide to patients with non-seminoma, while dosage

as high as AUC 10 can be given as a single agent to patients with seminoma. Further expansion of these studies is an urgent priority for the future with subsequent testing of the optimum dose in a randomized trial against radiation in early metastatic disease.

One other area that has been little investigated in prognostication of metastatic seminoma is the use of molecular markers to try and identify the subgroup with early evidence of transformation into non-seminoma phenotype (De Reise *et al.*, 1994; Ferreiro, 1994). Detailed studies of the histology from patients admitted to recently closed MRC TE12 carboplatin versus EP trial could provide interesting information on this issue.

6.7 SUMMARY AND CONCLUSIONS

For metastatic seminoma, the classical non-seminoma prognostic risk factors, i.e. tumor volume and tumor marker levels, provide a lesser degree of prognostic discrimination than the equivalent risk factors for non-seminoma. With more than 95% of metastatic seminoma cured by BEP chemotherapy, the cure rate is little different from that of good risk non-seminoma. As a consequence in a service setting this should be the standard treatment for all metastatic seminoma with the possible exception of patients without blood-borne metastasis who may be suitable for further studies aimed to reduce treatment toxicity using single agent platinum compounds.

New evidence from tissue culture, immunology and cytogenetic studies suggests that seminoma may be hormone responsive, subject to immune regulation and an intermediary stage in transformation from carcinoma *in situ* to non-seminoma, and that these observations are of prognostic significance in determining survival of patients with metastatic seminoma. This view is supported by three pieces of information. Firstly, there is increasing evidence that atrophy with loss of feedback inhibition of the pituitary and increased FSH is the final common pathway for development of both seminoma and non-seminoma, and elevated FSH has been associated with an increased risk for development of contralateral tumors and metastases for patients with stage I tumors. Secondly, spontaneous regression data and information on prognostic significance of lymphocyte infiltrate in seminoma, taken together with the lymphocytosis and thymic regeneration induced by testosterone withdrawal, suggests that temporary androgen blockade might be an effective therapy for testicular carcinoma *in situ* that could improve fertility of this subfertile group of patients and, thirdly, preliminary data shows that the incidence of metastases and overall cure of HIV-positive patients may be lower than in patients with a normal immune response. Approaches have been presented to explore the use of cellular immunotherapy as part of the treatment of such patients as has been successfully explored in treatment of lymphomas in immune-suppressed individuals.

For the future, with the increasing worries of late toxicity from radiation and etoposide, there is a need for more research on the biological basis of the prognostically significant difference in chemosensitivity of seminoma and non-seminoma as this may identify the subgroup of patients without blood-borne metastases in whom single agent platinum is offering considerable benefits over radiation and BEP combination therapy. Despite the recent problems arising from carboplatin studies, new data on dose escalation is giving greater confidence that there may be a safe dose for use of this clearly less toxic drug. However, there remain considerable problems as to how to sponsor the large scale trials necessary to prove this now that the drug companies have lost interest in the drug as it is nearly out of patent. A final area of interest for the future comes from reports that neoadjuvant use of chemotherapy may enable testis conservation to become routine in patients with metastases and possibly justify its use in patients with severe atrophy or absence of the contralateral testis.

REFERENCES

Ash, P. (1980) Influences of radiation on fertility in man. *Br. J. Radiol.*, **53**, 271–8.

Boshoff, C.B., Begent, R.H.J., Oliver, R.T.D. *et al.* (1995) Secondary tumours following etoposide containing therapy for germ cell cancer. *Ann. Onc.*, **6**, 35–40.

Buzelin, F., Karam, G., Moreau, A. *et al.* (1994) Testicular tumor and the acquired immunodeficiency syndrome. *Eur. Urol.*, **26**, 71–6.

Calvert, A.H., Newell, D.R. and Gumbrell, L.A. (1989) Carboplatin dosage: Prospective evaluation of a simple formula based on renal function. *J. Clin. Oncol.*, **7**, 1748–56.

Carlsen, E., Giwercman, A., Keiding, N. *et al.* (1992) Evidence for decreasing quality of semen during the past 50 years. *BMJ*, **305**, 609–12.

Childs, W.J., Nicholls, E.J. and Horwich, A. (1992) The Optimisation of carboplatin dose in carboplatin, etoposide and bleomycin combination chemotherapy for good prognosis metastatic non-seminomatous germ cell tumours of the testis. *Ann. Oncol.*, **3**, 291–6.

Chisholm, R.A., Dixon, A.K., Williams, M.V. *et al.* (1992) Bleomycin lung: the effect of different chemotherapeutic regimens. *Cancer Chemother. Pharmacol.*, **30**, 158–60.

Dalgleish, A., Woods, R. and Levi, J. (1984) Bleomycin pulmonary toxicity: its relationship to renal dysfunction. *Med. Paed. Onc.*, **12**, 313–17.

Damstrup, L., Daugaard, G., Gertstoft, J. *et al.* (1989) Effects of antineoplastic treatment of HIV positive patients with testicular cancer. *Eur. J. Cancer*, **25**, 983–6.

Dayan, A.D. and Marshall, A.M.E. (1964) Immunological reaction in man against certain tumours. *Lancet*, **2**, 1102–3.

De Riese, W.T., Albers, P., Walker, E.P. *et al.* (1994) Predictive parameters of biologic behaviour of early stage nonseminomatous testicular germ cell tumours. *Cancer*, **74**, 1335–41.

Dieckmann, K., Krain, J., Kuster, J. and Bruggeboes, B. (1996) Adjuvant carboplatin treatment for seminoma clinical stage I. *J. Cancer Res. Clin. Oncol.*, **122**(1), 63–6.

Ferreiro, J.A. (1994) Ber-H2 expression in testicular germ cell tumors. *Human Pathology*, **25**, 522–4.

Friedman, M. (1944) Supervoltage Roentgen Therapy at Walter Reed General Hospital. *Surg. Clin. North Amer.*, **24**, 1424–32.

Gold, E., Masters, T., Babbit, B. *et al.* (1996) Ex vivo activated memory T-lymphocytes as adoptive cellular therapy of human renal cell tumour targets with potentiation by *cis*-diamminedichloroplatinum (II). *Brit. J. Urol.*, in press.

Higby, D.J., Wallace, H.J., Albert, D.J. and Holland, J.F. (1974) Diaminodichloroplatinum: a phase I study showing responses in testicular and other tumors. *Cancer*, **33**, 1219–55.

Horwich, A. and Peckham, M. (1985) Etoposide and cisplatin for small volume non-seminoma. *Br. J. Cancer*, **49**, 135–7.

Horwich, A., Dearnaley, D., A'Hern, R. *et al.* (1992) The Activity of single-agent carboplatin in advanced seminoma. *Eur. J. Cancer*, **28A**, 1307–10.

Horwich, A. and Sleijfer, D. (1993) Carboplatin-based chemotherapy in good prognosis metastatic non seminoma of the testis (NSGCT): An interim report of an MRC/EORTC randomised trial. *Eur. J. Cancer Proc. ECCO 7*, **29A**, 1350 (Abstract).

Jacobsen, G.K., Henriksen, O.B. and von der Maase, H. (1981) Carcinoma in-situ of testicular tissue adjacent to malignant germ cell tumours. A study of 105 cases. *Cancer (Philadelphia)*, **47**, 2260–2.

Jodrell, D.I., Egorin, M.J. and Canetta, R.M. (1992) Relationships between carboplatin exposure and tumour response and toxicity in patients with ovarian cancer. *J. Clin. Oncol.*, **10**, 520–8.

Krain, J. and Dieckmann, K. (1994) Treatment of testicular seminoma in patients with HIV infection. Report of two cases. *Eur. Urol.*, **26**(2), 184–6.

Logothetis, C.J., Samuels, M.L. and Ogden, S.L. (1987) Cyclophosphamide and sequential cisplatin for advanced seminoma: Long term follow up of 52 patients. *J. Urol.*, **138**, 789–94.

Looijenga, L.H.J., Gillis, A.J.M., van Putten, W.L.J. *et al.* (1993) *In situ* numeric analysis of centrometric regions of chromosomes 1, 12, and 15 of seminomas, nonseminomatous germ cell tumors, and carcinoma in situ of human testis. *Laboratory Investigation*, **68**, 211–19.

Lyter, D., Bryant, J., Thackeray, R. *et al.* (1994) Incidence of Kaposi's sarcoma (KS), non-Hodgkin's lymphoma (NHL), and other malignancies in a cohort of gay men with human

immunodeficiency virus (HIV) infection. *Proc. Amer. Soc. Clin. Oncol.*, **13** (Abstract).

Marks, L.B., Rutgers, J.L., Shipley, W.U. *et al.* (1990) Testicular seminoma: clinical and pathological features that may predict para-aortic lymph node metastases. *J. Urol.*, **143**, 524–7.

Mead, G. and Stenning, S. (1995) International germ cell cancer collaborative group prognostic factor scoring system, in preparation.

Mencel, P.J., Motzer, R.J. and Mazumdar, M. (1994) Advanced seminoma: treatment results, survival and prognostic factors in 142 patients. *J. Clin. Oncol.*, **12**, 120–6.

Motzer, R.J. and Bosl, G.J. (1992) High-dose chemotherapy for resistant germ cell tumors: recent advances and future directions. *J. Natl. Cancer Inst.*, **84**, 1703–9.

Moyle, G., Hawkins, D.A. and Gazzard, B.G. (1991) Seminoma and HIV infections. *Int. J. STD. AIDS*, **2**, 293–4.

Murty, V.V.V.S., Houldsworth, B.J.G., Meyers, M. *et al.* (1994) Allelic loss and somatic differentiation in human male germ cell tumours. *Oncogene*, **9**, 2245–51.

Nouri, A.M.E., Hussain, R.F., Oliver, R.T.D. *et al.* (1993) Immunological paradox in testicular tumours: The presence of a large number of activated T cells despite the complete absence of MHC antigens. *Eur. J. Cancer*, **29A**, 1895–9.

Oliver, R.T.D. (1987) Limitations to the use of surveillance as an option in the management of stage I seminoma. *Int. J. Androl.*, **10**, 263–8.

Oliver, R.T.D. *et al.* (1988) Risking less treatment in cancer patients: lessons from germ-cell tumours, *Lancet*, **2**, 430–1.

Oliver, R.T.D. (1990) Clues from natural history and results of treatment supporting the monoclonal origin of germ cell tumours. *Cancer Surveys*, **9**, 332–68.

Oliver, R.T.D. and Gallagher, C.J. (1995) Intermittent endocrine therapy and its potential for chemoprevention of prostate cancer. *Cancer Surveys*, **23**, 191–207.

Oliver, R.T.D., Dhaliwal, H.S., Hope-Stone, H.F. *et al.* (1988) Short course etoposide, bleomycin and cisplatin in the treatment of metastatic germ cell tumours. Appraisal of its potential as adjuvant chemotherapy for stage I testis tumours. *Br. J. Urol.*, **61**, 53–8.

Oliver, R.T.D., Edmonds, P., Ong, J.Y.H. *et al.* (1994) Pilot studies of 2 and 1 course carboplatin as adjuvant for Stage I seminoma: should it be tested in a randomized trial against radiotherapy? *Int. J. Rad. Oncol. Biol. Phys.*, **29**, 3–8.

Oliver, R.T.D., Hope-Stone, H.F. and Blandy, J.P. (1984) Possible new approaches to the management of seminoma of the testis. *Br. J. Urol.*, **56**, 729–33.

Oliver, R.T.D., Leahy, M. and Ong, J. (1995) Combined seminoma/non-seminoma should be considered as intermediate grade germ cell cancer (GCC). *Eur. J. Cancer*, 1392–4.

Oliver, R.T.D., Love, S. and Ong, J. (1990) Alternatives to radiotherapy in management of seminoma. *Br. J. Urol.*, **65**, 61–7.

Oliver, R.T.D., Nouri, A.M.E., Crosby, D. *et al.* (1989) Biological significance of Beta hCG, HLA and other membrane antigen expression on bladder tumours and their relationship to tumour infiltrating lymphocytes (TIL). *J. Immunogenetics*, **16**, 381–90.

Oliver, R.T.D., Ong, J., Blandy, J. and Altman, D. (1996). Testis conservation studies in germ cell cancer justfied by improved primary chemotherapy response and reduced delay 1978–1994. In press.

Oosterhuis, J., Gillis, A., de Jong, B., and Looijenga, L.H.J., (1994) Interphase cytogenetics of testicular germ cell tumours: Clonal origin of seminoma and nonseminoma components in combined tumours, in *Germ Cell Tumours III* (ed. W.G. Jones, P. Harnden and I. Appleyard), Pergamon, Oxford, pp. 89–94.

Papadopoulos, E., Ladanyi, M., Emanuel, D. *et al.* (1994) Infusions of donor leukocytes to treat Epstein–Barr virus-associated lymphoproliferative disorders after allogeneic bone marrow transplantation. *New Engl. J. Med.*, **330**, 1185–91.

Peckham, M.J., Horwich, A. and Hendry, W.F. (1985) Advanced seminoma: treatment with cis-platinum-based combination chemotherapy or carboplatin (JM8). *Br. J. Cancer*, **52**, 7–13.

Schmoll, H.J., Harstrick, A., Bokemeyer, C. *et al.* (1993) Single-agent carboplatinum for advanced seminoma – a phase-II study. *Cancer*, **72**, 237–43.

Skakkebæk, N.E., Grigor, K.M., Giwercman, A. *et al.* (1993) Management and biology of carcinoma *in situ* and cancer of the testis. *Eur Urol.*, **23**, 1–256.

Timmerman, J.M., Northfelt, D.W. and Small, E.J. (1995) Malignant germ cell tumors in men infected with HIV: natural history and results of therapy. *J. Clin. Oncol.*, **13**, 1391–7.

Vaccher, E., Bernardi, D., Errante, D. *et al.* (1994) Treatments of testicular germ-cell tumours in patients with HIV infection: The GICAT experience. *Ann. Oncol.*, **5** (Abstract), 6.

van Leeuwen, F.E., Stiggelbout, A.M., Vandenbeltdusebout, A.W. *et al.* (1993) Second tumors after radiation treatment of testicular germ-cell tumors. *J. Clin. Oncol.*, **11**, 2286–7.

von der Maase, H., Specht, L., Jacobsen, G.K. *et al.* (1993) Surveillance following orchidectomy for stage I seminoma of the testis. *Eur. J. Cancer*, **29A**, 1931–4.

Williams, S.D., Birch, R., Einhorn, L.H. *et al.* (1987) Treatment of disseminated germ-cell tumours with cisplatin, bleomycin, and either vinblastine or etoposide. *New Engl. J. Med.*, **316**, 1435–40.

Zagars, G. (1993) Stage I testicular seminoma following orchidectomy – to treat or not to treat. *Eur. J. Cancer*, **29A**, 1923–4.

D.F. Bajorin

7.1 INTRODUCTION

The management of patients with non-seminomatous germ cell tumors (NSGCT) has made remarkable progress over the past two decades. Despite the success of cisplatin-based combination chemotherapy, however, approximately 20% of patients presenting with metastatic disease will die of their disease due either to tumor refractory to initial chemotherapy or to recurrence after attaining an initial complete response (CR). Two NSGCT groups can be distinguished on the basis of chemotherapy-induced CR and eventual survival. The first group, which includes the majority of patients, is likely to obtain an initial CR ('good risk' NSGCT). The focus of investigational trials in these patients is to reduce the toxicity of chemotherapy (Stoter *et al.*, 1987a; Bosl *et al.*, 1988a; Einhorn *et al.*, 1989). The second group consists of the minority of patients in whom the prognosis is poor due to refractory disease ('poor risk' NSGCT). The primary objective of investigational trials in this patient population is to improve the proportion of CR, and the chemotherapy programs for this group of patients are, in general, associated with greater toxicity. Therefore, modeling to allocate NSGCT patients to the appropriate trials based on prognostic variables is necessary to minimize toxicity to good risk patients and maximize therapy for the poor risk population.

The clinical factors reported to impact on the prognosis of NSGCT patients are variable. Extent or 'bulk' of disease, initial serum concentrations of alpha-fetoprotein (AFP), human chorionic gonadotrophin (HCG), lactate dehydrogenase (LDH), histology, time from diagnosis to treatment, time from symptoms to treatment, performance status, treatment protocol, age, visceral organ involvement, number of metastatic disease sites and primary site of disease have all been reported to affect survival.

The use of these factors in the criteria allocating patients to good and poor risk studies is substantial. As a consequence, the results of trials that use the various criteria may differ markedly depending on the criteria used. For example, the interim response rates of a randomized trial of cisplatin/etoposide/bleomycin (BEP) versus alternating cycles of BEP/PVB (cisplatin/vinblastine/bleomycin) performed by the European Organization for Research into Treatment for Cancer (EORTC) in poor risk patients resulted in 78 and 77% CR rates, respectively (Stoter, Kaye and Sleijfer, 1986). The chemotherapy in this trial was similar to a single arm trial of alternating vinblastine/cyclophosphamide/dactinomycin/bleomycin/cisplatin (VAB-6) and etoposide/cisplatin (EP) chemotherapy in which the eligibility criteria were different but the response rate was 51% (Bosl *et al.*, 1987).

Testicular Cancer: Investigation and management. Second edition. Edited by Professor A. Horwich.
Published in 1996 by Chapman & Hall. ISBN 0 412 61210 0.

Table 7.1 Factors constituting poor risk disease in published clinical trials

	Size/extent of disease			Organ sites			Extragonadal primaries*	Serum markers		
	RP	Mediastinum	Lung	CNS	Liver	Bone		AFP	HCG	LDH
MSKCC (Bosl et al., 1983)	>5 cm	Number of sites		No	No	No	Yes	No	Log	Log
EORTC (Stoter, Kaye and Sleijfer et al., 1986)	NS	NS	>2 cm	Yes	Yes	Yes	Yes	$>10^3$ ng ml^{-1}	$>10^4$ ng ml^{-1}	No
IU (Birch et al., 1986)	>10 cm; palp	50%	>3 cm; >10/lung	Yes	Yes	Yes	No	No	No	No
NCI (Ozols et al., 1988)	>10 cm; palp	5 cm	5 cm; >5/lung	Yes	Yes	NS	Yes	$>10^3$ ng ml^{-1}	$>10^4$ mIu m^{-1}	No
Cleveland Clinic (Bukowski, Smith and Montie, 1988)	>5 cm/palp	NS	>2 cm	NS	NS	NS	Yes	>40 ng ml^{-1}	$>10^5$ mIu ml^{-1}	> 3XN
Royal Marsden Hospital (Horwich et al., 1989)	>5 cm	Yes	>2 cm; >3/lung	NS	Yes	Yes	Yes	>500 kU l^{-1}	$>10^3$ IU l^{-1}	No
Istituto Tumori (Pizzocaro et al., 1985)	>10 cm	NS	>5 cm	Yes	Yes	Yes	NS	$>10^3$ ng ml^{-1}	$>5 \times 10^4$ mIU ml^{-1}	No
MD Anderson (Logothetis et al., 1986)	>10 cm	NS	>2 cm	Yes	Yes	NS	NS	No	No	No
GATTS (Chacon et al., 1985)	>10 cm	'Any'	'Extensive'	NS	Yes	NS	NS	NS	NS	NS
Finsen Institute (Daugaard, 1986)	>10 cm	>5 cm	>5 cm	NS	Yes	NS	Yes, + markers	No	$>10^5$ U l^{-1}	No
Dana Farber (Garnick and Richie, 1986)	NS	NS	NS	Yes	Yes	NS	Yes	No	$>2 \times 10^3$ ng	No
City of Hope (Blayney et al., 1986)	>8 cm	NS	NS	Yes	Yes	NS	Yes	$>2 \times 10^3$ ng ml^{-1}	$>10^4$ mIU ml^{-1}	No
U. Hannover (Schmoll et al., 1986)	>10 cm	5 cm	>2 cm; $n \geq 5$;	Yes	Yes	Yes	NS	NS	NS	NS
U. Essen (Kath et al., 1987)	>5 cm	>5 cm	>10 cm^3	Yes	Yes	Yes	NS	NS	NS	NS
Gustave-Roussy (Droz et al., 1989)	No	No	No	No	No	No	NS	√AFP	√HCG	No
U. Munich (Hartenstein, Clemm and Scheiber, 1988)	>10 cm	>10 cm	Mult. >5 cm	NS	Yes	NS	No	No	No	No
Hospital de la Croix-Rousse (Biron et al., 1989)	'Bulky'	NS	$n > 10$	NS	NS	NS	NS	'Very high'	'Very high'	No

*All extragonadal primaries constitute poor risk disease.
NCI, National Cancer Institute, USA. GATTS, Grupo Argentino de Tratemiento de los Tumores Solidos. IU, Indiana University. n, number. NS, not stated. +, elevated markers. RP, retroperitoneum. MSKCC, Memorial Sloan-Kettering Cancer Center. palp, palpable.

A summary of the published factors constituting poor risk NSGCT is outlined in Table 7.1. Two observations are readily apparent. Firstly, the two most frequently represented prognostic features are the extent or 'bulk' of disease and the use of serum tumor markers. Secondly, no general consensus exists in any one of the variables deemed significant. The purpose of this chapter is to summarize data regarding prognostic factors in NSGCT patients and to estimate their impact on reported results of clinical trials.

7.2 FACTORS INFLUENCING PROGNOSTIC MODELING

Several issues may impact on the factors considered significant in the prognosis of NSGCT patients.

1. *Serum tumor markers*. Both AFP and HCG are reported in varying units of measurement. Although AFP is predominantly reported in nanograms per ml, several analyses have been performed with AFP reported in kU l^{-1} (Newlands *et al.*, 1983; Medical Research Council, 1985). The variability of assays for HCG is substantial and, although most laboratories report values in milli-international units (mIU ml^{-1}), or IU l^{-1}, some are reported in mass units (ng ml^{-1}). A variety of commercial assays are available but the ratio of units (mIU) to nanograms is not standardized and varies from 2.5:1 to 14:3 (Nisselbaum, 1986). In practical terms, an HCG of 70 ng ml^{-1} may be equivalent to 175 mIU ml^{-1} (2.5:1) by another assay or 1000 mIU ml^{-1} (14.3:1) by a third. Any attempt to compare data among different institutions and studies is difficult in the absence of conversion factors. Assays for lactate dehydrogenase (LDH) are equally variable with normal values differing by a substantial degree depending on the assay used (Vogelzang, 1987; Rustin and Volgelzang, in press).
2. *Extent of disease*. The significance of the

extent of disease may vary according to the manner in which it is scored. Bulk of disease has taken the form of tumor volume, largest diameter of a specific site of disease, number of metastases per lung(s), visceral organ(s) involved, and total number of disease sites regardless of size. Although staging systems are used in a number of studies, the lack of a common staging system results in different assessments of extent of disease.

3. *The use of variables*. The definition of each variable in the data set may affect the outcome of the analysis. An example of such diversity and its subsequent impact on modeling is demonstrated by the use of serum tumor markers. These values may be incorporated in the form of discrete or continuous variables. The Memorial Sloan-Kettering Cancer Center (MSKCC) and Institut Gustav-Roussy models use the LDH, HCG or AFP as continuous variables; other studies performed by the EORTC and Medical Research Council (MRC) Working Party on Testicular Tumours use discrete categories of values such as HCG less than or greater than 1000 ng ml^{-1} or 1000 IU l^{-1}, respectively (Medical Research Council, 1985; Stoter *et al.*, 1987b). Marker variables may be statistically significant when entered in one form and not significant if used in another. Serum markers are easier to use when employed as discrete variables but are inherently more powerful when utilized as continuous variables.

The eventual criteria developed are dependent on the number of variables available for inclusion and analysis in the model. For example, if a particular data set does not include the serum LDH or number and measurement of lung metastases, the eventual prognostic model will differ from those in which these parameters are included. Furthermore, many of the prognostic factors determined in retrospective analyses may be interrelated.

An example is the observation of chorio-carcinoma coinciding with that of an elevated HCG value. In order to exclude the impact of the interrelationship of these factors, careful multivariate analyses are required.

4. *Distribution of data.* The values of the serum markers LDH, HCG and AFP are generally 'skewed' with the majority of values in the normal range. In order to analyze these skewed data, transformation of the data to a normally distributed pattern is often performed. In general, this takes the form of a logarithmic or square root function.

5. *Patient selection.* Most studies include all patients treated at the respective institution. Various analyses may or may not include patients with extragonadal primaries. Some studies include only a subset of patients, i.e. patients with retroperitoneal masses >10 cm or with evidence of lung metastases which will directly affect the resulting model. The number of patients included for analysis may impact on the model if the power is insufficient to detect a significant variable.

6. *Change in prognosis over time.* Changes in diagnostic and clinical factors over time can favorably affect the prognosis of NSGCT patients independent of treatment effect, a phenomenon referred to as 'stage migration' (Feinstein, Sosin and Wells, 1985; Bosl, Geller and Chan, 1988). The MRC observed an improvement in survival over time that was independent of treatment, staging or marker distribution (Medical Research Council, 1985). This effect was also observed in sequential studies using PVB in patients treated at Indiana University. Initial trials reported cure rates of 57%, which increased to 80% in subsequent studies despite a decrease in the vinblastine dose and the deletion of maintenance vinblastine (Einhorn, 1986). Similarly, an increase in the pretreatment probability of response has been observed in successive poor risk NSGCT trials at MSKCC (Pfister *et al.*, 1989). Bosl, Geller and Chan, (1988) observed a significant decrease in the pretreatment values of serum tumor markers, the number of metastatic sites and the proportion of patients with lung metastases, and an increase in the probability of CR in patients treated between 1975 and 1982. In a multivariate logistic regression analysis, time was found to be an independent significant variable (Bosl, Geller and Chan, 1988).

7. *Endpoint of interest.* The endpoint and its definition impacts on the final prognostic model. A particular variable may not impact substantially on the attainment of CR but may impact on relapse (Stoter *et al.*, 1987b). The use of CR as an endpoint of interest is not uniform among studies since the definition of CR is variable. Complete response may be defined as only patients with residual fibrosis, necrosis and mature teratoma in resected specimens after chemotherapy (Birch *et al.*, 1986; Stoter *et al.* 1987b) or may include patients who have residual malignant elements in the resected specimen but in whom the resection has been complete (Bosl *et al.*, 1983). These differences may influence the significance of the prognostic variables, their relative contribution to a multivariate model, or both.

8. *Statistical methodology.* The most common method of evaluating prognostic features is the use of multivariate analysis to determine independent prognostic factors. The endpoint of interest affects the type of analysis used. Stepwise logistic regression is employed to determine the contribution of the variables in achieving the desired endpoint of a CR, or the Cox regression method if the endpoint of interest is survival. Confirmation on an independent data set is essential to validate the model.

9. *Unknown factors.* Certain clinical factors recently discovered or as yet unknown may play a role in prognosis. Examples

include multiple copies of the chromosome *i*(12p) in patients with refractory disease but considered good risk by both MSKCC and Indiana University (IU) criteria (Bosl, 1989) or the ability to repair platinum–DNA adducts (Reed, Ozols and Tarone, 1988).

7.3 MULTIVARIATE ANALYSES

There have been ten studies in germ cell tumor (GCT) patients in which the prognosis has been evaluated using the technique of multivariate analysis. The first study was reported by von Eyben *et al.* (1982) in which the outcome of 39 patients treated with vinblastine and bleomycin was analyzed. Since achieving CR and survival in GCT patients is directly related to cisplatin-based therapy, only those studies performed on patients receiving standard dose therapy will be considered further. The studies will be evaluated for patient selection, factors included for analysis, desired endpoint, verification of the model in an independent data set and the model's use in prospective trials.

The first multivariate analysis was published by Bosl *et al.* (1983). This was a retrospective study evaluating 171 GCT patients with testicular primaries treated from 1972 to 1981 with three chemotherapy regimens employing standard dose cisplatin (120 mg m^{-2}). Variables considered in this analysis included AFP, HCG, LDH, carcinoembryonic antigen (CEA), treatment protocol, histopathology exclusive of yolk sac tumor, prior treatment, palpable abdominal disease and the number of sites of metastases. Patients with extragonadal (EGN) NSGCT were considered poor risk and not included for analysis. The endpoint of interest was that of an initial CR. Significant factors included the $\log_{10}$ (LDH + 1), $\log_{10}$ (HCG + 1) and the total number of metastases (TOTMET) defined as 0 (markers only), 1' site and 2 or more sites of disease exclusive of the size or number of metastases at any particular site. The value of 1 is added

to the HCG since the $\log_{10}$ of zero does not exist. Alpha-fetoprotein approached but did not attain statistical significance. The probability of patient *i* (*Pi*) attaining a CR took the form of an equation:

$$Pi = \exp Hi/(1 + \exp Hi) \qquad (7.1)$$

where $Hi = 8.514 - 1.973 \log (\text{LDH} + 1) - 0.53 \log (\text{HCG} + 1) - 1.111 \text{ TOTMET}$. Human chorionic gonadotrophin was expressed in mass units (ng ml^{-1}). The negative coefficients indicate a decreasing likelihood of obtaining CR with increasing values of LDH, HCG and the number of metastatic sites of disease.

Good risk assignment was equated with values of *Pi* ≥ 0.5 whereas patients with a *Pi* < 0.5 were considered poor risk. This model was tested on an independent data set of 49 GCT patients and correctly predicted 84% of all CR and 71% of nonresponding patients. The predictive ability of this model has been used to allocate over 300 patients with NSGCT treated at MSKCC since 1982. In two successive poor risk trials the CR rates were 51 and 40% and the durable CR rates were 33 and 26%, respectively (Bosl *et al.*, 1987; Pfister *et al.*, 1989). A randomized trial of VAB-6 versus EP in patients considered good risk resulted in CR rates of 96 and 93%, respectively (Bosl *et al.*, 1988a). The model has also been verified over time with the prognostic importance of the values of LDH, HCG and the number of sites of metastases confirmed with an additional 100 patients (Bosl, Geller and Chan 1988). Some expertise is required in its use for clinical trials; conversion of the HCG to mass units, conversion of the LDH to MSKCC values and a calculator are needed in order to predict response.

Newlands *et al.* (1983) analyzed 69 patients treated between 1979 and 1982 at the Charing Cross Hospital with the sequential chemotherapy regimen cisplatin/vincristine/methotrexate/bleomycin/etoposide/dactinomycin/cyclophosphamide (POMB/ACE) and included patients with gonadal and extragonadal origin. Patients were staged according to the Royal Marsden

Table 7.2 Royal Marsden Hospital staging classification for testicular germ cell tumors

Stage		Definition
I		No evidence of metastases
IM		Rising serum markers with no other evidence of metastases
II		Abdominal node metastases
	A	<2 cm in diameter
	B	2–5 cm in diameter
	C	>5 cm in diameter
III		Supradiaphragmatic node metastases
	M	Mediastinal
	N	Supraclavicular/cervical/axillary
	O	No abdominal node metastases
	ABC	Abdominal nodes defined in Stage II
IV		Extralymphatic metastases
	Lung	
	L1	≤3 Metastases
	L2	>3 Metastases all <2 cm in diameter
	L3	>3 Metastases, one or more >2 cm in diameter
	H+	Liver metastases
	Br+	Brain metastases
	Bo+	Bone metastases

Hospital staging classification (Table 7.2). The overall survival of these patients was 83%. Analysis confirmed that the serum concentration of HCG (>50 000 IU l^{-1}) and/or AFP (>500 kU l^{-1}) were greater determinants of survival than advanced retroperitoneal masses (>5 cm), advanced lung disease (L3 disease), or both. No validation of the findings in an independent population was reported.

The Medical Research Council (1985) Working Party on Testicular Tumours reviewed 458 patients treated between 1976 and 1982 at six British centers. Patients treated at the Charing Cross Hospital were included in the analysis and all patients were staged according to the Royal Marsden Hospital staging classification. The AFP and HCG levels were identified pretreatment and measured in kU l^{-1} and IU l^{-1}, respectively. The serum LDH was not evaluated and patients with EGN NSGCT were not considered. The endpoint of interest was survival and the contribution of factors was assessed using the Cox regression method. Factors portending poor survival were para-aortic nodes >5 cm, L3 lung disease, liver or bone metastases, the number of sites of metastases, age >30 years, AFP >500 kU l^{-1} and HCG >1000 IU l^{-1}. In contrast to earlier findings in the Charing Cross Hospital patients, the level of serum tumor markers and tumor bulk together were more powerful in evaluation prognosis than either factor alone. On the basis of these factors, three prognostic groups were identified with 3-year survival rates of 91, 74 and 47%, respectively. The worst prognosis was that of patients having very large volume (defined as L3 pulmonary disease or involvement of liver, bone or the central nervous system) and high marker disease as defined above. Validation of the findings was not performed on an independent data set. These criteria are currently being used to allocate patients to poor risk trials (Horwich *et al.*, 1989).

Horwich *et al.* (1987) reported on 93 patients treated from 1979 to 1981 at the Royal Marsden Hospital in whom no prior therapy other than orchidectomy had been performed. The study included patients with EGN primaries; some patients had been included in the MRC study. Treatment regimens included PVB, BEP and bleomycin/etoposide/vinblastine/cisplatin (BEVIP). Cox regression analysis of relapse-free survival showed AFP (>1000 µg l^{-1}) and bulk of disease to be independent significant factors. Pretreatment HCG levels did not adversely affect relapse but this may have been influenced by the small number of patients with high HCG levels in this series. This study validated the findings of the MRC study within an individual contributing institution.

Birch *et al.* (1986) examined the pretreatment characteristics of 180 patients treated with PVB ± doxorubicin. The ability to achieve CR was related to the various prognostic variables using logistic regression. Six models were derived using either clinical assess-

Table 7.3 The Indiana University classification system

Stage	Definitions
Minimal disease	
1	Elevated HCG and/or AFP only
2	Cervical nodes (± non/palpable retroperitoneal nodes)
3	Unresectable, but non/palpable, retroperitoneal disease
4	Minimal pulmonary metastases – less than five per lung field and the largest <2 cm (± non/palpable abdominal disease)
Moderate disease	
5	Palpable (≥10 cm) abdominal mass as only disease
6	Moderate pulmonary metastases – five to ten pulmonary metastases per lung field and the largest <3 cm or a mediastinal mass >50% of the intrathoracic diameter or a solitary pulmonary metastasis >2 cm (± non-palpable abdominal disease)
Advanced disease	
7	Advanced pulmonary metastases – mediastinal mass >50% of the intrathoracic diameter or greater than ten pulmonary metastases per lung field or multiple pulmonary metastases, largest >3 cm (± non/palpable abdominal disease)
8	Palpable abdominal mass plus pulmonary metastases 8.1–minimal pulmonary 8.2–moderate pulmonary 8.3–advanced pulmonary
9	Hepatic, osseous, or CNS metastases

ment of tumor bulk, elevated serum tumor markers, or both. The use of tumor bulk alone using the IU staging system (Table 7.3) predicted a good prognosis group of patients with a CR rate of 96% for minimal and moderate disease and a poor risk category (advanced disease) with a 58% response rate and was found superior to the model using the M.D. Anderson clinical staging system. When logistic regression of the IU staging system serum markers and the M.D. Anderson system were considered simultaneously, the M.D. Anderson system did not enter the model. A second model using only the pretreatment values of LDH, HCG and AFP was remarkably similar to the MSKCC model. The probability of CR was calculated using Equation 7.1 in which the linear function took the form:

$$Hi = 10.087 - 1.142 \log (LDH + 1) - 0.204 \log (AFP + 1) - 0.14 \log (HCG + 1) \qquad (7.2)$$

In two additional models, the use of serum tumor markers added to the predictive ability of the IU clinical staging in patients with advanced disease.

The above models were validated in 112 patients treated with PVB or BEP equating poor risk with $Pi < 0.5$. The various models are consistent with the added predictive power of serum tumor markers when used in conjunction with bulk of disease.

The IU staging system has been applied in good risk patients in a prospective trial of three versus four cycles of BEP; CR rates were 98 and 97% and disease-free survival 92 and 92%, respectively (Einhorn, 1986). Its use in two randomized poor risk trials is ongoing.

Stoter *et al.* (1987b) performed a multivariate linear logistic regression analysis in 163 patients treated with PVB. Patients differed only in the amount of vinblastine per cycle, 0.4 versus 0.3 mg kg^{-1} (Stoter *et al.*, 1986). Attainment of CR was the endpoint of the study. Significant variables included trophoblastic elements in the primary tumor, serum markers, size of infradiaphragmatic metastases, size and number of metastases and the number of sites of metastases. The probability was calculated using Equation 7.1 where the linear function took the form:

$$Hi = 1.9381 - (2.1327 \times TROPH) - (2.2723 \times ALPH(AFP)) + (4.87 \times LUNG) - (2.3212 \times SIXNB) \qquad (7.3)$$

where the assigned values were:

TROPH (trophoblastic elements in primary): 0 = no or possible, 1 = yes;

ALPH (AFP): $0 < 1000$, $1 \geqslant 1000$;

LUNG: 0 = no, 1 = yes;

SIXNB (size + number of lung metastases): 0 = none, 1 = 1 to 3 and $\leqslant 3$ cm, 2 = 4 to 19 and $\leqslant 3$ cm, or 1 to 3 and $\geqslant 3$ cm, 3 = $\geqslant 20$ or 4 to 19 and > 3 cm.

Tumor bulk was analyzed to a greater degree than other studies. The model did not retain the prognostic importance of HCG because of the high correlation with other variables, especially trophoblastic elements in the primary site and the size and number of lung metastases. The sensitivity was 81%, specificity was 82% and the misallocation rate was 37% (37% of patients predicted not to respond actually achieved CR) when applied to the same patient population. This model differs from others in that the histology of the primary lesion was important and patients with one to three lung metastases have a better prognosis than patients who have no lung metastases. The latter phenomenon may be explained by the number of patients with no lung metastases but in whom retroperitoneal metastases in excess of 5 cm were present. The findings were self-validated within the same data set and independent validation is pending.

Droz *et al.* (1988) evaluated 84 patients treated on three cisplatin-based regimens between 1978 and 1985. Forty-one patients were treated with cisplatin doses less than 100 mg m^{-2} per course of therapy, which may have had a deleterious impact on the response rate. Complete response was the endpoint for

identifying prognostic factors and the definition of CR was similar to that of Stoter *et al.* This study differed from those previously discussed in that only patients with 'advanced disease' were considered for analysis. They were defined as patients with retroperitoneal masses >10 cm and/or distant metastases. Factors significant in the univariate analysis were the HCG (in mIU ml^{-1}), AFP, the presence of an abdominal mass and visceral metastases other than pulmonary disease. Serum LDH was not examined owing to the small number of patients with this parameter obtained prior to therapy. All variables were examined using the likelihood ratio test and only the AFP and HCG values were retained as significant. The linear function took the form:

$$Hi = 1.90 - 0.033 \sqrt{AFPi} - 0.021 \sqrt{HCGi} + 0.033 \, HCGi/1.00 \qquad (7.4)$$

This model correctly predicted 77% of CR in an independent group of 29 patients and 69% of nonresponders when a *Pi* of 0.7 was used to discriminate between good and poor risk. The prognostic significance of the AFP and HCG values was retained when survival was used as the outcome of interest. This model is being used in prospective allocation of patients to a poor risk trial employing high dose chemotherapy and autologous bone marrow transplantation (Droz *et al.*, 1989).

Scheulen *et al.* (1984) reported the evaluation of prognostic factors for 71 consecutive patients treated with alternating therapy of vinblastine/bleomycin and doxorubicin/cisplatin. All patients had pulmonary involvement. Complete response was the endpoint of interest, but it was not defined in the abstract. Factors analysed included pulmonary tumor volume, number of pulmonary metastases, extent of retroperitoneal and liver involvement, histology, pretreatment and serum levels of AFP, HCG and LDH. All parameters found significant on univariate analysis were found to be dependent on the pretreatment value of LDH in the multi-

Table 7.4 Modification of Samuels' staging criteria for advanced disease

Stage	Definitions
IIIA	Disease confined to supraclavicular nodes
IIIB$_1$	Either one or more biomarker elevated or gynecomastia, unilateral or bilateral; both may be present together; no demonstrable mass
IIIB$_2$	Minimal pulmonary disease: up to five nodules in each lung field, and the largest diameter of any single lesion no greater than 2.0 cm (total tumor volume does not exceed 40 cm^3)
IIIB$_3$	Advanced pulmonary disease: presence of any mediastinal or hilar mass, neoplastic pleural effusion, or intrapulmonary mass greater than 40 cm^3
IIIB$_4$	Advanced abdominal disease, defined as abdominal mass greater than 10 cm
IIIB$_5$	Visceral disease (excluding lung), most often liver but also gastrointestinal tract and brain

variate analysis. No verification in an independent population has been published.

Logothetis *et al.* (1986) evaluated 100 patients treated with the cyclophosphamide/doxorubicin/cisplatin/vinblastine/bleomycin (CISCA$_{II}$/VB$_{IV}$) regimen. Both gonadal and extragonadal tumors were included in the analysis. Tumor bulk was evaluated using the modified Samuels' staging criteria (Table 7.4). Factors considered in the analysis included AFP as a discrete variable above 500 ng ml^{-1}, HCG $> 50\,000$ mIU ml^{-1}, obstructive uropathy, hepatic metastases, extragonadal origin, Stage IIIB$_5$ disease, choriocarcinoma and the clinical stage of disease. Using stepwise logistic regression, HCG was the only prognostic factor to determine outcome. The clinical staging system, extragonadal origin and choriocarcinoma entered the model only after HCG was excluded from the analysis.

7.4 COMPARISONS OF ELIGIBILITY CRITERIA FOR GOOD AND POOR RISK TRIALS

A comparison of the criteria used by the EORTC, Indiana University, the National Cancer Institute and MSKCC was performed in 118 consecutive NSGCT patients treated on MSKCC protocols reported by Bajorin *et al.* (1988). All patients were treated with standard dose cisplatin-based therapy between 1982 and 1986. Patients had been prospectively allocated to good and poor risk groups by the

MSKCC criteria outlined above. Retrospective allocation to good or poor risk status by the other three sets of criteria demonstrated marked differences in risk assignment. The allocations of patients to either good or poor risk categories by all four sets of criteria were concordant in only 66 patients (56%). All criteria were successful in predicting CR with response rates ranging from 88 to 95% and the corresponding survival distributions were favorable.

Major differences occurred in patients considered poor risk; patients allocated to the poor risk group by the four sets of criteria ranged from 31 to 72%. Complete response rates ranged from 38 to 62% in patients deemed poor risk by the various criteria and similar differences were evident in the survival distributions. Substantial variation in CR rate occurred in patients in whom the risk assignment was discordant; patients considered poor risk by one set of criteria but good risk by another had CR rates as high as 87%.

Marked variance occurred when the various criteria were examined for sensitivity, specificity and overall predictive value (Table 7.5). Sensitivity was defined as the correct prediction of CR, specificity as the correct prediction of nonresponders and overall predictive value as the correct prediction of both responders and nonresponders. Criteria designed to capture the greatest number of nonresponders (increase specificity) resulted in

Table 7.5 Classification, response, sensitivity, specificity and overall predictive value in 118 non-seminomatous germ cell tumors of the testis patients treated with standard dose cisplatin (Bajorin *et al.*, 1988)

	MSKCC	IU	NCI	EORTC
1. Good risk (%)	81 (69)	74 (63)	60 (51)	43 (39)
2. Poor risk (%)	37 (31)	44 (37)	58 (49)	72 (61)
3. Sensitivity*	0.85	0.74	0.65	0.49
	(77/89)	(65/89)	(57/89)	(43/89)
4. Specificity†	0.76	0.72	0.93	0.93
	(23/29)	(21/29)	(27/29)	(27/29)
5. Correct overall prediction	0.81	0.74	0.72	0.60
6. Nonresponders	23	21	27	27
7. Good risk patients in poor risk group	14	23	31	45

* Correct prediction of responders.
† Correct prediction of nonresponders.
MSKCC, Memorial Sloan-Kettering Cancer Center; IU, Indiana University; NCI, National Cancer Institute; EORTC, European Organisation for Research and Treatment of Cancer.

inclusion of a greater number of patients who achieved CR in the poor prognosis category. For, example, EORTC criteria had the highest specificity (0.93) but this resulted in 61% of all patients allocated to the poor risk category and a correct overall prediction of only 60% of patients. In direct comparison to MSKCC criteria, 31 more patients were allocated to the poor risk group resulting in only four additional nonresponders.

Bosl *et al.* (1988*b*) compared the MSKCC and IU classifications in 205 NSGCT patients treated at MSKCC. Substantial agreement occurred in the two sets of criteria for patients classified as good risk. Of the 133 patients classified as good risk by both criteria, 95% achieved CR. Major variation occurred in patients allocated to the poor risk category. The MSKCC criteria allocated 20% of all patients to the poor risk category, whereas 32% of this population were considered poor risk by IU criteria. Each IU subgroup was evaluated for the ability to predict CR. In IU group 7, 26/32 (81%) patients achieved CR. For subgroups 8 and 9, the proportion achieving CR was 50%. In the latter two subgroups, 15/34 (44%) patients were classified as good risk by MSKCC criteria. Thirteen of these 15 patients (87%) achieved CR. This is consistent with the findings of Birch *et al.* (1986) that the

use of serum tumor markers enhanced the prognostic capabilities of this classification system in patients with advanced disease.

Bajorin *et al.* (1994) evaluated 796 patients treated on Memorial Sloan-Kettering Cancer Center germ cell tumor chemotherapy protocols over the 15-year period from 1975 to 1990. Treatment regimens included: five-drug regimens consisting of cisplatin, cyclophosphamide, vinblastine, bleomycin and dactinomycin (VAB-4, VAB-5 and VAB-6); etoposide and carboplatin (EC); etoposide and cisplatin (EP); etoposide, carboplatin and bleomycin (EBC); and VAB-6 alternating with EP. Mediastinal primary, seminomatous histology, LDH, HCG and the number of metastases were independently significant for both CR and event-free survival. The variable 'bone, brain or liver' metastases was found comparable to the number of metastases as an independent variable. The prediction of CR could also be made using the ratio of the measured value to the upper limits of normal of the assay for both LDH and HCG, making the use of these variables more universally applicable.

Based on the lack of international consensus on prognostic factors and risk stratification in patients with advanced disease, the International Germ Cell Cancer Collaborative

Table 7.6 Prognostic classification system recommended by the International Germ Cell Cancer Collaborative Group. LDH is expressed as the ratio of the laboratory value to the upper limit of normal for that assay, e.g. a value of 400 using an assay with an upper limit of normal of 200 would be 2.0

Serum tumor marker categories			
	LDH ratio	*HCG (IU l⁻¹)*	*AFP (ng ml⁻¹)*
Good	<1.5	<5000	<1000
Intermediate	1.5–10	5000–50 000	>1000–10 000
Poor	>10	>50 000	>10 000

Classification status
Good Risk
    Seminoma, any primary, no evidence of nonpulmonary visceral metastases, any marker
    NSGCT, testis or retroperitoneal primary, no evidence of nonpulmonary visceral metastases, good markers
Intermediate Risk
    Seminoma, any primary, evidence of nonpulmonary visceral metastases, any marker
    NSGCT, testis or retroperitoneal primary, no evidence of nonpulmonary visceral metastases, intermediate markers
Poor Risk
    NSCGT, testis or retroperitoneal primary, with either evidence of nonpulmonary visceral metastases or poor markers
    NSGCT, mediastinal primary regardless of marker levels or nonpulmonary visceral metastases

Group (IGCCCG) was formed, comprised of investigators from Europe, North America, New Zealand and Australia. A data base was established consisting of 5202 patients with advanced NSGCT and seminoma treated with cisplatin- and carboplatin-based chemotherapy to determine independently significant prognostic factors. Mead (1995), on behalf of the IGCCCG, reported that a mediastinal primary, elevated serum tumor markers AFP, HCG and LDH, and the presence of nonpulmonary visceral metastases were significantly associated with adverse survival. This allowed the establishment of an internationally accepted prognostic classification system that could be used in clinical practice and provide standardization of good, intermediate and poor risk categories for both risk-directed therapy and stratification for clinical trials. Risk categories defined by these criteria are outlined in Table 7.6.

7.5 CONCLUSIONS

The studies performed to determine statistically significant prognostic variables in NSGCT differ markedly in the factors analyzed, patients considered for analysis, year of therapy, regimen and methodology. These explain the differences in the conclusions of the multivariate analyses and provide a better understanding of the variation of reported response rates in poor risk trials.

Despite these differences, several observations are apparent. The biological markers HCG, LDH and AFP clearly play a major role in determining prognosis (Table 7.7). Both HCG and AFP are dominant variables in six of nine studies despite the lack of standardization in measurement and use. The independent significance of the pre-treatment value of LDH has now been established with the IGCCCG study (Mead, 1995).

Extent of disease appears of equal but not greater importance. The early observation that palpable retroperitoneal disease is a poor prognostic feature appears misleading; palpable or 'bulky' retroperitoneal disease in and of itself is not necessarily poor risk when controlled for other prognostic factors (Bosl *et al.*, 1983, 1988a; Birch *et al.*, 1986). The number of sites of disease are important in

Table 7.7 Prognostic factors determined to be of significance in multivariate analysis

	BULK	Number metastatic sites	Specific sites of metastases	LDH	HCG	AFP	Histology
MSKCC	−	+	−	+	−	−	−
Charing Cross	−	−	−	NE	+	+	−
MRC	+	+	+	NE	+	+	−
Royal Marsden	+	NS	+	NE	−	+	−
Indiana Univ.	+	+	+	+	+	+	NS
EORTC	+	+	+	−	−	+	+
Gustave-Rossy	+	NE	+	NE	+	+	−
MD Andersen	−	−	−	NE	+	−	−
Univ. Essen	−	−	−	+	−	−	−
MSKCC	−	+	+	+	+	−	+
IGCCCG	−	−	+	+	+	+	+

Abbreviations: +, statistically significant; −, not statistically significant; NE, not evaluated; NS, not stated; MSKCC, Memorial Sloan-Kettering Cancer Center; MRC, Medical Research Council; EORTC, European Organisation for Research and Treatment of Cancer; IGCCCG, International Germ Cell Cancer Collaborative Group; LDH, lactate dehydrogenase; HCG, human chorionic gonadotrophin; AFP, alpha-fetoprotein.

the two largest studies and specific sites of disease such as liver and bone metastases have less prognostic value when controlled for other variables (Bosl *et al.*, 1983, 1988a; Birch *et al.*, 1986). The specific sites of disease, expressed as either nonpulmonary visceral metastases or metastases to liver, brain, or bone, can replace the number of sites of metastases (Bajorin *et al.*, 1994; Mead, 1995).

The data overwhelmingly support the observation that the use of biological markers and extent or bulk of disease together are more predictive of response and survival than either one alone. Their combined use results in a smaller percentage of the NSGCT population allocated to poor risk trials, minimizes exposure to toxicity of good risk patients and maintains a high response rate in the good risk population.

Studies comparing treatment results with those of other trials or historical controls should be viewed with extreme caution owing to the impact of diverse eligibility criteria and stage migration. The efficacy of any particular regimen must be made in the context of a randomized trial with contemporary standard therapy in order to determine any definitive improvement in response rates and survival. Despite this, randomized trials in patients with poor risk disease will continue to be scrutinized for the definition of poor risk NSGCT employed in the trial. The inclusion of patients considered good risk by more rigorous criteria may result in the conclusion of the 'new' regimen as superior when the greater response rate and survival may be a consequence of an imbalance of prognostic features in the treatment arms.

Differences in definitions of risk have been resolved as a result of the effort by the IGCCCG to establish an international classification system (Mead, 1995). This cooperative effort has lead to a more thorough understanding of the prognostic importance of these factors and has resulted in the development of standardized criteria for good, intermediate and poor risk GCT trials.

ACKNOWLEDGEMENT

Supported in part by grant CA-05826 and contract CM-57732 from the National Cancer Institute.

REFERENCES

Bajorin, D., Katz Chan, E. *et al.* (1988) Comparison of criteria assigning germ cell tumor patients to 'good risk' and 'poor risk' studies. *J. Clin. Oncol.*, **6**, 786–92.

Bajorin, D.F., Mazumdar, M., Motzer, R.J. *et al.* (1994) Model comparisons predicting germ cell tumor (GCT) response to chemotherapy. *Proc. Am. Soc. Clin. Oncol.*, **13**, 232.

Birch, R., Williams, S., Cone, A. *et al.* (1986) Prognostic factors for favorable outcome in disseminated germ cell tumors. *J. Clin. Oncol.*, **4**, 400–7.

Biron, P., Brunat-Montigny, M., Bayle, J.Y. *et al.* (1989) Cisplatinum-VP 16 and ifosfamide (VIC) + autologous bone marrow transplantation (ABMT) in poor prognostic nonseminomatous germ cell tumors (NSGCT). *Proc. Am. Soc. Clin. Oncol.*, **8**, 148.

Blayney, D.W., Goldberg, D.A., Leong, L.A. *et al.* (1986) High risk germ cell tumors (GCT) with severe toxicity with high dose (HD) platinum (P), vinblastine (Ve), bleomycin (B) and VP-16 (V): PVeBV. *Proc. Am. Soc. Clin. Oncol.*, **5**, 101.

Bosl, G.J. (1989) *i*(12p): a specific karyotypic normality in germ cell tumors (GCT). *Proc. Am. Soc. Clin. Oncol.*, **8**, 131.

Bosl, G.J., Geller, N.L., Bajorin, D. *et al.* (1988a) A randomized trial of etoposide + cisplatin versus vinblastine + bleomycin + cisplatin + cyclophosphamide + dactinomycin in patients with good-prognosis germ cell tumors. *J. Clin. Oncol.*, **6**, 1231–8.

Bosl, G.J., Geller, N.L. and Chan E.Y.W. (1988) Stage migration and the increasing proportion of complete responders in patients with advanced germ cell tumors. *Cancer Res.*, **48**, 3524–7.

Bosl, G.J., Geller, N.L., Cirrincione, C.C. *et al.* (1983) Multivariate analysis of prognostic variables in patients with metastatic testicular cancer. *Cancer Res.*, **43**, 3404–7.

Bosl, G.J., Geller, N.L., Penenber, D. *et al.* (1988b) A comparison of the Memorial Hospital and Einhorn classifications of germ cell tumor (GCT) patients (PTS). *Proc. Am. Soc. Clin. Oncol.*, **7**, 121.

Bosl, G.J., Geller, N.L., Vogelzang, N.J. *et al.* (1987) Alternating cycles of etoposide plus cisplatin and VAB-6 in the treatment of poor-risk patients with germ cell tumors. *J. Clin. Oncol.*, **5**, 436–40.

Bukowski, R.M., Smith, G.W. and Montie, J.E. (1988) Combination chemotherapy including VP-16 for poor prognosis germ cell neoplasms. *Urology*, **21**, 403–7.

Chacon, P.R.D., Estevez, R.A., Cedaro, L. *et al.* (1985) Treatment of poor prognosis (PP) germ cell tumors (GCT) with alternating cycles of cisplatin, (P), bleomycin, (B), vinblastine (v) and VP-16. *Proc. Am. Soc. Clin. Oncol.*, **4**, 111.

Daugaard, G. (1986) High dose cisplatin and VP-16 with bleomycin, in the management of advanced metastatic germ cell tumors. *Eur. J. Cancer Clin. Oncol.*, **22**, 477–85.

Droz, J.P., Kramar, A., Ghosn, M. *et al.* (1988) Prognostic factors in advanced non-seminomatous testicular cancer. A multivariate logistic regression analysis. *Cancer*, **62**, 564–8.

Droz, J.P., Pico, J.L., Ghosn, M. *et al.* (1989) High complete remission (CR) and survival rates in poor prognosis (PP) non seminomatous germ cell tumors (NSGCT) with high dose chemotherapy (HDCT) and autologous bone marrow transplantation (ABMT). *Proc. Am. Soc. Clin. Oncol.*, **8**, 130.

Einhorn, L.H. (1986) Have new aggressive chemotherapy regimens improved results in advanced germ cell tumors? *Eur. J. Cancer Clin. Oncol.*, **22**, 1289–93.

Einhorn, L.H., Williams, S.D., Loehrer, P.J. *et al.* (1989) Evaluation of optimal duration of chemotherapy in favourable-prognosis disseminated germ cell tumors: a Southeastern Cancer Study Group Protocol. *J. Clin. Oncol.*, **7**, 387–91.

von Eyben, F.E. *et al.* (1982) Multivariate analysis of risk factors in patients with metastatic testicular germ cell tumors treated with vinblastine and bleomycin. *Invasion Metastasis*, **2**, 125–35.

Feinstein, A.R., Sosin, D.M. and Wells, C.K. (1985) The Will Rogers phenomenon. Stage migration and new diagnostic techniques as a source of misleading statistics for survival in cancer. *N. Engl. J. Med.*, **312**, 1604–8.

Garnick, M.B. and Richie, J.P. (1986) Intensive alternating chemotherapy with cisplatin (P)-vinblastine (V)-bleomycin (B) (PVB) with P-etoposide (E)-B (PEB) for poor prognosis germ cell and undifferentiated tumors. *Proc. Am. Soc. Clin. Oncol.*, **5**, 101.

Hartenstein, R., Clemm, C. and Scheiber, H. (1988) Poor prognosis nonseminomatous germ cell tumors (NSGCT): intensive chemotherapy with etoposide, cisplatin, bleomycin and cyclophosphamide (ECBC). *Proc. Am. Soc. Clin. Oncol.*, **7**, 127.

Horwich, A., Brada, M., Nicholls, J. *et al.* (1989) Intensive induction chemotherapy for poor risk non-seminomatous germ cell tumors. *Eur. J. Cancer Clin. Oncol.*, **25**, 177–84.

Horwich, A., Easton, D., Husband, J. *et al.* (1987) Prognosis following chemotherapy for metastatic malignant teratoma. *Br. J. Urol.*, **59**, 578–83.

Kath, R., Wandl, U., Schumacher, G. *et al.* (1987) Treatment of high-risk non-seminomatous testicular cancer (NSTC) with cisplatinum, ifosfamide and bleomycin (PIB). *Proc. Am. Soc. Clin. Oncol.*, **6**, 109.

Logothetis, C.J., Samuels, M.L., Selig, D.E. *et al.* (1986) Cyclic chemotherapy with cyclophosphamide, doxorubicin, and cisplatin plus vinblastine and bleomycin in advanced germinal tumors. *Am. J. Med.*, **81**, 219–28.

Mead, G.M. (1995) International consensus prognostic classification for metastatic germ cell tumours treated with platinum based chemotherapy: final report of the International Germ Cell Cancer Collaborative Group (IGCCCG). *Proc. Am. Soc. Clin. Oncol.*, **14**, 235.

Medical Research Council Working Party Report on Testicular Tumours (1985) Prognostic factors in advanced nonseminomatous germ-cell testicular tumours: results of a multicentric study. *Lancet*, **i**, 8–11.

Newlands, E.S., Rustin, G.J.S., Begent, R.H.J. *et al.* (1983) Further advances in the management of malignant teratomas of the testis and other sites. *Lancet*, **i**, 948–51.

Nisselbaum, J.S. (1986) Argument in favor of using mass units to calibrate and report concentrations of human choriogonadotropin. *Clin. Chemother.*, **32**, 198–200.

Ozols, R.F., Ihde, D.C., Linehan, W.M. *et al.* (1988) A randomized trial of standard chemotherapy versus a high-dose chemotherapy regimen in the treatment of poor prognosis nonseminomatous germ-cell tumors. *J. Clin. Oncol.*, **6**, 1031–1040.

Pfister, D.G., Cooper, K., Motzer, R. *et al.* (1989) Treatment of poor risk nonseminomatous germ cell tumor (NSGCT) patients (PTS) with carboplatin (CBDCA) + etoposide (E) + bleomycin (B). *Proc. Am. Soc. Clin. Oncol.*, **8**, 131.

Pizzocaro, G., Piva, L., Salvioni, R. *et al.* (1985) Cisplatin, etoposide, bleomycin as first-line therapy and early resection of residual tumor in far-advanced germinal testis cancer. *Cancer*, **56**, 2411–15.

Reed, E., Ozols, R.F. and Tarone, R. (1988) The measurement of cisplatin-DNA adduct levels in testicular cancer patients. *Carcinogenesis*, **9**, 1909–11.

Rustin, G.J.S. and Vogelzang, N.J. (1990) Consensus statement on evaluating tumor markers and staging of patients with germ cell tumors in *Prostate Cancer and Testicular Cancer, EORTC Genitourinary Group Monograph 7*, Wiley–Liss, New York.

Scheulen, M.E., Pfeiffer, R., Hoffken, K. *et al.* (1984) Long-term survival (LTS) and prognostic factors (PF) in patient (pts) with disseminated testicular cancer (DTC). *Proc. Am. Soc. Clin. Oncol.*, **3**, 163.

Schmoll, H.J., Arnold, A., Bergmann, T. *et al.* (1986) Effective chemotherapy in testicular cancer with bulky disease: platinum ultra high dose/VP16/bleomycin. *Proc. Am. Soc. Clin. Oncol.*, **5**, 102.

Stoter, G., Sleijfer, D.T., ten Bokkel Huining, W.W. *et al.* (1986) High-dose versus low-dose vinblastine in cisplatin-vinblastine-bleomycin combination chemotherapy of non-seminomatous testicular cancer: a randomized study of the EORTC Genitourinary Tract Cancer Cooperative Group. *J. Clin. Oncol.*, **4**, 1199–206.

Stoter, G., Kaye, S. and Sleijfer, D. (1986) Preliminary results of BEP (bleomycin, etoposide, cisplatin) versus an alternating regimen of BEP and PVB (cisplatin, vinblastine, bleomycin) in high volume metastatic (HVM) testicular non-seminomas. An EORTC study. *Proc. Am. Soc. Clin. Oncol.*, **5**, 106.

Stoter, G., Sylvester, R., Sleijfer, D.T. *et al.* (1987b) Multivariate analysis of prognostic factors in patients with disseminated nonseminomatous testicular cancer: results from a European Organization for Research and Treatment of Cancer multi-institutional phase III study. *Cancer Res.*, **47**, 2714–18.

Stoter, G., Kaye, S., Jones W. *et al.* (1987a) Cisplatin (P) and VP16 (E) +/– bleomycin (B) (BEP vs EP) in good risk patients with disseminated non-seminomatous testicular cancer; a randomized EORTC GU group study. *Proc. Am. Soc. Clin. Oncol.*, **6**, 110.

Stoter, G. *et al.* (1990) Prognostic factors in metastatic germ cell tumors, in *Prostate Cancer and Testicular Cancer, EORTC Genitourinary Group Monograph 7*, Wiley–Liss, New York.

Vogelzang, N.J. (1987) Prognostic factors in metastatic testicular cancer. *Int. J. Androl.*, **10**, 225–37.

G.K. Zagars

8.1 INTRODUCTION

Stage I seminoma is defined as seminoma confined to the testis or extending into the epididymis, tunica vaginalis, scrotum or spermatic cord without clinical or radiographic evidence of lymphatic or hematogenous dissemination. As shown in Table 8.1, approximately three-quarters of patients with seminoma have Stage I disease. For over 60 years it has been more or less routine to deliver postorchidectomy radiotherapy to the para-aortic and pelvic regions of such patients (Desjardins, Squire and Morton, 1929; Boden and Gibb, 1951). The exceptionally good outcome following this treatment approach is well documented and all series report cure rates in excess of 95% (Section 8.5). Furthermore, the recently demonstrated efficacy of platinum chemotherapy (Logothetis *et al.*, 1987; Horwich *et al.*, 1989) suggests that the few patients who relapse following orchidectomy and radiotherapy are very likely to be salvaged. Two recent studies on a total of 382 patients with Stage I disease reported that only seven (1.8%) relapsed following radiotherapy and all but one were salvaged for a total seminoma mortality of 0.3% (Thomas, 1985; Hamilton *et al.*, 1986).

With cure rates approaching 100% it is no longer possible to improve the prognosis for the patient with Stage I seminoma. Any improvements in management must be sought in possible detoxification of treatment and in improving the cost-effectiveness of medical care for these patients.

Routine postorchidectomy radiotherapy has a low morbidity rate (Section 8.6). Further reduction in morbidity might be achieved by selecting the lowest effective dose and by technical refinements in dose delivery. The ultimate detoxification, however, may consist of

Table 8.1 Incidence of Stage I disease in seminoma series

Series	Total number of patients	Number in Stage I (%)
Jackson *et al.* (1980)	229	151 (66)
Dosoretz *et al.* (1981)	171	135 (79)
Thomas *et al.* (1982)	444	338 (76)
Sause (1983)	108	84 (78)
Schultz *et al.* (1984)	554	424 (77)
Willan and McGowan (1985)	188	149 (79)
Thomas (1985)	178	150 (84)
Lester, Morphis and Hornback (1986)	54	33 (61)
Duncan and Munro (1987)	152	103 (68)
Babaian and Zagars (1988)	240	165 (69)
Ellerbroek, Tran and Selch (1988)	103	76 (74)
Bayens *et al.* (1992)	184	132 (72)
Total	2605	1940 (74)

Testicular Cancer: Investigation and management. Second edition. Edited by Professor A. Horwich.
Published in 1996 by Chapman & Hall. ISBN 0 412 61210 0.

postorchidectomy surveillance with treatment administered only to those patients who unequivocally demonstrate that they have metastatic disease (as discussed in Chapter 9). Surveillance for seminoma, however, does pose problems from both medical and cost-effectiveness viewpoints. This chapter will review the arguments for continuing with a policy of routine postorchidectomy radiotherapy, discuss radiotherapy techniques and doses to minimize morbidity and present the results and complications following such treatment.

8.2 RATIONALE FOR RADIOTHERAPY

Radiotherapy for seminoma became widespread when it was realized that this tumor was exquisitely radiosensitive and that the outlook for patients was substantially improved following irradiation (Desjardins, Squire and Morton, 1929). With the introduction of a staging system for this disease in 1951, it was shown that patients in Stage I fared extremely well if given prophylactic postorchidectomy radiotherapy (Boden and Gibb, 1951). In the absence of any curative alternative and with the continuing demonstration of high success rates with low morbidity, postorchidectomy irradiation became firmly established as standard care for seminoma.

Over the years, progressive refinements in retroperitoneal staging have more accurately assigned patients to their true stage, but faith in lymphangiography was never sufficient to risk disease progression by withholding radiotherapy from patients with Stage I disease. Moreover, retroperitoneal lymph node dissection, with its attendant morbidity, was not indicated in this disease, and so the true incidence of micrometastatic nodal disease in Stage I seminoma was never elucidated in any large series of unselected patients. Indeed, it would have been unwise in the absence of any reliable alternative treatment to abandon so successful a treatment as postorchidectomy radiotherapy, and surgical staging would only have been meddlesome curiosity.

Today, the situation has changed, and surveillance is being investigated as discussed in Chapter 9. Nevertheless radiotherapy has the advantage of a 'track record' extending over many decades resulting in cure rates exceeding 95%. The acute morbidity of radiation is acceptable, consisting of 3 weeks of mild-to-moderate nausea. The pretreatment evaluation of Stage I patients destined to have radiation is simple and cost-effective (Section 8.3). Following radiotherapy, repeated evaluations of the abdomen with computed tomography (CT) are unnecessary: for the vast majority of patients a history, physical examination and chest X-ray repeated at 6-monthly intervals for 3 years, and yearly thereafter, are all that is required (Babaian and Zagars, 1988). The occasional patient with elevated pretreatment serum human chorionic gonadotrophin should have this checked at each follow-up consultation.

After reviewing arguments for and against surveillance or radiotherapy, it become perhaps a philosophical question as to where the balance truly lies. However, this author is decisively swayed by the intrinsic problems that potentially complicate surveillance. In the final analysis, it seems exceedingly difficult to justify departing from a treatment strategy – orchidectomy and radiotherapy – that regularly cures more than 95% of patients with minimal morbidity.

8.3 INVESTIGATION AND STAGING EVALUATION

The specific evaluation of a patient with testicular seminoma begins after pathological diagnosis of the orchidectomy specimen. However, blood should be taken before orchidectomy for determination of alpha-fetoprotein (AFP) and beta-human chorionic gonadotrophin (BHCG) levels.

The importance of a full history and complete physical examination cannot be over emphasized. Important facts to be elucidated include a history of cryptorchidism, orchidopexy, prior ipsilateral inguinal herniorrhaphy, or prior scrotal surgery, since, when present, these are likely to need modifications in radiotherapy technique. Prior fertility and future intentions regarding paternity are important. Patients desiring a future family should be referred to a sperm-banking facility for evaluation and possible cryopreservation of semen.

Physical examination should include an appraisal of the orchidectomy scar. The correct surgical approach to orchidectomy for a testicular tumor is through an inguinal incision. Any trans-scrotal approach to the tumor, including needle biopsy, must be noted. Surgical violation of the scrotum, particularly if the tunica albuginea was incised or punctured in situ, is an indication for hemiscrotal radiation. Although testicular tumors rarely metastasize to inguinal nodes, there are circumstances such as prior scrotal or inguinal surgery which may reroute testicular lymph to the ipsilateral groin, and the inguinal regions should be examined.

Evaluation of the orchidectomy specimen requires not only examination of multiple sections to exclude the diagnosis of non-seminomatous germ cell tumor but should include an assessment of patterns of invasion. Although pathological features are not major determinants of outcome and treatment, the pathologist should note whether the tumor invades the epididymis, the spermatic cord or transgresses the tunica albuginea, and the cut end of the spermatic cord should be evaluated for tumor.

The most important aspect of the evaluation of a patient with seminoma is the search for demonstrable metastatic disease. In this regard it is important to guard against routine overinvestigation. It is all too easy to request a lymphangiogram (LAG), scans of the chest, abdomen and pelvis, intravenous pyelography, AFP, BHCG, lactate dehydrogenase (LDH) and placental-like alkaline phosphatase (PLAP) determinations on all patients at presentation. When the treatment philosophy is to use routine postorchidectomy radiotherapy for patients with Stage I disease, not all of these investigations are needed for the vast majority of seminoma patients and contribute only to medical expense.

The occurrence of detectable hematogenous or mediastinal nodal metastases at initial presentation in the absence of demonstrable retroperitoneal lymphadenopathy is virtually unknown with testicular seminoma. Thus, the retroperitoneal nodes are of primary importance in the staging of testicular seminoma. The bipedal LAG in conjunction with intravenous urography was the traditional mainstay of retroperitoneal staging (Wallace and Jing, 1970). However, at the M.D. Anderson Cancer Center (MDACC) the LAG has been abandoned in favour of the abdominal–pelvic CT scan for patients with seminoma (Babaian and Zagars, 1988). The LAG may have some advantage over the CT scan in detecting small volume metastases (Dunnick and Javadpour, 1981; Ehrlichman, Kaufman and Siegelman, 1981; Heiken, Balfe and the McClennan, 1984), although this has never been proven in seminoma. There is, therefore, a risk that some patients classified as having Stage I disease by CT scan may actually have Stage II disease by LAG. However, the relevant issue is whether the doses commonly used in elective radiotherapy for seminoma would be adequate to control nodal disease of a volume below the resolution of CT scanning. The question of dose control is extensively discussed below. Here it suffices to note that virtually no patients develop in-field recurrences following 25 to 35 Gy for LAG-staged Stage I disease, and that in the large experience reported from the Princess Margaret Hospital in which fewer than one-quarter of Stage I patients had a LAG, abdominal–pelvic recurrences occurred in only seven of 338 patients (2%) given 21 to 30 Gy (Thomas *et al.*, 1982). It was not reported whether these seven relapses were inside or outside the radiation fields. In the Patterns of Care Study

(Hanks, Herring and Kramer, 1981) a group of 33 patients nominally in Stage I, but without LAG or CT evaluation, had no instance of abdominal relapse. These data strongly suggest that doses of radiation routinely used for Stage I seminoma will dependably eradicate nodal disease of a volume just below the resolution of CT scanning.

The patient with testicular seminoma who has a negative abdominal–pelvic CT scan requires little else by way of specific investigation if he is to have radiotherapy. A chest X-ray, presumably performed as part of the preanaesthetic assessment before orchidectomy, should be reviewed, but lung tomograms and thoracic CT scans are unnecessary. A complete blood count and routine blood biochemistry are evaluated. If the patient had preorchidectomy AFP and BHCG levels measured and they were normal, then there is no need to repeat these. Patients whose AFP is elevated without an alternative cause should be regarded as having a non-seminomatous germ cell tumor. If the preorchidectomy BHCG was elevated, this should be repeated prior to radiotherapy. If no markers were measured preorchidectomy, then these should be determined postorchidectomy. The possible significance of elevated BHCG in seminoma is discussed later, but has no proven deleterious effect on prognosis in Stage I seminoma.

In summary, for routine postorchidectomy radiotherapy the evaluation of patients with Stage I seminoma is simple and straightforward, and consists of a history, physical examination, CT scan of the abdomen and pelvis, serum marker estimations, chest X-ray, complete blood count, routine biochemical screen and a review of the pathology.

Prior to commencing radiation, the patient and, if married, his spouse, should be offered a brief session of psychosexual counseling to allay a variety of anxieties that these patients may have (Schover, Gonzales and von Eschenbach, 1986).

8.4 RADIOTHERAPY

8.4.1 STANDARD TARGET VOLUME

Testicular seminoma pursues a characteristic and predictable pattern of local growth and metastatic spread. The primary tumor rarely invades through the tunica albuginea, the incidence of such invasion being less than 5% (Sandeman and Matthews, 1979; Zagars and Babaian, 1987). Extension to the epididymis via the rete testis occurs more frequently and is seen in 8–15% of cases (Sandeman and Matthews, 1979; Zagars and Babaian, 1987). Involvement of the spermatic cord either by direct infiltration or by embolism or permeation of lymphatics occurs in 10–15% of patients with Stage I disease (Zagars and Babaian, 1987). Of these various modes of local spread, extension of tumor through the tunica albuginea or further invasion of the scrotal wall are indications for elective radiotherapy of the hemiscrotum.

Metastatic spread of seminoma begins via testicular lymphatics. Hematogenous dissemination in the absence of demonstrable lymph node metastasis is virtually nonexistent. The lymphatic drainage of the testicle has been fully delineated by anatomical dissection (Rouvière, 1938), testicular lymphangiography (Busch and Sayegh, 1963, 1965; Chiappa *et al.*, 1966) and by the distribution of surgically documented lymph node metastases in patients with non-seminomatous germ cell tumors of the testis (Ray, Hajdu and Whitmore, 1974; Donohue, 1984). All the lymphatics of the testicle, including those from the tunica albuginea, leave the posterosuperior border of the organ as four to eight vessels that run in the spermatic cord. At the internal inguinal ring these blood vessels leave the cord, accompany the testicular vessels through the retroperitoneum, curve medially and terminate in the lumbar lymph nodes (see Fig. 8.1). On the right side the collecting lymph vessels terminate in interaortocaval, precaval and preaortic nodes predominantly

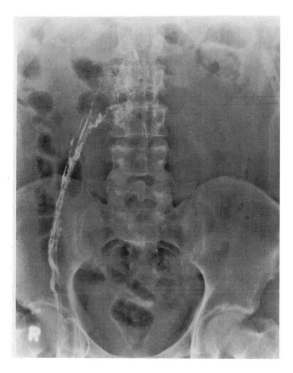

Fig. 8.1 Right testicular lymphangiogram showing the termination of testicular hymphatic vessels in the lumbar lymph nodes.

between the levels of the renal vessels superiorly and the aortic bifurcation inferiorly. Lymphatics from the right testicle exhibit a tendency to cross midline and may terminate in nodes lying to the left of midline. Collecting lymphatic vessels from the left testicle terminate in left lateral para-aortic, preaortic and intcraortocaval nodes mainly between the same superior and inferior levels as right-sided lymph vessels. Left testicular lymphatic vessels, however, do not cross the midline to the right. Although the majority of testicular lymph vessels terminate in nodes at or below the level of the renal hilae, occasional lymphatics have been shown to terminate in nodes as high as the eleventh thoracic vertebra (Busch and Sayegh, 1963, 1965). In the design of radiotherapy portals it is important to note the relationship between the first echelon testicular nodes and vertebral bony landmarks. Normal-sized testicular lymph nodes opacified by testicular lymphangiography do not project laterally further than the tip of the widest lumbar transverse process, usually that of the third lumbar vertebra.

Although the major first echelon lymph nodes for the testis are located in the lumbar nodal group, there are connections between testicular lymph vessels and ipsilateral iliac nodes (Rouvière, 1938). A collecting vessel from the testicle departs its fellows at the internal inguinal ring and passes posteriorly and superiorly to terminate in an external iliac node in front of the common iliac bifurcation. This node also receives some of the lymph vessels from the epididymis. In keeping with this anatomical fact is the finding that approximately 10% of solitary nodal metastases from non-seminomatous germ cell tumors of the testis occur in iliac nodes (Ray, Hajdu and Whitmore, 1974). Contralateral iliac drainage from the testicle has not been reported and contralateral iliac nodal metastases in the absence of bulky para-aortic disease are exceedingly rare (Ray, Hajdu and Whitmore, 1974; Donohue, 1984).

Thus, for the usual case of Stage I seminoma the nodal volume for radiotherapy extends from the level of the eleventh thoracic vertebra superiorly, encompasses the para-aortic region just wide of the widest lumbar transverse process, and follows the ipsilateral hemipelvis to include the external iliac nodes. However, opinions appear to be divided on the need to irradiate the ipsilateral lymphatic vessels from the cut end of the spermatic cord to the lumbar nodes. As visualized by testicular lymphangiography, the testicular lymphatic vessels often pursue a course quite lateral to the vertebral column (Fig. 8.1), and would require radiotherapy portals to be considerably widened ipsilaterally to assure adequate coverage in all patients. In radical retroperitoneal lymph node dissection for non-seminomatous germ cell tumors, the spermatic cord remaining after inguinal orchidectomy is removed and the ipsilateral testicular vessels (including the lymphatics) are removed (Ray, Hajdu and Whitmore, 1974; Donohue, 1984). For Stage I seminoma some authorities appear to attempt irradiation of the ipsilateral lymphatic vessels as shown by the ipsilateral widening of treatment portals below the kidney (Dosoretz *et al.*, 1981; Gibb and Read, 1985; White and Maier, 1987), while others do not attempt such coverage (Ytredal and Bradfield, 1972; Dobbs and Barrett, 1985; Zagars and Babaian, 1987). Since intercalated nodes have not been described along the path of the spermatic vessels and since infradiaphragmatic relapse rates are low in all series regardless of whether a systematic attempt is made to irradiate these vessels or not, one can conclude that such wide-field irradiation is not indicated in Stage I disease.

There is also no unanimity regarding the need to irradiate the inguinal orchidectomy scar routinely. Some authorities routinely irradiate the scar (Schultz *et al.*, 1984; Zagars and Babaian, 1987) and even bolus it (Duncan and Munro, 1987); others explicitly state that they do not attempt to irradiate the scar routinely (White and Maier, 1984) or imply that they do not (Dobbs and Barrett, 1985; Hamilton *et al.*, 1987). Since recurrences in the scar have not been reported when the scar is not routinely treated (Hamilton *et al.*, 1987), such irradiation does not appear necessary. In practice, however, the additional volume irradiated when the scar is included is small. The scar should be treated if the spermatic cord was involved by tumor.

Thus, for the majority of patients with Stage I seminoma the target volume for radiotherapy extends from the level of the eleventh thoracic vertebra superiorly, encompasses the para-aortic region just wide of the lumbar transverse processes and extends into the ipsilateral hemipelvis to include the external iliac nodes. There is no need to attempt irradiation of all ipsilateral testicular lymphatic vessels and irradiation of the orchidectomy scar is not routinely indicated, although

little extra volume is involved in including the scar.

8.4.2 MODIFIED TARGET VOLUME

A number of circumstances may be encountered for which the radiation target volume needs modification relative to the standard. The following situations require discussion: prior ipsilateral herniorrhaphy, prior orchidopexy, scrotal incision and seminoma in maldescended pelvic or inguinal testis.

A history of prior ipsilateral herniorrhaphy is not uncommon in patients with testicular tumors and occurred in 14 of 165 patients (8.5%) with Stage I seminoma in the M.D. Anderson Cancer Center (MDACC) study (Zagars and Babaian, 1987). Disruption of lymphatic vessels in the spermatic cord during herniorrhaphy establishes anastomoses between testicular lymphatic vessels and regional lymph vessels destined for ipsilateral inguinal and iliac nodes. Rerouting of lymph flow under these circumstances has been demonstrated by testicular lymphangiography (Busch and Sayegh, 1965) and by the occurrence of iliac–inguinal nodal metastases in patients developing testicular tumors following herniorrhaphy (Herr, Silber and Martin, 1973; Klein *et al.*, 1984). Although the incidence of ipsilateral iliac–inguinal nodal metastasis under these circumstances is unknown, the conventional tumor volume for seminoma should be extended to encompass the herniorrhaphy scar and ipsilateral iliac–inguinal nodes. The inferior border of the treatment portal should be several centimeters below the level of the lesser trochanter of the femur. For this situation many authors have recommended the irradiation of iliac–inguinal nodes bilaterally (Ytredal and Bradfield, 1972; Dosoretz *et al.*, 1981; White and Maier, 1984; Lester Morphis and Hornback, 1986) and this was standard practice at the MDACC for many years (Hussey, 1980; Zagars and Babaian, 1987). Although at least one patient has been reported to have relapsed in the contralateral groin (Sause, 1983), the likelihood of this occurrence in Stage I seminoma would seem to be very remote and contralateral pelvic irradiation is unnecessary in this setting.

Because of the well-defined relationship between cryptorchidism and subsequent testicular tumor development, seminoma patients occasionally present after a prior orchidopexy. Approximately 2–4% of patients with seminoma will have a history of prior orchidopexy. Like herniorrhaphy, orchidopexy reroutes some testicular lymph to the ipsilateral iliac–inguinal nodes (Busch and Sayegh, 1965). The incidence of iliac–inguinal node metastasis from testicular tumors following orchidopexy or other scrotal operations such as varicocoelectomy or vasectomy is not well defined but has been estimated to lie between 3 and 10% (Batata *et al.*, 1980; Klein *et al.*, 1984). Most authors recommend that patients with seminoma who have a history of prior scrotal surgery should receive elective irradiation to the ipsilateral hemiscrotum and iliac–inguinal regions (Hussey, 1980; Dosoretz *et al.*, 1981; Klein *et al.*, 1984; Hamilton *et al.*, 1986; Ellerbroek, Tran and Selch, 1988).

Since the early years of this century inguinal orchidectomy has been the standard surgical approach to the management of testicular tumors. In the early days, trans-scrotal orchidectomy often included *in situ* biopsy of the tumor with consequent tumor spillage and contamination of the hemiscrotum. Under these circumstances Dean (1929) reported that approximately one-quarter of patients developed scrotal recurrence. However, if a trans-scrotal orchidectomy is accomplished without incision of the tunica albuginea, then it is unlikely that scrotal recurrence could occur and rerouting of lymphatics would be irrelevant. This may account for the low incidence of scrotal or inguinal relapses after scrotal orchidectomy in recent series even when the inguinal–scrotal regions received no adjuvant treatment (Herr, Silber and Martin, 1973; Thomas *et al.*, 1982; Klein *et al.*, 1984). Unfortunately, it is not always possible

to ascertain with certainty what transpired during a scrotal operation for testicular tumor and one study revealed that relapse rates in patients with Stage I seminoma who underwent scrotal orchidectomy were higher than in patients having inguinal orchidectomy, although the sites of relapse were not specified (Ozen *et al.*, 1988). It is wise to regard every scrotal incision during the course of orchidectomy for a testicular tumor as an error, and to deliver radiation to the ipsilateral hemiscrotum and iliac–inguinal region.

In summary, the indications for extending the conventional radiotherapy target volume in Stage I seminoma to include the hemiscrotum are: (a) any prior trans-scrotal surgery including orchidopexy, varicocoelectomy, vasectomy; (b) trans-scrotal orchidectomy or trans-scrotal biopsy; (c) tumor extension through the tunica albuginea. Whenever the hemiscrotum is to be irradiated, then the ipsilateral inguinal nodes also require irradiation. In addition, a history of prior ipsilateral herniorrhaphy is an indication for ipsilateral groin irradiation.

We now turn to seminoma arising in an undescended testicle. Some 5–11% of patients with testicular seminoma have a history of cryptorchidism (Jackson *et al.*, 1980; Hamilton *et al.*, 1986; Zagars and Babaian, 1987; Ellerbroek, Tran and Selch, 1988). In the majority of these patients the cryptorchidism is corrected (surgically, hormonally or spontaneously) by the time they present with seminoma (Batata *et al.*, 1980). In some patients, however, a testicular tumor may develop in a pelvic or an inguinal testis. The higher the location of the undescended testis, the more likely it is that the tumor will be a seminoma. In one series, 93% of pelvic testicle tumors were seminomas, 63% of inguinal testicle tumors were seminomas, and 30% of corrected cryptorchid testicle tumors were seminomas (Batata *et al.*, 1980). At MDACC we have encountered 13 patients with pelvic seminoma. Patients with pelvic seminomas tend to have larger primary tumors than do patients with scrotal disease (Batata *et al.,* 1980) and a higher proportion have demonstrable lymph node metastases. Two of 13 patients with this syndrome in our series were in Stage I (Babaian and Zagars, 1988). The nondescended testis appears to acquire abundant lymphatic connections with ipsilateral iliac nodes in addition to the usual lumbar connections, and iliac node metastasis is a significant threat under these circumstances (Jonsson *et al.,* 1978). Guidelines for postsurgical radiotherapy in cases of inguinal or pelvic seminoma Stage I have not been described. Based on the MDACC experience with 13 patients, mostly in Stage II, who received postsurgical radiotherapy to wide fields and none of whom subsequently relapsed (Babaian and Zagars, 1988), it is recommended that in addition to the standard para-aortic volume, the whole pelvis and ipsilateral inguinal nodes be irradiated.

More recently, the need for extending the irradiation field beyond the para-aortic area has been questioned, based on the patterns of recurrence seen with a policy of surveillance as described in Chapter 9. The UK Medical Research Council has conducted a prospective randomized trial comparing a para-aortic field with the more standard policy of para-aortic plus ipsilateral pelvic fields. At present, analysis is available on more than 500 patients with minimum of 1 year follow-up (Fosså *et al.* for the MRC Testicular Tumour Working Party, 1995). Patients on both arms of the trial were treated to a dose of 30 Gy in 15 fractions over 3 weeks. There is no overall difference in recurrence rate and there have only been two recurrences in pelvic nodes. This result is supported by a single center pilot study from the Christie Hospital based on 94 patients treated between 1991 and 1993 with a para-aortic field to a dose of 20 Gy in eight fractions (Read and Johnston, 1993). No in-field recurrences occurred.

8.4.3 RADIOTHERAPY TECHNIQUES

Perusal of some standard textbooks of radiotherapy reveals that a variety of techniques can be employed for postorchidectomy irradiation of testicular seminoma (Hussey, 1980; Dobbs and Barrett, 1985; Gibb and Read, 1985; White and Maier, 1987; Cox, 1989). Although strong opinions have been expressed on what constitutes the optimal technique, sufficient evidence to support a particular position in this regard is lacking. Relapse-free survival rates following postorchidectomy radiotherapy for Stage I seminoma treated by various techniques and with various nuances in tumor volume are so similar that a therapeutic advantage for any specific approach cannot be demonstrated. There may be economic advantages to certain techniques, but this issue has not been addressed. This section will describe the technique used at MDACC. Details of other techniques can be found in the textbooks referred to above and in the articles referred to in Table 8.2.

Virtually all patients are treated with 6 MeV linear accelerator photons. The para-aortic region is treated with parallel-opposed anterior–posterior rectangular portals measuring 9 to 11 cm in width on the skin and extending from the top of the tenth thoracic vertebra to the bottom of the fifth lumbar vertebra. These fields are centred at midline and field shaping is not used. Each field is treated at 100 cm source-to-skin distance and the patient is supine for the anterior field and prone for the posterior. The tumor dose for these fields is specified at midline along the central axis and is equally weighted from both sides. The ipsilateral hemipelvis is treated via only one anterior field. Superiorly, this field matches the lower border of the para-aortic fields at the bottom of the fifth lumbar vertebra, resulting in a 2–3 cm skin gap on the lower anterior abdomen. Medially, the field extends 1 cm over midline to the contralateral side; laterally, the iliac crest is shielded; inferiorly, the orchidectomy scar is

Table 8.2 Average total dose and fraction number used in Stage I seminoma patients

Series	Number of patients	Average total dose (cGy)	Number of fractions
Dosoretz *et al.* (1981)	135	2500	13
Sause (1983)	84	3000	15–17
Willan and McGowan (1985)	149	2750	15–20
Hamilton *et al.* (1986)	232	3000	15–18
Lester, Morphis and Hornback (1986)	33	2569	15
Zagars and Babaian (1987)	161	2475	15
Duncan and Munro (1987)	103	3000	20
Lederman *et al.* (1989)	79	3000	–
Schultz *et al.* (1984)	424	3300–3500	16–20
Fosså, Aass and Kaalhus (1989a)	365	3600–4000	18–20
Lai *et al.* (1994)	95	2500	14–20
Giacchetti *et al.* (1993)	184	210	8

covered (without bolus). The lower medial corner of this field is shielded to exclude the root of the penis and to place the direct beam of radiation further from the opposite testicle. This field is treated at 100 cm source-to-skin distance. The tumor dose is specified at a point 3 cm anterior to midline along the central axis. If the scrotum and inguinal region require treatment the hemipelvic field is simply extended inferiorly and the scrotum is placed on the device described by Harter *et al.* (1976). Simulation films of typical para-aortic and hemipelvic fields are shown in Fig. 8.2 and the anterior skin marks drawn on a patient are shown in Fig. 8.3. Because the para-aortic and pelvic fields are matched at the bottom of L5, a skin gap of 2–3 cm occurs between these two fields. These fields should **never** abut on skin. Lateral laser marks are used to position the patient correctly. In practice, the anterior portals are treated sequentially with the patient supine and then the posterior para-aortic field is treated with the patient prone.

8.4.4 TUMOR DOSE

Seminoma is exquisitely sensitive to radiation. Bulky metastases can be regularly eradicated with doses of 35–40 Gy (Hanks, Herring and Kramer, 1981; Thomas *et al.*, 1982; Sause, 1983; Lester, Morphis and Hornback, 1986; Babaian and Zagars, 1988). The minimal dose needed to eradicate microscopic disease dependably has not been defined, but is certainly less than 30 Gy. Table 8.2 is a compilation of approximate doses employed by various centres for postorchidectomy radiation in Stage I seminoma. The ten series in this table include 1765 patients and only two patients were reported to have failed in the irradiated volume. In one case the total dose was 15 Gy (Lester, Morphis and Hornback, 1986) and in the other case the total dose was 21 Gy in 22 fractions over 35 days (Dosoretz *et al.*, 1981). The almost universal local control in 976 patients in the upper portion of the table argues strongly that there is no need to deliver more than 30 Gy in Stage I seminoma. Indeed, several of the studies reveal that 25 Gy in 15 fractions over 3 weeks is adequate (Dosoretz *et al.*, 1981; Lester, Morphis and Hornback, 1986; Zagars and Babaian, 1987).

A recent report from Christie Hospital in Manchester was based on 94 patients treated to a dose of 20 Gy in eight fractions to the para-aortic region. With a minimum follow-up of 15 months (median 34 months), no patient has relapsed in the abdomen.

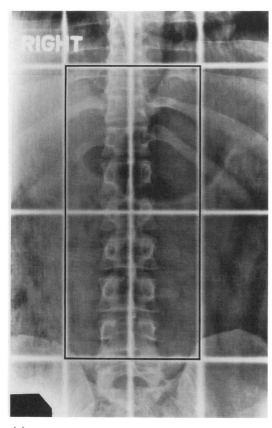

(a)

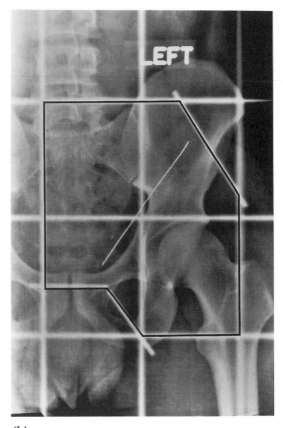

(b)

Fig. 8.2 (a) Simulation film of a para-aortic radiation portal. The field extends from the top of T10 to the bottom of L5 and measures 10 cm in width. (b) Simulation film of a left hemipelvic field. The orchidectomy scar is outlined with a wire.

8.5   RESULTS

The results for Stage I seminoma treated by orchidectomy and postorchidectomy radiotherapy are truly excellent. Table 8.3 is a compilation of 16 larger series reported since 1980 and shows that only 4.4% of 2603 patients sustained relapse of their tumor. Death from seminoma occurred in only 2.1% of patients. Although these series were reported within the last decade, patient accrual to many of them extended back several decades and the pretreatment work-up of such patients did not include estimations of serum markers (to exclude non-seminomatous germ cell tumors) or even retroperitoneal evaluation acceptable by current standards. It is the outcome in patients fully worked up that must be compared with those under surveillance. The report by Thomas (1985) on 150 patients with Stage I seminoma accrued between 1977 and 1985 and fully evaluated prior to treatment revealed that only two relapsed (1.3%) and that both of these were salvaged, leading to no seminoma mortality.

The low relapse rate after radiotherapy for Stage I seminoma requires that many series must be pooled to reasonably establish patterns of failure. Table 8.4 summarizes sites

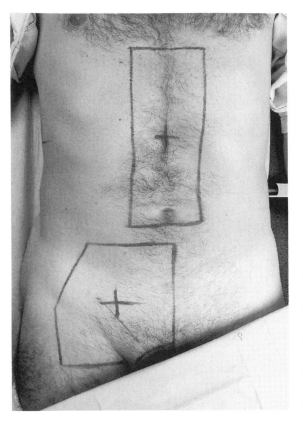

Fig. 8.3 Photograph of the anterior fields for a right-sided seminoma marked on the skin.

of first relapse in series where these data were given. Of all relapses, hematogenous spread accounts for approximately 40% (about 2% of all patients treated) and mediastinal–supraclavicular nodal spread accounts for approximately one-third (about 1.5% of all patients treated). Abdominal relapse is about one-half as common as hematogenous relapse and occurs in 1% of all patients treated. The abdominal failures are mostly described as 'marginal', occurring at or just beyond the radiation portal margin. Approximately one-half of the hematogenous relapses are in lung and the rest occur in a variety of unpredictable sites including liver, bone and soft tissue.

The median time to relapse has not been well documented but seems to lie between 12 and 24 months (Hamilton *et al.*, 1986; Lester, Morphis and Hornback, 1986; Zagars and Babaian, 1987; Lederman *et al.*, 1989). In the MDACC series the median time to relapse was 17 months and this was significantly longer than the median time to relapse for Stage II seminoma (Babaian and Zagars, 1988). Relapses after 3 years are not rare but relapses beyond 5 years are uncommon.

As shown in Table 8.3, 61 of 116 patients (53%) who relapsed were successfully salvaged. In the series presented in this table, the majority of relapses occurred at a time when *cis*-platinum-based chemotherapy regimens were unavailable and salvage consisted of further radiotherapy or other chemotherapy. Today, the long-term disease-free survival for patients with advanced or recurrent seminoma is of the order of 90% following treatment incorporating *cis*-platinum (Fosså *et al.*, 1987; Logothetis *et al.*, 1987). Thus, treatment with *cis*-platinum-based chemotherapy appears to be the best form of salvage therapy for the patient with Stage I seminoma who relapses after radiotherapy. There would be no argument with this for the patient with hematogenous relapse. For the patient with mediastinal–supraclavicular nodal relapse, however, some authors report very high salvage rates with radiotherapy (Willan and McGowan, 1985; Hamilton *et al.*, 1986). Unfortunately not all reports have had such favorable outcomes with radiation salvage in this situation. Only two of six such patients were salvaged in the report by Thomas *et al.* (1982) and no such patient was salvaged by radiation in the MDACC report (Zagars and Babaian, 1987). Thus, it seems best to recommend *cis*-platinum-based chemotherapy to all patients who relapse after radiotherapy.

For Stage I seminoma treated with radiotherapy unequivocal prognostic factors have not been demonstrated. Cryptorchidism or prior herniorrhaphy are not prognostically significant (Zagars and Babaian, 1987). Scrotal incision is not adverse if correctly managed

Table 8.3   Relapses and tumor deaths in Stage I seminoma patients after orchidectomy and radiotherapy

	Number of patients	Number relapsed	Number salvaged
Dosoretz et al. (1981)	135	7	3
Thomas et al. (1982)	338	20	6
Sause (1983)	84	3	2
Huben et al. (1984)	24	2	0
Schultz et al. (1984)	424	13	9
Willan and McGowan (1985)	149	11	8
Thomas (1985)	150	2	2
Lester, Morphis and Hornback (1986)	54	4	1
Hamilton et al. (1986)	232	5	5
Zagars and Babaian (1987)	163	7	3
Duncan and Munro (1987)	103	12	5
Ellerbroek, Tran and Selch (1988)	76	7	0
Lederman et al. (1989)	79	2	1
Fosså, Aass and Kaalhus (1989a)	365	13	9
Bayens et al. (1992)	132	6	5
Lai et al. (1994)	95	2	2
Total	2603	116	61

Seminoma relapses 116/2603 (4.4%).
Seminoma deaths 55/2603 (2.1%).

Table 8.4   Sites of first relapse in Stage I seminoma patients after orchidectomy and radiotherapy

Series	Total number of patients	Number of patients relapsed	Mediastinum supraclavical	Abdomen pelvis	Scrotum	Hematogenous
Dosoretz et al. (1981)	135	7	0	3	1	3*
Hanks, Herring and Kramer (1981)	262	11	4	2	0	5
Thomas et al. (1982)	338	20	6	6	1	7*
Sause (1983)	108	3	1	2	0	0
Huben et al. (1984)	24	2	0	0	0	2*
Schultz et al. (1984)	424	13	4	3	3	3*
Willan and McGowan (1985)	149	11	5	1	0	5*
Hamilton et al. (1986)	232	5	3	0	0	2*
Lester, Morphis and Hornback (1986)	54	4	1	1	0	2*
Zagars and Babaian (1987)	163	7	3	1	0	3*
Duncan and Munro (1987)	103	12	6	2	0	4*
Ellerbroek, Tran and Selch (1988)	76	7	1	1	0	5*
Fosså, Aass and Kaalhus (1989a)	365	13	7	0	0	6*
Bayens et al. (1992)	132	6	4	0	0	2*
Lai et al. (1994)	95	2	1			1*
Total	2660	123	46	22	5	50

* 20 of 38 (53%) hematogenous relapses were in the lung.

(Zagars and Babaian, 1987). A number of pathological factors, including tumor size, seminoma type, tumor necrosis, mitotic index, vascular invasion and extent of local spread, have been evaluated for possible prognostic significance. Some of these factors have occasionally been reported to be prognostically significant in seminoma series of all stages combined. However, when prognostic factor analysis is confined to Stage I patients receiving radiotherapy the following pathological factors are of no prognostic significance: primary tumor size, seminoma subtype (classic versus anaplastic), tumor necrosis, mitotic index, tumor extension to the epididymis, tumor extension through the tunica albuginea, tumor involvement of the spermatic cord, vascular invasion (Vaeth *et al.*, 1984; Zagars and Babaian, 1987).

The potential significance of elevated serum BHCG levels in patients with seminoma has received considerable attention. It is well documented that pure seminoma may produce HCG and that the cells responsible for this abnormal production are syncytiotrophoblast giant cells within the tumor (Morgan *et al.*, 1982; Butcher *et al.*, 1985). Unfortunately, an accurate estimate of the occurrence of this type of seminoma is impossible since the reported incidence of patients with elevated serum BHCG varies widely among different series. For Stage I seminoma the incidence of elevated serum BHCG prior to orchidectomy has been reported as 5.3% (Nørgaard-Pedersen *et al.*, 1984), 22.7% (Lange *et al.*, 1980), 36.4% (Peckham *et al.*, 1987), or 40% (Fosså and Fosså, 1989). Postorchidectomy elevations of serum BHCG in Stage I seminoma are reported to occur with an incidence of 0% (Vaeth *et al.*, 1984; Fosså and Fosså, 1989), 9% (Thomas, 1985), or 25% (Zagars and Babaian, 1987). The reasons for these wide discrepancies are unknown but different sensitivity/specificity of various commercial assays for BHCG probably plays a significant role (Catalona, Vaitukaitis and Fair, 1979). It has been shown that some assays

cross-react with luteinizing hormone (LH) and may give a falsely elevated BHCG value, especially after orchidectomy when serum LH levels may be raised (Catalona, Vaitukaitis and Fair, 1979; Lange *et al.*, 1980). Modest elevations of BHCG after orchidectomy in seminoma patients should be viewed with scepticism.

In the presence of such wide variation in the reported incidence of BHCG-positive seminoma, the prognostic significance of an elevated serum BHCG is difficult to evaluate unequivocally. There are reports concluding that seminoma with elevated BHCG is more aggressive than typical seminoma and is associated with a worse prognosis (Lange *et al.*, 1980; Morgan *et al.*, 1982; Schultz *et al.*, 1984; Butcher *et al.*, 1985) and should perhaps be managed as a non-seminomatous germ cell tumor with retroperitoneal lymph node dissection as part of the treatment (Pritchett *et al.*, 1985). On the other hand, there are reports that elevated BHCG is of no prognostic significance in seminoma and calls for no special change in treatment (Swartz, Johnson and Hussey, 1984; Mirimanoff *et al.*, 1985; Thomas, 1985; Peckham *et al.*, 1987; Zagars and Babaian; 1987). Until BHCG assays become standardized and the incidence of BHCG-producing seminoma is better delineated, the prognostic significance of such tumors remains somewhat uncertain, but as summarized in Table 8.5, patients in Stage I with preorchidectomy elevations in BHCG have an extremely good prognosis following radiotherapy and these data do not suggest that therapeutic modifications are indicated in this circumstance. Further evidence that preorchidectomy elevation in serum BHCG is of no prognostic significance in Stage I comes from the surveillance report of Peckham *et al.* (1987), where none of eight patients with elevated levels relapsed, whereas one of 14 patients with normal levels had relapsed. It should be noted that in the vast majority of patients with seminoma who have elevated serum BHCG levels, the levels are only

Table 8.5 Relapse rates in Stage I seminoma patients with preorchidectomy serum human chorionic gonadotrophin (HCG) elevation treated by radiotherapy

Series	Number of patients with elevated HCG	Number relapsed
Javadpour *et al.* (1978)	4	0
Mauch, Weichselbaum and Botnick (1979)	5	0
Lange *et al.* (1980)	8	1
Dosoretz *et al.* (1981)	3	0
Vaeth *et al.* (1984)	8	0
Total	28	1

modestly above normal, with values in the range 20–50 mIU ml^{-1}.

Sometimes the first serum BHCG value is obtained after orchidectomy. In Stage I the expectation is that elevation would be extremely uncommon and due only to BHCG production by nodal micrometastases. Some series indeed report that no patient with Stage I seminoma had elevated postorchidectomy BHCG (Vaeth *et al.*, 1984; Fosså and Fosså, 1989). There are, however, several reports of postorchidectomy elevation in serum BHCG. The elevations reported are typically modest (Zagars and Babaian, 1987) and the majority probably represent false elevations due to cross-reaction with LH. In three reports (Mirimanoff *et al.*, 1985; Thomas, 1985; Zagars and Babaian, 1987) a total of 31 patients with Stage I seminoma had elevated postorchidectomy BHCG. Only three of these patients relapsed after radiotherapy, suggesting that modest elevations of BHCG postorchidectomy are of little prognostic significance in such patients.

8.6 COMPLICATIONS

8.6.1 ACUTE COMPLICATIONS

The acute morbidity of para-aortic–iliac radiotherapy, although not serious, has not been well documented. At MDACC, the major morbidity during treatment is nausea with or without vomiting. Some degree of nausea occurs in the majority of patients and approximately one-fifth develop vomiting. In the worst cases symptoms of the acute radiation syndrome (Danjoux, Rider and Fitzpatrick, 1979) can occur: after a latent period of 1 to 1.5 hours the patient suddenly develops intense nausea and vomiting lasting for approximately 0.5 hours and followed by a period of rest or sleep. A second bout of nausea and vomiting can occur some 6 hours later. Although severe nausea and vomiting are uncommon, it is our practice to prescribe antiemetics for all patients beginning on the evening before the first treatment. Patients are counseled to have a light meal approximately 30 minutes prior to each treatment. With this regimen the vast majority of patients continue their normal daily activities during the course of radiation. A minority of patients develop diarrhea, which is easily controlled with antidiarrheal medication. Significant hematological depression is uncommon with a reported incidence of 1.8–3.3% (Duncan and Munro, 1987; Coia and Hanks, 1988).

8.6.2 DELAYED INTRA-ABDOMINAL COMPLICATIONS

Following radiotherapy at doses customary for seminoma, long-term complications involving intra-abdominal organs are uncommon. Hepatic, renal, urinary bladder, large bowel and spinal cord complications occur in fewer than 1% of patients (Coia and Hanks, 1988; Fosså, Aass and Kaalhus, 1989b). The only complications reported with any frequency occur in the stomach and small bowel. Peptic ulceration, mostly duodenal, has been documented in 6–9% of patients following para-aortic irradiation to doses of 30–45 Gy (Hamilton *et al.*, 1986, 1987; Coia and Hanks, 1988; Fosså, Aass and Kaalhus, 1989b). These ulcers typically appear between 10 and 40 weeks after completion of radiation and the majority heal with conservative medical management. The etiological role of radiation in the genesis of these ulcers has not been unequivocally established since none of the reports provides an entirely adequate control group with which to compare this incidence. One study attempted to provide a control group of patients by comparing the incidence of peptic ulcers in two similar groups of men with Stage I non-seminomatous germ cell tumors, one group being under surveillance and the other receiving 40–45 Gy to the para-aortic region (Hamilton *et al.*, 1987). While the incidence of subsequent ulcer disease was significantly higher in the irradiated group, some patients in the irradiated group had a history of prior ulcer disease, whereas none had such a history in the control group. When patients with prior ulcer disease are excluded from analysis the difference in incidence of ulcer disease between those irradiated and those non-irradiated does not achieve statistical significance. Furthermore, there are significant inconsistencies among different reports regarding pretreatment factors potentially influencing the development of these ulcers following relatively lowdose irradiation. One report found a significant correlation between prior abdominal surgery and occurrence of later peptic ulceration (Hamilton *et al.*, 1986), whereas another report did not (Hamilton *et al.*, 1987). Some reports (Hamilton *et al.*, 1987; Fosså, Aass and Kaalhus, 1989b) found a significant correlation between prior peptic ulceration and subsequent ulceration, whereas another report did not (Coia and Hanks, 1988). For doses in the range 30–45 Gy, no correlation has been documented between dose and ulcer incidence. These considerations weaken the argument for an etiological relationship between para-aortic irradiation to doses of 30–45 Gy and subsequent duodenal ulceration. Nevertheless, the possibility of such a relationship argues for the use of the smallest dose consistent with adequate tumor eradication.

Doses of 10–20 Gy have been extensively used in the management of peptic ulceration in years gone by and were not documented to induce any deleterious long-term effects on the stomach (Clayman, Palmer and Kirsner 1968). Thus, the dose recommended for Stage I disease in this chapter (25 Gy in 15 fractions) is likely to offer the least likelihood of subsequent ulcer disease with excellent long-term disease control.

In addition to peptic ulceration a diverse group of other gastrointestinal complications have been reported to occur. Diarrhea, dyspepsia, heartburn and small bowel obstruction have been documented to occur following doses of 25–45 Gy to the para-aortic region (Coia and Hanks, 1988; Fosså, Aass and Kaalhus 1989b). The incidence of these complications is clearly related to dose and serious grades of these complications occur in fewer than 1% of patients at doses of <35 Gy and are not observed at doses <25 Gy (Coia and Hanks, 1988). This is further reason to limit the para-aortic dose to 25 Gy.

8.6.3 REPRODUCTIVE COMPLICATIONS

The median age of patients with seminoma is between 30 and 40 years, and potentially adverse effects of irradiation on future fertility are of concern to a proportion of these men. Testicular germinal epithelium is exquisitely sensitive to the cytotoxic effects of ionizing radiation. Although the remaining testis is not intentionally irradiated, the small amount of scattered radiation reaching that organ causes significant acute depression of spermatogenesis, which poses a potential threat to later fertility. An additional concern is the theoretical risk of genetic abnormalities among the offspring of these patients.

Before considering the effects of radiation on spermatogenesis, however, it is important to realize that many patients with testicular tumors, including seminoma, have significant abnormalities in spermatogenesis that antecede any postorchidectomy radiation therapy. In three large series of patients with testicular tumors evaluated after unilateral orchidectomy but before additional treatment (Berthelsen and Skakkebæk, 1983; Hendry *et al.*, 1983; Fosså, Abyholm and Aakvaag, 1984) it was found that approximately three-quarters of these men had severe depression of spermatogenesis. Aspermia occurred in 15–20%, oligospermia ($<20 \times 10^6$ sperm ml^{-1} ejaculate) occurred in about one-third, and nearly one-half of those with satisfactory sperm counts had significant impairment of sperm motility. Serum follicle-stimulating hormone (FSH) level was elevated in 10–20% and serum testosterone level was moderately subnormal in 20–25%. Routine biopsy of the contralateral testicle in 81 consecutive men with Stage I seminoma revealed the Sertoli cell-only pattern in nine (11%), spermatogenic arrest in eight (10%), hyalinization of seminiferous tubules in 12 (15%), spermatogenic cell depletion in 16 (20%) and carcinoma *in situ* in eight (10%) (Berthelsen and Skakkebæk, 1983). The defect in spermatogenesis did not correlate with tumor type (seminoma versus non-seminomatous germ cell tumor) nor with the stage of disease. The cause of this defective spermatogenesis is unknown. The well-known correlation between cryptorchidism, testicular atrophy, infertility and testicular germ cell tumor (Pryor *et al.*, 1983) is unlikely to be the only factor in most cases since approximately 25% of men documented to be aspermic after unilateral orchid-ectomy have fathered children in the years preceding diagnosis of their testicular tumor (Hendry *et al.*, 1983; Fosså, Abyholm and Aakvaag, 1984). Furthermore, similar defects in spermatogenesis have been found in a similarly high proportion of young men following the diagnosis of Hodgkin's disease, but before any therapeutic intervention (Chapman, Sutcliffe and Malpas, 1981; Hendry *et al.*, 1983; Reed, Sander and Armitage, 1986). The natural history of this disorder is poorly defined, but in many men it appears to be reversible as evidenced by their eventual achievement of sperm counts above baseline despite radiation or chemotherapy (Fosså *et al.*, 1986, Hansen *et al.*, 1989). In some cases, however, the changes seen on testicular biopsy are of such severity that recovery would seem unlikely (Berthelsen and Skakkebæk, 1983). The preirradiation depression of spermatogenesis not only complicates the evaluation of the effects of radiation on fertility but also limits the usefulness of cryopreservation of semen (Fosså *et al.*, 1986; Reed, Sander and Armitage, 1986). One large study revealed that only about 25% of men with testicular tumors had semen of adequate quality to make sperm banking a worthwhile undertaking (Hendry *et al.*, 1983).

The effects of single radiation doses on normal human spermatogenesis have been documented in a series of studies on normal human volunteers (Rowley *et al.*, 1974; Clifton and Bremner, 1983). Table 8.6 summarizes

Table 8.6   Effects of single radiation exposures on normal human spermatogenesis

Testicular radiation dose (cGy)	Spermatogonial survival (% of baseline)	Minimal sperm count (% of baseline)	Time to minimal sperm count (weeks)	Time to increase of spermatogonia (weeks)	Time to increase in sperm count (weeks)
7.5–10	40–80	100	–	15	–
10–50	10–40	1–50	20–40	26–27	30–40
50–100	≈7.5	0–0.5	≈15	25–29	40–60
100–200	≈3	0	10–15	≈29	≈60
200–300	≈1.5	0	≈10	≈29	60–80
300–600	<1	0	≈10	≈29	80–120+

Data from Rowley *et al.* (1974) and Clifton and Bremner (1983).

Table 8.7 Effects of scattered radiation over 15–30 fractions* on human spermatogenesis in patients with pretreatment sperm counts $\geq 10^6$ ml^{-1}

Total testicular dose (cGy)	Effect
15–50	Temporary oligospermia†, recovery to $\geq 20 \times 10^6$ in all by 20–80 weeks
50–150	Aspermia in virtually all; recovery to $\geq 20 \times 10^6$ in majority by 90 weeks
150–300	Aspermia in all; recovery in some by 5 years
300–400	Long-term, possibly permanent aspermia in all

* Dose per fraction 3–20 cGy.
† Doses between 30 and 50 cGy may produce temporary aspermia in patients with sperm counts $<10^6$ ml^{-1}.
Data from Sandeman (1966); Speiser, Rubin and Casarett (1973); Hahn *et al.* (1982); Freund *et al.* (1987); Schlappack *et al.* (1988); Kinsella *et al.* (1989).

some of the results. The spermatogonium, especially the type B cell, is the most radio-sensitive cell in the human germinal epithelium. A single dose of 9.7 cGy causes a 50% depletion of this cell type (Clifton and Bremner, 1983). Spermatocytes are an order of magnitude more resistant. In view of the length of normal spermatogenesis there is a delay of some weeks between irradiation and fall in sperm counts. Single doses <50 cGy do not produce aspermia in normal men, although sperm counts are drastically reduced. At approximately 50 cGy aspermia is observed in some men and is universal after doses ≥100 cGy. The time to reach minimal sperm counts is inversely related to dose, with a minimal time of 10 weeks at high doses. After doses in the range 7.5 to 600 cGy, all normal men eventually recover spermatogenesis and achieve sperm counts equivalent to baseline. The time to spermatogenic recovery is directly related to dose and recovery after ≥200 cGy may take longer than 5 years. It is interesting that spermatogonial recovery antecedes sperm count recovery by many weeks or months. These studies also showed that serum testosterone levels did not change significantly after irradition, but that serum FSH levels did rise and mirrored the depression in sperm count.

Data on the effects of fractionated radiation on human spermatogenesis are confined to reports on men receiving scattered testicular radiation incidental to radiotherapy for testicular tumors, Hogkin's disease or soft tissue sarcomas. Table 8.7 summarizes the effects of scattered radiation to the testis over 15–30 fractions. It should be noted that men with severe preirradiation oligospermia ($<10^6$ sperm ml^{-1} may become aspermic after doses as low as 30 cGy (Sandeman, 1966). The relationship between total dose and the incidence of aspermia seems little different when comparing single with fractionated radiation and the time to aspermia is also approximately the same. However, recovery of sperm counts appears to take longer in these patients than in the normal volunteers. Whether this difference reflects a difference in the response of germinal epithelium to fractionated irradiation, or whether the original defect in spermatogenesis in these patients is a factor, cannot be decided. Similar to the findings for single doses, fractionated radiation has been shown to cause elevation of serum FSH and to have no significant effect on serum testosterone (Shapiro *et al.*, 1985; Fosså *et al.*, 1986).

Table 8.7 presents a range of doses from 15 to 400 cGy. During postorchidectomy radiation of seminoma the contralateral testicle receives doses at the lower end of this spectrum. The actual testicular dose delivered will depend on the tumor dose, on the energy of radiation, on whether the scrotum is irradiated and on the type of testicular shielding employed (Harter *et al.*, 1976; Kubo and Shipley, 1982). At MDACC thermoluminescent dosimetry was performed on 29 patients with seminoma irradiated according to the technique outlined earlier. For 16 patients whose hemiscrotum was not irradiated total testicular dose ranged from 18 to 66 cGy, with a mean of 36 cGy and a median of 34 cGy. For 13 patients who received hemiscrotal irradiation using the shield described by Harter *et al.* (1976), total testicular dose ranged from 33 to 126 cGy, with a mean of 65 cGy and a median of 60 cGy. The latter doses were statistically significantly higher than those delivered without hemiscrotal radiation. These testicular doses are within the 30–120 cGy range reported by others for patients with seminoma (Hahn *et al.*, 1982; Schlappack *et al.*, 1988). Thus, the patient with Stage I seminoma receiving postorchidectomy irradiation will experience temporary oligospermia or aspermia but can expect recovery of his sperm count by 18 months after treatment. The patient must be warned not to rely on irradiation as a contraceptive since there are several reports of conception during the first year, even within the first 3 months, after radiotherapy (Sandeman, 1966; Smithers, Wallace and Austin, 1973).

There are numerous reports of successful paternity after irradiation (Smithers, Wallace and Austin, 1973; Fosså *et al.*, 1986; Schover,

Gonzales and von Eschenback, 1986; Fried *et al.*, 1987), but the incidence of infertility has not been accurately determined. Two surveys (Berthelsen, 1987; Fosså, Aass and Kaalhus, 1989b) indicated that approximately two-thirds of men wishing to father children were able to do so. Fortunately, despite the induction of chromosomal abnormalities in human sperm by radiation (Martin *et al.*, 1986), there has been no evidence of an increased incidence of genetic handicaps among offspring of men irradiated for seminoma (Sandeman, 1966; Smithers, Wallace and Austin, 1973; Fried *et al.*, 1987). It is customary to counsel patients against conception for at least 1 year after irradiation to allow for loss of possibly mutated gametes.

8.6.4 SECOND MALIGNANT TUMORS

In considering second malignant tumors a distinction has to be made between subsequent testicular tumors that reflect a tumor diathesis, and subsequent nontesticular tumors, some of which may result from radiation. Table 8.8 summarizes the crude incidence of second testicular tumors reported in seven recent radiotherapy series. The average incidence is approximately 3%. However, the incidence percentages quoted are

Table 8.8 Incidence of second malignant testicular tumors following postorchidectomy radiotherapy for seminoma

Series	*Total number of seminoma patients*	*Number of second testicular tumors (%)*	*Time interval between seminoma and second tumor (years)*
Jackson *et al.* (1980)	334	8 (2.4)	2–18
Dosoretz *et al.* (1981)	171	4 (2.3)	6–18
Hamilton *et al.* (1986)	232	12 (5.2)	0–6
Duncan and Munro (1987)	152	4 (2.6)	NA
Babaian and Zagars (1988)	240	3 (1.3)	2–15
Ellerbroek, Tran and Selch (1988)	103	6 (5.8)	2–18
Fosså, Aass and Kaalhus (1989a)	365	6 (1.6)	NA
Total	1597	43* (2.7)	

* Approximately 50% are seminomas.
NA, not available.

only approximate estimates of risk since the duration of patient follow-up in these series was variable. The relatively long period at risk is noteworthy. The predisposition of a patient with one testicular tumor to develop a subsequent one in the contralateral testis is well documented. The clearest evidence that these second testicular tumors are a manifestation of an underlying diathesis rather than iatrogenic is the finding of carcinoma *in situ* in the contralateral testis in approximately 5% of patients with unilateral germ cell tumors prior to any postorchidectomy treatment (von der Maase *et al.*, 1986; Reinberg, Manivel and Fraley, 1989).

Although the carcinogenic potential of radiation is well documented, radiation delivered in therapeutic doses does not dramatically increase the risk of developing a second malignant tumor. One study of 232 patients with Stage I seminoma treated with post-orchidectomy irradiation and followed for up to 20 years reported five second nontesticular malignancies compared with an expected number of 5.2 based on age-standardized incidence rates (Hamilton *et al.*, 1986). Another study addressing the incidence of leukemia following treatment of germ cell tumors found that radiation alone was not associated with a significantly increased risk of leukemia (Redman *et al.*, 1984). Similarly, another study on radiotherapy for seminoma failed to find any case of leukemia among 362 patients receiving radiotherapy (Jackson *et al.*, 1980). However, Hay, Duncan and Kerr (1984) did find a significantly enhanced risk for second solid tumors in 547 patients with testicular tumors treated with radiation and followed for an average of 15.4 years. Excluding contra-lateral testicular tumors, the major enhanced risk for solid tumors appeared at 15–19 years after treatment and the observed-to-expected ratio for this period was 2.90. In this study, although the risk of developing a second cancer was significantly greater than expected, the excess risk was still low. No increase in incidence of leukemia was noted.

In summary, the available data indicate that postorchidectomy irradiation does not significantly increase the risk of leukemia, but that some increase in solid tumors may occur at times beyond 15 years after irradiation. The absolute risk seems small but additional studies are warranted.

8.7 CONCLUSIONS

The routine management of patients with Stage I testicular seminoma consists of orchidectomy followed by para-aortic and ipsilateral hemipelvic radiotherapy to a dose of 25 Gy in 3 weeks. The work-up of a patient with Stage I disease who is to receive radiotherapy, when based on an understanding of this disease and its outcome, is simple, relatively devoid of expensive medical technology and capable of accurately identifying that 75% of all seminoma patients who will have better than 95% chances for cure. In essence the work-up consists of a history, physical examination, pathological review of the orchidectomy specimen, a CT scan of the abdomen and pelvis, a chest X-ray, serum AFP and BHCG estimations, and routine blood counts and chemistries.

A variety of techniques is available for adequate irradiation. Common to all techniques is a tumor volume that encompasses the lumbar nodes from the eleventh thoracic vertebra downward and along the ipsilateral pelvic nodal groups. The text describes a simple technique used at MDACC for 30 years which has effectively controlled all para-aortic disease. The radiotherapist should be aware of circumstances that require modifications to standard treatment fields to encompass the ipsilateral hemiscrotum and inguinal regions. Prior ipsilateral inguinal surgery is an indication to include the ipsilateral inguinal nodes in the radiation volume. Tumor extension through the tunica albuginea, prior trans-scrotal surgery or current trans-scrotal orchidectomy are indications for hemiscrotal and inguinal treatment. The minimal effective radiation dose for subclinical seminoma has not been defined but extensive experience proves that 25 Gy in 15 fractions (1.67 Gy per fraction) over 3 weeks will control subclinical disease in all patients and higher doses are unnecessary.

The follow-up evaluation of treated patients is simple. Patients should be seen at 6-monthly intervals for 3 years, and yearly thereafter, with a history, physical examination and chest X-ray as the only essential requirements. Routine blood work is usually also performed. Only those patients whose BHCG was elevated at some time need to have this repeated. After the fifth year relapse is exceedingly rare and further follow-up is required only to monitor the contralateral testis and document any unlikely long-term problems such as second malignancies.

The results for patients managed as above are outstanding. Fewer than 5% will ever relapse and those who do fail will mostly be rescued with platinum-based chemotherapy. Mortality from seminoma is expected in fewer than 1% of patients.

Morbidity of radiotherapy is low and a significant incidence of delayed complications does not occur. There may be a low risk (approximately 5%) for peptic ulcer disease, which argues for the lowest radiation dose compatible with cure. Scattered radiation to the contralateral testicle is expected to produce temporary oligospermia or aspermia, but sperm counts recover within 2 years. Approximately two-thirds of men desiring to have children will succeed in this. In view of the known association between infertility and testicular tumor development, it is likely that radiation contributes relatively little to subsequent infertility. There is sufficient evidence that radiation for seminoma does not increase the risk of leukemia. The evidence in relation to solid tumor induction by radiotherapy for seminoma is conflicting. If there is an enhanced risk it is small and delayed for at least 15 years.

REFERENCES

Babaian, R.J. and Zagars, G.K. (1988) Testicular seminoma: the M.D. Anderson experience. An analysis of pathological and patient characteristics and treatment recommendations. *J. Urol.*, **139**, 311–14.

Batata, M.A., Whitmore, W.F., Chu, F.C.H. *et al.* (1980) Cryptorchidism and testicular cancer. *J. Urol.*, **124**, 382–7.

Bayens, Y.C., Helle, P.A., Van Putten, W.L. and Mali, S.P. (1992) Orchidectomy followed by radiotherapy in 176 stage I and II testicular seminoma patients: Benefits of a 10-year follow-up study. *Radiother. Oncol.*, **25**(2), 97–102.

Berthelsen, J.G. (1987) Testicular cancer and fertility. *Int. J. Androl.*, **10**, 371–80.

Berthelsen, J.G. and Skakkebæk, N.E. (1983) Gonadal function in men with testis cancer. *Fertil. Steril.*, **39**, 68–75.

Boden, G. and Gibb, R. (1951) Radiotherapy and testicular neoplasms. *Lancet*, **ii**, 1195–7.

Busch, F.M. and Sayegh, E.S. (1963) Roentgenographic visualization of human testicular lymphatics: a preliminary report. *J. Urol.*, **89**, 106–10.

Busch, F.M. and Sayegh, E.S. (1965) Some uses of lymphangiography in the management of testicular tumors. *J. Urol.*, **93**, 490–5.

Butcher, D.N., Gregory, W.M., Gunter, P.A. *et al.* (1985) The biological and clinical significance of HCG-containing cells in seminoma. *Br. J. Cancer*, **51**, 473–8.

Catalona, W.J., Vaitukaitis, J.L. and Fair, W.R. (1979) Falsely positive specific human chorionic gonadotropin assays in patients with testicular tumors: conversion to negative with testosterone administration. *J. Urol.*, **122**, 126–8.

Chapman R.M., Sutcliffe, S.B. and Malpas, J.S. (1981) Male gonadal dysfunction in Hodgkin's disease. *JAMA*, **245**, 1323–8.

Chiappa, S., Uslenghi, C., Galli, G. *et al.* (1966) Lymphangiography and endolymphatic radiotherapy in testicular tumors. *Br. J. Radiol.*, **39**, 498–512.

Clayman, C.B., Palmer, W.L. and Kirsner, J.B. (1968) Gastric irradiation in the treatment of peptic ulcer. *Gastroenterology*, **55**, 403–7.

Clifton, D.K. and Bremner, W.J. (1983) The effect of testicular x-irradiation on spermatogenesis in man. A comparison with the mouse. *J. Androl.*, **4**, 387–92.

Coia, L.R. and Hanks, G.E. (1988) Complications from large field intermediate dose infradiaphragmatic radiation: an analysis of the patterns of care outcome studies for Hodgkin's disease and seminoma. *Int. J. Radiat. Oncol. Biol. Phys.*, **15**, 29–35.

Cox, J.D. (1989) The testicle, in *Radiation Oncology Rationale, Technique, Results*, (eds W.T. Moss and J.D. Cox), C.V. Mosby, St. Louis, pp. 468–76.

Danjoux, C.E., Rider, W.D. and Fitzpatrick, P.J. (1979) The acute radiation syndrome. *Clin. Radiol.*, **30**, 581–4.

Dean, A.L. 1929 The treatment of teratoid tumors of the testis with radium and the Roentgen ray. *J. Urol.*, **21**, 83–91.

Desjardins, A.U., Squire, F.H. and Morton, S.A. (1929) Radiotherapy for tumors of the testis. *Am. J. Roentgenol.*, **22**, 137–46.

Dobbs, J. and Barrett, A. (1985) *Practical Radiotherapy Planning. Royal Marsden Hospital Practice* Edward Arnold, London, pp. 192–8.

Donohue, J.P. (1984) Metastatic pathways of non-seminomatous germ cell tumors. *Sem. Urol.*, **11**, 217–19.

Dosoretz, D.E., Shipley, W.U., Blitzer, P.D. *et al.* (1981) Megavoltage irradiation of pure testicular seminoma: results and patterns of failure. *Cancer*, **48**, 2184–90.

Duncan, W. and Munro, A.J. (1987) The management of testicular seminoma: Edinburgh 1970–1981. *Br. J. Cancer*, **55**, 443–8.

Dunnick, N.R. and Javadpour, N. (1981) Value of CT and lymphangiography: distinguishing retroperitoneal metastases from nonseminomatous testicular tumors. *Am. J. Roentgenol.*, **136**, 1093–9.

Ehrlichman, R.J., Kaufman, S.L., Siegelman, S.S. (1981) Computerized tomography and lymphangiography in staging testis tumors. *J. Urol.*, **126**, 179–81.

Ellerbroek, N.A., Tran, L.M., Selch, M.T. (1988) Testicular seminoma: a study of 103 cases treated at UCLA. *Am. J. Clin. Oncol.*, **11**, 93–9.

Fosså, S.D., Aass, N. and Kaalhus, O. (1989a) Radiotherapy for testicular seminoma stage I: treatment results and long-term post-irradiation morbidity in 365 patients. *Int. J. Radiat. Oncol. Biol. Phys.*, **16**, 383–8.

Fosså, S.D., Aass, N. and Kaalhus, O. (1989b) Long-term morbidity after infradiaphragmatic radiotherapy in young men with testicular cancer. *Cancer*, **64**, 404–8.

Fosså, S.D., Abyholm, T. and Aakvaag, A. (1984) Spermatogenesis and hormonal status after orchidectomy for cancer and before supplementary treatment. *Eur. Urol.*, **10**, 173–7.

Fosså, S.D., Abyholm, T., Normann, N. and Jetne, V. (1986) Post-treatment fertility in patients with testicular cancer. III. Influence of radiotherapy in seminoma patients. *Br. J. Urol.*, **58**, 315–19.

Fosså, S.D., Borge, L., Aass, N. *et al.* (1987) The treatment of advanced metastatic seminoma: experience in 55 cases. *J. Clin. Oncol.*, **5**, 10771–7.

Fosså, A. and Fosså, S.D. (1989) Serum lactate dehydrogenase and human choriogonadotrophin in seminoma. *Br. J. Urol.*, **63**, 408–15.

Fosså, S.D., Horwich, A., Russel, J.M., Roberts, J.P., Jakes, R., MRC Testicular Working Party (1995) Optimal field size in adjuvant treatment of stage I seminoma. *Eur. J. Cancer*, **31A**, Supplement 5, p.S188, Abst no. 902.

Freund, I., Zenzes, M.T., Muller, R-P. *et al.* (1987) Testicular function in eight patients with seminoma after unilateral orchidectomy and radiotherapy. *Int. J. Androl.*, **10**, 447–55.

Fried, P., Steinfeld, R., Casileth, B. and Steinfeld, A. (1987) Incidence of developmental handicaps among the offspring of men treated for testicular seminoma. *Int. J. Androl.*, **10**, 385–7.

Giacchetti, S., Raoul, Y., Wibault, P. *et al.* (1993) Treatment of stage I testis seminoma by radiotherapy: Long-term results – a 30-year experience. *Int. J. Radiat. Oncol. Biol. Phys.*, **27**(1), 3–9.

Gibb, R. and Read, G. (1985) Testis, in *The Radiotherapy of Malignant Disease* (eds E.C. Easson and R.C.S. Pointon), Springer-Verlag, Berlin, pp. 331–5.

Hahn, E.W., Feingold, B.S., Simpson, L. and Batata, M. (1982) Recovery from aspermia induced by low-dose radiation in seminoma patients. *Cancer*, **50**, 337–40.

Hamilton, C., Horwich, A., Bliss, J.M. and Peckham, M.J. (1987) Gastrointestinal morbidity of adjuvant radiotherapy in stage I malignant teratoma of the testis. *Radiother. Oncol.*, **10**, 85–90.

Hamilton, C., Horwich, A., Easton, D. and Peckham, M.J. (1986) Radiotherapy for stage I seminoma testis: results of treatment and complications. *Radiother. Oncol.*, **6**, 115–20.

Hanks, G.E., Herring, D.F. and Kramer, S. (1981) Patterns of care outcome studies: results of the national practice in seminoma of the testis. *Int. J. Radiat. Oncol. Biol. Phys.*, **7**, 1413–17.

Hansen, P.V., Trykker, H., Andersen, J. and Helkjaer, P.E. (1989) Germ cell function and hormonal status in patients with testicular seminoma. *Cancer*, **64**, 1956–61.

Harter, D.J., Hussey, D.H., Delclos, L. *et al.* (1976) Device to position and shield the testicle during irradiation. *Int. J. Radiat. Oncol. Biol. Phys.*, **1**, 361–4.

Hay, J.H., Duncan, W. and Kerr, G.R. (1984) Subsequent malignancies in patients irradiated for testicular tumors. *Br. J. Radiol.*, **57**, 597–602.

Heiken, J.P., Balfe, D.M. and McClennan, B.L. (1984) Testicular tumors: oncologic imaging and diagnosis. *Int. J. Radiat. Oncol. Biol. Phys.*, **10**, 275–7.

Hendry, W.F., Stedronska, J., Jones, C.R. *et al.* (1983) Semen analysis in testicular cancer and Hodgkin's disease: pre- and post-treatment findings and implications for cryopreservation. *Br. J. Urol.*, **55**, 769–73.

Herr, H.W., Silber, I. and Martin, D.C. (1973) Management of inguinal lymph nodes in patients with testicular tumors following orchidopexy, inguinal or scrotal operations. *J. Urol.*, **110**, 223–4.

Horwich, A., Dearnaley, D.P., Duchesne, G.M. *et al.* (1989) Simple nontoxic treatment of advanced metastatic seminoma with carboplatin. *J. Clin. Oncol.*, **7**, 1150–6.

Huben, R.P., Williams, P.D., Pontes, E. *et al.* (1984) Seminoma at Roswell Park, 1970 to 1979. An analysis of treatment failures. *Cancer*, **53**, 1451–5.

Hussey, D.H. (1980) Testis, in *Textbook of Radiotherapy*, 3rd edn, (ed. G.H. Fletcher), Lea and Febiger, Philadelphia, pp. 867–76.

Jackson, S.M., Olivotto, I., McLoughlin, M.G. and Coy, P. (1980) Radiation therapy for seminoma of the testis: results in British Columbia. *Can. Med. Associ. J.*, **123**, 507–12.

Javadpour, N., McIntyre, K.P., Waldman, T.A. and Bergman, S.M. (1978) The role of alpha-fetoprotein and human chorionic gonadotropin in seminoma. *J. Urol.*, **120**, 687–90.

Jonsson, K., Wallace, S., Jing, B.S. *et al.* (1978) Lymphangiography in patients with malignancy in a non-descended testicle. *J. Urol.*, **119**, 614–17.

Kinsella, T.J., Trivette, G., Rowland, J. *et al.* (1989) Long-term follow-up of testicular function following radiation therapy for early-stage Hodgkin's disease. *J. Clin. Oncol.*, **7**, 718–24.

Klein, F.A., Whitmore, W.F., Sogani, P.C. *et al.* (1984) Inguinal node metastases from germ cell testicular tumors, *J. Urol.*, **131**, 497–500.

Kubo, H. and Shipley, W.U. (1982) Reduction of the scattered dose to the testicle outside the radiation treatment fields. *Int. J. Radiat. Oncol. Biol. Phys.*, **8**, 1741–5.

Lai, P.P., Bernstein, M.J., Kim, H. *et al.* (1994) Radiation therapy for stage I and IIA testicular seminoma. *Int. J. Radiat. Oncol. Biol. Phys.*, **28**(2), 373–9.

Lange, P.H., Nochomovitz, L.E., Rosai, J. *et al.* (1980) Serum alpha-fetoprotein and human chorionic gonadotrophin in patients with seminoma. *J. Urol.*, **124**, 472–8.

Lederman, G.S., Herman, T.S., Jochelson, M. *et al.* (1989) Radiation therapy of seminoma: 17-year experience at the Joint Center for Radiation Therapy. *Radiother. Oncol.*, **14**, 203–8.

Lester, S.G., Morphis, J.G. and Hornback, N.B. (1986) Testicular seminoma: analysis of treatment results and failures. *Int. J. Radiat. Oncol. Biol. Phys.*, **12**, 353–8.

Logothetis, C.J., Samuels, M.L., Ogden, S.L. *et al.* (1987) Cyclophosphamide and sequential cisplatin for advanced seminoma: long-term follow-up in 52 patients. *J. Urol.*, **138**, 789–94.

von der Maase, H., Rørth, M., Walbom-Jorgensen, S. *et al.* (1986) Carcinoma *in situ* of contralateral testis in patients with testicular germ cell cancer: study of 27 cases in 500 patients. *BMJ*, **293**, 1398–401.

Martin, R.H., Hildebrand, K., Yamamoto, J. *et al.* (1986) An increased frequency of human sperm chromosomal abnormalities after radiotherapy. *Muta. Res.*, **174**, 219–25.

Mauch, P., Weichselbaum, R. and Botnick, L. (1979) The significance of positive chorionic gonadotropins in apparently pure seminoma of the testis. *Int. J. Radiat. Oncol. Biol. Phys.*, **5**, 887–9.

Mirimanoff, R.O., Shipley, W.U., Dosoretz, D.E. and Meyer, J.E. (1985) Pure seminoma of the testis: the results of radiation therapy in patients with elevated human chorionic gonadotropin titers. *J. Urol.*, **134**, 1124–6.

Morgan, D.A.L., Cailland, J.M., Bellet, D. and Eschwege, F. (1982) Gonadotrophin-producing seminoma: a distinct category of germ cell neoplasm. *Clin. Radiol.*, **33**, 149–53.

Nørgaard-Pedersen, B., Schultz, H.P., Arends, J. *et al.* (1984) Tumour markers in testicular germ cell tumours. Five-year experience from the DATECA study 1976–1980. *Acta Radiol. Oncol.*, **23**, 287–94.

Ozen, H., Altug, N., Bakkaloglu, M.A. and Remzi, D. (1988) Significance of scrotal violation in the prognosis of patients with testicular tumors. *Br. J. Urol.*, **62**, 267–70.

Peckham, M.J., Hamilton, C.R., Horwich, A. and Hendry, W.F. (1987) Surveillance after orchidectomy for stage I seminoma of the testis. *Br. J. Urol.*, **59**, 343–7.

Pritchett, T.R., Skinner, D.G., Selser, S.F. and Kern, W.H. (1985) Seminoma with elevated human chorionic gonadotropin. The case for retroperitoneal lymph node dissection. *Urology*, **25**, 344–6.

Pryor, J.P., Cameron, K.M., Chilton, C.P. *et al.* (1983) Carcinoma *in situ* in testicular biopsies from men presenting with infertility. *Br. J. Urol.*, **55**, 780–4.

Ray, B., Hajdu, S.I. and Whitmore, W.F. (1974) Distribution of retroperitoneal lymph node metastases in testicular germinal tumors. *Cancer*, **33**, 340–8.

Read, G. and Johnston, R.J. (1993) Short duration radiotherapy in stage I seminoma of the testis: Preliminary results of a prospective study. *Clin. Oncol. R. Coll. Radiol*, **5**(6), 364–6.

Redman, J.R., Vugrin, D., Arlin, Z.A. *et al.* (1984) Leukemia following treatment of germ cell tumors in men. *J. Clin. Oncol.*, **2**, 1080–7.

Reed, E., Sander, W.G. and Armitage, J.O. (1986) Results of semen cryopreservation in young men with testicular cancer and lymphoma. *J. Clin. Oncol.*, **4**, 537–9.

Reinberg, Y., Manivel, J.C. and Fraley, E.E. (1989) Carcinoma *in situ* of the testis. *J. Urol.*, **142**, 243–7.

Rouvière, H. (1938) *Anatomy of the Human Lymphatic System*, Edwards Brothers, Ann Arbor, Michigan, pp. 221–3.

Rowley, M.J., Leach, D.R., Warner, G.A. and Heller, C.G. (1974) Effect of graded doses of ionizing radiation on the human testis. *Radiat. Res.*, **59**, 685–8.

Sandeman, T.F. (1966) The effects of x-irradiation on male human fertility. *Br. J. Radiol.*, **39**, 901–7.

Sandeman, T.F. and Matthews, J.P. (1979) The staging of testicular tumors. *Cancer*, **43**, 2514–24.

Sause, W.T. (1983) Testicular seminoma – analysis of radiation therapy for stage II disease. *J. Urol.*, **130**, 702–3.

Schlappack, O.K., Kratzik, C., Schmidt, W. *et al.* (1988) Response of the seminiferous epithelium to scattered radiation in seminoma patients. *Cancer*, **62**, 1487–91.

Schover, L.R., Gonzales, M. and von Eschenbach, A.C. (1986) Sexual and marital relationships after radiotherapy for seminoma. *Urology*, **27**, 117–23.

Schultz, H.P., von der Maase, A., Rørth, M. *et al.* (1984) Testicular seminoma in Denmark 1976–1980. *Acta Radiol. Oncol.*, **23**, 263–70.

Shapiro, E., Kinsella, T.J., Makuch, R.W. *et al.* (1985) Effects of fractionated irradiation on endocrine aspects of testicular function. *J. Clin. Oncol.*, **3**, 1232–9.

Smithers, D.W., Wallace, D.M. and Austin, D.E. (1973) Fertility after unilateral orchidectomy and radiotherapy for patients with malignant tumours of the testis. *BMJ*, **4**, 77–9.

Speiser, B., Rubin, P. and Casarett, G. (1973) Aspermia following lower truncal irradiation in Hodgkin's disease. *Cancer*, **32**, 692–8.

Swartz, D.A., Johnson, D.E. and Hussey, D.H. (1984) Should an elevated human chorionic gonadotropin titer alter therapy for seminoma? *J. Urol.*, **131**, 63–5.

Thomas, G.M. (1985) Controversies in the management of testicular seminoma. *Cancer*, **55**, 2296–302.

Thomas, G.M., Rider, W.D., Dembo, A.J. *et al.* (1982) Seminoma of the testis: results of treatment and patterns of failure after radiation therapy. *Int. J. Radiat. Oncol. Biol. Phys.*, **8**, 165–74.

Thomas, G.M., Sturgeon, J.F., Alison, R. *et al.* (1989) A study of post-orchidectomy surveillance in stage I testicular seminoma. *J. Urol.*, **142**, 243–7.

Vaeth, M., Schultz, H.P., von der Maase, H. *et al.* (1984). Prognostic factors in testicular germ cell tumours. *Acta Radiol. Oncol.* **23**, 271–5.

Wallace, S. and Jing, B-S. (1970) Lymphangiography: Diagnosis of nodal metastases from testicular malignancies. *JAMA*, **213**, 94–6.

White, R.L. and Maier, J.G. (1984) Treatment techniques of testis tumors, in *Technological Basis of Radiation Therapy: Practical Clinical Applications*, Lea and Febiger, Philadelphia, pp. 271–7

White, R.L. and Maier, J.G. (1987) Testis tumors, in *Principles and Practice of Radiation Oncology*, (eds C.A. Perez and L.W. Brady), J.B. Lippincott, Philadelphia, pp. 899–911.

Willan, B.D. and McGowan, D.G. (1985) Seminoma of the testis: a 22-year experience with radiation therapy. *Int. J. Radiat. Oncol. Biol. Phys.*, **11**, 1769–75.

Ytredal, D.O. and Bradfield, J.S. (1972) Seminoma of the testicle: prophylactic mediastinal irradiation versus periaortic and pelvic irradiation alone. *Cancer*, **30**, 628–33.

Zagars, G.K. and Babaian, R.J. (1987) Stage I testicular seminoma: rationale for postorchidectomy radiation therapy. *Int. J. Radiat. Oncol. Biol. Phys.*, **13**, 155–62.

A. Horwich

9.1 INTRODUCTION

The conventional management of Stage I seminoma of the testis is by adjuvant retro-peritoneal node irradiation, as fully described in Chapter 8. This policy is highly successful and it is unlikely that any alternative management policies would reduce the recurrence rate further. At the same time it seems likely that a substantial proportion of patients were cured by their orchidectomy and a valid question is whether overall treatment morbidity may be less with a policy of close surveillance, reserving treatment only for those few who relapse.

The side-effects of adjuvant radiotherapy are not severe because of the low doses of radiotherapy required in this context. Many patients suffer mild nausea during the course of their treatment although this is usually for only 1 to 2 hours per treatment day and is rarely associated with vomiting. Of more concern is the possibility of later radiation damage leading to peptic ulceration (Hamilton et al., 1986; Hamilton, et al., 1987; Coia and Hanks, 1988). The impact of radiation on the incidence of ulceration has been assessed in Stage I testicular cancer by comparison of an irradiated group and a surveillance group (Table 9.1) This complication would appear to affect about 5% of patients and is mainly seen within the first year after radiotherapy and in those with a prior history of abdominal surgery or peptic ulceration.

A second issue is whether adjuvant radio-therapy might lead to second malignancies. Though there is extensive literature reporting increased cancer risk following exposure to low doses of ionizing radiation, including children irradiated *in utero* (Bithell and Stewart, 1975) the survivors of atomic bombs (Bizzozero, Johnson and Ciocco, 1966) and those given therapeutic radiation for ankylos-

Table 9.1 Peptic ulceration after radiotherapy for Stage I testicular non-seminomatous germ cell tumors (8# = fractions)

		Peptic ulceration after radiotherapy for Stage I testicular NSGCT		
Date	*No. of patients*	*Treatment*	*Ulcers within 2 years of orchidex*	
<1979	142	Adjuvant RT 40 Gy, 20#, 4 wks	7	$p = 0.05$
>1979	106	Surveillance	0	

Data from Hamilton *et al.* (1987).

Testicular Cancer: Investigation and management. Second edition. Edited by Professor A. Horwich. Published in 1996 by Chapman & Hall. ISBN 0 412 61210 0.

ing spondylitis (Court Brown and Doll, 1957; Smith and Doll, 1982), the risks following high dose radiotherapy are less evident (Kapp, *et al.*, 1982; Lee, *et al.*, 1982). Hay, Duncan and Kerr (1984) analyzed second cancer risk in 547 patients treated with radiotherapy for tumors of the testis between 1950 and 1969. The population base for this study was the case records of five Scottish radiotherapy centers. There were two cases of leukemia observed (expected 0.51 – not significant), but both were chronic lymphocytic leukemia. Within the high dose radiation volume there were 19 tumors observed (expected 9.81 $p<0.05$), but this relative risk was not higher than in nonirradiated areas. The in-field excess risk was confined to transitional cell carcinomas of the genitourinary tract and tumors of unknown primary located within the gastrointestinal tract. The peak time of the urinary and gastrointestinal tumors was in the period 15 to 19 years after irradiation.

More recently, cancer registry studies have been reported (Coleman, Bell and Fraser, 1987; Kaldor, *et al.*, 1987). The South Thames Cancer Registry study of 2013 patients with testicular cancer (not only seminoma) registered between 1961 and 1980 found a relative risk of second malignancy of 0.7 (90% confidence intervals 0.5 to 1.0, observed 27, expected 36). Two cases of acute leukemia were observed (expected 0.80). Kaldor, *et al.* (1987), reported risk of second cancers from collaborative studies among 11 population-based cancer registries that included 17 730 patients with testicular tumors registered between 1945 and 1984. Apart from tumors of the second testis there was an increased incidence of cancer of the rectum (29 observed versus 21 expected), of connective tissue tumors (7 observed versus 2.3 expected), of malignant melanomas (16 observed versus 8.9 expected), of non-Hodgkin's lymphomas (28 observed versus 10 expected) and of acute leukemia (9 observed versus 4.4 expected). If the first 10 years of follow-up was excluded an excess second cancer risk remained, pre-

dominantly cancer of the rectum. It should be emphasized that these studies were not confined to seminoma of the testis and the population-based studies were not restricted to patients treated with radiotherapy alone.

In considering radiotherapy for testicular seminoma the carcinogenic risk remains unclear. Fosså, Aass and Kaalhus (1989) reported long-term follow-up after radiotherapy in 365 patients treated with radiotherapy for Stage I seminoma; no cases of leukemia were observed and though there were in total 15 second non-germ cell cancers, the only subtype in excess was lung cancer, with four observed, 1.66 expected ($p = 0.05$). We also performed analysis of second cancers following radiotherapy for pure seminoma (Horwich and Bell, 1994). Of 859 patients treated between 1961 and 1985, 42 developed second cancers and there were 20 deaths from second cancer (expected 22.1 – non significant). The only subtype with significant excess was leukemia (four cases observed, 0.64 expected; relative risk 6.2, 95% confidence intervals 2.7–14.8). These were cases of acute undifferentiated or acute myeloid leukemia occurring 3–11 years after irradiation.

It is clear that certain types of chemotherapy, especially alkylating agents, are associated with secondary leukemia and that cyclophosphamide may lead to transitional cell carcinoma of the bladder (IARC, 1981). When risk estimates are based on reports from individual institutions of patients with Stage I seminoma treated entirely by infradiaphragmatic radiotherapy, the period of follow-up has usually included the time period 0–5 years when the peak incidence of secondary leukemia would be expected. Since reports of this are so rare it seems unlikely that leukemia is a consequence of radiotherapy in this context. However, these reports rarely contain significant follow-up for more than 15 years after radiotherapy and therefore the issue of whether second solid tumors may be induced remains open, although it does seem clear from population-based registries that the risk of solid tumor induction by adjuvant radiotherapy must be extremely small.

Conventional field arrangements associated with techniques of scrotal shielding reduce scattered irradiation of the contralateral testis to doses of the order of 0.5 Gy. This leads to temporary oligospermia but also to the possibility of genetic damage such that patients are counseled to avoid conception for 2 years. The majority of patients have recovered their pretreatment sperm count by 2 to 3 years after radiotherapy (Hahan, *et al.*, 1982; Fosså, *et al.*, 1986). However, impairment of spermatogenesis may be much more severe when the radiation field is more extensive and especially when part of the scrotum has been irradiated (Thomas *et al.*, 1977). The policy of surveillance for Stage I non-seminoma has been discussed extensively elsewhere in this volume (see Chapter 13). It has appeared from both single center (Hoskin, *et al.*, 1986) and multicenter (Freedman *et al.*, 1987) studies that this policy can be safely explored when a successful salvage treatment is available.

The background to surveillance in seminoma includes therefore the possibility of reducing toxicity, the desirability of documenting the number of patients with clinical Stage I seminoma who have subclinical metastases at presentation and the availability of highly successful treatments for overt metastatic disease.

9.2 THE SURVEILLANCE MANAGEMENT POLICY FOR STAGE I SEMINOMA

The management policy is influenced by the absence of a sensitive serum tumor marker and by the relatively slow natural history of the tumor. Thus surveillance need not be so intensive as with Stage I non-seminoma; however, it must be prolonged and include radiological assessments of abdominal lymph nodes up to at least 5 years from diagnosis. The Royal Marsden Hospital policy is illustrated in Fig. 9.1. It should be noted that

patients were staged both with a computed tomography (CT) scan of thorax and abdomen and with a lymphogram, the latter enabling both sensitive examination of the presentation pattern of abdominal lymph nodes and also the possibility of frequent radiological follow-up during the first year. Outpatient visits on surveillance were every 2 months for the first year following orchidectomy, and abdominal CT scanning is carried out once a year.

All patients who entered the Royal Marsden Hosital study had histological verification of pure seminoma on review, although it is recognized that combined tumors may occur and that the sections prepared for review might not reflect the full range of tumor heterogeneity. Patients with raised serum alpha-fetoprotein (AFP) prior to orchidectomy are excluded.

The intensity of surveillance represents a compromise between the desire to detect recurrence as sensitively as possible and the desire to minimize both hospital visits for the patients and the use of scarce or expensive resources such as CT scanning. It is anticipated that the method of surveillance will be modified once more experience of the policy has accumulated. In particular it may be more desirable to perform more frequent scans to reduce the risk of large volume abdominal node relapse or, alternatively, should a useful serum tumor marker be developed then radiological assessment may need to be performed much less frequently.

It has been proposed that serum placental alkaline phosphatase (PLAP) may be a useful tumor marker for seminoma (Lange *et al.*, 1982). A number of variants of this enzyme have been distinguished by monoclonal antibodies and thus a variety of assays are under investigation. The antibody H17E2, which had been raised against term placental membranes, appears to reflect the presence of metastatic seminoma reliably (Horwich, Tucker and Peckham, 1985). However, false positive results were obtained in subjects who smoked cigarettes, and even in patients with gross

Month	1	2	3	4	5	6	7	8	9	10	11	12	18	24	30	36
OPD	+		+		+		+		+		+	)				
Markers	+		+		+		+		+		+	)		Then as below		
CXR	+		+		+		+		+		+	)				
Abd.XR	+		+		+		+		+		+	)				
CT Scan											+			+		+
U/S Abd.													+		+	

Year 2	OPD q 2/12	U/S @ 18/12	CT @ 24/12
Year 3	OPD q 3/12	U/S @ 30/12	CT @ 36/12
Year 4	OPD q4/12		
Year 5	OPD q6/12		CT@60/12

Fig. 9.1 Logistics of the Royal Marsden Hospital stage 1 seminoma surveillance policy (1983–89). Abd. XR, abdominal X-ray; CT, computed tomography; U/S Abd., abdominal ultrasound; OPD, clinic visit; CXR, chest X-ray; q, every (q^3/12 = every 3 months).

metastatic disease the serum concentration of PLAP was close to the normal range. Our surveillance policy incorporates regular assays of serum HCG. This serum marker is less sensitive in assessment of seminoma than of non-seminomatous germ cell tumors. Patients with metastatic seminoma rarely have serum HCG concentrations of more than 50 units per liter and elevations are usually seen only in the presence of gross metastatic disease. The marker hardly qualifies therefore as a sensitive measure of relapse.

9.3 RESULTS OF SURVEILLANCE FOR STAGE I SEMINOMA

Surveillance for stage I seminoma has been explored in a limited number of centers. The major series are those from the Princess Margaret Hospital, Toronto (Warde *et al.*, 1993), the Danish National Study (von der Maase *et al.*, 1993) and the Royal Marsden

Hospital. Some variation in results between these centers would be expected, depending upon the staging investigations and the technique of monitoring.

The Royal Marsden Hospital (RMH) series is based on patients with Stage I seminoma registered between 1983 and 1988 (Peckham *et al.*, 1987; Duchesne *et al.*, 1990). One hundred and thirteen patients were registered and after a median follow-up period of 33 months the pattern of relapse is illustrated in Fig. 9.2, which is confined to the 103 patients who had institutional histology review. The probability of recurrence by 1 year was 6.2% (95% confidence intervals 4.5%), the probability of relapse by 2 years was 12.1% (95% confidence intervals 6.3%), and the probability of relapse by 3 years was 14.9% (95% confidence intervals 7.1%). This is in close accord with the Danish National Study (von der Maase *et al.*, 1993), which was based on

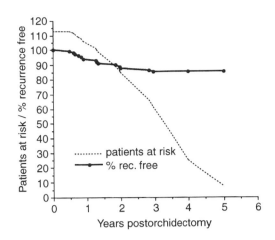

Fig. 9.2 Stage I seminoma surveillance: relapse-free survival in 113 patients. Data from the Royal Marsden Hospital, 1983–9.

261 patients registered between 1985 and 1988 with a median follow-up of 48 months. Forty-eight patients had relapsed and the median time to relapse was 12 months (2.5–38.5 months). At first a somewhat lower risk of recurrence was found in the Princess Margaret Hospital series (Thomas *et al.*, 1989). Of 81 patients followed for 3–43 months (median 19 months) only three had relapsed at 3, 5 and 18 months after orchidectomy. The Princess Margaret Hospital experience has now been extended to 140 patients on surveillance and the number of relapses has risen to 23 (Warde *et al.* 1993) as shown in Table 9.2

The sites of relapse in the three series are shown in Table 9.3. Patients were staged at relapse with a CT scan of the thorax and abdomen. Eight-five percent of recurrences were restricted to the para-aortic region. In two Royal Marsden Hospital cases the para-aortic recurrence was 6 cm in diameter and therefore was managed with chemotherapy (single agent carboplatin (Horwich *et al.*, 1989)) followed by para-aortic radiotherapy. Other Royal Marsden Hospital recurrences were with small volume para-aortic lymph-

adenopathy; however, one was managed with carboplatin chemotherapy because of prior radiotherapy for a previous testicular tumor. Twelve recurrences were treated with retroperitoneal node irradiation using a standard 'dog leg' technique to para-aortic and ipsilateral pelvic lymph nodes to a dose of 30 Gy in 15 to 17 fractions over 3 weeks followed by a para-aortic field boost to a further 5 Gy in three fractions. Four of these patients relapsed again. These second relapses were in mediastinal (three) or supraclavicular (one) nodes at 5, 6, 10 and 19 months after retroperitoneal node irradiation. All were managed with carboplatin chemotherapy and in three cases the site of relapse was treated with radiotherapy also. At present all patients are disease free and the cause-specific survival on the RMH study is 100%.

A similar pattern was seen in the Princess Margaret Hospital study with 20 of 21 recurrences being in retroperitoneal region alone and in the Danish series with 41 or 49 recurrences in para-aortic nodes.

In the three series a total of 68 patients suffered nodal relapse in the para-aortic area and were treated with radiotherapy alone and, as shown in Table 9.4, 11 of these (16%) suffered a further relapse out of the radiation field and, taken with the one patient in each series suffering an initial supradiaphragmatic relapse on surveillance, a total of 14 of the 512 Stage I patients managed by surveillance developed supradiaphragmatic disease.

It is of interest to question whether the delay in treating those patients who presented with Stage I seminoma, but had untreated subclinical metastases, led to a greater proportion of patients developing more widespread metastases; however, there is no evidence from this analysis of surveillance that this proportion (14 of 512 = 2.7%) is greater than the supradiaphragmatic relapse pattern observed in series of Stage I seminoma treated initially with adjuvant radiotherapy (Chapter 8).

Table 9.2   Relapse in Stage I seminoma patients

Institute	Series	N	Period	Median FU (months)	Relapse	4–5 yr % RFS
RMH	Horwich *et al.*, 1992	103	83–88	62	17	82
PMH	Warde *et al.*, 1993	148	84–91	47	23	81
Denmark	von der Maase *et al.*, 1993	261	85–88	48	49	80

Table 9.3   Initial relapse sites in Stage I seminoma patients on surveillance

Institute*	N	R	PA nodes	Pelvic/inguinal nodes	Supradiag nodes	Lung	Only PA nodes
RMH	103	17	17	1		1	15
PMH	148	23	21	3	1		20
Denmark	261	49	41	7		1	41
Total	512	89	79	11	1	2	76

- 85% of relapses were in PA nodes alone.
* See Table 9.2.
N = Patients survived. R = Patients relapsing. PA = Para-aortic.

Table 9.4   Relapses from treatment with radiotherapy alone

Series	RMH	PMH	Denmark	Total
Node relapse treated with radiotherapy alone	12	19	37	68
Further relapse	4	3	4	11 (16%)
Initial supradiaphragmatic relapse	1	1	1	3

- 14 of 512 (2.7%) Stage I patients developed supradiphragmatic disease.

9.3.1   PROGNOSTIC FACTORS ANALYSIS

Clearly it would be useful if a subgroup at high risk of recurrence could be selected for adjuvant treatment. All three series have performed prognostic factor analyses. The Royal Marsden Hospital analysis (Horwich *et al.*, 1992) was confined to histopathological factors since these were so helpful in identifying recurrent risk in non-seminoma. A higher risk of relapse was found in those with lymphatic and vascular invasion within the primary tumor. The Princess Margaret series found that the most significant factor predicting relapse was age at diagnosis (Warde *et al.*, 1993). In those aged 34 years or less the 5-year relapse-free survival was 70%, compared with 91% in those aged more than 34 years.

The Danish series found that the diameter of the primary tumor was the most significant predictor of relapse (von der Maase *et al.*, 1993). In 68 patients whose primary tumor diameter was less than 3 cm the 4-year relapse-free survival was 94%. In 124 patients whose primary tumor diameters were between 3 and 6 cm the 4-year relapse-free survival was 82%, and in the 67 patients whose primary tumor diameters were >6cm the 4-year relapse-free survival was only 64%. It seems likely that the younger patient with large primary tumor and demonstrated vascular invasion in the primary should be considered at high risk, but more accurate quantitation of relative risk of these quantitation factors should emerge from a combined analysis of the series.

Table 9.5 Surveillance postorchidectomy for Stage I seminoma patients

Advantages	*Disadvantages*
80–85% require no treatment	Radiotherapy associated with only 2% relapse rate
Avoid acute and late side-effects of radiotherapy	Very low dose radiotherapy is effective (25–30 Gy)
Fertility	
GI tract	
? 2nd tumor	
	Surveillance difficult (markers negative, abdominal nodes hard to palpate) and stressful in some
Relapse can be treated successfully	
	Relapse may be late
	2nd relapse may be a consequence of delay in treating abdominal nodes
	Patients may abscond from follow-up

9.4 CONCLUSIONS

Studies over the last 6 years have suggested that surveillance may be an alternative to adjuvant retroperitoneal irradiation in the management of stage I seminoma following orchidectomy. This innovation must be judged with extreme caution since a wealth of experience with radiotherapy would suggest this policy is safe, effective and nontoxic. Nevertheless it is unsatisfactory to employ adjuvant radiotherapy in a setting where the proportion of patients who benefit has not been established and a major contribution of the surveillance policies has been to elucidate the natural history of Stage I seminoma. Where radiotherapy is contraindicated it is established that surveillance offers a safe alternative; however, a number of possible disadvantages of surveillance may be considered (Table 9.5). The practice is difficult and labor intensive for the physician. It would be rendered considerably more facile if a sensitive serum marker were available. Surveillance may also be extremely stressful for the patient, and the slow natural history of seminoma requires monitoring of the possibility of recurrence to at least 5 years following orchidectomy and thus stress may be quite prolonged.

A further possible disadvantage of surveillance might be that delay in treating retro-peritoneal node metastases could lead to further dissemination of the disease. This concern was raised particularly by the Royal Marsden Hospital study in which four of 11 patients treated with radiotherapy for retroperitoneal recurrence subsequently had supradiaphragmatic nodal recurrence. This contrasts with five of 232 recurrences in patients treated initially with adjuvant radio-therapy (Hamilton *et al.*, 1987). The difference is not significant, and the larger number of patients in the Danish National Study has reduced concern over secondary metastases from untreated retroperitoneal nodes.

A further problem in surveillance is the patient who fails to attend for follow-up appointments. When this possibility can be identified prospectively surveillance would be contraindicated. Of the 17 patients who recurred in the Royal Marsden Hospital series, one was a persistent nonattender and his recurrence was with large volume para-aortic lymphadenopathy (6 cm in diameter). He required treatment with chemotherapy.

In comparing the policy of routine adjuvant retroperitoneal irradiation with the policy of surveillance, it is extremely unlikely that a survival difference could be demonstrated and choice of management should therefore be based on morbidity. Surveillance will avoid specific anticancer treatment following orchidectomy in approximately 85% of patients; however, for the patients who recur there is a risk that their treatment becomes more intensive than might otherwise have been needed. In the Royal Marsden Hospital series seven patients required chemotherapy.

In Stage I non-seminoma (Chapter 13) analysis of the primary tumor histopathology has allowed a prediction of the risk of recurrence from Stage I disease. Prognostic factor analysis has also been performed in Stage I seminoma so that adjuvant treatment can be given selectively. However, there is as yet no international agreement on how this selection should be decided, as discussed above. Surveillance of the remainder would be greatly facilitated by use of a serum marker. In the meantime surveillance should be considered to be a research protocol rather than a standard management option.

REFERENCES

Bithell, J.F. and Stewart, A.M. (1975) Pre-natal irradiation and childhood malignancies: A review of British data from the Oxford survey. *Br. J. Cancer*, **31**, 271–87.

Bizzozero, O.J., Johnson, K.G. and Ciocco, A. (1966) Radiation-related leukaemia in Hiroshima and Nagasaki 1946–1964. 1. Distribution, incidence and appearance time. *N. Engl. J. Med.*, **274**, 1096–101.

Coia, L.R. and Hanks, G.E. (1988) Complications from large field intermediate dose in infradiaphragmatic radiation: An analysis of the patterns of care outcome studies for Hodgkin's disease and seminoma. *Int. J. Radiat. Oncol. Biol. Phys.*, **15**, 29–35.

Coleman, M.P., Bell, C.M.J. and Fraser, P. (1987) Second primary malignancy after Hodgkin's disease, ovarian cancer and cancer of the testis: A population-based cohort study. *Br. J. Cancer*, **56**, 349–55.

Court Brown, W.M. and Doll, R. (1957) *Leukaemia and Aplastic Anaemia in Patients Irradiated for Ankylosing Spondylitis*, HMSO, London.

Duchesne, G.M., Horwich, A., Dearnaley, D. *et al.* (1990) Orchidectomy alone for stage I seminoma of the testis. *Cancer*, **65**(5), 1115–18.

Fosså, S.D., Aass, N. and Kaalhus, O. (1989) Radiotherapy for testicular seminoma stage I: treatment results and long-term post-irradiation morbidity in 365 patients. *Int. J. Radiat. Oncol. Biol. Phys.*, **16**(2), 383–88.

Fosså, S.D., Abyholm, T., Norman, N. and Jetne, V. (1986) Post-treatment fertility in patients with testicular cancer. III Influence of radiotherapy in seminoma patients. *Br. J. Urol.*, **58**, 315–19.

Freedman, L.S., Parkinson, M.C., Jones, W.G. *et al.* (1987) Histopathology in the prediction of relapse of patients with stage I testicular teratoma treated by orchidectomy alone. *Lancet*, **ii**, 294–8.

Hahan, E.W., Feingold, S.M., Simpson, L. and Batata, M. (1982) Recovery from aspermia induced by low dose radiation in seminoma patients. *Cancer*, **50**, 337–40.

Hamilton, C., Horwich, A., Easton, A. and Peckham, M.J. (1987) Radiotherapy for stage I seminoma testis: Results of treatment and complications. *Radiother. Oncol.*, **6**, 115–20.

Hamilton, C.R., Horwich, A., Bliss, J.M. and Peckham, M.J. (1987). Gastrointestinal morbidity of adjuvant radiotherapy in stage I malignant teratoma of the testis. *Radiother. Oncol.*, **10**, 85–90.

Hay, J.H., Duncan, W. and Kerr, G.R. (1984) Subsequent malignancies in patients irradiated for testicular tumours. *Br. J. Radiol.*, **57**, 597–602.

Horwich, A., Alsanjari, N., A'Hern, R. *et al.* (1992) Surveillance following orchidectomy for stage I testicular seminoma. *Br. J. Cancer*, **65**, 775–8.

Horwich, A. and Bell, J. (1994) Mortality and cancer incidence following radiotherapy for seminoma of the testis. *Radiother. Oncol.*, **30**(3), 193–8.

Horwich, A., Brada, M., Nicholls, J *et al.* (1989) Intensive induction chemotherapy for poor risk non-seminomatous germ cell tumours. *Eur. J. Cancer*, **25**(2), 177–84.

Horwich, A., Tucker, D.F. and Peckham, M.J. (1985) Placental alkaline phosphatase as a tumour marker in seminoma using the H17E2 monoclonal antibody assay. *Br. J. Cancer*, **51**, 625–9.

Hoskin, P., Dilly, S., Easton, D. *et al.* (1986) Prognostic factors in stage I non seminomatous germ cell testicular tumours managed by orchidectomy and surveillance: implications for adjuvant chemotherapy. *J. Clin. Oncol.*, **4**, 1031–6.

IARC (1981) *Monographs on the Evaluation of the*

Carcinogenic Risk of Chemicals to Humans, IARC, Lyon.

Kaldor, J.M., Day, N.E., Band, P *et al.* (1987) Second malignancies following testicular cancer, ovarian cancer and Hodgkin's disease: an international collaborative study among cancer registries. *Int. J. Cancer*, **39**(5), 571–85.

Kapp, D.S., Fischer, D., Grady, K.J. and Schwartz, P.E. (1982) Subsequent malignancies associated with carcinoma of the uterine cervix: including an analysis of the effect of patient and treatment parameters on incidence and sites of metachronous malignancies. *Int. J. Radiat. Oncol. Biol. Phys.*, **8**, 197–205.

Lange, P.H., Millan, J.L., Stigbrand, T. *et al.* (1982) Placental alkaline phosphatase as a tumour marker for seminoma. *Cancer Res.*, **42**, 3244–7.

Lee, J.Y., Perez, C.A., Ettinger, N. and Fineberg, B.B. (1982) The risk of second primaries subsequent to irradiation for cervix cancer. *Int. J. Radiat. Oncol. Biol. Phys.*, **8**, 207–11.

Peckham, M.J., Hamilton, C.R., Horwich, A. and Hendry, W.F. (1987) Surveillance after orchidectomy for stage I seminoma of the testis. *Br. J. Urol.*, **59**, 343–7.

Smith, P.G. and Doll, R. (1982) Mortality among patients with ankylosing spondylitis after a single treatment course with X-rays. *BMJ*, **284**, 449–60.

Thomas, G.M., Sturgeon, J.F., Alison, M. *et al.* (1989) A study of post-orchidectomy surveillance in stage I testicular seminoma. *J. Urol.*, **142**(2), 313–16.

Thomas, P.R.M., Mansfield, M.D., Hendry, W.F. and Peckham, M.J. (1977) The implications of scrotal interference for the preservation of spermatogenesis in the management of testicular tumours. *Br. J. Surg.*, **64**, 352–4.

von der Maase, H., Specht, L., Jacobsen, G.K. *et al.* (1993) Surveillance following orchidectomy for stage I seminoma of the testis. *Eur. J. Cancer*, **29A**(14), 1931–4.

Warde, P.R., Gospodarowicz, M.K., Goodman, P.J. *et al.* (1993) Results of a policy of surveillance in stage I testicular seminoma. *Int. J. Radiat. Oncol. Biol. Phys.* **27**(1), 11–15.

RADIOTHERAPY IN THE MANAGEMENT OF METASTATIC SEMINOMA

G.M. Thomas

10.1 INTRODUCTION

Using the currently available radiological tests and serum tumor markers, approximately 75% of patients with seminoma appear to have disease confined to the testicle. The sensitivity of the staging methods that are currently available is relatively high, at approximately 85%. Thus, of all patients presenting with pure seminoma of the testicle, it is estimated that 25% will require some form of initial therapy for overt disease beyond the testicle, while the 15% with occult disease not detected by available staging methods are usually included in a group that are treated with adjuvant radiation therapy in the Stage I setting.

Historically, prior to the availability of cisplatin-containing chemotherapy, radiation therapy was used for the treatment of all stages and extents of disease. Because of the exquisite radiosensitivity of seminoma, orchidectomy and postoperative radiation therapy to all sites of known disease yielded cure rates of the order of 85% (Thomas *et al.*, 1982).

In recent years, it has been shown that seminomas are also highly sensitive to the same chemotherapeutic agents as the non-seminomatous germ cell tumors of the testis (NSGCTT) (Loehrer *et al.*, 1987). Thus when there are two highly effective treatment modalities available for this disease, it has become important to define the appropriate roles for each of these modalities in the treatment armamentarium.

This chapter will address the role of radiation therapy in the management of Stage II, III and IV disease, as well as its role in the management of residual or recurrent masses after primary chemotherapy. Despite the continued publication of articles relating the use of radiation therapy in Stage II seminoma, relatively few new insights have led to changes in practice over the past 5 years.

For the purposes of this discussion, the staging system to be used will be a modification of the Royal Marsden Hospital staging system as adopted by the Consensus Conference on the Management of Testicular Seminoma 1989 (Thomas, 1990) (Table 10.1).

Table 10.1 Seminoma staging system

Stage	Description
I	No evidence of metastases
II	Metastases confined to nodes
	A: Maximum diameter ≤2 cm
	B: Maximum diameter >2–5 cm
	C: Maximum diameter >5–10 cm
	D: Maximum diameter >10 cm
III	Supra- and infradiaphragmatic nodes
	Abdominal status: A, B, C or D
IV	Extralymphatic metastases

Testicular Cancer: Investigation and management. Second edition. Edited by Professor A. Horwich. Published in 1996 by Chapman & Hall. ISBN 0 412 61210 0.

10.2 STAGE II

The Stage II category clearly encompasses a wide range of disease extent. The A, B, C and D categories reflect our current understanding of the prognostic significance of the bulk of retroperitoneal disease. Prior to the availability of computed axial tomography (CT scanning) and lymphography, which more precisely define the bulk of retroperitoneal disease, we relied on the intravenous pyelogram and a physical examination to separate patients into two groups by their disease bulk, i.e. those with and without palpable abdominal masses, previously called Stage IIA and IIB, respectively (Thomas *et al.*, 1982; Zagars and Babaian, 1987). Even with this imprecise division of patients, it was clear that following routine postorchidectomy irradiation, the 5-year survival was dependent on disease bulk. For those without a mass it was significantly better, at 87%, than for those with a mass, at 62% (Thomas *et al.*, 1982).

Computed tomography scanning has allowed a more precise definition of the volume of retroperitoneal disease. Most recent publications on the outcome of patients with Stage II disease have used the largest transverse diameter of the mass as a measure of retroperitoneal bulk. Arbitrarily these reports usually document treatment results for patients with masses less than 2 cm in diameter, from 2 to 5 cm, from 5 to 10 cm and greater than 10 cm, corresponding to the current A, B, C and D categories (Ball, Barrett and Peckham, 1982; Evensen *et al.*, 1985; Zagars and Babaian, 1987; Mason and Kearsley, 1988). Presumably a spectrum of outcome exists which is a continuum through all volumes of retroperitoneal disease.

Since most recent treatment results are reported in the literature, using the A, B and C categories, this same classification will be used to discuss the role of radiation therapy in Stage II disease.

Using up-to-date staging methods, approximately 15% of patients fall into the Stage II category (Fosså *et al.*, 1987). This represents the majority of patients who have disease disseminated beyond the testicle and attests to the fact that pure seminoma spreads in an orderly fashion through the first echelon of draining lymphatics in the retroperitoneum and only later to the lymph nodes in the mediastinum and supraclavicular fossa and very rarely subsequently disseminates hematogeneously. Careful surgical dissection has clearly outlined the first site of lymphatic drainage from the testicle as the retroperitoneal lymph glands between the levels of T11 and L4, but mainly at the level of L1 to L3. The nodes lie in relation to the aorta and vena cava with extensive intercommunicating lymphatic channels. By lymphography, crossover from the right side to the left side is constant, whereas crossover from the left to the right side is rare and occurs after the primary nodes are filled. Involvement of the pelvic nodes is relatively rare, at less than 5%. Theoretically previous inguinal surgery may disrupt the draining lymphatics and redirect lymph drainage through the subcutaneous lymphatics of the anterior abdominal wall and into bilateral iliac nodes. The lymphatic drainage of the skin and subcutaneous tissues of the scrotum is into the inguinal and iliac nodes. From the retroperitoneal lumbar nodes drainage occurs through the thoracic duct to lymph nodes in the mediastinum and supraclavicular fossa.

Radiation therapy has been delivered to patients with Stage II disease using radiation volumes to encompass the known pattern of drainage to the retroperitoneal and pelvic nodes. A division of opinion developed as to whether the next echelon of nodes in the mediastinum and supraclavicular fossa should receive prophylactic irradiation (Thomas, 1985). This review of the role of radiation therapy in the management of Stage II disease will focus on several aspects of its utility: local control of disease in the abdomen, prevention of the development of subsequent mediastinal relapse and overall and disease-free survival results.

10.2.1 STAGE IIA AND IIB

The data on the specific results of radiation therapy in the management of Stage A, i.e. those patients whose disease is considered to be less than 2 cm in maximum transverse diameter, are scanty. Generally, the CT scan is not helpful in defining disease of less than 2 cm in diameter and therefore these patients have often been included in reports of patients with tumor masses less than 5 cm in diameter, or earlier they were included in reports of patients with non-palpable retroperitoneal disease identified by lymphography. There are, however, two specific reports relating to this subgroup. Data from the Royal Marsden Hospital (Ball, Barrett and Peckham, 1982) indicate that, between 1963 and 1979, 32 patients with Stage IIA were treated with radiation therapy in a dose of 30 Gy to the para-aortic and ipsilateral pelvic nodes. From the reports, it appears that 12 of these patients also received prophylactic mediastinal irradiation (PMI). Subsequently, three patients relapsed. One had received infra-diaphragmatic irradiation only, and relapsed in supradiaphragmatic nodes and also in the stomach or adrenal gland. This patient died of his disease as attempts to cure him with appropriate combination chemotherapy failed. One other patient who had infradiaphragmatic irradiation only failed in supradiaphragmatic nodes, but was rendered disease free with surgery. One other patient who had

both infradiaphragmatic irradiation and PMI failed in both treated sites and also in the scrotum and lung. His attempted salvage therapy with further radiation and cyclophosphamide failed. Thus in total 11% (three of 28) relapsed following initial radiation therapy and 7% (two of 28) died of recurrent seminoma (Mason and Kearsley, 1988).

The report from the M.D. Anderson Hospital describes 36 patients in whom the diameter of the abdominal disease could be measured (Zagars, 1989). There were four patients with masses less than 2 cm in diameter. None of the four patients relapsed following radiation therapy. Further data from the Norwegian Radium Hospital show that, of 73 patients with Stage II disease, six had disease less than 2 cm in diameter and none of the six have relapsed (Evensen *et al.*, 1985).

Thus in the literature, of the 38 reported cases with disease identified as less than 2 cm in diameter, only three from one series or 8% have relapsed and 5% (two of 38) have died of disease, one of these prior to the era of the use of cisplatin-based chemotherapy.

Considerably more data exist describing the outcome for patients with masses less than 5 cm in diameter, i.e. including both Stage A and B (Table 10.2). In four large series a total of 106 patients with masses less than 5 cm received either infradiaphragmatic or infra-diaphragmatic and prophylactic mediastinal irradiation. In total 7.5% (eight of 106) relapsed following primary irradiation and 3% (three of 106) died of disease, one prior to the era of cisplatin-containing chemotherapy. The anomalous result of the survival of those

Table 10.2 Outcome following radiation therapy for patients with Stage IIA, IIB disease (abdominal mass <5 cm in diameter)

Reference	Number patients	Number relapsing	Dead of disease
Mason and Kearsley (1988)	25	1	0
Evensen *et al.* (1985)	24	1	0
Zagars (1989); Zagars and Babaian (1987)	18	1	1 (?)
Gregory and Peckham (1986)	39	5	2
Total	106	8 (8%)	3 (3%)

with Stage A disease being slightly less than those of Stage A and B together is undoubtedly explained by the small number of patients in the relevant reports.

For patients with retroperitoneal disease of less than 5 cm in diameter, the expectation of disease-free survival is 93% and that of overall survival is 95%.

Some specific data are available pertaining to patients with masses stated to be between 2 and 5 cm in diameter who have been treated with primary radiation therapy. These reports specifically refer to the results of radiation by the size of the retroperitoneal mass but it is important to recognize that without CT scanning there was considerable difficulty in measuring the size of retroperitoneal masses. The stated sizes must therefore be viewed as estimates. Nevertheless, within the constraints of estimates, some data on outcome for patients with masses between 2 and 5 cm are available. In the report from the Royal Marsden Hospital, of patients treated between 1970 and 1974, there were 11 Stage IIB patients, three of whom were treated with infradiaphragmatic radiation and eight of whom received infradiaphragmatic radiation and PMI (Ball, Barrett and Peckham, 1982). One patient relapsed from each treatment group, a relapse rate of 18%. The patient receiving infradiaphragmatic irradiation relapsed only in the supraclavicular nodes and/or mediastinum and was treated with carboplatin and rendered disease free. The other patient who relapsed did so in the scrotum and lung. He received some further radiation therapy and unknown chemotherapy but died of disease. Thus, primary radiation therapy given either to the infradiaphragmatic or infra- and supradiaphragmatic nodes yielded 82% progression free. Only one of 11 patients died and that patient did not apparently receive cisplatin-containing chemotherapy. In the series from the Norwegian Radium Hospital, 18 patients were estimated to have Stage IIB disease and received primary radiation therapy (Evensen *et al.*, 1985). It is un-

clear from the report what percentage received PMI in addition to infradiaphragmatic irradiation, but approximately 70% of patients with Stage IIA or IIB disease did so. One of 18 patients suffered a subsequent relapse and his final outcome is not available.

In the M.D. Anderson Hospital series between 1960 and 1982, 48 patients with Stage II testicular seminoma received definitive irradiation (Zagars and Babaian, 1987). Thirty-six of the 48 patients had radiographs available from which disease dimensions could be measured and of these 14 had Stage IIB disease. After primary radiation therapy, which is presumed to have included PMI, one of 14 patients relapsed and his final outcome is unclear. Thus in three series in which the outcome of patients with Stage IIB disease is available, 39 of 43 (91%) were rendered disease free by primary irradiation. In the Princess Margaret Hospital series, 16 Stage II patients had radiologically identified nonpalpable infradiaphragmatic nodal disease (Thomas, 1985). Nonpalpable disease probably corresponds in most cases to what is currently called Stage IIA or IIB. Following infradiaphragmatic irradiation only one in 16 relapsed in the abdomen, mediastinum and lung and died of disease. He had a previous embryonal carcinoma, and did not receive chemotherapy at relapse. The disease-free and overall survival for this group was 94%.

These results justify the continued use of primary irradiation for Stage IIA and IIB disease with the expectation of disease-free survival being approximately 95%. Only 5% of patients will require subsequent salvage chemotherapy, yielding an expected overall survival for Stage IIA and IIB disease of the order of 98%. Many reports in the literature show no apparent survival benefit for PMI (Ball, Barrett and Peckham, 1982; Thomas *et al.*, 1982; Herman, Sturgeon and Thomas, 1983; Evensen *et al.*, 1985). Despite these reports there are still some advocates for its continued use, particularly in the USA. Such advocates suggest that PMI may prevent

Table 10.3 Relapse following radiation therapy* for patients with Stage IIC disease (abdominal mass >5–10 cm in diameter)

Reference	Number of patients	Number relapsing
Zagars (1989); Zagars and Babaian (1987)	10	0
Evensen *et al.* (1985)	20	2
Mason and Kearsley (1988)	12†	2
Smalley *et al.* (1985)	3	0
Green *et al.* (1985)	3	0
Total	48	4 (8%)

* Majority received intradiaphragmatic radiotherapy plus prophylactic mediastinal irradiation.
† Some also received platinum/vinblastine/bleomycin (PVB).

mediastinal relapse, but they have not addressed the question of whether preventing such a relapse leads to improved survival, nor the cost of that unnecessary treatment to the majority of patients who will derive no benefit from it. Where infradiaphragmatic radiation only has been given to small volume, nonpalpable Stage II disease, compiled data show mediastinal relapse in only 3% (8 of 250) of patients (Doornbos, Hussey and Johnson, 1975; Dosoretz *et al.*, 1981; Ball, Barrett and Peckham, 1982; Herman, Sturgeon and Thomas, 1983; Huben *et al.*, 1984; Thomas, 1985). Seven of the eight patients were salvaged with radiation at the time of relapse. Thus the possible additional survival benefit attributable to PMI is 0.4% (1 in 250). The lack of a substantial survival advantage and the toxicity associated with PMI (see below and Hanks, Peters and Owen, 1992) cannot justify its continued use, particularly now that effective curative cisplatin-based chemotherapy is available as salvage therapy (Thomas, 1985).

A range of radiation doses have been used to treat the para-aortic and ipsilateral pelvic nodes. Total doses have varied between 20 and 40 Gy in 15 to 30 fractions. Only occasional in-field relapses have been reported on any of the dose regimens employed. There appears to be no evidence that total doses in excess of 25 Gy are necessary for the treatment of non-bulky disease. The Leeds Consensus Conference accepted 25 Gy as the recommended treatment dose (Thomas, 1990). A discussion of dose control information follows in Section 10.2.2, but it is unclear whether higher doses of radiation are necessary for any bulk of disease and if they are, for what size of mass the higher dose should be used.

10.2.2 STAGE IIC

Several series in the literature (Green *et al.*, 1983; Evensen *et al.*, 1985; Smalley *et al.*, 1985; Zagars and Babaian, 1987; Mason and Kearsley, 1988; Zagars, 1989) have reported specific outcome results for patients estimated to have masses between 5 and 10 cm in diameter treated with radiation (Table 10.3). Considerable other data are available for all patients with masses in excess of 5 cm in diameter, but do not specifically look at the Stage IIC subset. The results of radiation in this group of patients are critical to our understanding of the role of radiation therapy in bulky abdominal disease.

There continues to be major controversy centered around the issue of the maximum size of mass above which patients with Stage II disease should be treated with primary chemotherapy rather than primary irradiation. Many investigators have chosen to use primary chemotherapy for those with retroperitoneal masses equal to or greater than 5 cm in maximum transverse diameter.

The five series provide data pertinent to the controversy. In total, 48 patients received primary irradiation. It would appear that almost all received both infradiaphragmatic irradiation and PMI, although the specific numbers are unavailable. In one series (Evensen *et al.*, 1985) a few patients may have also received adjuvant combination cisplatin-containing chemotherapy. Four of 48 patients relapsed following radiation therapy. Thus primary irradiation yielded 92% of patients progression free.

This cumulated progression-free survival of 92% from the five series suggests that the risk of relapse after initial radiation therapy for those with masses between 5 and 10 cm is very low. This is in contradistinction to the report from the Royal Marsden Hospital (Ball, Barrett and Peckham, 1982), in which four out of 14 patients treated with initial radiation had a subsequent relapse. It was initially projected that as many as 50% of patients treated only with abdominal irradiation for palpable abdominal disease would subsequently relapse (Thomas, 1985). Those projections were formulated using data from a group of patients treated without the benefits of sensitive radiological tests for assessing the retroperitoneum, without CT guided radiation therapy planning and often without the benefit of serum tumor markers by which non-seminomatous elements could be excluded. In that era when bulky palpable abdominal disease was treated with radiation, it was expected that approximately 20% of patients would develop a subsequent mediastinal relapse and in 25% disease would either progress in the abdomen or develop through hematogenous spread, usually as pulmonary metastases. However, the measurement of alpha-fetoprotein (AFP) and beta-subunit of human chorionic gonadotrophin (BHCG) has substantially decreased the risk of relapse or failure related to the presence of previously unidentified occult non-seminomatous elements. The availability of CT scanning to delineate retroperitoneal disease has also decreased the risk of abdominal failure due to geographical missing of tumor. These factors plus the use of PMI probably

account for the high progression-free rate (92%) reported from the five series where primary radiation therapy has been used for patients with masses between 5 and 10 cm in diameter.

In patients with Stage IIC disease, it is impossible to resolve completely the issue of whether prophylactic mediastinal irradiation should be used. Clearly, the risk of mediastinal relapse in Stage IIC disease patients is higher than in patients with Stage IIA, IIB disease. Prophylactic mediastinal irradiation does decrease the risk of mediastinal relapse. The projected mediastinal relapse rate for patients with palpable disease being 20% compared with none that occurred in the five series. It is unclear, however, whether this prophylactic mediastinal irradiation actually improved cure rates since the majority of patients relapsing after infradiaphragmatic irradiation will be cured with subsequent platinum-containing chemotherapy. Several retrospective analyses have recently appeared indicating significant cardiopulmonary toxicity from elective mediastinal irradiation. Hanks *et al.* have recently updated their Patterns of Care Survey to include 15-year follow-up on 387 patients (Hanks, Peters and Owen, 1992). They reported a 13% actuarial rate of cardiac deaths at 15 years for patients who received elective mediastinal irradiation. In this retrospective analysis there were 5.5% cardiac deaths among those patients who had received mediastinal irradiation versus 1% among those who did not. Peckham and McElwain also reported a significant incidence of death among those patients who received mediastinal irradiation (13.5%) as compared with those who did not (2.5%) (Peckham and McElwain, 1974). In another recent retrospective analysis, Lederman *et al.*, found postradiation cardiac complications in 10% of those patients who received mediastinal irradiation (Lederman *et al.* 1987). Since elective mediastinal irradiation does place the patient at increased risk of potential lethal cardiac damage and possibly compromises

Table 10.4 Results of primary chemotherapy in 'bulky' Stage II seminoma

Reference	Number of patients	Survival progression free (%)	Other therapy: radiotherapy, surgery (%)
Friedman *et al.* (1985)	12	100	64
Peckham *et al.* (1982, 1985)	17	88	?
Fosså *et al.* (1987)	21	92	100
Schuette *et al.* (1985)	15	93	47
Zagars (1989); Zagars and Babaian (1987)	14	86	14
Schmoll *et al.* (1993)	27	74	24

chemotherapeutic salvage for radiation therapy failures, and has been shown to offer no significant disease-free survival benefits, there would appear to be no indication for its routine use in patients with Stage II disease.

To summarize the dilemma with respect to PMI: it may contribute about 20% to relapse-free but not overall survival while treating 80% unnecessarily. It may significantly impair the necessary salvage therapy for the 8 or 10% of patients who relapse after such treatment and produce unacceptable cardio-thoracic morbidity. If PMI is withheld, approximately 20% more patients will require salvage chemotherapy which can be safely delivered after infradiaphragmatic irradiation only.

A recent review of patients treated at the M.D. Anderson Hospital for retroperitoneal disease less than 10 cm in diameter indicated that three of 16 patients relapsed in the supraclavicular fossa (Dosmann and Zagars, 1993). For this reason the authors suggested elective irradiation of the left supraclavicular fossa for all patients with disease less than 10 cm in diameter. This treatment however, would constitute unnecessary therapy in 13 of 16 such patients, and is difficult to justify despite its low morbidity. Since platinum-based chemotherapy successfully salvaged 18 of 19 patients with Stage II disease who relapsed, isolated supraclavicular radiation would be hard to justify even for patients with masses between 5 cm and 10 cm where two of three patients sustained isolated supraclavicular relapse, compared with only two of 13 with retroperitoneal masses less than 5 cm in diameter.

The alternative approach to the treatment of 'bulky Stage II seminoma' is to use primary cisplatin-containing chemotherapy. Table 10.4 shows the results of such an approach in an accumulated 79 patients from five literature series. The progression-free survival using primary chemotherapy for undefined bulks of abdominal disease ranges between 86 and 100%, but how much of this is achieved by chemotherapy alone is uncertain in view of the fact that between 14 and 100% of patients also received additional therapy with radiation or surgery.

It appears that for patients with masses between 5 and 10 cm acceptable initial approaches to treatment include primary infradiaphragmatic irradiation or primary chemotherapy. The role of radiation as consolidation treatment of residual masses will be discussed below.

Most investigators appear to have quoted the size of the mass in the abdomen as the single criterion for selecting primary radiation or primary chemotherapy. In practice, outside of a study setting the decision to use one modality instead of the other should be based on factors. Clearly, the expertise of the available oncologists is important. Also if the primary modality chosen is such that the risk of subsequent relapse and necessary salvage therapy may be higher, it is mandatory to be able to follow the patient clinically and with the necessary radiological investigations. The other factor that needs to be considered in deciding whether to use initial abdominal irradiation is the location of the retroperitoneal mass. If a mass between 5 and 10 cm in diameter is centrally located, it is possible to deliver the necessary doses of irradiation without substantial risk of renal or hepatic damage. This lack of risk is related to the dose of radiation used and also to the volume of the organs irradiated. When the mass lies centrally, it should be encompassed by the field without encroaching on more than the medial third of the kidneys. If, however, the mass lies in such a position that the radiation volume will encompass a substantial proportion of the kidneys or the liver, the risk of radiation damage to those organs increases significantly. In those circumstances it would be more appropriate to use primary chemotherapy rather than primary irradiation.

Where primary radiation is used for Stage IIC disease, there would appear to be no information in the literature to support total doses in excess of 3500 cGy. The available dose control information in the literature with respect to seminoma is difficult to interpret. Several investigators have quoted abdominal failure rates and related them to a range of radiation doses employed (Ball, Barrett and Peckham 1982; Thomas *et al.*, 1982; Lester, Morphis and Hornback, 1986). The difficulties in interpreting these data stem from the fact that abdominal control rates were quoted for patients with all extents of Stage II disease. Also, they do not specifically correlate the dose of radiation used with the size of mass. Lastly, because most of the reports came from an era when CT scanning was unavailable, geographical missing could be responsible for some of the observed abdominal failures. In the Royal Marsden Hospital experience as reported by Ball, Barrett and Peckham (1982) the abdominal failure rate was 36% (five of 14) after a dose of 30 to 40 Gy. The data from the Princess Margaret Hospital were similar, showing no

increase in abdominal control rates whether or not the dose was greater or less than 30 or 35 Gy (Thomas *et al.*, 1982). In contradistinction, Lester's (1986) data from Indianapolis suggested that no abdominal failure occurred using a dose of over 30 Gy (seven of seven patients), while with a dose of less than 30 Gy 33% failed (four of 12). Three of the four relapsing patients in this series had retroperitoneal disease less than 5 cm in diameter, thus it is difficult to understand that the explanation for these failures is related to the use of a too-low radiation dose. Many series report almost 100% local control for doses of 25 Gy to 30 Gy for masses less than 5 cm in diameter. Most investigators arbitrarily now use a total dose of 35 Gy in 25 to 35 fractions as an acceptable regimen for patients receiving radiation for 'bulky' seminoma. Usually the initial large volume of radiation includes the retroperitoneum and either the ipsilateral or bilateral pelvic nodes. Some investigators have elected to treat the pelvic nodes bilaterally to cover the risk of retrograde spread from large retroperitoneal masses to the contralateral pelvis. There are no data to support or refute this practice. The initial volume is treated to 2500 cGy in 20 fractions. A repeat abdominal CT scan when the patient has received 18 to 20 Gy will usually show significant decrease in the size of the mass. A boost dose of 10 Gy may then be delivered to a relatively small volume.

The late toxicity of infradiaphragmatic irradiation in doses of 25 to 35 Gy is acceptable. Little precise prospective data on acute toxicity is available, but acute side-effects usually consist of some degree of fatigue, minor amounts of anorexia, nausea and occasional vomiting, and rarely depression of white blood cell and platelet counts. Late gastrointestinal morbidity is dose related. Fosså, Aass and Kaalhus (1989) observed significant dyspepsia in 6% and frank peptic ulceration in 3% of patients after radiation doses of 35 to 40 Gy in 2 Gy fractions. Similar data from the Royal Marsden Hospital (Hamilton *et al.*, 1986) confirm a 6%

incidence of peptic ulceration after retroperitoneal irradiation. Data from the US Patterns of Care Study observed a 6% incidence of hemorrhagic gastritis of doses of 40 to 45 Gy, while the incidence of intestinal obstruction and peptic ulceration decreased to 2% with doses between 25 and 35 Gy. Radiation may cause a potential reduction in fertility related to the dose scattered to the remaining testicle. The dose received by the remaining testicle is determined by physical treatment factors including the radiation dose prescribed, the adequacy of the testicular shielding and particularly the proximity of the testis to the edge of the radiation field (i.e. the placement of the inferior border). With adequate shielding the dose to testicle can be reduced to 1% of the prescribed midplane radiation dose (Kubo and Shipley, 1982). Available data suggest that if the dose received by the testis is 100 cGy to 600 cGy, all patients will become azoospermic, at least transiently. Recovery to baseline levels will usually occur within 3 to 10 years of therapy (Hahn, Feingold and Niscle, 1976; Fossa et al., 1986).

Several authors have suggested that infradiaphragmatic radiation may induce second malignancies (Hamilton et al., 1986; Coia and Hanks, 1988; Fosså, Aass and Kaalhus, 1989). Data from the Scottish Registry suggested a doubling of the risk of second malignancies within the radiation volume (19 observed versus 9.8 expected; $p < 0.05$). The excess risk was for transitional cell carcinomas of the genitourinary tract and for unknown primaries within the gastrointestinal tract (Hay, Duncan and Kerr, 1984). Similar data from the Norwegian Radium Hospital suggest an increased relative risk of second malignancies from infradiaphragmatic radiation (Fosså et al., 1987). Other data suggest increased incidences of leukemia when follow-up is sufficiently protracted (Osterland, Rørth and Prener, 1985).

10.2.3 STAGE IID

The Stage IID category of disease was formulated at the 1989 Seminoma Consensus Conference at Leeds in the UK (Thomas, 1990). This subcategory of Stage II was designated to account for a group of patients with infradiaphragmatic disease whose prognosis appears to be different from that of the Stage IIC category. While some series suggest that the prognosis after radiation is the same regardless of size over 5 cm (Ball, Barrett and Peckham, 1982), three series in the literature separate out patients with masses larger than 10 cm in diameter and show that this is a more unfavorable group (Evensen et al., 1985; Mason and Kearsley, 1988; Zagars, 1989). In the three series (Table 10.5), a total of 49 patients received primary irradiation either with infradiaphragmatic or infra- and supradiaphragmatic treatment. Seventeen of the 49 patients, or 35%, relapsed following this treatment. It is unclear how many of these patients survived with salvage chemotherapy. These relapse rates plus the fact that radiation volumes of necessity would probably include large volumes of the renal or hepatic parenchyma suggest that patients with Stage IID disease would be more appro-

Table 10.5 Relapse following radiation therapy for patients with Stage IID disease (abdominal mass >10 cm in diameter)

Reference	Number of patients	Number relapsing
Zagars (1989); Zagars and Babaian et al. (1985)	8	4
Mason and Kearsley (1988)	12	4
Evensen et al. (1985)	29	9
Total	49	17 (35%)

priately managed with initial combination chemotherapy. Unfortunately, there are few data pertinent to the use of chemotherapy alone in patients with such bulky disease, and it is not as yet known how many of these patients treated with initial chemotherapy actually need subsequent consolidation radiation therapy or therapy for relapse. Schmoll *et al.* (1993) have reported on the use of single agent carboplatin in 11 patients with Stage IID disease. Eighty-two per cent (nine of 11) remain continuously free from relapse or progression, but four of the nine achieved this state with additional surgery. When we know more precisely how many patients with Stage IID disease fail after chemotherapy alone we will be better able to compare its utility to that of initial radiotherapy which produces a progression-free rate of 65%.

It is highly likely that overall cure rates will be comparable, regardless of the choice of initial therapy. The utility of the alternative approaches will need to be evaluated by accurate observation of the associated toxicities and accompanying quality of life for the patient.

10.3 MARKER-POSITIVE PURE SEMINOMA

Up to 20% of patients, in whom the primary tumor has been carefully examined and reported as histologically pure seminoma, will have postorchidectomy elevations of beta human chorionic gonadotrophin (BHCG) or alpha-fetoprotein (AFP) (Javadpour, 1980; Thomas, 1985). It is unclear how many have preorchidectomy elevations. Elevations of BHCG may occur because of the presence of syncytiotrophoblastic cells admixed with pure seminoma, or may be due to the presence of occult NSGCTT. Marked elevation with pure seminoma is rare. It is, however, impossible to set an upper limit beyond which the probability of occult NSGCTT is high enough to justify treatment as if for NSGCTT. Most investigators have reported that elevation of BHCG in pure seminoma does not confer a

poorer prognosis on patients treated with primary radiotherapy, nor should it alone influence treatment decisions (Evensen *et al.*, 1985; Thomas, 1985; Gregory and Peckham, 1986).

Elevations of AFP occurring in pure seminoma have been accepted by most as signifying the presence of occult NSGCTT (Javadpour, 1980). This interpretation has resulted in the generally accepted practice of treating as for a similar stage of NSGCTT. Two reports in the literature suggest that cells which are morphologically pure seminoma may have surface characteristics of NSGCTT and produce AFP (Raghaven *et al.*, 1982; Srigley *et al.*, 1988). Regardless of whether such tumors are labelled as seminoma or NSGCTT, these tumors appear to have a poorer prognosis than pure seminoma and should be treated as for NSGCTT.

Thus, BHCG elevations alone in the absence of Stage IID, III or IV disease should not proscribe the use of initial radiation therapy, whereas an elevation of AFP should.

10.4 RESIDUAL MASSES AFTER CHEMOTHERAPY

Considerable controversy has arisen as to the role of radiation therapy in treating patients who have residual masses after initial treatment with chemotherapy. Several authors (Peckham, Horwich and Hendry, 1985; Motzer *et al.*, 1987; Zagars and Babaian, 1987) have reported that following chemotherapy relapse in almost all cases involves the site of previous bulky disease. The reported incidence of residual masses varies with the time at which the patient is assessed after completion of chemotherapy and with the initial volume of disease. Peckham, Horwich and Hendry (1985) report that one in 11 patients (9%) with nonbulky disease initially had a residual mass 1 month after chemotherapy. By contrast, 78% (29 in 33) of patients treated with chemotherapy for bulky disease had a residual mass 1 month after chemotherapy.

Thus in total in that series, 32% (14 out of 44 patients) had a residual mass 1 month following chemotherapy. A number of reports in the literature have documented surgical procedures carried out on residual masses either with therapeutic or diagnostic intent. The incidence of apparently viable seminoma cells will vary somewhat in relation to the time after chemotherapy that the surgical procedure was performed and the size of the initial mass. Reports have documented that residual masses may be densely fibrotic and the surgery associated with significant toxicity or even death (Friedman *et al.*, 1985; Fosså *et al.*, 1987). In data available from the literature, the overall incidence of residual tumor appears to be 12% (eight out of 60). Only the series from the Memorial Sloan-Kettering Hospital documents an unusually high incidence of residual disease (Motzer *et al.*, 1987). In their experience with surgery performed 1 month after the completion of chemotherapy, 36% (five of 14) appear to have viable tumor present in the mass if the residual mass was greater than 3 cm in diameter. While the risk of viable residual disease is probably slightly higher for large rather than for small masses (Motzer *et al.*, 1987), the available data on relapse do not suggest that all such patients will recur.

The overall average risk of 12% having residual microscopic disease appears to agree with the available data on the incidence of relapse in patients with residual masses after chemotherapy. Two series suggest that the risk of relapse was 11% and 7%, respectively (Peckham, Horwich and Hendry, 1985; Stomper *et al.*, 1986). This risk of persistent viable tumor in residual masses has caused some investigators to recommend routine postchemotherapy radiation treatment to all residual masses (Fossa *et al.*, 1987; Zagars, 1989). This approach of routine irradiation would treat patients with viable disease slightly earlier than if patients are simply observed until there is overt evidence of tumor progression. However, it implies that over 85% of patients would be treated unnecessarily since only 12–15% of patients do have viable tumor present in residual masses. Furthermore, it has been reported (Zagars and Babaian, 1987) that three of four patients who relapsed after chemotherapy by regrowth of disease in sites of initial bulky disease were successfully salvaged by radiation therapy. The toxicity of postchemotherapy irradiation, particularly of residual masses in the mediastinum, is not insubstantial. It would therefore seem appropriate to recommend that patients with residual masses postchemotherapy are simply observed and treated only if there are signs of progressive disease. This approach will spare the majority of patients unnecessary radiation therapy, but patients with postchemotherapy residual masses need to be observed at frequent intervals with repeated CT scanning to ensure that residual masses are not increasing in size.

10.5 STAGES III AND IV

Collected results from the literature on radiation therapy for Stages III and IV disease show a survival of 36% (136 out of 375) (Doornbos, Hussey and Johnson, 1975).

Analysis of data from the Princess Margaret Hospital (Thomas *et al.*, 1982) shows that those likely to be cured with radiation therapy alone are patients with supradiaphragmatic nodal disease, without bulky abdominal disease or visceral metastases. Occasional patients have been reported in whom cures have been obtained in pulmonary or even bony metastases from pure seminoma. The hematogenous dissemination of pure seminoma is an extremely rare event and Stage IV patients are uncommon (Thomas, 1985). Because treatment with radiation therapy involves at least infra- and supradiaphragmatic fields to cover sites of known disease and because the risk of relapse and thus the need for salvage chemotherapy is high, initial systemic therapy is obviously preferable in such patients. The use of initial radiation therapy in Stage III and

IV disease has been supplanted by the use of cisplatin-based chemotherapy (Einhorn and Williams, 1980; Fosså *et al.*, 1987; Loehrer *et al.*, 1987).

10.6 METASTATIC DISEASE

Death from uncontrolled pure seminoma is a very rare event. Nevertheless, occasionally patients with disseminated seminoma have disease that is uncontrolled by any of the available chemotherapeutic combinations. In these patients, worthwhile palliation of symptoms and occasionally significant prolongation of life or cure may be obtained with the use of relatively low-dose radiation therapy to sites of disease. Radiation therapy may be useful for the treatment of spinal cord compression from extradural seminoma. It may be useful for the relief of pain from bony metastases. It may also be potentially curative in the very rare patient who develops central nervous system metastases from pure seminoma.

10.7 CONCLUSIONS

In summary, radiation therapy is still a highly effective modality for the management of seminoma disseminated beyond the testicle. It is effective as the sole agent for the cure of Stage IIA, IIB and IIC disease. It may be curative in the treatment of progressive disease in large masses following chemotherapy. It may offer significant palliation and prolongation of life to the occasional patients who have failed systemic chemotherapy. It is important to remember that the response rates of pure seminoma to relatively low-dose radiation therapy closely approach 100%.

REFERENCES

Ball, D., Barrett, A. and Peckham, J. (1982) The management of metastatic seminoma testis. *Cancer*, **50**, 2289–94.

Coia, L.R. and Hanks, G.E. (1988) Complications from large field intermediate dose infradiaphragmatic radiation: An analysis of the patterns of care outcome studies for Hodgkin's disease and seminoma. *Int. J. Radiat. Oncol. Biol. Phys.*, **15**, 29–31.

Doornbos, J.F., Hussey, D.H. and Johnson, D.E. (1975) Radiotherapy for pure seminoma of the testis. *Radiology*, **116**, 401–4.

Dosmann, M.A. and Zagars, G.K. (1993) Post-orchidectomy radiation therapy for Stage I and II testicular seminoma. *Int. J. Radiat. Oncol. Biol. Phys.*, **26**, 381–90.

Dosoretz, D.E., Shipley, W.U., Blitzer, P.H. *et al.* (1981) Megavoltage irradiation for pure testicular seminoma. *Cancer*, **48**, 2184–90.

Einhorn, L.H. and Williams, S.D. (1980) Chemotherapy of disseminated seminoma. *Cancer Clin. Trials*, **3**, 307–13.

Evensen, J.F., Fosså, S.D., Kjellevold, K. and Lien, H.H. (1985) Testicular seminoma: analysis of treatment and failure for Stage II disease. *Radiother. Oncol.*, **4**, 55–61.

Fosså, S., Aass, N. and Kaalhus, O. (1989) Radiotherapy for testicular seminoma stage I: treatment results and long-term post-irradiation morbidity in 365 patients. *Int. J. Radiat. Oncol. Biol. Phys.*, **16**, 383–8.

Fosså, S.D., Abyholm, T., Normann, N. *et al.* (1986) Post-treatment fertility in patients with testicular cancer III: Influence of radiotherapy in seminoma patients. *Br. J. Urol.*, **58**, 315–19.

Fosså, S., Borge, L., Aass, N. *et al.* (1987) The treatment of advanced metastatic seminoma: experience in 55 cases. *J. Clin. Oncol.*, **5**, 1071–7.

Friedman, E.L., Garnick, M.B., Stomper, P.C. *et al.* (1985) Therapeutic guidelines and results in advanced seminoma. *J. Clin. Oncol.*, **3**, 1325–32.

Green, N., Broth, E., George, F. *et al.* (1983) Radiation therapy in bulky seminoma. *Urology*, **21**, 467–9.

Gregory, C. and Peckman, M.J. (1986) Results of radiotherapy for Stage II testicular seminoma. *Radiother. Oncol.*, **6**, 285–92.

Hahn, E.W., Feingold, S.M. and Niscle, L. (1976) Aspermia and recovery of spermatogenesis in cancer patients following incidental gonadal irradiation during treatment. A progress report. *Radiology*, **119**, 223–5.

Hahn, E.W., Feingold, S.M., Simpson, L. and Batata, M. (1982) Recovery from aspermia induced by low-dose radiation in seminoma patients. *Cancer*, **50**, 337–40.

Hamilton, C., Horwich, A., Easton, D. and

Peckham, M.J. (1986) Radiotherapy for stage I seminoma testis: results of treatment and complications. *Radiother. Oncol.*, **6**, 115–20.

Hanks, G.E., Peters, T. and Owen, J. (1992) Seminoma of the testis: long term beneficial and deleterious results of radiation. *Int. J. Radiat. Oncol. Biol. Phys.*, **24**, 1913–19.

Hay, J.H., Duncan, W. and Kerr, G.R. (1984) Subsequent malignancies in patients irradiated for testicular tumours. *Br. J. Radiol.*, **57**, 597–602.

Herman, J.G., Sturgeon, J. and Thomas, G.M. (1983) Mediastinal prophylactic irradiation in seminoma. *Proc. Am. Soc. Clin. Oncol.*, **2**, 133.

Huben, R.P., Williams, P.D., Pontes, J.E. *et al.* (1984) Seminoma at Roswell Park, 1970 to 1979. An analysis of treatment failures. *Cancer*, **53**, 1451–5.

Javadpour, N. (1980) Management of seminoma based on tumour markers. *Urol. Clin. N. Am.*, **7**, 773–89.

Kubo, H.D. and Shipley, W.U. (1982) Reduction of the scatter dose to the testicle outside the radiation treatment fields. *Int. J. Radiat. Oncol. Biol. Phys.* **8**, 1741–5.

Lederman, G.S., Sheldon, T.A., Chafey, J.T. *et al.* (1987) Cardiac disease after mediastinal radiation for seminoma. *Cancer*, **60**, 772–6.

Lester, S.G., Morphis, J.G. and Hornback, N.B. (1986) Testicular seminoma: analysis of treatment results and failures. *Int. J. Radiat. Oncol. Biol. Phys.*, **12**, 353–8.

Loehrer, P.J., Birch, R. Sr, Williams, S.D. *et al.* (1987) Chemotherapy of metastatic seminoma: the Southeastern Cancer Study Group experience. *J. Clin. Oncol.*, **5**, 1212–20.

Mason, B.R. and Kearsley, J.H. (1988) Radiotherapy for Stage II testicular seminoma: the prognostic influence of tumour bulk. *J. Clin. Oncol.*, **6**, 1956–62.

Motzer, R., Bosl, G., Heelan, R. *et al.* (1987) Residual mass: an indication for further therapy in patients with advanced seminoma following systemic chemotherapy. *J. Clin. Oncol.*, **5**, 1065–70.

Osterland, A., Rørth, M. and Prener, A. (1985) Second cancer following cancer of the male genital system in Denmark, 1943–1980. *Natl. Cancer Inst. Monogr.* **68**, 341–7.

Peckham, M.J. and McElwain, T.J. (1974) Radio-therapy of testicular tumors. *Proc. R. Soc. Med.* **67**, 300–3.

Peckham, M.J., Horwich, A. and Hendry W.F. (1985) Advanced seminoma: treatment with cisplatinum based combination chemotherapy or carboplatin (JM8). *Br. J. Cancer*, **52**, 7–13.

Peckham, M.J., Husband, J.E., Barrett, A. and Hendry, W.F. (1982) Orchidectomy alone in testicular Stage I non-seminomatous germ cell tumours. *Lancet*, **ii**, 678–80.

Raghaven, D., Sullivan, A.L., Peckham, M.J. and Neville, A.M. (1982) Elevated serum alpha feto-protein and seminoma. *Cancer*, **50**, 982–9.

Schmoll, H.J., Harstrick, A., Bokemeyer, C. *et al.* (1993) Single-agent carboplatinum for advanced seminoma. *Cancer*, **72**, 237–43.

Schuette, J., Niederle, N., Schuelen, M.E. *et al.* (1985) Chemotherapy of metastatic seminoma. *Br. J. Cancer*, **51**, 467–72.

Smalley, S.R., Evans, R.G., Richardson, R.L. *et al.* (1985) Radiotherapy as initial treatment for bulky Stage II testicular seminomas. *J. Clin. Oncol.*, **3**, 1333–8.

Srigley, J.R., MacKay, B., Toth, P. and Ayala, A. (1988) The ultrastructure and histogenesis of male germ neoplasia with emphasis on seminoma with early carcinomatous features. *Ultrastruct. Pathol.*, **12**, 67–82.

Stomper, P.C., Jochelson, M.S., Friedman, E.L. *et al.* (1986) CT evaluation of advanced seminoma treated with chemotherapy. *Am. J. Roentgenol.*, **146**, 745–8.

Thomas, G.M. (1985) Controversies in the management of testicular seminoma. *Cancer*, **55**, 2296–302.

Thomas, G.M. (1990) Consensus statement on the investigation and management of testicular seminoma 1989. Prostate Cancer and Testicular Cancer EORTC Genito-Urinary Group Monograph 7.

Thomas, G.M., Rider, W.D., Dembo, A.J. *et al.* (1982) Seminoma of the testis: results of treatment and patterns of failure after radiation therapy. *Int. J. Radiat. Biol. Phys.*, **8**, 165–74.

Zagars, G.K. (1989) The role of radiotherapy in advanced abdominal metastases from testicular seminoma. *Syst. Ther. GU Cancers*, **38**, 292–7.

Zagars, G.K. and Babaian, R.J. (1987) The role of radiation in Stage II testicular seminoma. *Int. J. Radiat. Oncol. Biol. Phys.*, **13**, 163–70.

CHEMOTHERAPY FOR METASTATIC SEMINOMA

L.Y. Dirix and A.T. Van Oosterom

11.1 INTRODUCTION

The curative treatment of seminoma staged as IIB or more consists essentially of chemotherapy, either alone or in combination with surgery and/or radiotherapy. The development of chemotherapy strategies for metastatic seminoma has in general followed those for non-seminomatous germ cell tumors. With the increased awareness of combined seminoma and teratoma, and the more frequent use of tumor marker assays, it is probably less common nowadays that combined tumors are inadvertently included in a series of pure seminomas. Serum chorionic gonadotrophin is raised in 10 to 20% of seminomas. However, 10% of patients with pure seminoma have an elevated beta-chorionic gonadotrophin (BHCG) subunit, which is often associated with the presence of syncytiotrophoblastic cells. In patients with bulky Stage II, Stage III or Stage IV disease these levels can indeed be elevated. Whether these BHCG-producing seminomas are distinct from nonBHCG-producing seminomas in terms of prognosis and treatment is still subject to some controversy (Butcher *et al.*, 1985; Motzer *et al.*, 1988). This could have implications regarding optimal chemotherapeutic strategies.

Another important problem in reporting results of chemotherapy in patients with bulky abdominal or metastatic seminoma is the frequent observation of residual masses after completion of treatment (Motzer *et al.*, 1987; Fosså *et al.*, 1987; Schultz *et al.*, 1989). The majority of these masses tend to resolve spontaneously and this has led to the reporting of disease-free survival or actuarial survival figures, rather than response data.

The overall excellent long-term survival figures of all stages of seminoma following orchidectomy and radiotherapy are largely the reflection of the early stage of presentation, the slow rate of progression and the predictability of the metastatic pathway. The overall survival figures using this approach are of the order of 85%+. These figures rapidly decline for bulky Stage II, Stage III and Stage IV disease. Only 20–40% of patients presenting with Stage III disease are cured with radiotherapy alone (Chapter 10).

11.2 HISTORY OF CHEMOTHERAPY IN METASTATIC SEMINOMA

11.2.1 SINGLE AGENT ACTIVITY IN THE PREPLATINUM ERA

Based on the exquisite radiosensitivity of seminomas, alkylating agents were the first drugs to be selected for the treatment of metastatic disease as a result of their radiomimetic properties. Initial studies from Russia, first reported by Blokhin and later updated by

Testicular Cancer: Investigation and management. Second edition. Edited by Professor A. Horwich.
Published in 1996 by Chapman & Hall. ISBN 0 412 61210 0.

Chebotareva, with phenylalanine mustard (melphalan), reported a response rate of 90%, with 38 out of 42 patients responding. Twenty-five patients died and 16 of the 17 remaining patients remained alive more than 3 years after treatment. In the USA other alkylating drugs have been used with similar results (Golbey, 1970).

Using cyclophosphamide as a single agent, Calman reported six complete responses and four partial responses in 19 treated patients, with a response rate of 53% (Calman, Peckham and Hendry, 1979). Ifosfamide was invest-igated in several Phase II trials but none of them was disease oriented. Niederle used a 5-day regimen with a daily 4-hour infusion of 60–80 mg kg^{-1} in six patients and observed two CR and three PR (Niederle *et al.*, 1983). In a recent literature survey by Schmoll, nine out of 12 patients responded to single agent ifosfamide, suggesting a similar response rate to that achieved by single agent cyclophos-phamide (Schmoll, 1989). These promising results have stimulated the application of ifosfamide in combination chemotherapy (Schuette *et al.*, 1985; Clemm *et al.*, 1994; Amato *et al.*, 1992).

11.2.2 COMBINATION CHEMOTHERAPY IN METASTATIC SEMINOMA

Li and colleagues introduced the first major advance in the treatment of testicular carcin-oma with the combination of actinomycin-D, chlorambucil and methotrexate (Li *et al.*, 1960). These regimens resulted in an object-ive response rate of around 50%. Even more importantly, these responses resulted in the first durable remissions. The history of chemo-therapy regimens in teratocarcinoma changed again significantly with the introduction of vinblastine and bleomycin. Samuels combined both these drugs in his different VBI to III (VB$_1$, VB$_2$, VB$_3$) protocols and introduced the bleo-COMF (cyclophosphamide/vincristine/metho-trexate/5-fluorouracil) program (Samuels *et al.*, 1976).

With the vinblastine/bleomycin combination no durable CR was observed in any of seven treated patients with metastatic seminoma. Complete response was observed in ten out of 18 patients with bleo-COMF combination. However, five of these ten CR relapsed. Treat-ment results with the different VB protocols were better in non-seminomatous germ cell tumors, suggesting a distinct chemosensitivity pattern of seminomas and teratocarcinomas.

11.3 SINGLE AGENT DATA WITH CISPLATIN

Cisplatin (CDDP) was first introduced in clinical Phase I trials in 1972. Its remarkable activity in testicular carcinomas was reported as early as 1974 by Higby. He reported a CR in a patient with seminoma Stage IV disease relapsing after initial treatment with radio-therapy and progressive under actinomycin-D chemotherapy. A CR was achieved with-in 2 weeks after one course of CDDP, 50 mg m^{-2} d^{-1} for 2 days every 3 weeks (Higby *et al.*, 1974). In 1983, Oliver reported his first results with single agent CDDP at a dose of 50 mg m^{-2} twice every 3 weeks. He observed seven out of eight CR with one relapsing patient receiving successful salvage bleomycin/etoposide/cisplatin (BEP) combina-tion chemotherapy. In his latest report on 27 previously untreated patients receiving single agent CDDP, continuously disease-free survival was 77% (85% alive) after a follow-up of 5 years (Oliver, 1988). Long-term results are invariably less excellent in patients relapsing after prior radiotherapy; however, a majority of these were eventually salvaged with cisplatin/vinblastine/bleomycin (PVB) or BEP combination chemotherapy. Samuels has treated the majority of patients with advanced seminoma with a combination of cyclophosphamide and sequential cis-platin. However, he also reports his results with single agent CDDP by a weekly infusion of 100 mg^{-1} in eight patients. All eight remain free of disease (Logothetis *et al.*, 1987).

From these data it can be concluded that seminomatous germ cell tumors are exquisitely sensitive to cisplatin, achieving single agent response rates rarely observed with any solid tumor.

11.4 SINGLE AGENT DATA WITH CARBOPLATIN

Carboplatin (JM8, CBDCA) is one of several platinum analogues that have been tested clinically since 1981. It has several advantages over CDDP, including a less pronounced nephrotoxicity, ototoxicity and neurotoxicity, and better gastrointestinal tolerance. This in general allows for outpatient administration. On the other hand, myelosuppression, and more specifically thrombocytopenia, is more severe.

Since 1982, patients with metastatic seminoma have been treated at the Royal Marsden Hospital with single agent carboplatin 400 mg m^{-2} every 3–4 weeks for four to six courses. Between 1982 and 1990, 70 patients have been treated with a median follow-up at time of reporting of 3 years (Peckham, Horwich and Hendry, 1985; Horwich *et al.*, 1992). Sixteen patients had relapsed and 4 of these have died. Of the 16 patients that relapsed, 12 have been salvaged with combination chemotherapy. The risk of relapse was clearly reduced in the latter part of this study by introducing postchemotherapy radiotherapy to involved nodes. In 20 patients treated with postchemotherapy irradiation only one relapse was observed, versus a relapse in 11 out of 31 Stage II or III patients who had completed four cycles of carboplatinum and could have been treated with extended radiotherapy.

A similar approach was used in 21 patients with Stage IIA and IIB disease. They were treated with a single course of carboplatin 400 mg m^{-2} followed by radiotherapy. All patients achieved complete remission after a median follow-up of 34 months (Yao *et al.*, 1994). Another mature report is the study by Schmoll *et al.* whereby carboplatin 400 mg m^{-2} was given as an outpatient infusion in 42 patients with IIC+ seminoma (Schmoll *et al.*, 1993). All patients received six cycles unless CR was observed after the first cycle; in these patients five cycles were deemed sufficient. A CR or PR was achieved in 38 (90%) patients. Relapse occurred in eight of these, 5/30 with an initial CR and 3/8 with an initial PR. With carboplatin alone, 30 patients were continuously free from relapse or progression (71%). The overall survival after salvage therapy was 93% (40/42).

The conclusion of both these studies must be that between 70 and 80% of patients with advanced seminoma can be cured with single agent carboplatinum, and that the majority of those relapsing can be rescued with a cisplatinum-based combination regimen.

11.5 CISPLATIN-BASED COMBINATION CHEMOTHERAPY

Chemotherapy in metastatic seminoma has in general been based on regimens used in non-seminomatous testicular cancer. After the introduction of the different vinblastine and bleomycin combinations by Samuels, the group at the Memorial Sloan-Kettering Cancer Center (MSKCC) added actinomycin-D to the VB combination, giving birth to the first of six VAB schedules.

In the mid 1970s, it became obvious that the addition of cisplatin resulted in superior response rates in the treatment of teratocarcinomas. Different modifications of the initial VAB protocol resulted in 1979 in the VAB-6 regimen at MSKCC. As well as the three initial drugs in the VAB-1 scheme, cyclophosphamide and cisplatin were added. In their first seven patients with metastatic seminoma, a 100% CR rate was observed, with two patients relapsing, however (Vugrin and Whitmore, 1984). The activity of this regimen has been substantiated by follow-up studies and the Sao Paolo experience (Table 11.1)

Table 11.1 Results with vinblastine/actinomycin-D/bleomycin/cis-platin/cyclophosphamide in advanced seminoma

Author	n	CR (%)	Progression-free survival
Simon *et al.* (1983)	10	10 (100%)	10 (100%)
Mencel *et al.* (1994)	43	34 (70%)	34 (79%)

(Simon *et al.*, 1983; Bosl *et al.*, 1986; Motzer *et al.*, 1988; Mencel *et al.*, 1994).

Between 1977 and 1984, Samuels and Logothetis at M.D. Anderson treated 52 patients with advanced seminoma with cisplatin as single agent in eight patients and in combination with cyclophosphamide in the remaining 44 cases (Logothetis *et al.*, 1987). With chemotherapy alone 44 out of 52 (85%) achieved CR, with four other patients being salvaged with other chemotherapy regimens or radiotherapy. This adds up to an impressive CR rate of 92% with these 48 patients being alive with no evidence of disease with a median follow-up of well over 3 years. It is, however, impossible from their data to draw a conclusion concerning the contribution of cyclophosphamide to these results. It seems more probable that these excellent results are due to their intensive cisplatin regimen of 100 mg m^{-2} once a week for 3 weeks. This was not, however, associated with major toxicity, except for neurotoxicity in 16 patients. A recent update from their results and the Mexican data confirm the excellent activity of this peculiar regimen (Dexeus *et al.*, 1990, Zinser *et al.*, 1993).

Cisplatin was first introduced in combination chemotherapy against testicular cancer by Einhorn and Donehue (1977) with the combination of vinblastine and bleomycin (PVB) and PVB with Adriamycin (doxorubicin hydrochloride) (PVBA). In one of their first publications these combinations were applied to 19 patients with metastatic seminoma (Mendenhall *et al.*, 1981). A CR was observed in 12/19 (65%) with no relapses after at least 1 year's follow-up. These results were superior to all previously used regimens in metastatic sem-

inoma, and PVB was established as the first choice combination regimen for metastatic seminoma.

A multicenter study from the Netherlands, Spain and the USA applied this regimen in 80 patients with advanced seminoma. All but eight of these patients received PVB; those eight were treated with PVBA. In the latest update, Van Oosterom *et al.* (1986) reported 61 complete responses with chemotherapy alone, with six PR rendered CR after consolidation radiotherapy. Fifty-seven (71%) were alive with no evidence of disease. The best results were obtained in the group of 42 patients who had received no prior radio- or chemotherapy. The toxicity of this regimen, however, was considerable, and myelotoxicity was very pronounced in patients who received prior radiotherapy. Three patients died of neutropenic septicemia and two as a result of progressive pulmonary toxicity, giving five out of 80 treatment-related deaths.

Several other reports have corroborated these results. In many studies vinblastine was later replaced by etoposide, changing PVB into BEP. In most publications detailed analysis of results obtained with either PVB or BEP are lacking. It should, however, be evident from Table 11.2 that, from those studies where these details are given, results with BEP are at least as good as those with PVB. In an attempt to decrease acute and long-term toxicity of chemotherapy, modifications have been made to the original PVB regimen.

The first was the replacement of vinblastine with etoposide in order to decrease neurotoxicity. In a randomized study from the Southeastern Cancer Study Group, 244 evaluable

Table 11.2 Results with cisplatin/vinblastine/bleomycin (PVB) and/or bleomycin/etoposide/cisplatin (BEP or EP) in advanced seminoma

Author	Regimen	n	CR (%)	Survival (%)
Mendenhall *et al.* (1981)	PVB(A)	19	19 (63%)	–
Oliver *et al.* (1983)	PVB/BEP	12	10 (83%)	10 (83%)
Friedman *et al.* (1985)	PVB/BEP	20	18 (90%)	16 (80%)
Peckham, Horwich and Hendry (1985)	PVB	8	8 (100%)	7 (87%)
Peckham, Horwich and Hendry (1985)	BEP	25	25 (100%)	24 (96%)
Van Oosterom *et al.* (1986)	PVB(A)	80	67 (84%)	57 (71%)
Pizzocaro *et al.* (1986)	PVB/BEP	31	24 (78%)	23 (74%)
Fosså *et al.* (1987)	PVB/BEP	54	49 (90%)	42 (78%)
Loehrer *et al.* (1987)	PVB(A)/BEP	60	41 (68%)	37 (66%)
Gietema *et al.* (1991)	PVB+BEP	30	30 (100%)	26 (79%)
Mencel *et al.* (1994)	EP	60	51 (85%)	55 (92%)

patients were randomized between PVB and BEP (Williams *et al.*, 1987). The BEP regimen was equally myelotoxic, but less neurotoxic, and was capable of inducing a significantly greater proportion of complete remissions in patients with advanced disease. This difference was also significant in survival terms in this poor prognosis group. Responses for patients with seminoma, 19 treated with PVB and 22 treated with BEP, were similar. Pulmonary toxicity was identical in both treatment arms.

The second modification concerned the role of bleomycin. At MSKCC patients with seminoma have been treated with a combination of cisplatin and etoposide, omitting bleomycin altogether. In their latest update on 60 patients treated with etoposide and cisplatin, 55 of them achieved a durable response with that regimen as the sole treatment. This compares favorably with the experience with the VAB-6 and etoposide–carboplatin regimen used by the same group (Mencel *et al.*, 1994). These results indicate that the EP regimen is equally as effective as PVB or BEP, and because of its decreased toxicity it is currently accepted as the treatment of choice.

Others, however, have attempted to use alternating cycles of the PVB and the BEP regimen in an attempt to improve the complete response rate and survival. Gietema *et al.* (1991) have treated 33 patients, of whom 30 are evaluable for response, and observed 13 CRs (43%) and 17 PRs (57%) with three patients relapsing after a median follow-up of 28 months. The hematological toxicity was severe with Grade IV leuko- and or thrombocytopenia occurring in 61% of the patients. There were three treatment-related deaths. In total, 26 of 33 (79%) of patients are continuously disease free.

Other groups have used a cisplatin–ifosfamide combination up front, attempting to improve response rates and survival (Table 11.3). Clemm *et al.* (1986) have investigated the efficacy of the VIP combination with cisplatin 20 mg m^{-2} and ifosfamide 1.5 mg m^{-2} both from days 1–5, and vinblastine 6 mg m^{-2} on days 1 and 2. Later on vinblastine was substituted with etoposide 75 mg m^{-2} on days 1–5. This regimen was highly effective with 47 out of 51 evaluable patients reaching a CR, usually after four cycles. This regimen achieved a 92% (47 of 51) no evidence of disease status with a median follow-up of 50 months. Fosså *et al.* (1995) for the EORTC genitourinary group have investigated the HOP regimen with ifosfamide 1.2 gr m^{-2} and cisplatin 20 mg m^{-2} from days 1–5. This was combined with vincristine 2 mg on day 1 in an attempt to avoid excessive hematological toxicity in these often preirradiated patients. This regimen was investigated in 42 patients

Table 11.3   Results of ifosfamide/platinum combinations in advanced seminoma

Author	Regimen	n	CR (%)	PR (%)	Survival (%) disease-free
Schuette *et al.* (1985)	IP	7	7 (100%)	–	7 (100%)
Schuette *et al.* (1985)	EI	7	6 (85%)	1 (15%)	6 (85%)
Amato *et al.* (1992)	Carbo/Ifos (±S/RT)	28	15 (54%)	12 (43%)	27 (97%)
Fosså *et al.* (1994)	HOP	42	26 (65%)	11 (28%)	38 (90%)
Clemm *et al.* (1986)	VIP	16	14 (88%)	1 (6%)	15 (93%)

and was very active, with 26 CRs (65%) and 11 PRs (28%). Toxicity was substantial, with ten patients experiencing neutropenic fever.

11.6   CONCLUSIONS

The majority of patients with seminoma will continue to be treated successfully with orchidectomy and prophylactic (Stage I) radiotherapy. Many very active chemotherapeutic regimens have been identified to treat successfully the rare patient relapsing after this strategy. The treatment of choice for patients with locally advanced or metastatic disease is chemotherapy. The combination with etoposide and cisplatin continues to be the first line choice. The observations made with single agent carboplatinum with consolidation radiotherapy or surgery offers a reasonable alternative. Whether this is truly comparable with the etoposide–cisplatin combination is the subject of two different ongoing trials. The superior toxicity profile of monotherapy with carboplatinum has to be put into perspective against the obligation of more and longer surveillance because of the increased risk of relapse. At present because of lack of reliable prognostic factors other than bulk of disease, it remains impossible to tailor treatment regimens for individual patients.

REFERENCES

Amato, R., Adelman, K., Sella, R. *et al.* (1992) High cure rate (97%) with carboplatin (CBDCA) ifosfamide (IFX) and selective consolidation in advanced seminoma. *Proc. Am. Soc. Clin. Oncol.*, p. 202 (Abstract 623).

Bosl, G.J., Gluckman, R., Geller, N.L. *et al.* (1986) VAB-6: an effective chemotherapy regimen for patients with germ cell tumors. *J. Clin. Oncol.*, **4**, 1493–9.

Butcher, D.N., Gregory, W.M., Gunter, P.A. *et al.* (1985) The biological significance of HCG-containing cells in seminoma. *Br. J. Cancer*, **51**, 473–8.

Calman, F.M.B., Peckham, M.J. and Hendry, W.F. (1979). The pattern of spread and treatment of metastases in testicular seminoma. *Br. J. Urol.*, **51**, 154–60.

Clemm, Ch., Gerl, A., Hentrich, M. and Wilmanns, W. (1994). Combination chemotherapy in bulky seminoma. *Ann. Oncol.*, **5**(S8), p. 69 (Abstract 342).

Clemm, Ch., Hartenstein, R., Willich, N. *et al.* (1986) Vinblastine–ifosfamide–cisplatin treatment of bulky seminoma. *Cancer*, **58**, 2203–7.

Dexeus, F.H., Finn, L., Eftekhari, F. *et al.* (1990) Cyclophosphamide and cisplatin (CP) for advanced seminoma (S); follow-up and radiographic correlation of residual masses. *Proc. Am. Ass. Cancer Res.*, p 187 (Abstract 1113).

Einhorn, L.H. and Donohue, J.D. (1977) Cisdiamminedichloroplatinum, vinblastine and bleomycin combination chemotherapy in disseminated testicular cancer. *Ann. Intern. Med.*, **87**, 293–8.

Fosså, S.D., Borge, L., Aass, N. *et al.* (1987) The treatment of advanced metastatic seminoma: experience in 55 cases. *J. Clin. Oncol.*, **5**, 1071–7.

Fosså, S.D., Droz, J-P., Stoter, G. *et al.* (1995) Cisplatin, vincristine and ifosfamide combination chemotherapy of metastatic seminoma. *Brit. J. Cancer*, **71**, 619–24.

Friedman, E.L., Garnick, M.B., Stomper, P.C. *et al.* (1985) Therapeutic guidelines and results in advanced seminoma. *J. Clin. Oncol.*, **3**, 1325–32.

Gietema, J.A., Willemse, P.H.B., Mulder, N.H. *et al.* (1991) Alternating cycles of PVB and BEP in the treatment of patients with advanced seminoma. *Eur. J. Cancer*, **27**, 1376–9.

Golbey, R.B. (1970) The place of chemotherapy in the treatment of testicular tumors. *JAMA*, **213**, 101–3.

Higby, D.J., Wallace, H.J., Albert, D.J. and Holland, J.F. (1974) Diamminodichloroplatinum: a Phase I study showing responses in testicular and other tumours. *Cancer*, **33**, 1219–25.

Horwich, A., Dearnaley, D.P., A'Hern, R. *et al.* (1992) The activity of single-agent carboplatin in advanced seminoma. *Eur. J. Cancer*, **28**, 1307–10.

Li, M., Whitmore, W., Golbey, R. and Grabstald, H. (1960) Effects of combined drug therapy on metastatic cancer of the testis. *JAMA*, **174**, 1291–9.

Loehrer, P.J., Birch, R., Williams, S.D. *et al.* (1987) Chemotherapy of metastatic seminoma: the Southeastern Cancer Study Group experience. *J. Clin. Oncol.* **5**, 1210–20.

Logothetis, C.J., Samuels, M.L., Ogden, S.L. *et al.* (1987) Cyclophosphamide and sequential cisplatin for advanced seminoma: long-term follow-up in 52 patients. *J. Urol.*, **138**, 789–94.

Mencel, P., Motzer, R.J., Mazumdar, M. *et al.* (1994) Advanced seminoma: treatment results, survival, and prognostic factors in 142 patients. *J. Clin. Oncol.*, **12**, 120–6.

Mendenhall, W.L., Williams, S.D., Einhorn, L.H. and Donohue, J.P. (1981) Disseminated seminoma: re-evaluation of treatment protocols. *J. Urol.*, **126**, 493–6.

Motzer, R.J., Bosl, G.L., Geller, N.L. *et al.* (1988) Advanced seminoma: the role of chemotherapy and adjunctive surgery. *Ann. Intern. Med.*, **108**, 513–18.

Motzer, R., Bosl, G., Heelan, R. *et al.* (1987) Residual mass: an indication for further therapy in patients with advanced seminoma following systemic chemotherapy. *J. Clin. Oncol.* **5**, 1064–70.

Niederle, N., Scheulen, M.E., Cremer, M. *et al.* (1983) Ifosfamide in combination chemotherapy for sarcomas and testicular carcinomas. *Cancer Treat. Rev.*, **10**, 129–35 (Suppl. A).

Oliver, R.T.D. *et al.* (1983) Cisplatinum in combination or as single agent for metastatic seminoma of the testis or dysgerminoma of the ovary. *Proc. Am. Soc. Clin. Oncol.*, p. 144 (Abstract C-564).

Oliver, R.T.D. *et al.* (1988) Long term follow-up of single agent cisplatin in metastatic seminoma and surveillance for stage 1 seminoma. *Proc. Am. Soc. Clin. Oncol.*, p. 120, (Abstract C-463).

Van Oosterom, A.T., Williams, S.D., Cortes Funes, H. *et al.* (1986) The treatment of metastatic seminoma with combination chemotherapy, in *Germ Cell Tumours II* (eds W.G. Jones, A.M. Ward and C.K. Anderson), Pergamon Press, Oxford, pp. 229–33.

Peckham, M.J., Horwich, A. and Hendry, W.F. (1985) Advanced seminoma: treatment with cisplatinum-based combination chemotherapy or carboplatin (JM8). *Br. J. Cancer*, **52**, 7–13.

Pizzocaro, G., Salvioni, R., Oiva, L. *et al.* (1986) Cisplatin combination chemotherapy in advanced seminoma. *Cancer*, **58**, 1625–9.

Samuels, M.L., Lanzotti, V.J., Holoye, P.Y. *et al.* (1976) Combination chemotherapy in germinal cell tumours. *Cancer Treat. Rev.*, **3**, 185–204.

Schmoll, H.J. (1989) Ifosfamide in testicular cancer. *Sem. Oncol.*, **16**, 82–95.

Schmoll, H.J., Harstrick, A., Bokemeyer, C. *et al.* (1993) Single-agent carboplatinum for advanced seminoma. *Cancer*, **72**, 237–43.

Schuette, J., Niederle, N., Scheulen, M.E. *et al.* (1985) Chemotherapy for metastatic seminoma. *Br. J. Cancer*, **51**, 467–72.

Schultz, S.M., Einhorn, L.H., Conces, D.J. *et al.* (1989) Management of postchemotherapy residual mass in patients with advanced seminoma: Indiana University experience. *J. Clin. Oncol.*, **7**, 1497–503.

Simon, S.D., Srougi, M. and Goes, G.M. (1983) Treatment of advanced seminoma with vinblastine, actinomycin-D, cyclophosphamide and cis-platinum. *Proc. Am. Soc. Clin. Oncol.*, **132** (Abstract C-157).

Vugrin, D. and Whitmore, W.F. (1984) The VAB-6 regimen in the treatment of metastatic seminoma. *Cancer*, **53**, 2422–4.

Williams, S.D., Birch, R., Einhorn, L.H. *et al.* (1987) Treatment of disseminated germ-cell tumors with cisplatin, bleomycin and either vinblastine or etoposide. *N. Engl. J. Med.*, **316**, 1435–40.

Yao, W.Q., Fosså, S.D., Dearnaley, D.P. and Horwich, A. (1994). Combined single course carboplatin with radiotherapy in treatment of Stage IIA,B seminoma – a preliminary report. *Radioth. Oncol.*, **33**, 88–90.

Zinser, J.W., Mendoza, A., Gaona, R. *et al.* (1993). Advanced seminoma (S) treated with chemotherapy (CT). *Fourth International Congress on Anti-cancer Chemotherapy*, p. 103 (Abstract C-180).

RESPONSE EVALUATION IN SEMINOMA

12

S.D. Fosså

12.1 INTRODUCTION

Evaluation of response to treatment of any malignancy enables the clinician to estimate the necessity of further treatment and the intensity of follow-up, and allows comparison of treatment results. Response to treatment is, furthermore, often correlated with survival. In a strict sense, response to treatment can only be defined in patients with metastatic lesions that are measurable by clinical, radiological and, as far as tumor markers are concerned, by biochemical methods.

For measurable and evaluable metastatic lesions from testicular cancer the World Health Organization (WHO) criteria for objective response are usually applied (Miller *et al.*, 1981). The response criteria concerning serum tumor markers are not uniformly defined. In Phase II studies where the efficacy of a drug is evaluated a 90% reduction of serum tumor markers is sometimes regarded as a partial remission (PR) (Kaye *et al.*, 1988). Time to progression (PD) and survival are additional indicators for the effectiveness of a treatment.

The WHO criteria (Miller *et al.*, 1981) refer to measurements based on clinical and radiological examinations. They do not take into account histopathological changes that may develop during therapy. Complete necrosis of tumor tissue due to effective treatment (complete response, CR) does not always lead to disappearance or size reduction of the metastatic lesion. This is a frequent observation in advanced non-seminomatous testicular cancer (Donohue *et al.*, 1987; Fosså *et al.*, 1989b). On the other hand, a negative abdominal computed tomography (CT) scan after chemotherapy of non-seminoma does not preclude the possibility of residual malignant tumor tissue or mature teratoma (Fosså *et al.*, 1989a). In seminoma patients with initially large retroperitoneal tumor masses the persistence of residual masses after chemotherapy is the rule rather than the exception, although the clinical course and/or histological examination prove that about 80% of the residual masses are tumor free. These observations render the application of the WHO criteria especially problematic in advanced seminoma.

The present chapter deals firstly with specific problems of evaluation of treatment of advanced seminoma differing between biochemical response, clinical response, histopathological response, secondly with the need for postchemotherapy consolidation treatment, and thirdly with progression-free and overall survival.

12.2 BIOCHEMICAL RESPONSE

12.2.1 LACTATE DEHYDROGENASE

Serum lactate dehydrogenase (LDH) and especially its isoenzyme LDH-1, has frequently

Testicular Cancer: Investigation and management. Second edition. Edited by Professor A. Horwich.
Published in 1996 by Chapman & Hall. ISBN 0 412 61210 0.

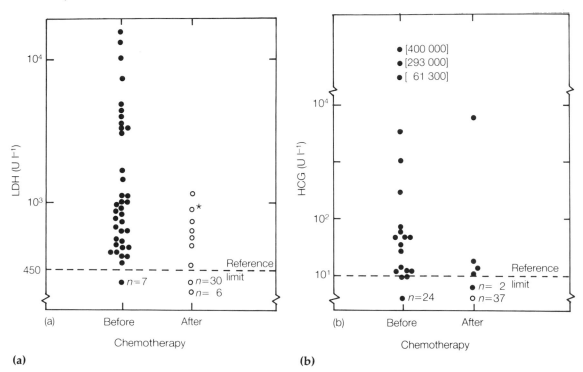

(a)   **(b)**

Fig. 12.1   (a) Serum lactate dehydrogenase (LDH) and (b) human chorionic gonadotrophin (HCG) in patients with advanced metastatic seminoma before and after chemotherapy. ●, patients with tumor manifestations; ○, patients without tumor manifestations. (Reproduced from Fosså and Fosså, 1989, *Br. J. Urol.*, **63**, 408, with permission of the Editor.)

been discussed as a tumor marker for seminoma. Lactate dehydrogenase is a glycolytic enzyme found in all living cells. Its activity in serum is increased in a number of malignant and nonmalignant diseases. Situations causing an increased leakage from cells or cell death lead to evaluated serum LDH levels. The reasons for the increase of LDH activity associated with cancer are still unknown (von Eyben, 1983; Taylor, Duncan and Horn, 1986; von Eyben *et al.*, 1988; Fosså and Fosså, 1989).

After orchidectomy and before further treatment LDH is elevated in about 80% of patients with metastases (Fig. 12.1a). During effective treatment serum LDH becomes normal in most patients, but about 15% of the tumor-free patients have slightly elevated LDH values immediately after chemotherapy (Fig.

12.1a). Thus, slight elevations of serum LDH do not count against complete response. Furthermore, during follow-up 7–25% of the seminoma patients without evidence of disease have temporarily slightly raised LDH serum levels (Taylor, Duncan and Horn, 1986; Fosså and Fosså, 1989) leading to a predictive value of elevated LDH of 83% (Table 12.1). In addition, during follow-up LDH remains normal in one-third of the relapsing seminoma patients (Table 12.2).

12.2.2   HUMAN CHORIONIC GONADOTROPHIN

Serum human chorionic gonadotrophin (HCG) elevations are found in 5–49% of seminoma patients (Paus *et al.*, 1988). The considerable interstudy variations are due to differences

Table 12.1 Specificity, sensitivity and predictive value of elevated lactate dehydrogenase (LDH) and human chorionic gonadotrophin (HCG) in seminoma

	HCG (%)	LDH (%)
Specificity	100	93.2
Sensitivity	31.9	46.7
Predictive value*	100	82.9

* Of positive tests.

Table 12.2 Serum lactate dehydrogenase (LDH) and human chorionic gonadotrophin (HCG) in seminoma patients at the time of diagnosis of recurrence of disease after previous cytotoxic treatment

LDH (IU l⁻¹)	HCG (U l⁻¹)			
	<10	10–<200	>200	Total
<450	5	1	1	7
450–<550	3	0	0	3
≥550	12	9	2	23
Total	20	10	3	33

between patient selection criteria with respect to tumor stage, prior treatment and time schedules for the HCG examinations, as well as differences in assay specificities. The use of a radioimmunoassay which measures intact as well as HCG split products yields a particularly high frequency of seminoma patients with HCG elevations (Paus *et al.*, 1988). Human chorionic gonadotrophin is a tumor marker with high specificity in patients with seminoma (Table 12.1), although other malignant diseases also occasionally lead to increased HCG serum levels. So far there is no evidence that slight or moderate serum HCG elevations in patients with histologically pure seminoma should alter the planned treatment (Swartz, Johnsen and Hussey, 1984; Mirimanoff *et al.*, 1985). Very high HCG levels are sometimes seen in patients with large metastases and indicate the presence of non-seminomatous elements.

Human chorionic gonadotrophin becomes

normal in all patients with advanced seminoma who respond completely to chemotherapy (Fig. 12.1b). During effective treatment of advanced seminoma transient elevations of serum HCG may occasionally occur as a result of tumor cell death and sudden release of large quantities of HCG (Paus *et al.*, 1987). Serum HCG is elevated in about half of the relapsing patients at the time of recurrence (Table 12.2).

12.2.3 PLACENTAL-LIKE ALKALINE PHOSPHATASE

Placental-like alkaline phosphatase (PLAP) is a polymorphic glycoprotein and can be demonstrated at trace amounts in the normal human testis.

Using polyclonal antisera, elevated serum levels of PLAP have been found in a number of malignancies (pancreas, lung, breast), but in particular in testicular cancer and ovarian cancer (Wahren, Holmgren and Stigbrand, 1979; Lange *et al.*, 1982; Javadpour, 1983; Nørgaard-Pedersen *et al.*, 1984; Horwich, Tucker and Peckham, 1985). Using a monoclonal antibody (Millán *et al.*, 1982) 80–100% of the patients with active seminoma displayed raised PLAP serum levels. However even monoclonal antibodies cross-react with PLAP-like proteins, which are frequently elevated in smokers (Epenetos *et al.*, 1985, Tucker *et al.*, 1985). Currently, there is no monoclonal antibody for PLAP available which discriminates between patients with active seminoma and healthy nonsmokers. Development of such a specific antibody against the 'germ cell alkaline phosphatase' may represent a step to higher accuracy of PLAP estimation (Millán and Manes, 1988). Today the high frequency of false positive values limits the clinical use of serum PLAP for response evaluation and during follow-up.

Nevertheless, elevated levels of serum PLAP in a patient with a history of seminoma, especially if the levels gradually increase, should always lead to the suspicion of disease activity, even in the absence of other signs of tumor manifestations (Lange *et al.*, 1982; Tucker *et al.*, 1985).

12.2.4 NEURON-SPECIFIC ENOLASE

Neuron-specific enolase (NSE) has been claimed to be a valuable marker for response of seminoma (Kuzmits, Schernthaner and Krisch, 1987). Increased serum NSE activity was measured in 73% of the patients with metastatic seminoma. Elevated serum NSE became normal during effective chemotherapy. Fosså, Klepp and Paus (1992) have confirmed the usefulness of serum NSE as a response monitor in individual patients with advanced seminoma. From a practical point of view, NSE determination is recommended, if a clinical situation leaves any doubt about disease activity in a patient with seminoma.

12.2.5 COMBINATION OF MARKERS

In an individual patient discordant behavior of serum markers for seminoma can be observed both at the time of diagnosis or at response evaluation and at the time of relapse (Table 12.2). Treatment for relapse diagnosed by serum marker elevation should only be initiated if **repeated** serum samples have shown elevated and preferably increasing values.

12.2.6 SUMMARY

In summary, in clinical practice LDH and especially HCG are useful tumor markers in biochemical response evaluation of the treatment of advanced seminoma. A complete response requires a normal serum HCG level. Serum LDH can occasionally be slightly elevated in tumor-free patients. In nonsmokers, PLAP determined by monoclonal radioimmunoassays may have a role for response monitoring. NSE may occasionally be useful in a clinically doubtful situation.

12.3 CLINICAL RESPONSE

The response category of major interest is complete response (CR) consisting of the complete disappearance of tumor manifestations. The clinician should be aware that normal retroperitoneal lymph nodes may be visible by abdominal CT up to a size of 15 mm (Lien *et al.*, 1983). Complete response of retroperitoneal tumor therefore means that there is no visible mass at all or that the size of any residual mass should not exceed 15 mm on a transverse CT plane. After chemotherapy of advanced seminoma the clinical CR rate is 10–25%, dependent on the bulk of the initial tumor (Peckham, Horwich and Hendry, 1985; Fosså *et al.*, 1989c) (Fig. 12.2). Sometimes it is difficult to define the clinical response category based on CT: not infrequently a diffuse thickening of the retroperitoneal structures without any discrete mass can be seen after treatment for advanced seminoma (Fig. 12.3). The significance of a clinically assessed partial remission (PR) in seminoma remains unknown in the individual patient. In 50–70% of the cases residual masses are seen immediately after chemotherapy for advanced seminoma (Fig. 12.4). One-third of the masses persist for several months after subsequent radiotherapy (Fosså *et al.*, 1989c).

The categories 'no change' and 'progression' based on measurements of metastatic lesions are rare in previously untreated seminoma patients. Loehrer *et al.* (1987) combined these two response categories into a 'no-response' category.

12.4 HISTOPATHOLOGICAL RESPONSE

The optimal means to demonstrate a CR is the histopathological confirmation of the absence of tumor tissue after treatment. This requires a complete resection of the residual masses. It is not considered to be sufficient to do multiple biopsies as small tumor foci may be missed. However, in seminoma patients

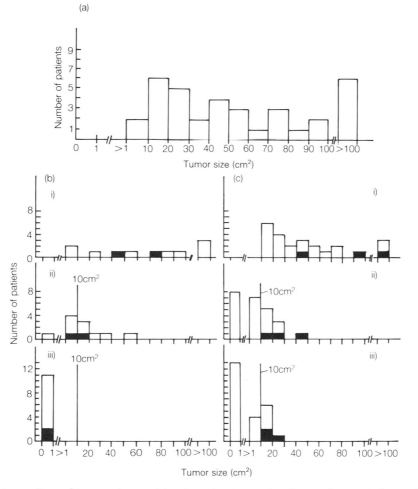

Fig. 12.2 Retroperitoneal tumor size and treatment outcome in advanced metastatic seminoma. (a) All retroperitoneal tumors before treatment (*n* = 35). (b) Retroperitoneal tumors with postchemotherapy surgery (*n* = 11). (c) Retroperitoneal tumors with postchemotherapy radiotherapy (*n* = 24). (i) Before treatment, (ii) 3–4 weeks after chemotherapy, (iii) 8–12 weeks after consolidation treatment. ■, patients with chemotherapy failure. (Reproduced from Fosså *et al.* 1989c, *Br. J. Urol.*, **64**, 530, with permission of the Editor.)

postchemotherapy surgery, for example, retroperitoneal lymph node dissection, is difficult from a technical point of view due to pronounced fibrotic changes (Friedman *et al.*, 1985; Fosså *et al.*, 1987; Loehrer *et al.*, 1987). Such surgery inherits a greater risk of major postoperative complications than is usually seen in non-seminoma patients. In addition, only 10–20% of resected lesions contain resid-

ual malignant tumor (Table 12.3). According to Motzer *et al.* (1988) lesions with a diameter less than 3 cm are less likely to contain vital seminoma than larger ones. This is in agreement with Fosså *et al.* (1989c) who showed that patients with residual retroperitoneal masses ≥10 cm^2 are more likely to relapse than those with smaller lesions (Fig. 12.3). However, neither Schultz *et al.* (1988) nor Horwich *et al.*

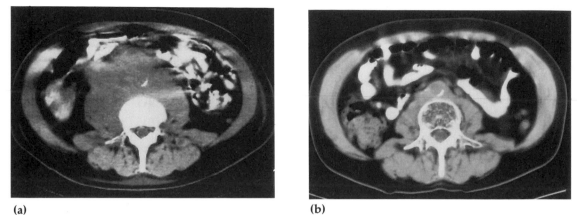

(a)   **(b)**

Fig. 12.3 Diffuse thickening of the retroperitoneal structures 3 years after treatment for advanced seminoma. (a) Before treatment. (b) After treatment.

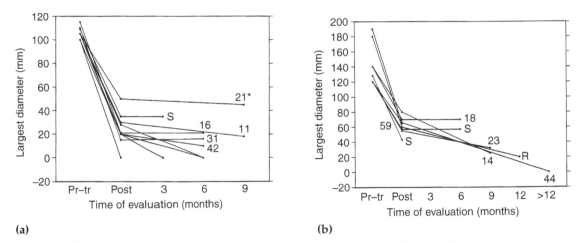

(a)   **(b)**

Fig. 12.4 Size changes in non-irradiated metastatic lymph nodes in patients with advanced seminoma treated with combination chemotherapy (ifosphamide, vincristine, cisplatin). (a) Infradiaphragmatic lesions 100–19 mm before chemotherapy. (b) Infradiaphragmatic lesions ≥ 120 mm before chemotherapy. S, consolidation surgery; R, consolidation radiotherapy; * Observation time (in months) without consolidation treatment after the last measurement of residual masses. (Reproduced from Fosså *et al.*, 1995, *Br. J. Cancer*, **71**(3), 619–24, with permission of the Editor.)

(1989) could find such relationship between the size of the residual mass and chemotherapy failure.

With the background of the low risk of residual malignant tumor and the high risk of postoperative complications, the need for surgical consolidation treatment has been questioned. Today most authors recommend not performing postchemotherapy resection routinely (Peckham, Horwich and Hendry, 1985; Loehrer *et al.*, 1987). As only 10–20% of the patients have residual seminoma, it also seems unjustifiable to apply radiotherapy to *all* patients with CT-visible tumor masses immediately after chemotherapy. If chemotherapy subsequently proves to be necessary

Table 12.3 Postchemotherapy histology

Reference	Number of patients	Fibrosis/necrosis	Vital malignant tumor
Peckham, Horwich and Hendry (1985)	4	4	0
Stanton *et al.* (1985)	10	9	1
Friedman *et al.* (1985)	3	3	0
Pizzocaro *et al.* (1986)	14	13	1
Fosså *et al.* (1987)	12	9	3
Loehrer *et al.* (1987)	13	10	3
Soo *et al.* (1981)	2	2	0
Jones *et al.* (1982)	1	0	3
de Kernion and Lupu (1977)	2	1	1
Simon, Srougi and de Góes (1983)	7	7	0
Oliver *et al.* (1983)	7	4	3
Ellison, Mostofi and Flanagan (1988)	1	0	1
Wilkinson, Read and Magee (1988)	3	3	0
Motzer *et al.* (1987; 1988)	24	18	6
Clemm *et al.* (1989)	9	9	0
Srougi, Simon and de Góes (1985)	7	7	0
Total	119	99	20 (17%)

this may be difficult because of the increased risk of myelosuppression due to the previous radiotherapy. Furthermore, the effect of post-chemotherapy consolidation treatment must be balanced against the observation that patients with advanced seminoma, recurring after primary chemotherapy, not infrequently relapse at sites not identical with the initial tumor manifestations (Fosså *et al.*, 1989c). In addition, there is evidence that long-term toxicity increases after combined chemo- and radiotherapy (Aass *et al.*, 1990).

As advanced seminoma is rare it is extremely difficult to perform randomized trials which can definitely decide on the necessity and timing of optimal postchemotherapy consolidation treatment. In this situation, and with the present knowledge of the tumor biology of advanced seminoma, it is recommended that patients with residual masses after chemomotherapy should be observed for several months rather than resect the tumor immediately. If large tumors persist and there are no significant contraindications against major surgery, resection of residual masses may be considered after 6–10 months.

If such surgery is not possible and the compliance to attend frequent follow-up examinations is questionable, radiotherapy may be applied in cases of residual masses.

12.5 PROGRESSION-FREE SURVIVAL AND OVERALL SURVIVAL

Owing to the clinical difficulties in defining complete remission in seminoma patients, many authors and protocols for advanced seminoma use progression-free survival as the principal endpoint of treatment, regardless of whether the patients obtain a clinical CR or PR. About 10% of the patients will progress after having developed a remission on primary chemotherapy (Peckham, Horwich and Hendry 1985; Fosså *et al.*, 1987; Loehrer *et al.*, 1987). Although most of the recurrences in advanced seminoma are detected within the first 3 years after cytotoxic treatment, late recurrences may be seen occasionally and indicate the necessity for long-term follow-up in these patients (Borge *et al.*, 1988). Only a few patients with advanced seminoma who relapse after adequate

Table 12.4 Overall survival after cisplatin-based chemotherapy

Reference	Total	Number of patients surviving
van Oosterom *et al.* (1986)	80	57
Peckham, Horwich and Hendry (1985)	33	31
Srougi, Simon and de Góes (1985)	10	10
Oliver *et al.* (1983)	26	23
Fosså *et al.* (1987)	55	43
Motzer *et al.* (1988)	62	53
Loehrer *et al.* (1987)	62	39
Clemm *et al.* (1989)	24	21
Schultz *et al.* (1989)	28	23
Fosså *et al.* (1995)	42	37
Total	443	351 (79%)

cisplatin-based chemotherapy are cured by salvage treatment, ending up with an overall survival rate of about 80% (Table 12.4).

In summary, the strict application of the WHO criteria for response is not very meaningful in patients with metastatic seminoma receiving chemotherapy. Histologically, 80–85% of the patients with residual masses are tumor free. In patients with residual masses after chemotherapy, frequent follow-up examinations are recommended followed by resection in cases of large masses persisting for several months. If these approaches are not possible, radiotherapy should be considered. Given the background of difficulties with regard to strict response evaluation in advanced seminoma, the estimation of progression-free survival and overall survival seems to represent a clinically more useful tool for evaluating treatment efficacy than evaluation of CR and PR.

REFERENCES

Aass, N., Kaasa, S., Lund, E. *et al.* (1990) Long-term somatic side effects and morbidity in testicular cancer patients. *Br. J. Cancer*, **61**, 151–5.

Borge, N., Fosså, S.D., Ous, S. *et al.* (1988) Late recurrence of testicular cancer. *J. Clin. Oncol.*, **6**, 1248–53.

Clemm, C., Hartenstein, R., Willich, N. *et al.* (1989) Combination chemotherapy with vinblastine, ifosfamide and cisplatin in bulky seminoma. *Acta Oncol.*, **28**, 231–5.

de Kernion, J.B. and Lupu, A.N. (1977) The response of metastatic retroperitoneal seminoma to chemotherapy. *J. Urol.*, **117**, 736–8.

Donohue, J.P., Rowland, R.G., Kopecky, Y. *et al.* (1987) Correlation of computerized tomographic changes and histological findings in 80 patients having radical retroperitoneal lymph node dissection after chemotherapy for testis cancer. *J. Urol.*, **137**, 117–9.,

Ellison, M.F., Mostofi, F.K. and Flanagan, R.C. (1988) Treatment of the residual retroperitoneal mass after chemotherapy for advanced seminoma. *J. Urol.*, **140**, 618–20.

Epenetos, A.A., Munro, A.J., Tucker, D.F. *et al.* (1985) Monoclonal antibody assay of serum placental alkaline phosphatase in the monitoring of testicular tumours. *Br. J. Cancer*, **51**, 641–4.

Fosså, S.D., Aass, N., Ous, S. *et al.* (1989b) Histology of tumour residuals following chemotherapy in patients with advanced non-seminomatous testicular cancer. *J. Urol.*, **142**, 1239–42.

Fosså, S.D., Borge, L., Aass, N. *et al.* (1987) The treatment of advanced metastatic seminoma. Experience in 55 cases. *J. Clin. Oncol.*, **5**, 1071–7.

Fosså, S.D., Droz, J.P., Stoter, G. *et al.* (1995) Cisplatin, vincristine and ifosfamide combination chemotherapy of metastatic seminoma: results of EORTC trial 30874. *Br. J. Cancer*, **71**(3), 619–24.

Fosså, A. and Fosså, S.D. (1989) Serum lactate dehydrogenase and human choriogonadotropin in seminoma. *Br. J. Urol.*, **63**, 408–15.

Fosså, S.D., Klepp, O. and Paus, E. (1992) Neuron-specific enolase – a serum tumour marker in seminoma? *Br. J. Cancer*, **65**, 297–9.

Fosså, S.D., Kullmann, G., Lien, H.H. *et al.* (1989c) Chemotherapy of advanced seminoma: Clinical significance of radiological findings before and after treatment. *Br. J. Urol.*, **64**, 530–4.

Fosså, S.D., Ous, S., Lien, H.H. and Stenwig, A.E. (1989a) Post-chemotherapy lymph node histology in radiologically normal patients with metastatic nonseminomatous testicular cancer. *J. Urol.*, **141**, 557–9.

Friedman, E.L., Garnick, M.B., Stomper, P.C. *et*

al. (1985) Therapeutic guidelines and results in advanced seminoma. *J. Clin. Oncol.*, **3**, 1325–32.

Horwich, A., Dearnaley, D.P., Duchesne, G.M. *et al.* (1989) Simple nontoxic treatment of advanced metastatic seminoma with carboplatin. *J. Clin. Oncol.*, **7**, 1150–6.

Horwich, A., Tucker, D.F. and Peckham, M.J. (1985) Placental alkaline phosphatase as a tumour marker in seminoma using the H17 E2 monoclonal antibody assay. *Br. J. Cancer*, **51**, 625–9.

Javadpour, N. (1983) Multiple biochemical tumour markers in seminoma. A double-blind study. *Cancer*, **52**, 887–9.

Jones, B.M., Newlands, E.S., Begent, R.H. *et al.* (1982) The role of abdominal surgery in the treatment of advanced testicular germ cell tumours. *Brit. J. Surg.*, **69**, 4–6.

Kaye, S.B., Stoter, G., von Oosterom, A.T. *et al.* (1988) Joint phase II study of high dose epirubicin in patients with progressive measurable metastatic non-seminomatous germ cell tumours, including extragonadal tumours, in *EORTC Protocol 30883. EORTC Protocol 16881.*

Kuzmits, R., Schernthaner, G. and Krisch, K. (1987) Serum neuron-specific enolase. A marker for response to therapy in seminoma. *Cancer*, **60**, 1017–21.

Lange, P.H., Millán, J.L., Stigbrand, T. *et al.* (1982) Placental alkaline phosphatase as a tumour marker for seminoma. *Cancer Res.*, **42**, 3244–7.

Lien, H.H., Fosså, S.D., Ous, S. and Stenwig, A.E. (1983) Lymphography in retroperitoneal metastases in non-seminoma testicular tumour patients with normal CT-scan. *Acta Radiol.*, **24**, 319–22.

Loehrer, P.J., Birch, R., Williams, S.D. *et al.* (1987) Chemotherapy of metastatic seminoma: The Southeastern Cancer Study Group Experience. *J. Clin. Oncol.*, **5**, 1212–20.

Millán, J.L. and Manes, T. (1988) Seminoma-derived Nagao isozyme is encoded by a unique alkaline phosphatase gene. *Proc. Natl. Acad. Sci. USA*, **85**, 27–31.

Millán, J.L., Stigbrand, T., Ruoslahti, E. and Fishman, W.H. (1982) Characterization and use of an allotype-specific monoclonal antibody to placental alkaline phosphatase in the study of cancer-related phosphatase polymorphism. *Cancer Res.*, **42**, 2444–9.

Miller, A.B., Hoogstraten, B., Staquet, M. and Winkler, A. (1981) Reporting results of cancer treatment. *Cancer*, **47**, 207–14.

Mirimanoff, R.O., Shipley, W.V., Dosoretz, D.E. and Meyer, J.E. (1985) Pure seminoma of the testis: the results of radiation therapy in patients with elevated human chorionic gonadotropin titers. *J. Urol.*, **134**, 1124–6.

Motzer, R.J., Bosl, G.J., Geller, N.J. *et al.* (1988) Advanced seminoma: The role of chemotherapy and adjunctive surgery. *Ann. Int. Med.*, **108**, 513–8.

Motzer, R.J., Bosl, G.J., Heelan, R. *et al.* (1987) Residual mass: an indication for further therapy in patients with advanced seminoma following systemic chemotherapy. *J. Clin. Oncol.*, **5**, 1064–70.

Nørgaard-Pedersen, B., Schultz, H.P., Arends, J. *et al.* (1984) Tumour markers in testicular germ cell tumours. Five-years experience from the DATECA Study 1976–1980. *Acta Rad. Oncol.*, **23**, 287–94.

Oliver, R.T.D., Blandy, J.P., Hendry, W.F. *et al.* (1983) Evaluation of radiotherapy and/or surgicopathological staging after chemotherapy in the management of metastatic germ cell tumours. *Brit. J. Urol.*, **55**, 764–8.

Paus, E., Fosså, A., Fosså, S.D. and Nustad, K. (1988) High frequency of incomplete human chorionic gonadotropin in patients with testicular seminoma. *J. Urol.*, **139**, 542–4.

Paus, E., Fosså, S.D., Risberg, T. and Nustad, K. (1987) The diagnostic value of human chorionic gonadotropin in patients with testicular seminoma. *Brit. J. Urol.*, **59**, 572–7.

Peckham, M.J., Horwich, A. and Hendry, W.F. (1985) Advanced seminoma: Treatment with cisplatinum-based combination chemotherapy or carboplatin (JM8). *Br. J. Urol.*, **52**, 7–13.

Pizzocaro, G., Salvioni, R., Piva, I. *et al.* (1986) Cisplatin combination chemotherapy in advanced seminoma. *Cancer*, **58**, 1625–9.

Schultz, S.M., Einhorn, L.H., Conces, D.Y. *et al.* (1989) Management of post-chemotherapy residual mass in patients with advanced seminoma: Indiana University Experience. *J. Clin. Oncol.*, **7**, 1497–503.

Simon, S.D., Srougi, M. and de Góes, G.M. (1983) Treatment of advanced seminoma with vinblastine (VBL), actinomycin D (AcD), cyclophosphamide (CTX), bleomycin (BLEO) and cisplatinum (CPDD). *Proc. Am. Soc. Clin. Oncol.*, **2**, 132, (abstract C-517).

Soo, C.S., Bernardino, M.E., Chuang, V.P. and Ordones, N. (1981) Pitfalls of CT findings in post-therapy testicular carcinoma. *J. Comput. Asst. Tomogr.*, **5**, 39–41.

Srougi, M., Simon, S.D. and de Góes, G.M. (1985) Vinblastine, actinomycin-D, bleomycin, cyclophosphamide and cisplatinum for advanced germ cell testis tumours: Brazilian experience. *J. Urol.*, **134**, 65–9.

Stanton, G.F., Bosl, G.J., Whitmore, W.F. Jr. *et al.* (1985) VAB-6 as initial treatment of patients with advanced seminoma. *J. Clin. Oncol.*, **3**, 336–9.

Swartz, D.A., Johnsen, D.E. and Hussey, D.H. (1984) Should an elevated human chorionic gonadotropin titer alter therapy for seminoma? *J. Urol.*, **131**, 63–5.

Taylor, R.E., Duncan, W. and Horn, D.B. (1986) Lactate dehydrogenase as a marker for testicular germ-cell tumours. *Eur. J. Cancer Clin. Oncol.*, **22**, 647–53.

Tucker, D.F., Oliver, R.T., Trawers, R.S. and Bodmer, W.F. (1985) Serum marker potential of placental alkaline phosphatase-like activity in testicular germ cell tumours evaluated by H17E2 monoclonal antibody assay. *Br. J. Cancer*, **51**, 631–9.

van Oosterom, A.T., Williams, S.D., Cortes, H. *et al.* (1986) Treatment of advanced seminomas with chemotherapy, in *Germ Cell Tumours II* (eds W.G. Jones, A.M. Ward and C.K. Anderson), Pergamon Press, Oxford, 229–33.

von Eyben, F.E. (1983) Lactate dehydrogenase and its isoenzymes in testicular germ cell tumours: an overview. *Oncodevelop. Biol. Med.*, **4**, 395–414.

von Eyben, F.E., Blaabjerg, O., Petersen, P.H. *et al.* (1988). Serum lactate dehydrogenase isoenzyme 1 as a marker of testicular germ cell tumour. *J. Urol.*, **140**, 986–90.

Wahren, B., Holmgren, P.A. and Stigbrand, T. (1979) Placental alkaline phosphatase alphafetoprotein and carcino embryonic antigen in testicular tumours. *Int. J. Cancer*, **24**, 749–55.

Wilkinson, P.M., Read, G. and Magee, B. (1988) The treatment of advanced seminoma with chemotherapy and radiotherapy. *Br. J. Cancer*, **57**, 100–4.

MANAGEMENT OF STAGE I NON-SEMINOMA: SURVEILLANCE

13

M.H. Cullen and J.-P. Droz

13.1 HISTORICAL INTRODUCTION

Virtually all patients with early stage testicular cancer can now expect to be cured. At the beginning of this century the figure was about 10% (Oliver *et al.*, 1984). This change has come about because there have been improvements in tumor detection and staging, allowing more accurate definition of Stage I disease, as well as improvements in therapy. Between 1900 and 1960 cure rates for orchidectomy alone increased from around 10 to 30%, largely as a result of the introduction of routine chest X-ray which 'upstaged' some cases. Following this, routine prophylactic treatment to the abdominal para-aortic nodes was adopted and survival for early stage non-seminomatous germ cell tumors of the testis (NSGCTT) increased to around 60% by the mid-seventies. In the USA and much of Europe this prophylactic treatment took the form of retroperitoneal lymph node dissection. In the UK and Denmark radiotherapy was preferred. However, tumor detection and staging were also refined with lymphography, whole lung tomography, computed tomography (CT) scanning and tumor markers. Using these techniques half the patients considered as clinical Stage I are upstaged producing a concomitant, apparent improvement in the results of treatment. Consequently, by the late 1970s several centers were reporting survival close to 100% for Stage I testicular teratoma. None of these therapeutic or investigational improvements was independently evaluated, thus it is impossible to quantify their individual contribution to the results. Developments in retroperitoneal surgery for Stage I NSGCTT are discussed in Chapters 15 and 16. Radiotherapy in this setting, which is largely of historic interest, will be discussed briefly here.

13.2 RADIOTHERAPY

It is recognized that NSGCTT is less radio-responsive than seminoma and requires doses approaching tissue tolerance for tumor control. Before the introduction of cisplatin for salvage treatment of recurrences, the survival rate for clinical Stage I NSGCTT treated with radiation therapy ranged from 70 to 90%. Peckham *et al.* (1979) reported a 3-year survival of 100% in 28 clinical Stage I and small volume Stage II patients after the introduction of cisplatin. In a study carried out by the Danish Testicular Cancer Study Group (DATECA) (Rørth *et al.*, 1991), 73 patients were randomized to receive radiotherapy. Eleven patients relapsed with a median time to relapse of 6 months (with a range 5 to 42 months). Three patients had a second relapse. Two patients died from relapsing therapy-resistant disease.

Testicular Cancer: Investigation and management. Second edition. Edited by Professor A. Horwich.
Published in 1996 by Chapman & Hall. ISBN 0 412 61210 0.

All the other relapsing patients were disease free after chemotherapy. None of the relapses occurred in the retroperitoneum.

Abdominal irradiation increases the risk of gastrointestinal and bone marrow complications in those patients who later need chemotherapy. Local fibrosis and increased risk of secondary neoplasms are other possible long-term effects. The impact of radiotherapy on fertility has not been thoroughly evaluated, but apparently radiotherapy seldom induces permanent infertility (Bracken and Johnson, 1976). Toxic effects of radiotherapy also include peptic ulceration (Hamilton *et al.*, 1986).

The radiotherapy versus surgery debate hinged largely upon the unwanted effects of these procedures. Classical bilateral retroperitoneal lymph node dissection is associated with lack of seminal emission due to interference with autonomic innervation in the majority of cases (Whitmore, 1982). As already stated the most important late effect of abdominal–pelvic radiotherapy was a reduced marrow tolerance to subsequent chemotherapy in those patients who relapse (Glatstein, 1982). Indeed it was the sudden revolution in the treatment for advanced teratoma produced by the introduction of cisplatin in the late 1970s (Einhorn and Donohue, 1977) that effectively made the radiotherapy versus classical retroperitoneal lymph node dissection (RPLND) debate redundant. Suddenly it became reasonable to consider no treatment at all for carefully investigated and monitored cases of Stage I teratoma, since those with tumor recurrence should be curable with cisplatin combination chemotherapy.

13.3 SURVEILLANCE

In 1979 a number of groups embarked upon a programme of surveillance alone for Stage I patients with teratoma. The first report (Peckham *et al.*, 1982) appeared in 1982. Among 53 patients there were nine relapses (17%), eight of which occurred within 6 months of orchidectomy. All nine were alive and disease free after chemotherapy. The following year Read *et al.* (1983) reported 45 similar patients with 11 relapses, ten in the first year. Again, all relapse cases were salvaged. Data from both these studies were subsequently incorporated into multicenter studies coordinated by the Medical Research Council. These now form by far the largest group of cases of Stage I NSGCTT, managed consistently on a surveillance policy, in the world. A recent review has summarized the worldwide experience of the surveillance policy in the literature (Droz and Van Oosterom, 1993).

13.4 MEDICAL RESEARCH COUNCIL STUDIES

News of the early results of surveillance spread rapidly and several other centers in the UK began a similar policy early in the 1980s. The Medical Research Council (MRC) Testicular Tumour Working Party coordinated a collaborative study involving these centers in which data were collected retrospectively on all patients managed with this policy. At the same time (January 1984) a prospective study was initiated.

13.4.1 RETROSPECTIVE STUDY

Between January 1979 and December 1983, 259 patients had entered this study, which was first reported by Freedman *et al.* (1987). All had histologically verified Stage I teratoma (according to the Royal Marsden Hospital classification), and had been treated with orchidectomy alone. The median follow-up is now 54 months, and 90% of cases have been followed for more than 2 years. Seventy patients (27%) have relapsed, 53 within the first 12 months after orchidectomy. After 18 months the risk of relapse decreased to about 4% per year. The overall relapse-free rate at 4 years is 68% (95% CI 60–75) (Fig. 13.1).

The stage at relapse is shown in Table 13.1. There were three deaths. Two of these patients relapsed with marker negative Stage II

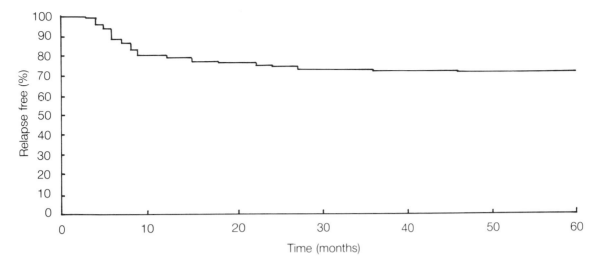

Fig. 13.1 Medical Research Council retrospective study of surveillance in Stage I non-seminoma germ cell tumor of the testis: overall relapse-free rate.

Table 13.1 Medical Research Council retrospective and prospective studies of surveillance in Stage I non-seminomatous germ cell tumors of the testis: stage at relapse

	Retrospective	*Prospective*	*Total*
Total relapses	70	100	170
Stage IM	14 (20%)	13 (13%)	27 (16%)
Stage IIA/B	23 (33%)	43 (43%)	66 (38%)
Stage IIC	3 (4%)	5 (5%)	8 (5%)
Stage II?	1 (1%)		1 (0.6%)
Stage IIIA/B	3 (4%)	6 (6%)	9 (5%)
Stage IIIC		1 (1%)	1 (0.6%)
Stage III?	1 (1%)		1 (0.6%)
Stage IVL1, L2, A/B	18 (26%)	20 (20%)	38 (22%)
Stage IVL1, L2, C		3 (3%)	3 (2%)
Stage IV, L3	1 (1%)		1 (0.6%)
Stage IV?	1 (1%)		1 (0.6%)
Stage IV liver, brain	1 (1%)	2 (2%)	3 (2%)
Scrotum/groin	3 (4%)	7 (7%)	10 (6%)
Contralateral testis*	1 (1%)	4 (2%)	5 (2%)

* These presumed second primaries are included for completeness.

disease, achieved complete response (CR) after chemotherapy but died later from further relapse. The other patient died shortly after relapsing with multiple organ metastases (including liver and brain).

The intensity of surveillance varied between centers, especially in the use of computed tomography (CT) scans. Approximately equal numbers of patients were seen at three groups of centers which used, on average, 3–5 scans per year, 1–2 scans per year and 0–1 scans per year in the first 2 years. There was no tendency for the centers doing scans frequently to detect relapses earlier or at a less advanced stage (Table 13.2). Table 13.3 shows the cumulative proportion of all recurrences

Table 13.2 Medical Research Council retrospective study of surveillance in Stage I non-seminomatous germ cell tumors of the testis: relapse according to frequency of computed tomography scanning

	Scans per year		
	3–5	1–2	0–1
Number of patients	96	70	93
Relapses (%)	28	30	24
Median time to relapse (wks)	25	26	24
Stage IM relapse (%)	22	33	19
Stage II (%)	37	43	38
Stage III and IV (%)	41	24	43

Table 13.3 Medical Research Council retrospective study of surveillance in Stage I non-seminomatous germ cell tumors of the testis: relapse detection according to procedure(s) first indicating relapse and computed tomography (CT) scanning frequency

Investigations	Frequency of CT scans			
	All	0–1	1–2	3–5
Examination only	17	23	14	15
Examination and markers	67	73	67	74
Examination and markers and chest X-ray	83	91	76	89
All tests	100	100	100	100

detected by clinical examination, markers, chest X-ray and all tests including CT scanning according to the frequency of scanning. Eighty-three per cent of all recurrences were detected by examination, markers and chest X-ray. Detailed histological review of these cases was undertaken and the resulting prognostic categories and their significance are discussed below in section 13.7.1.

13.4.2　PROSPECTIVE STUDY

In 1984 the MRC embarked upon a prospective surveillance study in which the collaborating centers elected to apply one of two different schemes of regular CT scanning assessment,

one being more intensive than the other. The results of this study were recently published (Read, 1992). The relapse data and overall survival are discussed here and the prospective application of the histological criteria generated in the retrospective study are expanded in section 13.7.2.

Three hundred and seventy-three eligible patients from 16 UK and one Norwegian centers entered the prospective study. Again all patients had histologically verified NSGCTT treated initially by orchidectomy alone in the 3 years from 1 January 1984. Follow-up attendances after staging investigations were at monthly intervals for the first year, two-monthly for the second and three-monthly in the third. Assessment consisted of clinical examination, alpha-fetoprotein (AFP) and human chorionic gonadotrophin (HCG) assay, and chest X-ray at each visit.

Marker investigations were performed more frequently if there was clinical need. Computed tomography scanning was performed at each centre according to one of two schedules. In schedule A, scanning of the thorax and abdomen was performed at alternate visits for the first 2 years. In schedule B, scanning was performed only at 2, 6, 8 and 12 months. The treatment of relapse was dependent on the stage and followed the usual practice for each participating center. The median follow-up for those patients who were relapse free when last seen was 5 years. A minimum of 2 years follow-up was available on all but five patients (currently lost to follow-up and censored at 4, 6, 19, 22 and 23 months after orchidectomy).

One hundred patients (27%) have relapsed (including two with presumed second primary tumors in the contralateral testes) of whom 78 (80%) were in the first 12 months following orchidectomy. The overall relapse-free curve is shown in Fig. 13.2. The curve is virtually identical to that for the retrospective study, and again the annual risk of relapse appears to drop sharply after the first 12 months following orchidectomy, and con-

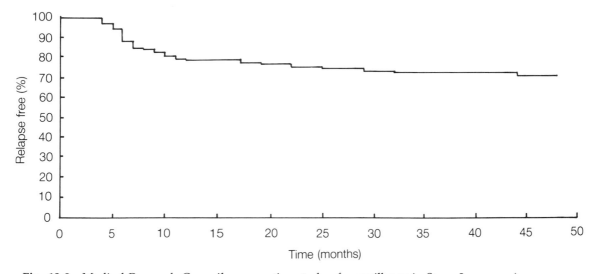

Fig. 13.2 Medical Research Council prospective study of surveillance in Stage I non-seminoma germ cell tumor of the testis: overall relapse-free rate.

tinues to decline in the second and subsequent years. The 2-year actuarial relapse-free rate is 75% (95% confidence interval 71–79%), dropping only to 72% 5 years after orchidectomy (95% confidence interval 67–77%). The latest relapse to have occurred in this group of patients was 44 months after orchidectomy.

The stages at relapse are shown in Table 13.1. Eighty-seven patients had 'small volume' disease, nine 'large volume' and two 'very large volume' by the criteria established in a previous MRC study.

Following relapse, chemotherapy was given according to the usual practice of the referring center. Residual masses after chemotherapy were removed surgically whenever possible, except for one center where radiotherapy was given routinely. Of all the patients who have relapsed, six are alive and disease free with a median follow-up after relapse of 52 months. Six patients have died after relapse and two more patients were alive with recurrent teratoma when last seen. A total of eight patients have died. One patient died from uncontrolled tumor; relapse was diagnosed 7 months after orchidectomy with one lung metastasis 2.5 cm in diameter. The

patient received cisplatin combination chemotherapy and achieved a complete response. He subsequently relapsed 12 months later with mediastinal and lung metastases and died despite further chemotherapy 3 months later. The second patient relapsed with Stage IIC disease after 18 months of surveillance. He achieved a complete response to carboplatin, vinblastine and etoposide (CVE) but relapsed and died 12 months later with widespread disease. The third patient relapsed with raised markers only, and entered complete response to four courses of BEP. He had a relapse 3 months later with increasing marker levels and small size retroperitoneal nodes. He achieved a second complete response to chemotherapy. He relapsed again, refused treatment and died 18 months after the first relapse. The fourth patient relapsed in the retroperitoneum with normal marker levels. He received four cycles of BEP and had a complete resection of residual tumor (malignant teratoma intermediate). Six months later, he relapsed with liver metastases and ascites and died 3 months later. One further patient died from bleomycin lung toxicity. His tumor markers were raised and a single lung metastasis 0.5 cm in diameter was detected 4 months after orchidectomy. The patient received four courses of chemotherapy with carboplatin, etoposide and bleomycin and achieved a complete response. Two months after the response evaluation the patient suffered a cardiorespiratory arrest from bilateral pneumothoraces. A further three patients have died from unrelated intercurrent events. The 4-year survival rate for mortality from all causes is 98%, and for tumor mortality is 99%.

The 2-year actuarial relapse-free rate of 75% (95% confidence interval 71–79%) is similar to the relapse-free rate of 74% reported in the retrospective study. This falls only to 72% 5 years after orchidectomy supporting the policy of intensive surveillance for the 2-year period following orchidectomy.

13.5 OTHER STUDIES OF SURVEILLANCE

Over 1000 patients have been reported from studies in which a surveillance policy has been adopted following orchidectomy for Stage I NSGCTT (Table 13.4). Over half the patients have been in MRC studies. The schedules of surveillance have not differed substantially from those employed in the MRC studies and the results have been remarkably similar. With median follow-up times of 30–40 months relapse rates have been 27% in both MRC studies and 28% in the other smaller series combined. Furthermore, complete response rates at the time of reporting were 96% in both MRC studies and 95% in the rest.

There have been a number of warnings of caution in the widespread adoption of surveillance in Stage I NSGCTT. Pizzocaro *et al.* (1986) pointed out that in some studies the minimum follow-up was rather short. The work cited has, in most cases, been updated and the shape of the relapse-free curves seem consistent and similar to the first MRC study, which has a median follow-up of 54 months. Although the vast majority of relapses occur

in the first 18 months from orchidectomy there continues to be a steady appearance of relapse up to 4 years. Pizzocaro also points out that, unlike lung metastases, the early clinical detection of retroperitoneal lymph node metastases is not easy. This is important since the retroperitoneum is the most common single site of recurrence, and several workers have described patients relapsing late with masses >5 cm when first detected (Pizzocaro *et al.*, 1986; Sogani and Fair, 1988; Rørth *et al.*, 1991). It must be assumed that this will have implications for the curability of these patients. For this reason Pizzocaro argues that surveillance should be conducted only in specialized centers, and that retroperitoneal lymphadenectomy should remain the standard treatment. Clearly, the new nerve-sparing retroperitoneal dissections must also be conducted in specialized centers, and, so far, not enough of these have been reported to be confident that they will always prevent retroperitoneal relapse (Donohue *et al.*, 1993. At all events there will continue to be 10–15% of patients who relapse elsewhere and careful follow-up of patients must continue following RPLND as well as of those having orchidectomy alone.

A number of investigators have pointed out that the principal disadvantage of a surveillance policy is that it requires a high degree of commitment by the institution operating it and a high degree of compliance by the patient (Young, 1991). Most patients are in their twenties and at a time in their lives when they are most likely to want to move, and are most affected by the disruption in career and social plans that is an inevitable part of careful surveillance programs. Young men can also have difficulty in coping with the monthly reminder of the possibility of relapse, and consequent need for intensive chemotherapy. Indeed, such is the anxiety generated by surveillance that for some patients the news of relapse can (ironically) be associated with a sense almost of relief that 'the waiting' is over and 'the

Table 13.4 Results of surveillance programs in Stage I non-seminomatous germ cell tumors of the testis

Series	Number of cases	Median follow-up (months)	Relapse number (%)	Complete response number (%)	Comments
MRC retrospective study					
Freedman *et al.* (1987)	259	54	70 (27)	67 (96)	2 patients died after 2nd relapse 1 patient died after multiple organ relapse (including brain)
MRC prospective study	373	37	98 (26)	92 (96)	1 patient died from
Read *et al.* (1992)					uncontrolled tumor 1 patient died from bleomycin toxicity
Princess Margaret Hospital					
Sturgeon *et al.* (1983)	30	14	12 (40)	12 (100)	
Auckland, NZ					
Thompson, Nixon and Harvey (1988)	36	36	12 (33)	11 (92)	4 second relapses, 1 died, 1 alive with disease, 2 in CR 57 and 18 months from salvage CT
Milan, Italy					
Pizzocaro *et al.* (1986)	59	30	18 (31)	17 (94)	2 second relapses, both disease free
M.D. Anderson, USA					
Dunphy *et al.* (1988)	93	34	28 (30)	?30 (97)	1 patient who relapsed died, 1 died before therapy, 1 suicide, 1 died after 2nd relapse
Memorial Sloan-Kettering Cancer Center, USA					
Sogani and Fair (1988)	102	40	25 (25)	22 (88)	3 patients never achieved CR
DATECA, Denmark					
Rørth *et al.* (1991)	77	64	23 (30)	23 (100)	
Gronigen, Netherlands					
Gelderman *et al.* (1987)	54	29 (mean)	11 (20)	11 (100)	
Bratislava					
Hornak, Zvara and Ondrus (1992)	100	36	35 (35)	31 (88)	
Princess Margaret Hospital					
Sturgeon *et al.* (1992)	105	60	37 (35)	36 (97)	
New Zealand					
Colls *et al.* (1992)	115	36	34 (29.5)	30 (88)	
Total	1403		403 (28.7)	382 (94.7)	

CR, complete response.

treatment' can begin. It has perhaps come as a surprise to many of us that the 'no-treatment' option of surveillance has not been viewed by many of the patients with the same enthusiasm that the oncologists practicing it had expected.

Moynihan (1987) has studied the psycho-social problems of 122 patients with testicular cancer, of whom 32 had Stage I disease and entered a surveillance program (Chapter 31). The Present State Examination (a standardized instrument for measuring anxiety and depression) was employed. Although the numbers involved were not sufficient to identify significant differences, one of the groups of patients experiencing the highest levels of psychological morbidity was those with Stage I disease who entered a surveillance program and relapsed within a year of diagnosis. Quoting from her study:

> Many of the men in the surveillance group described the tension they had experienced as they waited to be told the 'worst'. The words of one man were echoed by many: 'if I had had chemotherapy, the waiting would be all over by now.' It is interesting that 37% of the surveillance group were still worried about not receiving treatment at the time of interview.

Experiences like this have been observed in our own group, and have prompted the desire to look for prognostic factors that may allow patients at high risk of relapse to be identified and offered immediate adjuvant chemotherapy.

13.6 PROGNOSTIC FACTORS IN STAGE I NON-SEMINOMATOUS GERM CELL TUMORS OF THE TESTIS

13.6.1 HISTOLOGICAL SUBTYPE

Even before the cisplatin era the possibility of identifying high risk groups for adjuvant chemotherapy was considered. Johnson, Bracken and Blight (1976) observed that among 72 patients with clinical and pathological Stage I disease treated with RPLND only, the 5-year survival rate was 74.4% for embryonal carcinoma, 93% for teratocarcinoma and 100% for teratoma. The Royal Marsden Hospital (RMH) group (Hoskin *et al.*, 1986) noted that 44% of 43 patients with embryonal carcinoma relapsed in their surveillance program, compared with 20% of 66 patients with teratocarcinoma. An earlier report from this group (Raghavan *et al.*, 1982), in which the patients received adjuvant radiotherapy, found no difference. Javadpour *et al.* (1986) reported 60 cases of Stage I NSGCTT treated with RPLND. Eight of 10 patients who relapsed, or with tumor present in the RPLND specimen, had embryonal carcinoma. Similar conclusions were reached by Pizzocaro *et al.* (1986) in a surveillance study in which 50% of 18 cases of embryonal carcinoma relapsed against 23% of 39 cases of teratocarcinoma. There are other reports with trends suggesting an adverse effect of embryonal carcinoma (Gelderman *et al.*, 1987; Dunphy *et al.*, 1988; Fung *et al.*, 1988; Sogani and Fair, 1988; Rørth *et al.* 1991). The New Zealand study (Thompson *et al.*, 1988) found no significant difference, but the numbers in this report are small. The report from the Dana-Farber Cancer Institute in Boston (Fung *et al.*, 1988) suggested a **lower** rate of nodal metastases at RPLND in patients with endodermal sinus tumor elements in the primary tumor. This latter observation is also discussed in connection with the MRC studies, which are described in Section 13.7.

13.6.2 PRIMARY TUMOR STAGE

Local extension of the tumor into paratesticular structures is generally accepted as indicating a higher risk of regional and distant metastases in NSGCTT. The earlier (radiotherapy) study from the RMH (Raghavan *et al.*, 1982) reported an 18% relapse rate with T_1 tumors compared with 60% for T_{2-4} lesions. Moriyama *et al.* (1985) reported 46 and 81% respectively in their study from the Massachusetts General Hospital, whereas Fung *et al.* (1988) noted an 18% relapse rate for T_1 tumors and 52% for stage T_{2-4}, and in a Pizzocaro *et al.*'s (1986) series the corresponding figures were 14 and 47%. In the later RMH study (Hoskin *et al.* 1986) tumor involvement of the rete and epididymis was correlated with an increased risk of relapse, but involvement of the tunica albuginea and spermatic cord were not significant prognostic factors. Cases in this report were later included in the much more exhaustive MRC retrospective analysis discussed below.

13.6.3   TUMOR INVASION OF TESTICULAR LYMPHATICS AND VEINS

A number of authors have recorded the prognostic importance of tumor invasion of testicular lymphatics and veins. Rodriguez, Hafez and Messing (1986) reviewed the histological material on 120 NSGCTT patients of all stages paying particular attention to vascular invasion. Only 9% of patients with Stage I disease had vascular invasion, compared with 53% of those with metastatic disease. Moriyama *et al.* (1985) found metastases in 25 of 29 patients with vascular invasion, but in only three of 16 tumors with no such vessel involvement. In patients presenting with Stage I disease, Fung *et al.* (1988) reported a significant correlation between vascular invasions and nodal metastases found at RPLND. Both venous and lymphatic invasions had statistically significant associations with nodal deposits but the distinction between the two did not add to the power of the prediction. There was a suggestion that vascular invasion predicted a higher risk of relapse **following** RPLND but this did not reach statistical significance. In a retrospective study the presence of intratesticular small vessel invasion was demonstrated to be predictive of both retroperitoneal lymph node invasion and relapse in patients who were treated by either retroperitoneal lymph node dissection or surveillance respectively (Chraibi *et al.*, 1994). Both venous and lymphatic invasion were significantly associated with a higher relapse rate in the surveillance study reported by Hoskin *et al.* (1986), but in a multiple regression analysis lymphatic invasion and histological subtype (presence of embryonal carcinoma) were the only independent predictors. Lymphatic and/or venous invasion have also come out as indicators of higher relapse risk in the reports of Stage I NSGCTT from Javadpour *et al.* (1986), Pizzo-

caro *et al.* (1986), Dunphy *et al.* (1988), Sogani and Fair (1988) and Thompson, Nixon and Harvey (1988) and in the MRC studies discussed below.

13.6.4   OTHER CRITERIA

Many of the series quoted above looked at other possible prognostic criteria. Most are agreed that preorchidectomy marker levels (Moriyama *et al.*, 1985; Hoskin *et al.*, 1986; Pizzocaro *et al.*, 1986; Sogani and Fair, 1988; Thompson, Nixon and Harvey, 1988), primary tumor size (Raghavan *et al.*, 1982; Moriyama *et al.*, 1985; Hoskin *et al.*, 1986; Dunphy *et al.*, 1988; Fung *et al.*, 1988; Thompson, Nixon and Harvey, 1988) and side-effects (Raghavan *et al.*, 1982; Moynihan, 1987) are not significantly associated with risk of metastasis. Different studies were focused on different biological prognostic factors. The DNA content measured by flow cytometry may have independent prognostic value (Moul *et al.*, 1993). Conversely, the expression of the p53 gene protein appeared to have no prognostic significancy (Lewis *et al.*, 1994).

13.7   MEDICAL RESEARCH COUNCIL STUDIES OF PROGNOSTIC FACTORS

13.7.1   RETROSPECTIVE STUDY

The retrospective MRC study was concerned not only with relapse rates but it also involved a thorough histological review (by Dr Constance Parkinson). Each neoplasm was assessed (without knowledge of clinical outcome) with regard to histopathological staging and tumor classification, including all the criteria cited in previous studies and a number of others (Freedman *et al.*, 1987). The criteria included are given in Table 13.5. The relationship between 27 histological variables and the 2-year relapse-free rates was investigated. Fifteen variables were significantly related to relapse and these were subjected to a multivariate analysis assuming a proportional

Table 13.5 Medical Research Council studies of surveillance in Stage I non-seminomatous germ cell tumors of the testis: histological assessments

1. Pathological staging:

Sections examined for presence or absence of tumor infiltration of tunica albuginea, rete, epididymis, levels of cord, veins, lymphatics

Pathological staging systems

British Testicular Tumour Panel and Registry, UICC

2. Tumor classification

Sections assessed using WHO diagnostic criteria for presence or absence of:

Mature or immature somatic tissues, undifferentiated (embryonal) tissue, yolk sac tumor, trophoblastic tumor (choriocarcinoma), syncytiotrophoblastic giant cells, seminoma, 'carcinoma *in situ*' in surrounding tubules

Table 13.6 Medical Research Council retrospective study of surveillance in Stage I non-seminomatous germ cell tumors of the testis: results of stepwise selection of histological variables for a predictive index

Step	Variable included	χ^2 for inclusion	P	Regression coefficients at step 4
1	Veins testis	30.7	<0.001	1.5
2	Lymphatics testis	12.3	<0.001	0.9
3	Yolk sac	7.2	0.007	−0.8
4	Undifferentiated	5.7	0.02	1.4

hazards model. Variables were chosen for inclusion in the calculation by a stepwise, forward selection procedure. The most important independent predictor of relapse was tumor invasion of testicular veins, followed by invasion of testicular lymphatics, then came **absence** of yolk sac (endodermal sinus tumor) elements and finally the presence of undifferentiated tumor (Table 13.6). Although vessel invasion might have been an expected prognostic factor, the absence of yolk sac elements was more surprising. Similar findings have since been reported from Boston in

a small series of Stage I patients. Fung *et al.* (1988) found a lower rate of nodal metastases at RPLND in the presence of endodermal sinus tumor. The reason for this is not clear. It may reflect a greater accuracy in the staging of these patients since the greater propensity of tumors containing these elements to produce AFP would lead to a more reliable detection of metastases by the persistent elevation of tumor markers at diagnosis. Alternatively there may be other explanations related to more fundamental biological properties of tumors containing yolk sac components. For instance, they may confer a tendency to metastasize later, i.e. to exist as Stage I tumors for a greater part of their natural history.

The presence of undifferentiated tumor is not synonymous with malignant teratoma undifferentiated (MTU) (embryonal carcinoma), and requires clarification. Undifferentiated tumor was detected in the majority (85%) of specimens in the MRC series. It was just as common in malignant teratoma intermediate (MTI) tumors as in MTU tumors, and there was no evidence to support the finding of some that MTU histology tumors had a higher risk of relapse than MTI tumors. Instead, the explanation was that the **absence** of undifferentiated cells identified a small group of eight good prognosis patients with differentiated teratoma and another small group of eight good prognosis patients with MTU tumors containing yolk sac tumor but no undifferentiated cells. None of these patients relapsed.

A predictive index, employing the presence or absence (1 or 0, respectively) of each of the four independent variables in the MRC study and their regression coefficients was calculated as follows:

$$\text{Index} = (1.5 \times \text{veins}) + (0.9 \times \text{lymph}) - (0.8 \times \text{yolk}) + (1.4 \times \text{undifferentiated})$$

To simplify the predictive index for use in routine clinical practice each variable was given a weighting of 1 instead of the regres-

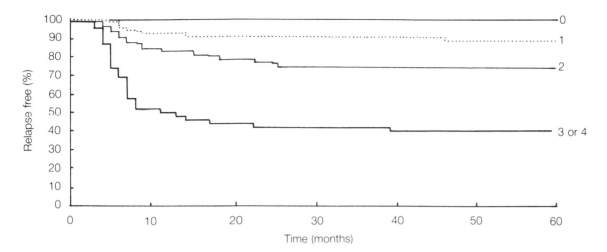

Fig. 13.3 Medical Research Council retrospective study of relapse-free rate for four groups according to number of risk factors.

sion coefficient. The resulting loss of predictive power was small. The simplified index was then defined as the number of the following features found by the pathologist:

1. invasion of testicular veins;
2. invasion of testicular lymphatics;
3. **absence** of yolk sac elements;
4. Presence of undifferentiated tumor.

Both the predictive index based on regression coefficients and the simplified index differentiated patients with very low rates of relapse from patients in a high risk group. Fig. 13.3 shows the relapse-free curve for four groups based on the simplified index. Group 1 (none of the four high risk features) had a 100% relapse-free rate at 2 years, but constituted only 3% of the cases. Group 2 (one high risk feature) had a 91% relapse-free rate at 2 years, and constituted 31.3% of the cases. Group 3 (any two high risk features) had a 75% relapse-free rate at 2 years, and constituted 34.4% of the cases. For Group 4 (any three or all four high risk features) the relapse-free rate at 2 years was only 42%. This 'high risk' group comprised 21.2% of the cases.

13.7.2 PROSPECTIVE STUDY

Having identified histological criteria with considerable prognostic significance the next step, clearly, was to verify these **prospectively** in a separate data set. The MRC prospective multicenter study of surveillance of Stage I NSGCTT, already discussed in Section 13.4.2, provided the opportunity to test the reliability of the criteria concerned. Histological sections from orchidectomy specimens of 366 out of 396 prospectively followed patients were again reviewed by the reference pathologist, Dr Constance Parkinson. The same simplified index was used to classify patients entered into the prospective study into prognostic groups. Fig. 13.4 shows the resulting survival curves for the same four groups of patients with 0, 1, 2 and 3 or all 4 high risk criteria. Inevitably the differentiation between the prognostic groups in the prospective study patients was less than that shown by the retrospective study since the index, by definition, was optimal for the latter group. However, it can be seen that it continues to work well in defining a group at high risk of relapse. In the prospective series,

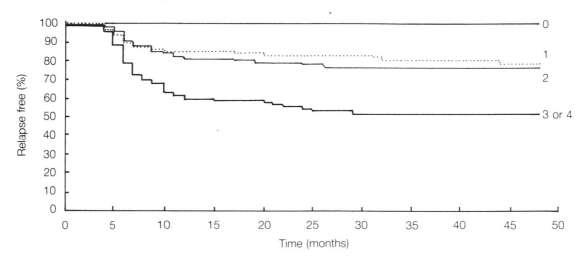

Fig. 13.4   Medical Research Council prospective study of relapse-free rate for four groups according to number of risk factors.

Table 13.7   Distribution of patients according to number of risk factors in Medical Research Council studies of surveillance

	Retrospective	*Prospective*	*Total*
Group 1 (No high risk features)	8 (3%)	9 (3%)	17 (3%)
Group 2 (Any 1 high risk feature)	81 (31%)	132 (35%)	213 (33%)
Group 3 (Any 2 high risk features)	89 (34%)	142 (37%)	231 (36%)
Group 4 (Any 3 or all 4 high risk features)	55 (21%)	83 (22%)	138 (22%)

the 'high risk' group again comprises just over 20% of all patients, and they show a 3-year relapse-free rate of 50% (95% confidence interval 38–62%). The proportional distribution of the other groups is also identical to that seen in the retrospective study (Table 13.7).

This series of 396 patients, the largest reported series of prospectively identified Stage I NSGCTT patients treated by orchidectomy alone, confirms the findings of the previous MRC report that a group of patients with a high probability of relapse comprising one-quarter of the total can be identified on histological criteria (Read *et al.*, 1992).

13.7.3   PATTERN OF RELAPSE IN MEDICAL RESEARCH COUNCIL HIGH AND LOW RISK GROUPS

The marked similarity in the results of the two MRC studies allows the data to be combined providing a unique population of carefully studied and uniformly managed cases of Stage I NSGCTT. Among a total of 632 patients, 168 relapses have been observed. Histological review has been conducted on 158 of these. The relapse cases have been divided according to presence or absence of each of the four high risk features, and also into 'low' (at most, two high risk features), and 'high' risk groups (any three or all

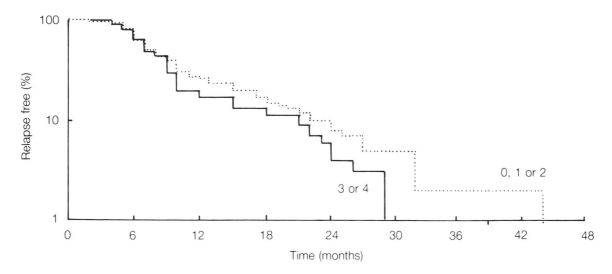

Fig. 13.5 Medical Research Council surveillance studies (combined) of time of relapse according to number of risk factors (semi-log plot).

four features). The following relapse features were then examined in relation to the above groupings:

1. (a) abdominal node relapse;
   (b) mediastinal node relapse;
   (c) supraclavicular node relapse;
   (d) at least one of the above;
2. (a) relapse with lung metastases;
   (b) relapse with liver, bone or brain metastases;
   (c) at least one of the above;
3. (a) relapse with raised AFP;
   (b) relapse with raised HCG;
   (c) relapse with either AFP or HCG or both raised;
4. (a) stage at relapse (IM vs.II vs.III vs.IV);
   (b) time of relapse.

The same trends were apparent in both retrospective and prospective studies and so combining the data was quite appropriate. There were very few statistically significant results from the numerous cross-tabulations performed. However, there was a significant negative association between invasion of testicular veins and abdominal node relapse (i.e. those patients **with** venous invasion

were less likely to relapse in abdominal or other nodes than those without). However, there was no increased tendency for patients with lymphatic invasion to relapse in abdominal nodes. There was a nonsignificant trend for patients with venous invasion to relapse more frequently in the lung than those without. As one might have predicted, patients with yolk sac elements in the primary tumor were significantly more likely to relapse with raised AFP. Interestingly there was no evidence of a different stage at relapse between the low and high risk groups, although there was a tendency for high risk patients to have fewer late (after 9 months) relapses (Fig. 13.5). The relapse rate over the first 9 months was very similar in low and high risk cases.

Thus it seems that there are very few, if any, clinically useful correlations available to facilitate the surveillance of Stage I NSGCTT. Consequently there is little room for tailoring surveillance programs more efficiently for different groups of patient. Given this, and the other drawbacks of surveillance policies already discussed, the need to evaluate adjuvant chemotherapy in high risk patients becomes more acute. A prospective MRC study of adjuvant chemotherapy was initiated in 1987 to determine whether two courses of chemotherapy given immediately after orchidectomy in patients with 'high risk' pathological features, when the volume of disease is minimal, will be sufficient to prevent relapse (Cullen *et al.*, 1996). This is discussed in Chapter 14.

13.8 CONCLUSIONS

In any formula describing the best treatment for early stage teratoma, the principal variables would be the accuracy of tumor detection and staging, and the efficacy and acceptability of treatment. To some extent these factors work in opposite directions. Clearly, if treatment is ineffective and toxic it is more important that detection and staging are accurate so that patients **not** requiring treatment are identified. Developments in tumor imaging and marker analysis have been important here. Conversely, as treatment has become very effective and recently less toxic (with fewer courses; etoposide substituting vinblastine; better antiemetic therapy) it has become arguably less important to identify patients not requiring treatment, because the consequences of receiving unnecessary therapy are less significant.

Retroperitoneal lymph node dissection for Stage I testicular non-seminoma is described in detail in Chapters 15 and 16. While the modified techniques reduce the incidence of ejaculatory dysfunction, they will ultimately be judged as cancer procedures based on local recurrence rates and survival when compared with other treatment strategies. Although the duration of follow-up to date has been insufficient to make definitive recommendations, one important factor must be considered; modified procedures will necessarily leave behind lymph nodes which, although admittedly rarely, may be involved microscopically with disease and ultimately result in an intra-abdominal relapse. Until

further follow-up defines the local relapse rate, it is prudent to perform routine radiographic visualization of the retroperitoneum, similar to patients followed up with surveillance only. Thus, although modified RPLND carried out in experienced centers has minimal acute morbidity and leads to preservation of ejaculatory function in the majority of patients, the relapse rate in patients subjected to this procedure will be 10–20%. Very few of these will occur in the retroperitoneum.

A surveillance policy for Stage I teratoma allows about two-thirds of patients to escape treatment and, in common with other management policies, survival is nearly, but not quite, 100%. However, there are drawbacks to surveillance. In particular, it requires good patient compliance, is inconvenient, and generates patient anxiety. Careful histological assessment can identify a group of patients (about 20% of the total) with a much higher chance of relapse. There is some evidence that short-course adjuvant chemotherapy would prevent this relapse in nearly every case, with acceptable short- and long-term toxicity. There is also a suggestion that most patients, given the choice, would prefer short-course adjuvant chemotherapy to surveillance with a 50/50 chance of needing more prolonged treatment. The MRC has recently addressed this important question in a non-randomized study (Chapter 14).

REFERENCES

Bracken, R.B. and Johnson, D.E. (1976) Sexual function and fecundity after treatment for testicular tumours. *Urology*, **7**, 35–8.

Chraibi, Y., Culine, S., Terrier-Lacombe, M.J., Kramar, A., Kattan, J. and Droz, J.P. (1994) Facteurs pronostiques d'atteinte extratesticulaire. *Bull. Cancer*, **81**, 311–17.

Colls, B.M., Harvey, V.J., Skelton, L., *et al.* (1992) Results of the surveillance policy in stage I nonseminomatous germ-cell testicular tumours. *Br. J. Urol.*, **70**, 423–8.

Cullen, M.H., Stenning, S.P. Parkinson, M.C., Fosså, S.D., Kaye, S.B., Horwich, A., Harland,

S.J., Williams, M.V. and Jakes, R. for the Medical Research Council Testicular Tumour Working Party (1996) Short-course adjuvant chemotherapy in high-risk stage I nonseminomatous germ cell tumours of the testis: A MRC report. *J. Clin. Oncol.*, **14**, 1106–13.

Donohue, J.P., Thornhill, J.A., Foster, R.S., Rowland, R.G. and Bihrle, R. (1993) Retroperitoneal lymphadenectomy for clinical stage A testis cancer (1965 to 1984): modifications of technique and impact on ejaculation. *J. Urol.*, **49**, 237–43.

Droz, J.P. and Van Oosterom, A.T. (1993) Treatment options in clinical stage I nonseminomatous germ-cell tumours of the testis: a wager on the future? A review. *Eur. J. Cancer*, **29A**, 1038–44.

Dunphy, C.H., Ayala, A.G., Swanson, D.A. *et al.* (1988) Clinical stage I nonseminomatous and mixed germ cell tumours of the testis: A clinicopathological study of 93 patients on a surveillance protocol after orchidectomy alone. *Cancer*, **62**, 1202–6.

Einhorn, L.H. and Donohue, J.P. (1977) Cis-diamminedichloroplatinum, vinblastine and bleomycin combination chemotherapy in disseminated testicular cancer. *Ann. Intern. Med.*, **87**, 293–8.

Freedman, L.S., Parkinson, M.C., Jones, W.G. *et al.* (1987) Histopathology in the prediction of relapse of patients with stage I testicular teratoma treated by orchidectomy alone. *Lancet*, **ii**, 294–8.

Fung, C.Y., Kalish, L.A., Brodsky, G.L. *et al.* (1988) Stage I nonseminomatous germ cell testicular tumour: Prediction of metastatic potential by primary histopathology. *J. Clin. Oncol.*, **6**, 1467–73.

Gelderman, W.A.H., Koops, H.S., Sleijer, D.T.H. *et al.* (1987) Orchidectomy alone in stage I nonseminomatous testicular germ cell tumours. *Cancer*, **59**, 578–80.

Glatstein, E. (1982) Optimal management of clinical stage I nonseminomatous testicular carcinoma: one oncologist's view. *Cancer Treat. Rep.*, **66**, 11–18.

Hamilton, C., Horwich, A., Easton, D. and Peckham, M.J. (1986) Radiotherapy for stage I seminoma testis: Results of treatment and complications. *Radiother. Oncol.*, **6**, 115–20.

Hornak, M., Zvara, V. and Ondrus, D. (1992) La surveillance des tumeurs non-séminomateuses du testicule. *Ann. Urol.*, **26**, 306–10.

Hoskin, P., Dilly, S., Easton, D. *et al.* (1986) Prognostic factors in stage I nonseminomatous germ cell testicular tumours managed by orchidectomy and surveillance: Implications for adjuvant chemotherapy. *J. Clin. Oncol.*, **4**, 1031–6.

Javadpour, N., Canning, D.A., O'Connell, K.J. and Young, J.D. (1986) Predictors of recurrent clinical stage I nonseminomatous testicular cancer. *Urology*, **27**, 508–11.

Johnson, D.E., Bracken, R.B. and Blight, E.M. (1976) Prognosis for pathologic stage I nonseminomatous germ cell tumours of the testis managed by retroperitoneal lymphadenectomy. *J. Urol.*, **116**, 63–5.

Lewis, D.J., Sesterhenn, I.A., McCarthy, W.F. and Moul, J.W. (1994) Immunohistochemical expression of p53 tumor suppressor gene protein in adult germ-cell testis tumors: clinical correlation in stage I disease. *J. Urol.*, **152**, 418–23.

Moriyama, N., Daly, J.J., Keating, M.A. *et al.* (1985) Vascular invasions as a prognosticator of metastatic disease in nonseminomatous germ cell tumours of the testis: Importance in 'Surveillance Only' protocols. *Cancer*, **56**, 2492–8.

Moul, J.W., Foley, J.P., Hitchcock, C.L., *et al.* (1993) Flow cytometric and quantitative histological parameters to predict occult disease in clinical stage I non-seminomatous testicular germ-cell tumors. *J. Urol.*, **150**, 879–83.

Moynihan, C. (1987) Testicular cancer: the psychosocial problems of patients and their relatives. *Cancer Surveys*, **6**, 477–510.

Oliver, R.T.D., Read, G., Jones, W.G. *et al.* (1984) Justification for a policy of surveillance in the management of stage I testicular teratoma, in *Controlled Clinical Trials in Urological Oncology* (eds L. Denis, G.P. Murphy, G.R. Prout and F. Schroder), Raven Press, New York, pp. 73–8.

Peckham, M.J., Barrett, A., McElwain, T.J. and Hendry, W.F. (1979) Combined management of malignant teratoma of the testis. *Lancet*, **ii**, 267–70.

Peckham, M.J., Barrett, A., Husband, J.E. and Hendry, W.F. (1982) Orchidectomy alone in testicular stage I non-seminomatous germ-cell tumours. *Lancet*, **ii**, 678–80.

Pizzocaro, G., Zanoni, F., Milani, A. *et al.* (1986) Orchidectomy alone in clinical stage I nonseminomatous testis cancer: A critical appraisal. *J. Clin. Oncol.*, **4**, 35–40.

Raghavan, D., Peckham, M.J., Heyderman, E. *et al.* (1982) Prognostic factors in clinical stage I nonseminomatous germ cell tumours of the testis. *Br. J. Cancer*, **45**, 167–73.

Read, G., Johnson, R.J., Wilkinson, P.M. and Eddleston, B. (1983) Prospective study of follow-up alone in stage I teratoma of the testis. *BMJ*, **287**, 1503–5.

Read, G., Stenning, S.P., Cullen, M.H., *et al.* (1992) Medical Research Council prospective study of surveillance for stage I testicular teratoma. *J. Clin. Oncol.*, **10**: 1762–8.

Rodriguez, P.N., Hafez, G.R. and Messing, E.M. (1986) Nonseminomatous germ cell tumour of the testicle: Does extensive staging of the primary tumour predict the likelihood of metastatic disease? *J. Urol.*, **136**, 604–8.

Rørth, M., Jacobsen, G.K., Van der Maas, H., *et al.* (1991) Surveillance alone versus radiotherapy after orchidectomy for clinical stage I non-seminomatous testicular cancer. *J. Clin. Oncol.*, **9**, 1543–8.

Sogani, P.C. and Fair, W.R. (1988) Surveillance alone in the treatment of clinical stage I non-seminomatous germ cell tumour of the testis (NSGCTT). *Sem. Urol.*, **6**, 53–6.

Sturgeon, J.F.G., Herman, J.G., Jewett, M.A.S. *et al.* (1983) A policy of surveillance alone after orchidectomy for clinical stage I non-seminomatous testis tumours. *Proc. Am. Soc. Clin. Oncol.*, **2**, 142.

Sturgeon, J.F.G., Jewett, M.A.S. and Alison, R.E. (1992) Surveillance after orchidectomy for patients with clinical stage I non-seminomatous testis tumours. *J. Clin. Oncol.*, **10**, 564–8.

Thompson, P.I., Nixon, J. and Harvey, V.J. (1988) Disease relapse in patients with stage I non-seminomatous germ cell tumour of the testis on active surveillance. *J. Clin. Oncol.*, **6**, 1597–603.

Whitmore, W.F. (1982) Surgical treatment of clinical stage I non-seminomatous germ cell tumors of the testis. *Cancer Treat. Rep.*, **66**, 5–10.

Young, B.J., Bultz, B.D., Russel, J.A. Trew, M.S. (1991) Compliance with follow-up of patients treated for non-seminomatous testicular cancer. *Br. J. Cancer*, **64**, 606–8.

ADJUVANT CHEMOTHERAPY IN HIGH RISK STAGE I NON-SEMINOMATOUS GERM CELL TUMORS OF THE TESTIS

14

M.H. Cullen

14.1 INTRODUCTION

In the last 30 years there have been important changes in the management of patients with Stage I non-seminomatous germ cell tumors of the testis (NSGCTT). Elective treatment of the retroperitoneal area with radiotherapy (in the UK and Denmark) or with surgery (in the USA and most of Europe) reduced the recurrence rate in this area, but disseminated relapse remained a problem. The advent of cisplatin-based combination chemotherapy in the early 1970s offered the real prospect of cure for all relapsing Stage I cases. However, the myelosuppression of chemotherapy in patients who had received radical para-aortic and pelvic radiotherapy was a significant problem, as was ejaculatory impotence in cases having elective retroperitoneal lymph node dissection (RPLND). This, plus the widespread use of CT scanning and tumor marker (AFP, HCG) assays to monitor disease recurrence, encouraged Peckham to suggest a policy of close surveillance in Stage I NSGCTT with chemotherapy at the first sign of relapse (Peckham *et al.*, 1982). The vast majority of cases are cured with this approach, despite a relapse rate of around 30% (Cullen, 1991).

14.2 DRAWBACKS OF SURVEILLANCE

On the face of it, surveillance would seem to be an almost perfect management policy in that the majority of cases escape treatment (other than orchidectomy) altogether, whilst the minority who relapse will be detected at an early stage and treated with curative chemotherapy. This had been my own view until sometime in 1986 when a patient of mine on surveillance, far from being disappointed to hear that his tumor markers were climbing and therefore required chemotherapy, was palpably relieved. 'At last I will be having some treatment instead of all these tests', was his comment. It was clear that the surveillance had been causing him significant stress by virtue of giving him monthly reminders of his diagnosis and the possibility of recurrence. It was preventing him from getting on with his life, and keeping him feeling tied to the hospital in case 'the worst' happened. Shortly after this a second patient expressed similar views. Hence this 'near-perfect' management strategy was distinctly unpopular with, at least some, patients.

Subsequently it became clear that this reaction to surveillance had been noted by

Testicular Cancer: Investigation and management. Second edition. Edited by Professor A. Horwich. Published in 1996 by Chapman & Hall. ISBN 0 412 61210 0.

others (Moynihan, 1987). Frequent examinations, CT scans and tumor marker analyses remind patients of their cancer history and of their continuing risk of relapse. This has been called the 'Damocles syndrome'.

There are other drawbacks to surveillance. The most important of these is that excellent patient compliance is essential. This may be a problem in a largely young population who may have less well-developed feelings of responsibility for their own health than older patients, and whose occupations may be less stable geographically. A recent population based study in Scotland revealed a defaulting rate of 35% amongst a group of Stage I teratoma patients, (Howard *et al.*, 1995). This explains only in part the rather high proportion of cases in which recurrent disease has been advanced at the time of detection (Sogani *et al.*, 1984; Vugrin *et al.*, 1984).

Surveillance is also costly and is not 100% effective. In the MRC prospective surveillance study, which is by far the biggest ever undertaken, the tumor-related mortality was 2% among 396 patients. In addition there can be significant morbidity associated with the event of relapse. Studies of surveillance alone show a consistent relapse rate around 30% (Peckham *et al.*, 1982).

14.3 ALTERNATIVES TO SURVEILLANCE

Retroperitoneal lymph node dissection is still widely practiced following orchidectomy in early stage NSGCTT. The relapse rate in patients with histologically negative retroperitoneal nodes is reduced from 30% to approximately 10%. Follow-up is still mandatory and 70–80% of clinical Stage I patients undergo unnecessary surgery (McLeod *et al.*, 1991).

Adjuvant chemotherapy is a clear alternative policy for Stage I NSGCTT, but the toxicity of chemotherapy is such that its applicability would be influenced by the proportion of patients who received treat-

ment unnecessarily. Clearly, adjuvant chemotherapy with significant toxicity would not be appropriate for a population of patients with a very small risk of recurrence. Arguably the most important information to emerge from the UK MRC Studies of surveillance is the histological prognostic scoring, allowing distinct categories of patients to be identified who have different risks of recurrence.

The UK MRC retrospective study of surveillance in 259 cases highlighted four histological factors within the primary tumor that carried independent prognostic significance (Freedman *et al.*, 1987). These were: tumor invasion of testicular veins, tumor invasion of testicular lymphatics, presence of undifferentiated cells and **absence** of yolk sac elements. The presence of any three or all four of these factors identifies a high risk group of Stage I NSGCTT patients with a chance of recurrence around 50%. A subsequent prospective study in 373 cases validated this prognostic index and allowed the identification of a group of patients to whom adjuvant chemotherapy might be offered (Read *et al.*, 1992). Data from surgically treated Stage II cases suggested that two courses of BEP would be sufficient adjuvant therapy (Williams *et al.*, 1987). Furthermore, the long-term toxicity of chemotherapy for NSGCTT seems to be related to total dose administered (Stuart *et al.* 1990). Hence just two courses were likely to be acceptable to a patient population where about half of those included would not be expected to develop metastatic disease.

14.4 MRC ADJUVANT CHEMOTHERAPY STUDY

Based on the above observations the UK MRC launched a study of adjuvant chemotherapy (BEP × 2) in October 1987 (Cullen *et al.*, 1996). Patients with newly diagnosed Stage I (i.e. CT scan of chest, abdomen and pelvis showing no metastases and normal AFP and HCG) NSGCTT were eligible if any three or all four of the high-risk histopathological features described above were present in the primary tumor.

A single pathologist in each participating center was responsible for assessing the number of risk factors and each had attended a workshop organized by the reference pathologist responsible for the original assessments on which the prognostic index was developed and tested. Hence it was possible to assess risk category rapidly in each collaborating center so that adjuvant chemotherapy could be offered and commenced promptly without necessitating the transfer of histopathological material to the reference pathologist.

14.4.1 CHEMOTHERAPY

Chemotherapy consisted of two courses of cisplatin, etoposide and bleomycin given in the following total doses, and repeated after 21 days:

Between days 1 and 5: cisplatin 100 mg m^{-2}IV, etoposide 120 mg m^{-2}IV × 3; bleomycin 30 mg IV infusion.
Day 8: bleomycin 30 mg IM/IV
Day 15: bleomycin 30 mg IM/IV

The second course was scheduled to commence on day 22.

14.4.2 TOXICITY ASSESSMENTS

In addition to standard short-term toxicity evaluation, longer-term toxicity problems were studied. These included fertility assessments, lung function studies and audiometry.

14.4.3 STATISTICS

In view of the fact that approximately 50% of patients would be receiving unnecessary chemotherapy, plus the unknown possibility of resistance to further chemotherapy in patients who relapse, it was felt that a recurrence rate of more than 5% would be unacceptable. Had a randomized trial against surveillance been conducted, an unacceptable relapse rate in the adjuvant arm would be sufficient justification for stopping, irrespective of the difference in relapse rate between the two arms. Consequently this was set up as a nonrandomized Phase II study with strict early stopping rules. One hundred patients were to be entered, enabling the final relapse rate to be estimated with a standard error of less than 5%. The trial was monitored using an early termination scheme in which the probability that the final relapse rate would exceed 5% was calculated, conditional on the current data, at the time of each relapse (Herson, 1979). Each patient in the trial at that time was weighted according to their follow-up time postorchidectomy, the weight being based on the known pattern of relapse in 'high risk' patients on surveillance. If this 'predictive probability' exceeded 95%, accrual would be stopped.

14.4.4 RESULTS

Between October 1987 and June 1994, 114 eligible patients are included with a median follow-up time of 4 years (range 7 months–7.3 years). One hundred and nine (97%) relapse-free patients had been followed up for at least one year; of these 93 (83%) had been followed up for at least 2 years and 75 (67%) for more than three years.

14.4.5 HISTOLOGY

Employing the British Testicular Tumour Panel classification, the histopathological diagnosis was MTU (malignant teratoma undifferentiated) in 73% of cases, MTI (malignant teratoma intermediate) in 23% of cases and MTT (malignant teratoma trophoblastic) in 3% of cases. Venous invasion was present in 96 cases, lymphatic invasion in 75, undifferentiated elements in 110 and yolk sac elements were **absent** in 90 cases (Table 14.1).

Table 14.1 Histological risk factors present

	Present		Absent		Not known
a. Venous invasion	96	85%	17	15%	1
b. Lymphatic invasion	75	66%	38	34%	1
c. 'Vascular' invasion (a or b)	114	100%	0	0%	0
d. Undifferentiated elements	110	97%	4	3%	0
e. Yolk sac elements	24	21%	90	79%	0

Table 14.2 Sperm density and motility before and maximum values on follow-up 9+ months after adjuvant chemotherapy. Number of cases in each band (%)

Density (million ml^{-1})			Motility (% motile forms)		
	Pre Rx	Max. on FU		Pre Rx	Max. on FU
<1	4 (10%)	4 (12%)	<10%	7 (18%)	4 (12%)
1–10	13 (32%)	8 (25%)	11–50%	14 (36%)	14 (44%)
11–20	9 (23%)	5 (16%)	>50%	18 (46%)	14 (44%)
>20	14 (35%)	15 (47%)			

Eighty-three patients (73%) had three high risk factors present and 30 (26%) had all four.

14.4.6 CHEMOTHERAPY DETAILS

The time from orchidectomy to the start of chemotherapy ranged from 14 to 104 days (median 37 days), with 90% of patients beginning chemotherapy within 2 months of orchidectomy.

14.4.7 LONG-TERM TOXICITY

14.4.7.1 Fertility

Forty patients had semen analysis carried out pretreatment. Twenty-four of these 40, plus a further seven without pretreatment results, had semen analysis on at least one occasion (>9 months) following treatment. Table 14.2 gives the sperm density in millions per milliliter and the percentage of motile forms pretreatment and the maximum values obtained in post treatment assessments. There are no significant differences between pre- and post-treatment values indicating no consistent reduction in these indices of fertility following two courses of BEP.

Table 14.3 Mean percentage of predicted values for lung function before, and minimum and maximum per cent of predicted values > 9 months after adjuvant chemotherapy

	Pretreatment (n = 19)	Min % predicted (n = 27)	Max % predicted (n = 27)
FVC	107%	106%	109%
FEV$_1$	109%	106%	110%
TLC*	108%	105%	111%
KCO	102%	89%	96%

* Pretreatment $n = 16$, min and max $n = 22$.

14.4.7.2 Lung function

Nineteen patients had pretreatment lung function test results; 16 of these patients, together with a further 11 patients without pretreatment test results, have had lung function tests on at least one occasion post-treatment. Table 14.3 shows the mean percentage predicted values pretreatment, and the minimum and maximum percentage of predicted values recorded at any point after completion of chemotherapy (all are at least 9 months post-chemotherapy). For patients with both pre- and post-treatment values the differences between pre- and minimum postchemotherapy values for FVC, FEV_1 and TLC were not statistically significant (paired *t*-test, mean differences FVC 4% ($p = 0.1$), FEV_1 2% ($p = 0.39$), TLC 4% ($p = 0.45$). However, 15 of the 16 patients (with pre- and postchemo results) showed a decrease in KCO (transfer factor coefficient). The decline in percentage predicted value ranged from 2 to 36% with an overall mean difference between pre- and minimum postchemotherapy values of 15% ($p = 0.002$). No patient had symptomatic respiratory dysfunction. The total dose of bleomycin administered to patients in this study was 180 mg.

14.4.7.3 Audiometry

Thirty-seven patients had a pretreatment audiogram. Twenty-two of these plus a further 12 (total 34) have had at least one postchemotherapy audiogram. Four patients (12%) had postchemotherapy audiograms showing typical high tone hearing loss of nerve conduction type, up to 60 dB at >4000 Hz.

14.4.8 PATIENT FOLLOW-UP RELAPSE AND SURVIVAL

The median follow up time is 4 years (range 7 months to 7.3 years). One hundred and nine (97%) relapse-free patients have been followed up for at least one year; of these 93 (83%) have been followed up for at least 2 years and 75 (67%) for more than three years. Two relapses have been reported:

1. The first relapse occurred seven months after the start of chemotherapy. At the time of the relapse detection the AFP was 62 kU l^{-1} and HCG 89 IU l^{-1}. There was retroperitoneal lymphadenopathy (max. diameter 4 cm), liver metastases and more than 30 pulmonary metastases (the largest was 1.9 cm). At this time the patient was treated with further conventional dose cisplatin-based chemotherapy ('C-BOP' regimen) incorporating carboplatin, cisplatin, vincristine and bleomycin in a rapidly cycling therapy, but progressed through this. He was then given high dose carboplatin and etoposide. Tumor markers normalized but small, residual abnormal shadows persisted in the liver, lungs and para-aortic area. Eighteen months later there was further progression with rising markers and liver metastases, and he was treated with paclitaxel and cisplatin. He again responded, but eventually died 27 months after the first recurrence.

2. The second patient was aged 59 at diagnosis. AFP and HCG were normal prior to orchidectomy and ever since. He relapsed in the groin after 18 months and subsequently experienced lung and further groin recurrences. He has had incomplete responses to more cisplatin based combination chemotherapy, and remains alive with progressive disease five years after orchidectomy. Central histopathological review of diagnostic material was undertaken by the reference pathologist without knowledge of clinical outcome. This was the only case among 104 reviewed where the diagnosis was thought not to be a germ cell tumor (GCT). Instead the most likely diagnosis was thought to be rete adenocarcinoma. Subsequent review of relapse material (inguinal nodes and scar) supported this view.

The relapse-free rate at two years is thus 98%, with a 95% lower confidence interval (CI) of 95%. The 95% confidence interval therefore excludes a true relapse rate of more than 5%. Within the group of patients reported by the reference pathologist to have a germ cell tumor with 3 or 4 risk factors present, one relapse has occurred. The estimated relapse free-rate is 98.4%, with a lower 95% CI of 95.2%. The estimated relapse-free rate in those 88 cases with confirmed germ cell tumor *and* vascular invasion is 98.8% with a lower 95% CI of 96.1%.

14.5   OTHER STUDIES OF ADJUVANT CHEMOTHERAPY

There have been three other studies of adjuvant chemotherapy in Stage I NSGCTT. These have all been very small studies. The study of Pont *et al.* (1990) included only 18 cases and is reported as an interim analysis. Patients were selected on the basis of vascular invasion alone, and received two courses of BEP. With a median follow-up of 27 months there had been two recurrences and one death from resistant tumor. No long-term toxicity data were reported. Oliver *et al.* (1992) reported a pilot study with 22 cases, which were selected using MRC criteria, but those with only two high risk factors (equivalent to a recurrence risk of less than 25%) were also eligible. There was one relapse and no late toxicity data. The study from Studer *et al.* (1993) has 43 patients selected on the basis of vascular invasion (five cases), $pT > 1$ (21 cases) and embryonal carcinoma (42 cases). The choice of these was based upon the findings of others, often in small retrospective comparisons that patients with these features had a higher risk of relapse than patients without them. They had not been validated in a separate series of patients prospectively (in the MRC surveillance studies (632 cases), embryonal carcinoma and $pT > 1$ were not independent prognostic variables), and it is not possible to estimate what the relapse rate, **without** chemotherapy would have been. After a median follow-up of 42 months there has been just one recurrence, and this consisted of mature teratoma that was treated surgically. Again no late toxicity data are reported.

14.6   OPTIONS PROJECT

The results of these studies of adjuvant chemotherapy, particularly the MRC study, suggested that two quite different management options, namely, surveillance with four courses of BEP for those who relapse, and adjuvant chemotherapy with two courses of BEP for all, produce similar high levels of cure in Stage I NSGCTT. We then embarked, in Birmingham, on a study to examine which of the two possible management options individuals would choose if they had Stage I NSGCTT (Cullen *et al.*, 1996, in press). To refine this in a quantifiable way we asked the subjects to imagine they had a newly diagnosed Stage I teratoma with a risk of recurrence of 10%, 20%, 30%, 40%, 50%, 70% and 90%. At each level of recurrence risk they were asked to select from:

1. adjuvant chemotherapy;
2. surveillance;
3. prefer decision to be made by doctor.

The options were described simply to the subjects by a trained oncology nurse, backed up by written information sheets covering the important aspects of each.

As well as canvassing 18 newly diagnosed stage I NSGCTT patients we also put the same 'hypothetical' scenario to 38 healthy males (firemen) within the NSGCTT age group (18–40), 56 medical students, 41 teratoma patients in remission who had direct, personal experience of surveillance, 38 patients in remission who had received BEP chemotherapy, and 5 who had experience of both surveillance and chemotherapy. The final group studied were the 'decision makers' themselves, namely 17 oncologist members of the MRC testicular tumor working party.

Figure 14.1 shows the number of newly diagnosed cases choosing each of the three options at the different hypothetical levels of recurrence risk. At the 50% level or greater, virtually all patients opted for adjuvant chemotherapy (AC). At the 40% level, about 60% chose AC and about 20% each chose surveillance (S) and 'doctor to decide' (DD). The preference for the decision to be made by the doctor increased at the lower levels of risk to 28% of cases at both the 20% and 10% levels. AC was still quite popular even at the 20% (28% of cases) and 10% (22% of cases)

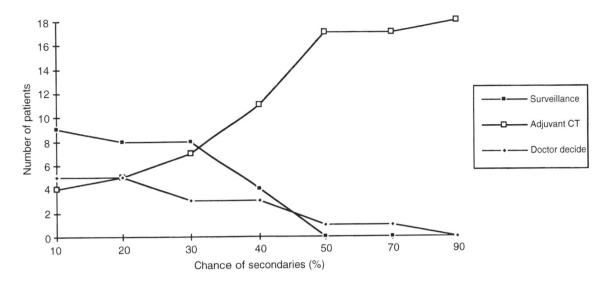

Fig. 14.1 Number of subjects selecting each option at specified risk levels: newly diagnosed Stage I NSGCTT (*n* = 18).

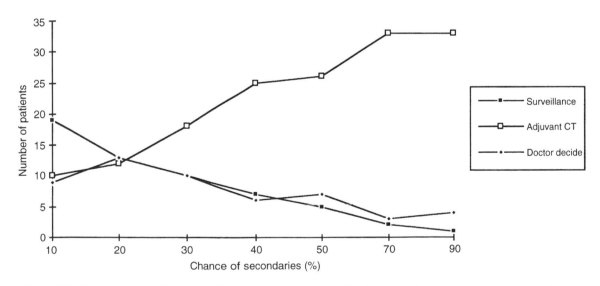

Fig. 14.2 Number of subjects selecting each option at specified risk levels: postchemotherapy patients – BEP (*n* = 38).

level of risk. Thirty-eight patients who had personal experience of BEP chemotherapy responded to the hypothetical scenario in similar general fashion (Fig. 14.2), except that the preference for adjuvant chemotherapy was clear at all risk levels above 20%. At 20% risk of recurrence almost identical numbers chose AC (12), S(13) and DD(13). At the lowest (10%) level of risk, still 26% of patients who had experience of BEP pre-

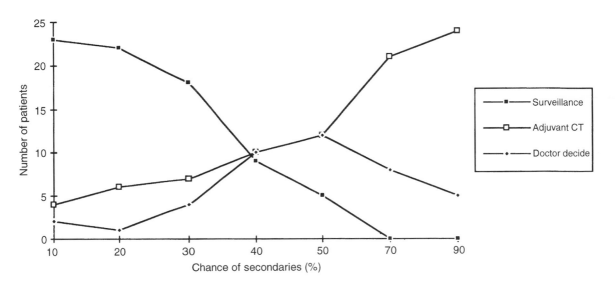

Fig. 14.3 Number of subjects selecting each option at specified risk levels: surveillance patients (*n* = 29).

ferred AC to S or DD. The picture for patients who have experience of surveillance is rather different (Fig. 14.3). Here the 'doctor to decide' option is much commoner in the higher 40–70% range and is even the choice of 17% of cases at the 90% recurrence risk level. Although surveillance is the most popular option at the 30% level and below, still a significant minority of patients chose AC (21% at the 20% level and 14% at the lowest 10% level). At the 40% cut off level the three groups are equally split between S, AC and DD.

The medical student and firemen control groups responded in almost identical fashion with the 'cross over' from S to AC occurring between 20% and 30% recurrence risk. The proportion of DDs was very low even in the lay control group of firemen, much lower than in the lay group of new patients (Fig. 14.4). This suggests that people with cancer are more likely to want the doctor to make the treatment decisions. In the final control group (oncologists specializing in testicular cancer) the 'cross over' from S to AC occurred at the slightly higher 30–40% risk level, with

even fewer opting for the doctor to decide (Fig. 14.5). Interestingly this was the only group with a significant proportion (12%, or two oncologists) opting for S at the 70% and 90% levels. Clearly these two oncologists are out of step with the vast majority of actual and potential patients (i.e. controls). The five patients who had experienced both S and then BEP on relapse, not surprisingly all favored AC since the S strategy had failed them.

This study seems to show that, given the options of surveillance or adjuvant chemotherapy, many patients would select adjuvant chemotherapy even at relatively low levels of risk of recurrence. This was true both for newly diagnosed Stage I NSGCTT patients and for those who had already experienced surveillance, chemotherapy or both. For the newly diagnosed cases it was a 'real life' decision, and for the others it was a hypothetical situation, but one based on real life experience of the options available. Of some concern is the finding that the testicular tumor specialist group expresses greater extremes of choice than all other groups.

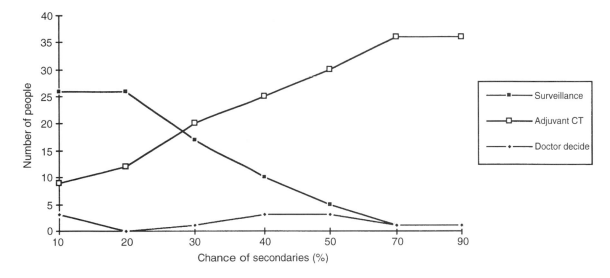

Fig. 14.4 Number of subjects selecting each option at specified risk levels: control group – Fire Service ($n = 38$).

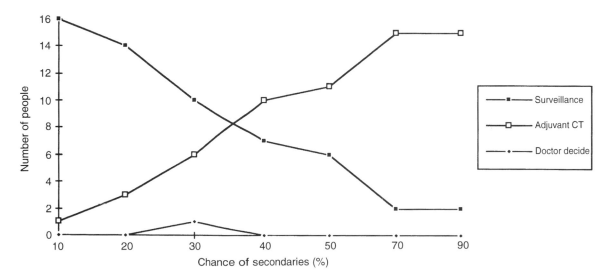

Fig. 14.5 Number of subjects selecting each option at specified risk levels: control group – testicular tumor specialists ($n = 17$).

14.7 CONCLUSIONS

When chemotherapy is used as adjuvant therapy in curable tumors, two endpoints other than recurrence are important. Firstly, it is crucial to have a clear understanding of the proportion of patients who are being treated unnecessarily. This information can only come from detailed prognostic factor analyses generated in large numbers of cases

cases and validated prospectively, as in the MRC studies forming the foundations of the present work. Secondly, it is vital to examine late toxicity since this is the enduring trade-off patients must accept for the avoidance of surveillance. The MRC adjuvant chemotherapy study shows that the main late toxicity problems associated with BEP chemotherapy, namely reduced fertility, impaired lung function and hearing, are absent or mild in the vast majority of cases following just two courses. This is as one would expect given the known correlation of these problems with total doses of drugs administered.

The principal areas of difficulty in identification of the histopathological high risk factors are the recognition that yolk sac tumor elements are not present, and distinguishing between venous and lymphatic invasion. In the current MRC adjuvant chemotherapy study, the population to whom adjuvant chemotherapy is offered are all those with 'vascular' invasion regardless of whether the vessel is thought to be a vein or a lymphatic. The other risk factors are ignored since this much simpler and reproducible criterion identifies a larger proportion of stage I patients with a recurrence risk only a little lower at 40%.

The ultimate aim of management in young people with malignant disease should be cure with minimal side-effects and follow-up. This last point is important since patients do not **feel** cured and experience the benefits of cure if their lives are interrupted frequently by hospital attendance and investigation. Clearly, careful surveillance was necessary in this study since the relapse rate was not known at the outset and strict early stopping rules based on relapse detection were incorporated. The policy of adjuvant chemotherapy as described in the MRC study does not guarantee 100% cure and hence discharge from follow-up immediately after chemotherapy. The relapse-free rate at 2 years was 98% and is most unlikely to increase with longer follow-up. However it is clear that a realistic alternative to intensive surveillance is not only available but may well be preferred by some patients.

REFERENCES

Cullen, M.H. (1991) Management of Stage I non seminoma: surveillance and chemotherapy; in *Testicular Cancer Investigation and Management* (ed. A. Horwich), Chapman & Hall, London, pp. 149–66.

Cullen, M.H., Billingham, L., Cook, J. and Woodroffe, C. (1996) Management preferences in stage I non-seminomatous tumours of the testis: an investigation among patients, controls and oncologists. *Brit. J. Cancer* (in press).

Cullen, M.H., Stenning, S.P., Parkinson, M.C., Fosså, S.D., Kaye, S.B., Horwich, A.H., Harland, S.J., Williams, M.V. and Jakes, J.R. (1996) Short course adjuvant chemotherapy in high risk Stage I non-seminomatous germ cell tumours of the testis (NSGCTT): An MRC study report. *J. Clin. Oncol.*, **14**, 1106–13.

Freedman, L.S., Parkinson, M.C., Jones, W.G., Oliver R.T.D., Peckham, M.J., Read, G., Newlands, E.S. and Williams, C.J., (1987) Histopathology in the prediction of relapse of patients with stage I testicular teratoma treated by orchidectomy alone. *Lancet*, **ii**, 294–8.

Herson, J. (1979) Predictive probability early termination plans for phase II clinical trials. *Biometrics*, **34**, 775–83.

Howard, G.C.W., Clarke, K., Elia, M.H., Hutcheon, A.W., Kaye, S.B., Windsor, P.M. and Yosef, H.M.A. (1995) A Scottish National Audit of current patterns of management for patients with testicular non-seminomatous germ-cell tumours. *Brit. J. Cancer*, **72**, 1303–6.

McLeod, D.G., Weiss, R.B., Stablein, D.M., Muggia, F.M., Paulson, D.F., Ellis., J.H., Spaulding, J.T. and Donohue, J.P. for The Testicular Cancer Intergroup Study (1991) Staging relationships and outcome in early stage testicular cancer. A report from the Testicular Cancer Intergroup Study. *J. Urol.* **145**, 1178–83.

Moynihan, C. (1987) Testicular cancer: the psychosocial problems of patients and their relatives. *Cancer Surveys*, **6**, 477–510.

Oliver, R.T.D., Raja, M.A., Ong, J. and Gallagher, C.J. (1992) Pilot study to evaluate impact of a policy of adjuvant chemotherapy for high risk stage I malignant teratoma on overall relapse rate of stage 1 cancer patients. *J. Urol.*, **148**, 1453–6.

Peckham, M.J., Barrett, A., Husband, J.E. and Hendry, W.E. (1982) Orchidectomy alone in testicular stage I non-seminomatous germ-cell tumours. *Lancet*, **ii**, 678–80.

Pont, J., Holtl, W., Kosak, D., Machacek, E., Kienzer, H., Julcher, H. and Honetz, N. (1990) Risk-adapted treatment choice in stage I non-seminomatous testicular germ cell cancer by regarding vascular invasion in the primary tumour: A prospective trial. *J. Clin. Oncol.*, **8**, 16–20.

Read, G., Stenning, S.P., Cullen, M.H., Parkinson, M.C., Horwich, A., Kaye, S.B. and Cook, P.A. (1992) Medical Research Council prospective study of surveillance for stage I testicular teratoma. *J. Clin. Oncol.*, **10**, 1762–8.

Sogani, P.C., Whitmore, W.F. Jr, Herr, H.W. *et al.* (1984) Orchidectomy alone in the treatment of clinical stage I nonseminomatous germ cell tumor of the testis. *J. Clin. Oncol.* **2**, 267–70.

Stuart, N.S.A., Woodroffe, C.M., Grundy, R. and Cullen, M.H. (1990) Long-term side-effects of chemotherapy for testicular cancer: The cost of cure. *Brit. J. Cancer*, **61**, 479–84.

Studer, U.E., Fey, M.F., Calderoni, A., Kraft, R., Mazzucchelli, L. and Sonntag, R.W. (1993) Adjuvant chemotherapy after orchidectomy in high-risk patients with clinical stage I non-seminomatous testicular cancer. *Eur. Urol.* **23**, 444–9.

Vugrin, D., Peckham, M.J., Pizzocaro, G. *et al.* (1984) Multinational experience with orchidectomy alone in the treatment of clinical stage I nonseminomatous tumours, in *Adjuvant Therapy of Cancer IV*, (eds S.E. Jones and S.E. Salmon), Grune & Stratton, Philadelphia, pp. 521–7.

Williams, S.D., Stablein, D.M., Einhorn, L.H., Muggia, F.M., Weiss, R.B., Donohue, J.P., Paulson, D.F., Brunner, K.W., Jacobs, E.M., Spaulding, J.T., De Wys, W.D. and Crawford, E.D. (1987) Immediate adjuvant chemotherapy versus observation with treatment at relapse in pathological stage II testicular cancer. *N. Engl. J. Med.*, **317**, 1433–8.

RATIONALE FOR LYMPHADENECTOMY IN STAGE I NON-SEMINOMA 15

G. Pizzocaro

15.1 INTRODUCTION

The management of clinical Stage I non-seminoma is controversial. In the past, the alternative was between high-energy irradiation and lymphadenectomy. In recent years it has been between surveillance and lymphadenectomy (Pizzocaro *et al.*, 1985) or adjuvant chemotherapy in high risk cases (Chapter 14).

The advantages of retroperitoneal lymph node dissection (RPLND) are a careful pathological staging and the definitive control of the retroperitoneal nodes. Both advantages are fully met only if the operation is performed carefully; then, morbidity is minimal and mortality is nil. Follow-up is simplified because only the serum tumor markers and the chest X-ray must be repeated at each clinical examination. With early recognition of distant metastases, virtually all patients with relapse can be salvaged with cisplatin combination chemotherapy, and the end cure rate can approach 100% (Pizzocaro, 1986).

The main disadvantage of RPLND is the possible loss of antegrade ejaculation, which occurs in approximately 70% of cases following a bilateral, radical operation. Loss of ejaculation is a very important issue in young patients with a very good outlook. It is not only a fertility issue; it can also become a psychological problem (Barbieri *et al.*, 1989). Therefore, surgeons have developed tech-niques in order to avoid dry ejaculation following RPLND (Hermaneck and Siegel, 1982; Fosså *et al.*, 1984; Pizzocaro, Salvioni and Zanoni, 1985; Donohue *et al.*, 1988; Jewett *et al.*, 1988). It is therefore important to discuss the pros and cons of RPLND in the management of clinical Stage I testicular non-seminoma.

15.2 PATHOLOGICAL VERIFICATION OF CLINICAL STAGING

Usually, surgical series are presented according to pathological staging (Table 15.1). The clinical false negative and false positive rates are not correctly reported. On the other hand, several radiologists reported sensitivity and specificity of single or combined radiographic examinations. Neither of these reports allows comparison of clinical and pathological staging. Only Pizzocaro (1986; Pizzocaro, Salvioni

Table 15.1 Pathological staging classification

Stage	Description
I	All nodes negative
IIA	Five or less metastatic nodes, no one ⩾2 cm, no extranodal spread
IIB	More than five metastatic nodes, at least one node >2 cm, any extranodal spread

Testicular Cancer: Investigation and management. Second edition. Edited by Professor A. Horwich.
Published in 1996 by Chapman & Hall. ISBN 0 412 61210 0.

and Nicolai, 1994) and the SWENOTECA (Klepp *et al.*, 1990) and Donohue *et al.* (1994) have reported results of RPLND in clinical Stage I non-seminoma.

Between January 1980 and August 1981, 36 consecutive patients underwent RPLND at the Istituto Nazionale Tumori for clinical Stage I non-seminoma (Pizzocaro, 1986). The main clinical investigations were postorchidectomy determination of serum alpha-fetoprotein (AFP) and human chorionic gonadotrophin (HCG), chest X-ray, bipedal lymphangiography (LAG) and abdominal ultrasound. Only eight patients had computed tomography (CT) scans. Retroperitoneal metastases were pathologically documented in eight cases (22.2%). Between August 1981 and December 1984, a surveillance study was performed at the Istituto Nazionale Tumori (Pizzocaro *et al.*, 1987). All patients had postorchidectomy half-life kinetics of serum AFP and HCG, chest X-ray and 'unequivocally normal' LAG and CT scans of the abdomen. After a 5-year follow-up, a total of 15 (17.6%) out of 85 evaluable patients developed retroperitoneal metastases: three with concomitant and one following distant dissemination. The median time to relapse in the retroperitoneal nodes was 1 year; two retroperitoneal relapses occurred after 3 years. Retroperitoneal metastases were >5 cm in seven cases when first recognized. It was then decided to end the surveillance study.

During the following 7 years (1985–1991 inclusive) 94 consecutive patients with clinical Stage I non-seminoma were submitted to RPLND (Pizzocaro, Salvioni and Nicolai, 1994). All patients had postorchidectomy normal or normalized AFP and HCG levels, chest X-ray, CT scan or magnetic resonance imaging (MRI) of the abdomen. Lymphangiography was not routinely performed and therefore it was not considered in the definition of clinical Stage I. Forty (20.6%) out of 194 cases had documented retroperitoneal lymph node metastases. The figure was even higher in other studies. Klepp *et al.* (1990) reported the results of RPLND in a total of 277 clinical Stage I non-seminoma operated in several centers in Norway between 1981 and 1986: 75 (27.1%) had pathologically documented retroperitoneal metastases. Donohue *et al.* (1993) reported retroperitoneal metastases in 112 (29.6%) of 378 clinical Stage I patients.

One could suppose that it was LAG that reduced the false negative clinical error in our surveillance study, but it is not completely true. In fact, 114 (58.8%) out of 194 clinical Stage I non-seminoma of our last series also had LAG (Pizzocaro *et al.*, 1992). It was pathological in nine (7.9%) cases, and six (66.7%) of them had documented retroperitoneal metastases. On the other hand, 20 (19.1%) of the 105 patients with negative LAG (negative CT scans and normal markers) had documented retroperitoneal metastases. So far, LAG has reduced the false negative error to only 19.1%. This figure is a little higher than the 17.6% found in the surveillance study at the Istituto Nazionale Tumori. When the radiologists were asked about the difference between the two series, they replied that they felt very committed and responsible during the surveillance study. Therefore, they considered normal only 'unequivocally' negative imaging when they knew that Stage I patients were entering surveillance. On the other hand, 40% false positive errors (negative histology) were reported in clinical Stage IIA patients operated on between 1980 and 1984 (Pizzocaro, 1987). Following the closure of the surveillance study, they felt much more relaxed, the negative criteria came back to normal, the false negative error increased for Stage I (19.1%) and the false positive error decreased for Stage IIA: 34.5% of the 29 patients operated on in the period 1985–91.

In conclusion, the false negative error in clinical Stage I non-seminoma can be estimated to be approximately 25% following 'normal' clinical staging. It means that one out of four patients with clinical Stage I non-seminoma actually has unrecognized retroperitoneal metastases.

15.3 THERAPEUTIC VALUE OF LYMPHADENECTOMY

It has been repeatedly stated by urological surgeons that 'retroperitoneal relapses following a properly executed RPLND are unlikely to occur'. Rørth *et al.* (1989) reviewed carefully the occurrence of retroperitoneal metastases following unilateral or nerve-sparing RPLND in clinical Stage I non-seminoma: Pizzocaro *et al.* reported no retroperitoneal recurrences in the first 61 cases (1985) and two out of the subsequent 194 patients (Pizzocaro, Salvioni and Nicolai, 1994). Boedefeld and Weissbach (1986) reported one out of 94 cases, Donohue *et al.* (1994) also reported three out of 378 patients, and Fosså *et al.* (1984) reported none in 53 cases. Overall, only six (0.7%) out of 780 patients who had undergone unilateral or nerve-sparing RPLND for clinical Stage I non-seminoma developed documented retroperitoneal recurrences. It is therefore confirmed that not only bilateral, radical RPLND, but also unilateral or nerve-sparing dissections can avoid retroperitoneal recurrences in over 99% of clinical Stage I non-seminoma. Furthermore, distant dissemination occurs in 10% of patients operated for negative nodes and in approximately 30% of those with positive histology not treated with adjuvant chemotherapy (Donohue *et al.*, 1994; Pizzocaro, Salvioni and Nicolai, 1994).

15.4 EVOLUTION OF SURGICAL SKILL

Donohue, Zachary and Maynard (1982) wrote a detailed and helpful paper on the distribution of retroperitoneal metastases in pathological Stage IIA and IIB (B_1 and B_2) non-seminoma. Not a single Stage IIA patient had suprahilar metastases, and the contralateral involvement was extremely rare. These data con-

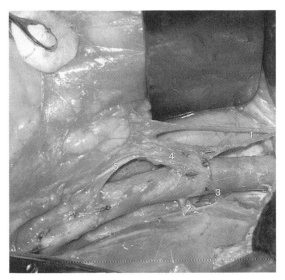

Fig. 15.1 Retroperitoneal sympathetic innervation on the left side. 1, Splanchnic nerves; 2, lumbar sympathetic chain; 3, postganglionic root of the third lumbar ganglion; 4, sympathetic plexus around the origin of the inferior mesenteric artery; 5, postganglionic trunk to hypogastric plexus.

firmed the reports by Hermaneck and Siegel (1982) in Germany and by Pizzocaro (1981) in Italy. Therefore, modified dissections were proposed in clinical Stage I non-seminoma, in order to decrease the incidence of postoperative dry ejaculation (Hermaneck and Siegel, 1982; Fosså *et al.*, 1984; Lange, Narayan and Fraley, 1984; Pizzocaro, Salvioni and Zanoni, 1985). Overall, approximately 90% of patients submitted to unilateral RPLND have been reported to maintain (or to recover) antegrade ejaculation postoperatively. The nerve-sparing RPLND (Figs 15.1, 15.2 and 15.3) was introduced late in the 1980s, and antegrade ejaculation can be maintained in approximately 98% of patients operated with this technique (Donohue *et al.*, 1988 and 1994; Jewett *et al.*, 1988). The development and surgical details of nerve-sparing RPLND are fully described in Chapter 16.

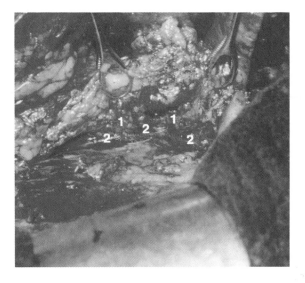

Fig. 15.2 Origin of the anterior roots. 1, From the lumbar sympathetic chain; 2, following medial mobilization of the left para-aortic nodes.

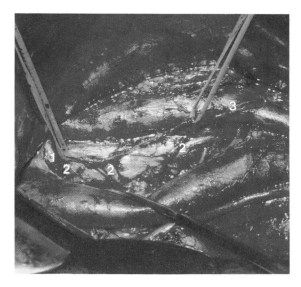

Fig. 15.3 Postganglionic fibers on the right side between the aorta and inferior vena cava. 1, Upper prerenal trunk; 2, lumbar roots; 3, preiliac trunk towards hypogastric plexus.

The major criticism about this sophisticated surgical technique is that 'patients should be referred to urologists who have experience in these procedures and, furthermore, CT scan of the retroperitoneal area is still recommended' (Rørth *et al.*, 1989). First of all, one should bear in mind that germ cell testicular tumors are very rare and highly curable neoplasms. Therefore, every patient with a germ cell testicular tumor 'must' be referred to a specialized center in order to achieve the maximum cure rate. The Irish experience is of paramount importance in this regard (Thornhill *et al.*, 1988). Secondly, Røth *et al.* (1989) reported only 0.7% retroperitoneal relapses following unilateral or nerve-sparing RPLND in the world literature. With such a low risk of relapse, repeated CT scans of the abdomen cannot be recommended. The much cheaper ultrasound is more than sufficient to follow the retroperitoneal area after surgery.

15.5 COMPARISON OF MEDICAL TREATMENTS AND LYMPHADENECTOMY

Any statistical comparison between surveillance and RPLND in the management of clinical Stage I non-seminoma cannot be done, because with a cure rate of over 95% several thousand patients would be necessary to carry out a randomized study. However, the two methods can be compared on the basis of simple and practical considerations.

The overall long-term relapse rate in the surveillance study is approximately 30%, with the majority of relapses occurring in the retroperitoneal area (Hoskin *et al.*, 1986, Friedman, *et al.*, 1987; Pizzocaro *et al.*, 1987; Rørth *et al.*, 1987; Read *et al.*, 1992). While distant dissemination usually occurs within the first-year follow-up (Pizzocaro *et al.*, 1987; Donohue, 1989), retroperitoneal metastases have been reported after 3 (Pizzocaro *et al.*, 1987), 4 (Hoskin *et al.*, 1986) and 5 years (Rørth *et al.*, 1987). Furthermore, in one study (Pizzocaro *et al.*, 1987), approximately 50% of retroperitoneal metastases were diagnosed when larger than 5 cm. With optimal chemotherapy at relapse over 90% of patients can be salvaged. However, the cure rate for patients with bulky retroperitoneal metastases is not so high. So far, with a 30% relapse rate, the cancer-related mortality in a surveillance study will be approximately 3% after a minimum 5-year follow-up. The cancer-related mortality can be even higher if the surveillance study is not carefully performed and metastases are diagnosed late. It can be considered that, in clinical Stage I non-seminoma, vascular invasions and the presence of undifferentiated cells (embryonal carcinoma) carry an increased risk of relapse (Hoskin *et al.*, 1986; Read *et al.*, 1992) or of (retroperitoneal) metastases (Klepp *et al.*, 1990). As two courses of adjuvant cisplatin vinblastine/bleomycin (PVB) have been shown to prevent relapses in patients who had undergone radical RPLND for pathologically documented retroperitoneal metastases (Williams *et al.*, 1987), medical oncologists suggest two courses of adjuvant chemotherapy for patients with clinical Stage I non-seminoma with a high risk of relapse (Medical Research Council, 1987; Rørth *et al.*, 1987) (see Chapter 14). These authors do not take into account that the results of the Testicular Cancer Intergroup Study (Williams *et al.*, 1987) demonstrated the ability of two courses of adjuvant PVB to prevent 'distant dissemination' following 'radical RPLND' not the ability to cure 'unrecognized retroperitoneal metastases in clinical Stage I'. It is known that, in good risk patients with metastatic disease, three courses of bleomycin/etoposide/cisplatin (BEP) are probably as good as four courses (Einhorn *et al.*, 1989). Furthermore, it may be that pulmonary metastases are more responsive to chemotherapy than retroperitoneal metastases. With two courses of adjuvant chemotherapy following orchidectomy alone in poor risk patients, a proportion of cases with unrecognized retroperitoneal metastases may be undertreated and will relapse, possibly with less responsive tumors, or mature tetratoma (Pont *et al.*, 1990).

On the other hand, with unilateral or nerve-sparing RPLND, the real situation concerning retroperitoneal nodes is immediately clear. The cost is zero mortality and minimal morbidity; the retroperitoneal relapse rate is less than 1% and the follow-up is simplified; the cure rate with surgery alone (Donohue *et al.*, 1994) is approximately 90% in patients with negative nodes and 70% in those with positive histology; with early (and easy) recognition of distant dissemination, nearly all patients with relapse will be cured with chemotherapy and the end cure rate will approach 99%. Only the occasional patient who will relapse with an unresponsive tumor will die of the disease. We lost only three (1.3%) out of 36 + 190 patients submitted to RPLND for clinical Stage I non-seminoma without any adjuvant chemotherapy: two out of 181 with negative and one out of 45 with positive nodes (Pizzocaro, 1986; Pizzocaro, Salvioni and Nicolai, 1994). Also Donohue *et al.* (1994) lost only three (0.9%) out of 330 clinical Stage I patients treated with RPLND alone: two out of 266 with negative nodes and one out of 64 with positive nodes not receiving adjuvant chemotherapy.

15.6 CONCLUSIONS

The surveillance study is very stimulating scientifically, but the same information can be obtained with RPLND if patients are carefully staged clinically (Klepp *et al.*, 1990; Donohue *et al.*, 1994; Pizzocaro *et al.*, 1994). Retroperitoneal lymph node dissection simplifies the management of clinical Stage I non-seminoma, while the surveillance program is potentially dangerous. With unilateral or nerve-sparing RPLND there is no contraindication to surgery. Furthermore, how can surgeons become skilful in performing RPLND in partial responders to chemotherapy if they are not allowed to do this very specialized surgery in early cases?

REFERENCES

Barbieri, A. *et al.*, (1989) Psychodynamic experience with patients undergoing treatment for germinal tumour of the testis. *Br. J. Sex. Med.*, **16**, 189–94.

Boedefeld, E.A. and Weissbach, L. (1986) Modified retroperitoneal lymph node dissection: ejaculation preserving approach in stage I NSGCT, in *Germ Cell Tumours II* (eds W.G. Jones, A.M. Ward and C.K. Anderson), Pergamon Press, Oxford, p. 457.

Donohue, J.P. (1989) Management of clinical stage I and II non-seminoma. The Indiana University approach, in *I Tumori Genito-Urinari* (eds U. Veronesi, G. Pizzocaro, E. Pisani and A. Santoro), CEA, Milano, pp. 319–22.

Donohue, J.P., Foster, R.S., Geier, G. *et al.* (1988) Preservation of ejaculation following nerve sparing retroperitoneal lymphadenectomy. *J. Urol.*, **139**, 206A (Abstract 176).

Donohue, J.P., Thornhill, J.A., Foster, R.S. *et al.* (1994) Retroperitoneal lymphadenectomy for clinical stage A testis cancer (1965 to 1989): modifications of technique and impact on ejaculation. *J. Urol.*, **149**, 237–43.

Donohue, J.P., Zachary, J.M. and Maynard, B.R. (1982) Distribution of nodal metastases in nonseminomatous testis cancer. *J. Urol.*, **128**, 315–20.

Einhorn, L.H., Williams, S.D., Loehrer, P.J. *et al.* (1989) Evaluation of optional duration of chemotherapy in favorable-prognosis disseminated germ cell tumors: a Southeastern Cancer Study Group Protocol. *J. Clin. Oncol.*, **7**, 387–91.

Fosså, S.D., Klepp, O., Ous, J. *et al.* (1984) Unilateral retroperitoneal lymph node dissection in patients with non-seminomatous testicular tumor in clinical stage I. *Eur. Urol.*, **10**, 17–22.

Friedman, L.S., Parkinson, M.C., Jones, W.J. *et al.* (1987) Histology in the prediction of relapse of patients with stage I testicular teratoma treated with orchidectomy alone. *Lancet*, **11**, 294–8.

Hermaneck, P. and Siegel, A. (1982) Necessary extent of lymph node dissection in testicular tumours. A histopathological investigation. *Eur. Urol.*, **8**, 135–44.

Hoskin, P., Dilly, S., Easton, D. *et al.* (1986) Prognostic factors in stage I non-seminomatous germ-cell testicular tumours managed by orchidectomy and surveillance: implications for adjuvant chemotherapy. *J. Clin. Oncol.*, **10**, 1031–6.

Jewett, M.A.S., Kong, Y.P., Goldberg, J.D. *et al.* (1988) Retroperitoneal lymphadenectomy for testis tumor with nerve sparing for ejaculation. *J. Urol.*, **139**, 1220–4.

Klepp, O., Olsson, A.M., Henrikson, H. *et al.* (1990) Prognostic factors in clinical stage I

testicular teratoma: multivariate analysis of a prospective multicentric study. *J. Clin. Oncol.*, **8**, 509–18.

Lange, P.H., Narayan, P. and Fraley, E.E. (1984) Fertility issue following therapy for testicular cancer. *Sem. Urol.*, **2**, 264–74.

Medical Research Council Urological Cancer Working Party, Testicular Subgroup (1987) Treatment of high risk stage I testicular teratomas. MRC Protocol, August.

Pizzocaro, G. (1981) The case for radical surgery and combined therapy in testicular non seminoma, in *Germ Cell Tumours* (eds L.K. Anderson, W.G. Jones and M.A. Ward), Taylor and Francis, London, pp. 315–27.

Pizzocaro, G. (1986) Retroperitoneal lymphadenectomy in clinical stage I non-seminomatous germinal testis cancer. *Eur. J. Surg. Oncol.*, **12**, 25–8.

Pizzocaro, G. (1987) Retroperitoneal lymph node dissection in clinical stage IIA and IIB non-seminomatous germ tumours of the testis. *Int. J. Androl.*, **10**, 269–75.

Pizzocaro, G., Nicolai, N., Salvioni. R. *et al.* (1992) Comparison between clinical and pathological staging in low stage nonseminomatous germ cell testicular tumours. *J. Urol.*, **148**, 76–9.

Pizzocaro, G., Salvioni, R. and Nicolai, N. (1994) Surgery in nonseminomatous germ cell tumours of the testis. In *Germ Cell Tumours III* (eds W.B. Jones, P. Harnden I. and Appleyard), Pergamon, London, pp. 311–17.

Pizzocaro, G., Salvioni, R. and Zanoni, F. (1985) Unilateral lymphadenectomy in intraoperative stage I non-seminomatous germinal testis cancer. *J. Urol.*, **134**, 485–89.

Pizzocaro, G., Salvioni, R., and Zanoni, F. *et al.* (1985) Surveillance or lymph node dissection in clinical stage I non-seminomatous germinal testis cancer? *Br. J. Urol.*, **57**, 759–62.

Pizzocaro, G., Zanoni, F., Salvioni, R. *et al.* (1987) Difficulties of a surveillance study omitting retroperitoneal lymphadenectomy in clinical stage I non-seminomatous germ cell tumors of the testis. *J. Urol.*, **138**, 1393–6.

Pont, J., Holtl, W., Kosak, D. *et al.* (1990) Risk-adapted treatment choice in stage I non-seminomatous testicular germ cell cancer by regarding vascular invasion in the primary tumour: a prospective trial. *J. Clin. Oncol.*, **8**, 16–20.

Read, G., Stenning, S.P., Cullen, M.H. *et al.* (1992) Medical Research Council prospective study of surveillance for stage I testicular teratoma. *J. Clin. Oncol.*, **10**, 1762–80.

Rørth, M. *et al.* (1989) Management of patients with non-seminomatous germ cell tumors stage I. A position paper. Consensus Conference on Prostate and Testis Cancer, Hull, 12–15 April.

Rørth, M., von der Maase, H., Nielson, E.S. *et al.* (1987) Orchidectomy alone versus orchidectomy plus radiotherapy in stage I nonseminomatous testicular cancer. A randomized study by the Danish Testicular Carcinoma Study Group. *Int. J. Androl.*, **10**, 255–62.

Thornhill, J.A. *et al.* (1988) An evaluation of prognostic factors for testis in Ireland. *Eur. Urol.*, **14**, 429–33.

Williams, S.D., Stablein, D.M., Einhorn, L.H. *et al.* (1987) Immediate adjuvant chemotherapy versus observation with treatment at relapse in pathological stage II testicular cancer. *N. Engl. J. Med.*, **317**, 1433–8.

RETROPERITONEAL LYMPHADENECTOMY IN STAGING AND TREATMENT: THE DEVELOPMENT OF NERVE-SPARING TECHNIQUES

J.P. Donohue and J.A. Thornhill

16.1 BACKGROUND TO DEVELOPMENTS IN RETROPERITONEAL LYMPHADENECTOMY

Two decades ago, the extended bilateral suprahilar retroperitoneal lymphadenectomy was described using special exposure techniques via the midline abdominal approach (Donohue, 1977). This wide template of dissection (Fig. 16.1) encompassed all the known sites of lymphatic drainage within the retroperitoneum. The rationale behind this somewhat extensive procedure was that it provided the best guarantee of removing all microscopic deposits of infradiaphragmatic metastatic disease in an era when relapse was often fatal owing to poor chemotherapy rescue. Results from that period justified this intensive surgical approach in non-seminomas; the lower relapse rate combined with improved survival was marginally better than prophylactic irradiation programs, the only other alternative treatment available at that time.

Since the mid 1960s we have performed retroperitoneal lymph node dissection (RPLND) operations at the Indiana University Medical Center. It is against this background of experience that we have gradually but consistently modified our surgical techniques. The initial impetus for modifying the type of operation we performed came from an improvement in our understanding of the specific sites of nodal metastases from testis cancer. Thus, the wide field of dissection in the suprahilar operation could be scaled without jeopardizing its potential for accurate staging or therapeutic benefit if nodes were involved. The other reason for wishing to modify our operative approach was that surgical morbidity became a significant factor to be taken into consideration when effective chemotherapy became available for non-seminomatous testis cancer (Einhorn and Donohue, 1977). In particular, both patients and surgeons alike focused on the loss of ejaculatory function as the principal area of concern because it invariably followed the standard bilateral lymphadenectomy (Donohue and Rowland, 1981). In this chapter we will trace the historical development of RPLND, including the downscaling of resection templates and the subsequent development of nerve-sparing techniques. The technique of nerve-sparing modified RPLND is then described in the manner that we perform these operations today. The

Testicular Cancer: Investigation and management. Second edition. Edited by Professor A. Horwich. Published in 1996 by Chapman & Hall. ISBN 0 412 61210 0.

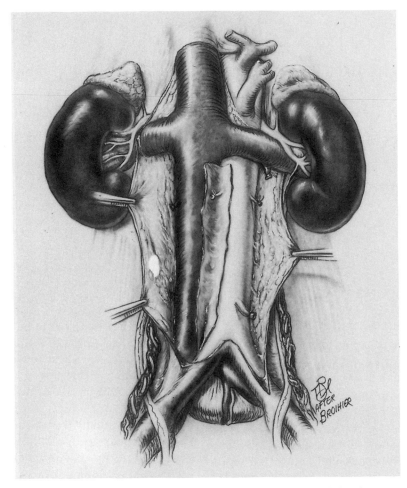

Fig. 16.1 The wide template of resection in the traditional bilateral suprahilar dissection is well above the renal vasculature. From the technical viewpoint, note how the lymphatic tissues are split and then rolled off the great vessels.

role of primary retroperitoneal lymphadenectomy and the choice between surgery or surveillance as the most appropriate management option in Stage I are not included as these are discussed in other chapters.

16.2 SEQUENTIAL MODIFICATIONS IN OPERATIVE TECHNIQUES

Our first modification to the traditional operation of bilateral suprahilar RPLND was omission of the suprahilar component of dissection. This reduction in the surgical template was considered appropriate when studies showed that the suprahilar lymph nodes were not a primary zone of metastatic spread in testis cancer unless there was gross involvement of the lower (infrahilar) para-aortic nodes (Ray, Hajdu and Whitmore, 1974). The safety of omitting a routine suprahilar dissection was confirmed by subsequent surgical series. In addition to the efficacy of the bilateral infrahilar approach, the operation gained popularity because it was technically less demanding than its predecessor and operative time was also reduced.

Considering the time period involved, the bilateral infrahilar RPLND was a safe and effective tool in the urologist's armamentarium against low stage cancer of the testis. The previous training for performing suprahilar dissections was not in vain and it became invaluable when operating for bulky disease in the postchemotherapy setting. However, the principal drawback of the bilateral infrahilar operation related to its morbidity, especially the loss of ejaculatory function, which occurred in all cases (Narayan, Lange and Fraley, 1982). This direct complication of surgery became of increasing importance when new developments in radiology and serum markers made it possible to evaluate disease stage more accurately using noninvasive methods. Also, the dawning of the era of chemotherapy with the introduction of cisplatin made it possible to rescue patients with relapse reliably. With this new emphasis on the morbidity of treatment, there was growing pressure to reject primary surgery in favor of surveillance in early stage non-seminomas, and this approach was adopted in several countries including the UK and Scandanavia. Meanwhile, surgical centers committed to RPLND further downscaled the boundaries of dissection in an effort to preserve postoperative ejaculation (Donohue, Zachary and Maynard, 1982; Pizzocaro, Salvioni and Zanoni, 1985; Donohue *et al.* 1988). Resulting modified unilateral templates (Fig. 16.2a and b) were based on prior knowledge of the zones of metastatic spread and a general recognition that the critical region in preserving ejaculation was the para-aortic tissues below the level of the inferior mesenteric artery (Richie and Garnick, 1987; Jewett *et al.*, 1988). This region contains the lumbar sympathetic chain and the postganglionic fibers from the ganglia L2 to L4 (Fig. 16.3). Studies of male sexual dysfunction following RPLND pointed to the injury of the sympathetic nerves as the key to this problem; further dissection work, both at Indiana University and elsewhere, elucidated the course of the sympathetic postganglionic

nerves (Lange, Chang and Fraley, 1987; Colleselli *et al.*, 1990). Travelling in the para-aortic tissues, these fibers decussate to form the so-called hypogastric plexus. The terminal nerve trunks from the plexus pass inferiorly to terminate in the ejaculatory apparatus of the seminal vesicles and ampullary portion of the vas.

These modified unilateral templates preserving sympathetic fibers were associated with greater preservation of ejaculation in the range 60 to 80%. This reduction in surgical morbidity has led to the adoption of unilateral modified RPLND by most surgical centers treating cancer of the testis. The benefits of a modified unilateral approach in combining a complete cancer operation with perhaps a better than even chance of ejaculatory preservation was a significant development in the management of early stage disease. This is particularly in view of the increasing number of relapse rates reported by centers using surveillance only (Hoskin *et al.*, 1986; Freedman *et al.*, 1987).

The modified template significantly reduced surgical morbidity, but it was felt that a more proactive role for the surgeon was indicated because the means of preserving the nerves in the modified unilateral operation relied simply on their exclusion from the dissected template. The results indicate that in about half of cases the nerves can be damaged using the modified template and, therefore, as long ago as 1978 we began our first efforts to identify prospectively sympathetic fibers in the course of RPLND. It was our belief that if dissection of the sympathetic fibers was done before lymphadenectomy then preservation of ejaculation might be preserved in virtually all RPLND patients. In carefully selected patients with low risk of recurrent disease we gradually introduced a nerve-sparing modification when performing a modified unilateral procedure. By 1984 we were convinced that some patients could have their postganglionic fibers identified and preserved during the course of an effective staging lymphadenectomy. The intermingling of sympathetic fibers

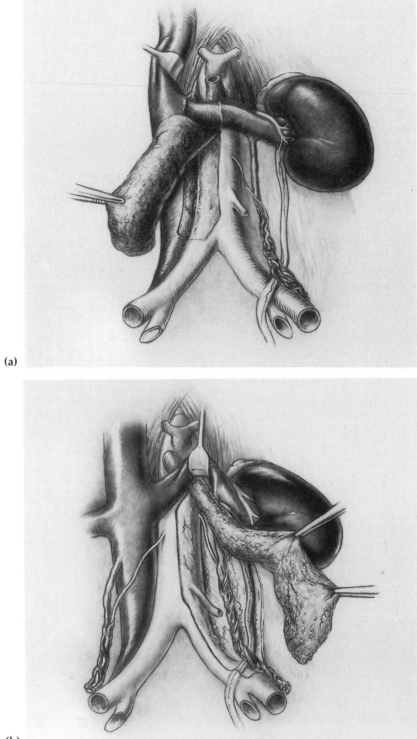

(a)

(b)

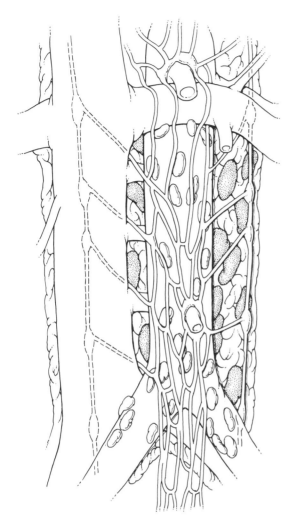

Fig. 16.3 A chematic diagram of the lumbar sympathetic nervous system and its relation to the great vessel. Note the sympathetic ganglia L2–L4, the hypogastric plexus and terminal nerve trunks.

with the lymphatic tissues is such that their preservation can be tedious and add significantly to operation time. However, as the results show (Section 16.4), we find that a

nerve-sparing procedure is not only feasible but removes the only remaining morbidity of primary RPLND.

16.3 THE SURGICAL TECHNIQUE OF NERVE-SPARING MODIFIED RETROPERITONEAL LYMPH NODE DISSECTION

As described earlier, the templates for resection are different for right- and left-sided testis tumors. Therefore, our operative approach varies according to the side of initial testis primary.

16.3.1 NERVE-SPARING MODIFIED RETROPERITONEAL LYMPH NODE DISSECTION FOR RIGHT-SIDED TUMORS

The retroperitoneum is exposed by incising the root of the small bowel from the cecum to the ligament of Treitz. The small bowel mesentery is separated from the anterior aspect of Gerota's fascia giving access to the great vessels. The gonadal veins are clearly visible. This exposure is maintained by the use of laparotomy pads and a large ring retractor.

Sometimes the terminal nerve trunks of the sympathetic hypogastric plexus are visible in the preaortic area near the origin of the right iliac artery, but in most patients these delicate strands are obscured by fat. Therefore, it is usually simplest to begin dissecting in the traditional manner at the level of the renal vein. The lymphatics on the anterior aspect of the left renal vein are divided; this dissection is carried medially and thence in a caudal direction to the crossing of the external iliac artery. Dissecting in the anterior midline of the cava (12 o'clock) avoids damaging the

Fig. 16.2 (a) The right-sided modified unilateral template in which the interaortacaval lymph nodes are included while the left para-aortic lymphatic tissue remains undisturbed. (b) The left-sided modified unilateral template includes the upper interaortacaval group and left para-aortic lymphatic tissues. The lower right para-aortic regions remains undisturbed.

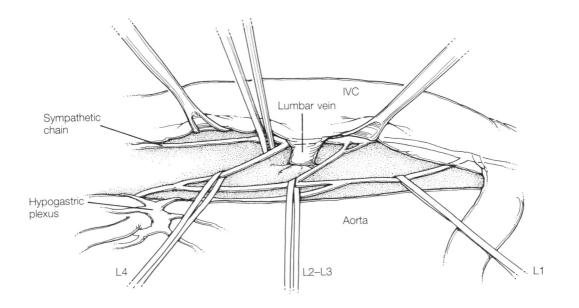

Fig. 16.4 The right postganglionic fibres L1–L4 arise from the right sympathetic trunk dorsal to the cava, emerge into the interaortacaval and pre-aortic area, where they co-mingle with splanchnic fibres in larger trunks. These are prospectively identified and isolated before lymphadenectomy.

nerve roots where they emerge medially from underneath the cava toward the aorta (Fig. 16.4). This anterior division of the lymphatics over the great vessels is called the 'anterior split'. The subsequent dissection of this package off the great vessels medially and laterally is called the 'roll' technique, hence, the term 'split and roll'. Using this technique, one can readily identify the nerve roots of L1, 2 and 3 in the packet of tissue that is rolled medially off the cava. A plastic vessel loop is placed around each nerve branch to make it more obvious and to permit gentle traction during subsequent dissection. Once the roots of L1, 2 and 3 are taped it is a simple matter to dissect distally and connect with the decussation of fibers that form the distal trunks of the hypogastric plexus as they pass anterior to the iliac vessels and down into the pelvis. In the course of this dissection, the anterior set of interaortocaval lymph nodes can be resected off the nerve roots, which lie posteriorly. The more substantial and difficult portion of the dissection follows and this involves mobilization of the remaining interaortocaval lymph nodes, which lie posterior to the nerve roots. These posterior interaortocaval nodes lie in a sulcus bounded by the nerve roots laterally, the anterior spinous ligaments and lumbar vessels posteriorly and the aorta medially. This package is delivered by sharp and blunt dissection from the overlying nerve roots, which are gently elevated in the vessel loops. This part of the dissection can be most tedious if the prepared nerve roots are to be preserved. Major lymphatics are secured by clips, especially distally and those against the posterior body wall. The cephalad limit of the dissection is the right renal artery. The L2 to L4 nerve roots lie inferior to the renal artery, but care must be taken when squaring out at the apex of the dissection so as not to catch the L1 nerve root as it passes to its ganglion just above and posterior to the renal artery. Ultimately the interaortocaval lymph node package is drawn out from under the nerve roots. Usually the specimen is removed *en bloc,* but sometimes this is difficult and nodal tissue must be removed in segments so as to preserve the nerves. There is a significant amount of nodal tissue between the aorta and nerve trunks along the posterior body wall and it may be necessary to divide the lumbar vessels during the course of removing these nodes. The right para-aortic sulcus is now clear and one can see the anterior spinous ligaments, aorta and nerve roots cleanly dissected.

The right-sided modified dissection is virtually complete, having removed the interaortocaval node group. The name 'interaortocaval' distinguishes these nodes from those on the opposite side of the vena cava (the right paracaval group). This latter group are rarely involved in primary testis tumors and are not of paramount importance when doing a nerve-sparing operation. However, they are easily stripped off the vena cava and the posterior body wall as a separate package. Again, care is taken to preserve the sympathetic chain and the branches of the genito-femoral and ilioinguinal nerve distally.

The interaortocaval node group (right para-aortic) is the central core of the modified template for right-sided tumors. The distal trunks below the inferior mesenteric artery and the contralateral L1 to L3 nerve roots are unlikely to be injured in such modified dissections if the zone of resection is limited to these interaortocaval parameters already mentioned. Therefore, even without ipsilateral nerve sparing, most patients should ejaculate when given a unilateral RPLND on this modified template.

Following dissection, the retroperitoneum is inspected and lymphatic leaks are clipped. The root of the small bowel is reapproximated with chromic catgut and the abdomen is closed without external drainage.

16.3.2 NERVE-SPARING RETROPERITONEAL LYMPH NODE DISSECTION FOR LEFT-SIDED PRIMARY TUMORS

As previously explained, the template for resection is different in left-sided primary tumors and we use an alternative method for exposing the retroperitoneum whereby the root of the small bowel is left intact. Instead, the left colon is elevated by dividing the left mesocolon from the level of the sigmoid up to and including the lienocolic ligament. The mesentery of the colon is separated from the underlying Gerota's fascia revealing the gonadal vein and great vessels. Retraction is set and the gonadal vein, which traverses the field, is divided where it enters the left renal vein. This exposes the underlying ureter, which forms the lateral boundary of the dissection template.

The initial step in a left-sided nerve-sparing technique is exposure of the lumbar sympathetic chain by dissecting posterolateral to the aorta. The L1 to L3 nerve roots are easily identified as they course medial and inferior, decussating with contralateral sympathetic branches and splanchnic sympathetic fibers, which course anterior to the aorta (Fig. 16.5). Occasionally the nerve roots are apparent initially when exposing the retroperitoneum. If so, they can be taped and dissected with the sympathetic chain and the ganglia can then be identified by dissecting along the nerve roots themselves. In either case, with the sympathetic chain and nerve roots identified the anterior set of nodes is easily dissected off them. These nodes are few in number compared with the posterior group, which is isolated from the overlying nerve roots using the same technique as described for right-sided primaries (Fig. 16.6). The nerve roots are dissected to permit their elevation off the nodal package lying in the sulcus bounded by the aorta medially, the spinous ligaments posteriorly, and the nerve roots themselves, which course ventrally over

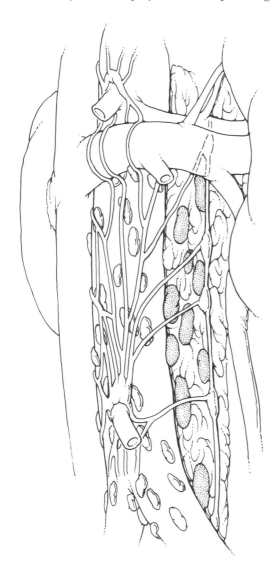

Fig. 16.5 The left sympathetic fibres from the L1–L4 ganglia of the sympathetic chain dorsal and left of the aorta join the pre-aortic decussation of nerve trunks, just as their right-sided (L1–L4) counterparts.

them. A combination of blunt and sharp dissection is useful. Again, it is critical not to incorporate the nerve roots inadvertently in the lymph node specimen when squaring off the package superiorly. Also, care should be taken to elevate the left renal vein and divide any lumbar vessels that drain into it to optimize exposure at the cephalad margin of the node package.

The left renal artery is the upper limit of dissection; the L1 to L3 nerve roots and the sympathetic chain course below this level. The node package can be dissected off the aorta with relative safety by keeping tension on the nerve roots in their plastic loops. The origin of the spermatic artery is divided and separated from the node package. As on the right, the interaortocaval nodes are drawn out from under the nerve roots while the lymphatic connections are clipped as they are encountered. Once this has been accomplished the nerve-sparing left-sided template is complete and the mesentery of the colon is reapproximated prior to closure.

16.4 THE RESULTS OF NERVE-SPARING MODIFIED RETROPERITONEAL LYMPH NODE DISSECTION

Several years ago, when reviewing 1180 RPLND operations performed at Indiana University Medical Center over the past 25 years, 140 patients have had primary RPLND using the nerve-sparing technique just described. At that time 73 patients had a median follow-up of 24 months (Donohue, Rowland and Bihrle, 1988). Fifty-nine patients were pathological Stage I, while the remaining 14 patients were found to have positive nodes by surgical/ pathological staging. Four patients had relapsed, of whom two cases had elevated serum markers only and another case developed chest metastases. These three cases received chemotherapy and are now disease free. Another patient who was shown to be Stage IIB by RPLND and who refused adjuvant chemotherapy developed both chest and abdominal metastases. He received combination chemotherapy and underwent a subsequent postchemotherapy resection of a residual suprahilar abdominal mass. This was found to

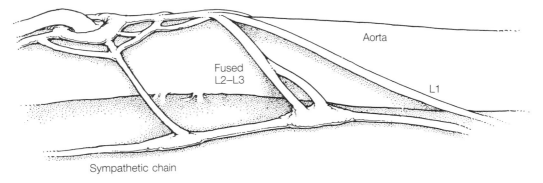

Hypogastric plexus

Aorta

Fused
L2–L3

L1

Sympathetic chain

Fig. 16.6 The left-sided nerve-sparing technique after clearance of the posterior set of lymph nodes. The ganglia of L2 and L3 may be fused or juxtaposed.

be scar and necrosis tissue. None of the 59 patients with pathological Stage I disease had relapse; this implied that modified RPLND did not miss any patient with positive nodes.

Seventy-two patients retained normal ejaculatory function after nerve-sparing RPLND. One single exception was time limited and resumed normal function several months later. In 1993, the group treated with NS-RPLND with more than 2-year follow-up numbered 167 (Donohue *et al.*, 1995).

An additional ten patients underwent nerve-sparing RPLND in the postchemotherapy setting. All had low volume disease (Stage IIA, IIB) and normal serology preoperatively. No case suffered local or distal relapse, while all these patients maintained normal ejaculatory function.

16.5 THE CONTRIBUTION OF NERVE-SPARING MODIFIED RETROPERITONEAL LYMPH NODE DISSECTION

The traditional aim of cancer surgery has been to achieve radical removal of the primary tumor with its regional zone of lymphatic drainage. As such, radical surgery offers the best chance of preventing a local recurrence and, if nodes are positive, then treatment has hopefully been early enough to prevent

further more distal relapse. However, this approach has long been known to produce considerable functional morbidity and in urological oncology today more emphasis is therefore put on combining good quality of life with the established concept of total tumor clearance.

Clearly, the ideal for patients with clinical Stage I cancer of the testis is to identify those who in fact have microscopic nodal disease so they can be treated expediently. Currently the most accurate way to achieve this aim is by RPLND. It can be therapeutic for those found to be Stage II and accurately directs further management. The combination of modern nerve-sparing techniques with a modified unilateral template means that this procedure can be performed without any long-term morbidity.

To conclude, it is perfectly reasonable to adopt nerve-sparing RPLND as appropriate management in early stage cancer of the testis considering the current state of the art in clinical staging. Similarly, the results with nerve-sparing RPLND in the postchemotherapy setting are most encouraging; it is in this latter group that the nerve-sparing procedure may well have the greatest future potential.

Our experience at Indiana University with clinical Stage A and B testis cancer has been

Table 16.1 Risk–benefit analysis of primary therapy (clinical Stage B NSGCT testis cancer)

1° RPLND surgery		1° chemotherapy
1/3	Failure rate (need for 2 Rx)	1/3
2%	Death rate	4%
0–1%	Late relapses (>2 yrs)	3–5%
1–10% (anejaculation)	Long-term toxicity	40–55% (infertility)
20%	Over treatment (clinical staging error)	Unreported est. 20%

Taken from *J. Urology* (January 1995) Vol. **153**, p. 88.

Table 16.2 Comparison of primary therapy: clinical Stage B NSGCT

Primary RPLND		Primary chemotherapy
2/3	Curative (as monotherapy)	2/3
1/3 (10–49%)	Failure rate as monotherapy	1/3 (20–40%)
98%	Overall survival incl. 2° therapy	96%
<1%	Late relapses	>3%
0–10%	Long-term toxicity	Unreported est. 10–30%

Taken from *J. Urology* (January 1995) Vol. **153**, p. 88.

recently reported in some detail (Donohue *et al.*, 1993, 1994, 1995; Baniel *et al.*, 1994). Cost–benefit and risk–benefit assessments of RPLND are now possible by virtue of this detailed analysis. This can be of practical value to physicians and patients alike as options of management are considered (Tables 16.1 and 16.2).

REFERENCES

Baniel, J., Foster, R.S., Rowland, R.G., Bihrle, R. and Donohue, J.P. (1994) Complications of primary retroperitoneal lymph node dissection. *J. Urol.*, **152**, 424–7.

Colleselli, K., Poisel, S., Schachtner, W. and Bartsch, G. (1990) Anatomic study and operative approach to nerve-sparing bilateral retroperitoneal lymphadenectomy. *J. Urol.*, **144**, 293.

Donohue J.P. (1977) Retroperitoneal lymphadenectomy: The anterior approach including bilateral suprarenal–hilar dissection. *Urol. Clin. North Am.*, **4**, 509.

Donohue, J.P., Foster, R.S., Geier, G. *et al.* (1988) Preservation of ejaculation following nerve-sparing retroperitoneal lymphadenectomy (RPLND). *J. Urol.*, **139**, 176.

Donohue, J.P., Foster, R.S., Geier, G. *et al.* (1990) Nerve-sparing retroperitoneal lympha-

denectomy with preservation of ejaculation. *J. Urol.*, **144**, 287.

Donohue, J.P. and Rowland, R.G. (1981) Complications of retroperitoneal lymphadenectomy. *J. Urol.*, **125**, 338.

Donohue, J.P., Rowland, R.G. and Bihrle, R. (1988) Transabdominal retroperitoneal lymph node dissection in diagnosis and management of genitourinary cancer, in *Genitourinary Cancer* (eds D.G. Skinner and G. Lieskowsky), W.B. Saunders, Philadelphia, Ch. 55, pp. 802–16.

Donohue, J.P., Zachary, J.M. and Maynard, S.D. (1982) Distribution of nodal metastases in nonseminomatous testicular cancer. *J. Urol.*, **128**, 315–20.

Donohue, J.P., Thornhill, J.A., Foster, R.S., Rowland, R.G. and Bihrle, R. (1995) The role of retroperitoneal lymphadenectomy in clinical stage B testis cancer: The Indiana University experience (1965 to 1989). *J. Urol.*, **153**, 85–9.

Donohue, J.P., Thornhill, J.A., Foster, R.S., Rowland, R.G. and Bihrle, R. (1994) Stage I nonseminomatous germ cell testicular cancer: Management options and risk–benefit considerations. *World J. Urol.*, **12**, 170–7.

Donohue, J.P., Thornhill, J.A., Foster, R.S., Rowland, R.G. and Bihrle, R. (1993) Primary retroperitoneal lymph node dissection in clinical stage A nonseminomatous germ cell testis cancer. *Brit. J. Urol.*, **71**, 326–35.

Donohue, J.P., Thornhill, J.A., Foster, R.S.,

Bihrle, R., Rowland, R.G. and Einhorn, L.H. (1995) The role of retroperitoneal lymphadenectomy in clinical stage B testis cancer: The Indiana University experience (1965–1989). *J. Urol.*, **153**, 85–9.

Einhorn, L.H. and Donohue, J.P. (1977) Improved chemotherapy in disseminated testicular cancer. *J. Urol.*, **117**, 65.

Freedman, L.S., Jones, W.G., Peckham, M.J. *et al.* (1987) Histopathology in the prediction of relapse of patients with stage I testicular teratoma treated by orchidectomy alone. *Lancet*, **2**, 294–8.

Hoskin, P., Dilly, S., Easton, D. *et al.* (1986) Prognostic factors in stage I nonseminomatous germ cell testicular tumors managed by orchidectomy and surveillance: Implications for adjuvant chemotherapy. *J. Clin. Oncol.*, **4**, 1031–6.

Jewett, M.A. *et al.* (1988) Retroperitoneal lymphadenectomy for testicular tumor with nerve-sparing for ejaculation. *J. Urol.*, **139**, 1220.

Lange, P.H., Chang, W.Y. and Fraley, E.E. (1987) Fertility issues in the therapy of nonseminomatous testicular tumors. *Urol. Clin. North Am.*, **14**, 731–45.

Narayan, P., Lang, P. and Fraley, E.E. (1982) Ejaculation and fertility after extended retroperitoneal lymph node dissection for testicular cancer. *World J. Urol.*, **127**, 685–8.

Pizzocaro, G., Salvioni, R. and Zanoni, F. (1985) Unilateral lymphadenectomy in intraoperative stage I nonseminomatous germinal testis cancer. *J. Urol.*, **134**, 485–9.

Ray, B., Hajdu, S.I. and Whitmore, W.F. Jr (1974) Distribution of retroperitoneal lymph node metastases in testicular germinal tumors. *Cancer*, **33**, 340–8.

Richie, J.P. and Garnick, M.B. (1987) Modified retroperitoneal lymphadenectomy for patients with clinical stage I testicular tumor. *J. Urol.*, **137**, 212A.

M.A.S. Jewett and E.D. Hirshberg

17.1 INTRODUCTION

The role for initial or primary retroperitoneal lymphadenectomy (RPL) as opposed to primary chemotherapy for clinical Stage II non-seminomatous testicular tumors remains controversial (Horwich *et al.*, 1994; Donohue *et al.*, 1995). Concerns about infertility after surgery due to loss of antegrade ejaculation have been addressed with the development of nerve-sparing techniques that have dramatically reduced this morbidity (Jewett *et al.*, 1988; Donohue *et al.*, 1990). The acute morbidity of both approaches is known and RPL is better tolerated than three to four courses of chemotherapy. The long-term morbidity of RPL is well defined and is very small, whereas for combination chemotherapy the long-term morbidity, particularly the risk of second malignancy and the loss of the spermatogenesis, appear to be greater (Baniel *et al.*, 1994; Bokemeyer and Schmoll, 1995; Travis, Curtis and Hankey, 1995). There is a small but persistent mortality rate with chemotherapy that is not reported with surgery (Horwich *et al.*, 1994).

Clinical staging of the retroperitoneum by imaging and markers in the presence of small volume metastases is not as accurate as we would desire, with a significant false positive rate (Donohue *et al.*, 1987; Pizzocaro *et al.*, 1992). Patients are at risk of overtreatment whichever primary modality is used. As the acute and chronic morbidity and mortality of 'unnecessary' chemotherapy appear to be greater than with RPL, many centers, particularly in North America where experience with surgery is greater, prefer to recommend initial surgery for staging as well as for treatment if the nodes are positive (Donohue *et al.*, 1995).

The current challenge is to minimize the overall morbidity of treatment while still achieving the high cure rates of more than 90%. While either modality is effective in most patients, additional treatment may be necessary. Adjuvant chemotherapy after RPL for prophylaxis is commonly prescribed but may not be necessary in selected cases (Pizzocaro and Piva, 1984; Hartlapp, 1987; Richie and Kantoff, 1991). Delayed treatment reserved for subsequent progression is a viable alternative management. Secondary RPL for residual retroperitoneal disease after primary chemotherapy is necessary in up to a third of patients, although a more limited 'lumpectomy' with laparotomy may be possible (Logothetis *et al.*, 1987). All of these possibilities may significantly increase the total burden of treatment. The sum of early and long-term treatment morbidity for all patients must be considered to determine the optimal first treatment.

There appears to be a role for RPL as the preferred initial treatment in skilled hands if the selected cases have a low risk of systemic

Testicular Cancer: Investigation and management. Second edition. Edited by Professor A. Horwich.
Published in 1996 by Chapman & Hall. ISBN 0 412 61210 0.

disease, and for primary chemotherapy where the risk of occult systemic disease is high. This chapter documents our overall experience with Stage II disease, as well as discussing the issues for the management of patients with clinical evidence of small volume retroperitoneal nodal metastases to support initial RPL in selected cases of clinical Stage II non-seminoma.

17.2   RISK OF OVERSTAGING

The first concern in the treatment of a patient with clinical evidence of retroperitoneal nodal metastases is the accuracy of the staging techniques used.

The accuracy of abdominal imaging remains at approximately 60–70% with false positive rates of at least 20% and false negative rates of 20–30% (Sternberg, 1993). This presents several problems. Firstly, this may result in overtreatment of the retroperitoneum in the patients with false positive CT scans, which is a risk that may be even higher than is generally appreciated (Aass *et al.*, 1990). This is of particular concern if chemotherapy is used as a primary modality. It has been suggested that equivocal scans be repeated in 6 weeks, which may well be useful but adds to patient anxiety and may allow disease progression. Secondly, the extent of disease may be underestimated and an RPL performed that is unlikely to be curative without adjuvant chemotherapy. This is more likely to occur when there are multiple smaller nodal metastases, which in our experience appear to be associated with a higher risk of occult systemic metastases that will require later chemotherapy for relapse (unpublished data). The pattern of retroperitoneal metastases has been well documented so that imaging can be interpreted with greater accuracy by the well informed (Ray, Hajdu and Whitmore, 1974; Donohue, Maynard and Zachary, 1982; Weissbach *et al.*, 1987). This knowledge should reduce false positives due to vascular anomalies and bowel as well as heighten suspicion of smaller nodes that may

be significant owing to their location. In our early experience with surveillance of clinical Stage I patients, we felt that our inexperience with interpretation of retroperitoneal imaging contributed to a higher relapse rate (Sturgeon *et al.* 1992). Presumably similar systematic errors can occur in clinical series reporting results with more advanced disease, which might bias results of treatment if surgical confirmation is not regularly obtained.

Bipedal lymphangiography (LAG) has been generally abandoned in the last few years because of its invasiveness, risks and lack of additional useful information in most patients (Wischnow, Johnson and Tenney, 1984). There is the occasional patient who may benefit because of equivocal findings on other imaging.

The tumor markers alpha-fetoprotein (AFP) and the beta subunit of human chorionic gonadotrophin (βHCG) have improved the accuracy of staging and monitoring of patients. The sensitivity for detection of retroperitoneal metastases for one or both of these markers is 70%, based on surgical series in which pathological staging was obtained (Sternberg, 1993). In our experience, the specificity of a persistently elevated marker level is high for metastatic disease after orchidectomy, although occult disease outside the retroperitoneum cannot be excluded particularly with high levels. Low but elevated levels, in the range of 5–15, should be followed serially and regarded with suspicion as a possible false positive.

Patients who have elevated markers as the only evidence of metastatic disease, i.e. with all imaging studies normal, pose a particular problem. Although most patients have predictable lymphatic pattern metastases to the retroperitoneum as the first site of spread, some may have hematogenous spread. Another possibility is small volume metastases in nodes that can't be imaged. The natural history of these patients is not well worked out and we do not really know what proportion need systemic therapy for cure. These patients are frequently treated with chemo-therapy initially.

17.3 TREATMENT WITH RETROPERITONEAL LYMPHADENECTOMY

The introduction of combination platinum-based chemotherapy provided both a safety net for failed patients after surgery and a useful adjuvant to surgery. Patients thought to be at risk of progression were given chemotherapy before clear identification and measurement of risk factors such as size of nodes, marker levels, etc. In fact we still do not have good information on the risks of progression after RPL by size of nodes or preoperative marker levels if adjuvant chemo-therapy is not used.

The history of RPL has been described (Heritz and Jewett, 1994). It is quite clear from the prechemotherapy experience that surgery alone was successful in curing some patients who presented with retroperitoneal lymphadenopathy. There was significant mor-bidity until nerve sparing was initially accom-plished by performing template lymphaden-ectomy. Sympathetic nerves were spared in zones that were unlikely to harbour meta-stases by not dissecting these areas. In 1988 we described 20 patients of various stages, including patients with masses, who had undergone full bilateral dissection with nerve identification and sparing. Follow-up using semen quality showed preservation of ante-grade ejaculation in 95% with a low risk of recurrence (Jewett *et al.*, 1988). This report, and the experience of others, stimulated re-newed interest in wider application of RPL as primary treatment as well as staging/prophy-laxis in patients with no evidence of retro-peritoneal disease (Stage I) as an alternative to surveillance (Donohue *et al.*, 1990). How-ever, the early literature was based on patients who were staged surgically and in whom some inoperable patients were excluded. Prior to the mid 1970s, CT scans were not in general use and imaging was limited to IVPs and

LAGs. Markers were not routinely done until this time as well. It is very difficult to extra-polate from this experience except to recognize that surgery alone was capable of curing some patients (Heritz and Jewett, 1994). This was more recently substantiated by the Inter-group Study in which 50% of patients were cured with surgery alone (Williams *et al.*, 1987). Reports of delayed adjuvant treatment also indicate that a majority of selected pa-tients may be cured with surgery alone (Richie and Kantoff, 1991).

Intraoperative nerve identification and stimulation makes sparing the important nerves even easier (Dieckmann, Huland and Gross, 1992; Recker and Tscholl, 1993). However, it is not routinely done in Stage II patients who have gross disease at the time of surgery because of the risk of leaving tumor. Reports of success are now appear-ing, however, and patients who have dis-ease in the left para-aortic region seem most suitable because the dominant nerves are usually on the right (Donohue *et al.*, 1995).

We have been performing nerve spar-ing for more than 10 years and have not routinely used adjuvant chemotherapy in patients who are carefully selected after orchidectomy and are found on imaging to have retroperitoneal nodal disease without supradiaphragmatic or visceral metastases. The size, extent and location of metastases, the tumor marker levels and histology of the primary may be useful in selecting the initial therapy. It is generally agreed that masses larger than 10 cm are best managed by initial chemotherapy. We have used 5 cm as our upper limit. One important issue is how size is reported. Firstly, bidimensional diameters on CT will sometimes under-state true size if the mass is cigar shaped or ovoid rather than spherical. The difference in volume will vary exponentially, leading to a gross underestimate of tumor volume and cell number. Secondly, there may be a number of nodal masses rather than one or two masses and we do not have a consistent system for reporting total volume. While it is reasonable to assume that the risk of progression after RPL is related to true total tumor burden in the retroperitoneum, we do not have clear evidence for this. Measurement inconsistencies may be one reason that the data are not available.

The relationship of marker levels to the extent of metastases is not documented, although in the Danish study high pre-orchidectomy levels heralded a 50 to 60% relapse (Rørth *et al.*, 1991). Our unpublished experience is that patients with normal or low marker levels have a lower incidence of systemic metatases. We therefore currently prefer to treat patients with one or more marker levels greater than 100 with initial chemotherapy, even if the imaging reveals limited disease in the retroperitoneum only.

Our technique of nerve identification and preservation while performing a full bilateral lymphadenectomy has been described (Jewett *et al.*, 1988; Jewett, 1990). We discovered that the nerves are predictably situated and that dissection of nodal disease can be complete with nerve preservation even in patients with advanced disease. The anatomical limits of dissection are the ureters laterally; 1–2cm above the renal arteries superiorly, and inferiorly to at least the midpoint of the ipsilateral external iliac artery and to the bifurcation of the contralateral common iliac artery including the aortic bifurcation. Posteriorly the anterior spinal ligament and psoas muscles are skeletonized.

Dissection is begun by incising the retroperitoneal tissue in the midline anterior to the inferior vena cava (IVC). The left side of the cava is exposed from the left renal vein to its origin at the left common iliac vein by peeling the adipose and lymphatic tissue medially, taking care to cauterise or ligate small vessels. The IVC is carefully rolled laterally with ligation and division of the left lumbar veins as required. The right sympathetic chain lies posterior to the midline of the cava immediately to the right of the ligated left lumbar

veins. From the fusiform ganglia, fine post-ganglionic nerve fibers can be seen coursing anteromedially and inferiorly to the right side of the aorta. These fibers are the lumbar splanchnic nerves and can be individually skeletonized from the underlying interaortocaval lymphatic tissue, which is ultimately mobilized posteriorly from the anterior spinal ligament and withdrawn inferiorly leaving the web of sympathetic nerves.

Before proceeding further, the left ureter is visualized by erecting a plane across the midline anterior to the retroperitoneal lymphatic tissue but behind the inferior mesenteric artery, mesocolic fat and other soft tissues. This dissection may require division of the inferior mesenteric artery, but it should be several centimeters distal to its origin. The left ureter can be exposed up to the perinephric tissue visualizing the left psoas muscle, leaving the left para-aortic retroperitoneal adipose tissue containing the lymph nodes intact. This bulk of tissue is carefully reflected medially to expose the left sympathetic chain. The lumbar vessels on the left are identified with this dissection as they course directly medial to the sympathetic chain. Again, as with the right-sided vessels, they are occasionally lateral or bifurcate around the chain. These vessels can be sacrificed as needed. The lumbar splanchnic nerves are identified as originating from the sympathetic ganglia coursing medially and anteriorly on to the side of the aorta. Superiorly, there may be a branch anterior to the renal artery coming from a higher ganglion, but this may be difficult to preserve.

At this point, the surgeon has a sense of the individual patient's sympathetic anatomy, which is variable. The aorta can now be exposed in the midline by mobilizing the left renal vein and splitting the soft tissue over it. Dissection is carried close to the aorta. The individual sympathetic nerve branches, having been identified on both right and left sides from preceding dissection, are seen on the anterior and lateral surfaces of the aorta. They are skeletonized, taking care to preserve those branches that form variable plexuses on the anterior aorta. This allows withdrawal of the interaortocaval lymphatic tissue and the left para-aortic tissue from between the anterior spinal ligament posteriorly and the nerves anteriorly. The plexus at and below the level of the inferior mesenteric artery condenses to form the two hypogastric nerves that pass over the aorta and proceed inferiorly into the pelvis. Identification and preservation of these two nerves allow all lymphatic tissue over the aortic bifurcation and common iliac veins down to the sacral promontory to be removed without sacrificing ejaculation. Inferiorly, it is our practice to limit the dissection to a point approximately midway along the ipsilateral external iliac artery and to the bifurcation of the contralateral common iliac artery. The remnant of the spermatic cord is removed ipsilaterally with as much of the vas deferens as is easily removable along with the spermatic vessels to their attachments in the retroperitoneum.

Frequently nodal metastases or tumor masses are immediately adjacent to or involve nerves. It is not necessary to preserve all postganglionic nerves to ensure ejaculation. Therefore, the surgeon should not hesitate to sacrifice nerves unilaterally or even in a limited manner bilaterally to ensure complete removal of disease. Nerve-sparing surgery has been more successful in patients with right-sided tumors, owing to preservation of the left para-aortic area below the aorta. Right-sided tumors rarely metastasized to this region. Preservation of seminal emission was not as favorable for left-sided tumors, although nerves could be preserved in some cases. Recently the use of intraoperative electrostimulation of individual sympathetic nerves with simultaneous observation of emission initially by transpelvic ultrasound and now by flexible cysto- and endoscopy has been added to our operative approach.

7.4 OUR RESULTS OF RETROPERITONEAL LYMPHADENECTOMY (RPL) FOR STAGE II NON-SEMINOMA

From 1977 to 1994, we have performed 164 RPLs for Stage II and III disease including those with residual masses after chemotherapy. Since 1984 when nerve sparing was begun, 83 of these cases have undergone full bilateral RPL with nerve-sparing, but in 34 cases it was not feasible in this same interval. This indicates that almost one in three of the cases with evidence of nodal disease will not be able to undergo nerve-sparing surgery safely. Cases who have disease anterior to the aortic bifurcation and in the lower interaortocaval area are more at risk of having the important sympathetic nerves sacrificed. Nineteen patients of our original twenty (95%) now report antegrade ejaculation (Jewett et al., 1988). Overall an 87% preservation rate of antegrade ejaculation has been achieved in the patients who have undergone nerve sparing to date. There was no clear dominance of any particular nerve fibers in preserving ejaculation, although intraoperative nerve stimulation studies suggest that the lower right sympathetic branches are dominant (Recker and Tscholl, 1993). Paternity has been achieved to date in 14 of 54 (26%) of patients who ejaculate. A significant number remain young and have not yet desired children.

All patients were staged by history and physical examination, serum tumor markers (AFP and BHCG), chest X-ray, computed tomography (abdomen, pelvis and possibly chest) and bilateral lymphangiography (until 1992). The staging classification system used was a modified Walter-Reed in which Stage II refers to disease clinically confined to the retroperitoneal nodes, with IIA for nodes less than 5 cm and IIB for nodes 5 cm or larger in the greatest of any of the three dimensions measured on CT. Only patients with Stage IIA disease who had preoperative marker levels plateaued or stabilized at less than 100 after orchidectomy underwent RPL. Our patients did not routinely receive adjuvant chemotherapy if nodes were positive unless there was a persistent marker elevation or histological evidence of aggressive tumor with extranodal tumor growth and none of these patients received adjuvant therapy. Stage IIB patients or those with higher markers underwent primary chemotherapy because of our impression that these were risk factors for occult systemic disease based on our early experience (unpublished data). All but two of 41 patients with IIB disease underwent chemotherapy first. One of these relapsed in the retroperitoneum, requiring chemotherapy, but the other is free of disease. All the remaining patients have come to surgery with only nine found to have necrosis/fibrosis. They are all alive free of disease without further treatment. The remaining 30 had either teratoma or carcinoma in the nodes and four have died or are alive with disease despite further treatment. The rest are free of disease, with an overall survival rate of 90%. Patients who underwent RPL for residual mass postchemotherapy for Stage III disease are not included in this analysis.

A total of 40 patients presented with clinical Stage IIA disease who met our criteria for primary RPL. There was no operative mortality and all patients have survived free of disease for a mean of 7.2 years (range 1–17 years). Our clinical staging accuracy was only 60% in these IIA patients, as opposed to the 100% accuracy in the IIB patients. In other words, 16 (40%) had negative nodes at surgery and all have remained free of disease, suggesting that the majority, if not all, were indeed node negative and free of other metastases. All had had a mass of less than 5 cm in diameter described on abdominal CT scan, although our bias is to upstage and operate on any patient with equivocal imaging findings as the alternative is surveillance for Stage I in our center. If these patients had received initial chemotherapy, there would hare been a similar but more morbid and potentially fatal overtreatment rate.

Of the remaining 24 patients with pathological Stage II disease, none received immediate adjuvant chemotherapy and seven (29%) have relapsed. The relapse pattern was marker elevation only in four and lung metastases in three, of whom one had a suggestion of retroperitoneal recurrence on CT scan. All seven have undergone chemotherapy and have remained disease free, with an overall 100% survival.

Therefore, the total burden of treatment was 40 RPLs and 21 cycles of chemotherapy. If we assume a similar survival for primary chemotherapy, the total therapy would have been 120–160 cycles of chemotherapy and 5–7 RPLs for residual disease (if we use 20–30% as the expected rate of residual mass after chemotherapy requiring surgery).

17.5   MODEL FOR STRATIFYING PATIENTS FOR TREATMENT

Selection of the initial treatment modality for Stage II patients should be made with the intent of minimizing the total morbidity while still achieving a high cure rate. While either surgery or chemotherapy is effective in the majority of patients, the addition of a second additional modality in the remaining patients has the potential to increase morbidity substantially. Immediate adjuvant chemotherapy after surgery as prophylaxis (often with reduced cycles or doses), delayed chemotherapy to detection of subsequent progression or surgery for residual retroperitoneal disease after primary chemotherapy may significantly increase the total burden of treatment. The sum of early and long-term treatment morbidity for all patients must be considered to determine the optimal first treatment.

There may be other strategies to reduce unnecessary initial treatment. For example, there is increasing experience with the use of laparoscopy in the staging of the retroperitoneum of men with possible nodal metastases (Gerber *et al.*, 1994; Klotz, 1994). The procedure can be done with minimal morbidity in experienced hands and may have a role to play in the management of early stage patients with Stage I and low volume Stage II disease. It is too early to predict whether the procedure will have a therapeutic role.

Future reports will hopefully provide better definition of risk factors for occult metastases in Stage II patients. We do know that the presence of teratoma in the primary testicular tumor increases the likelihood of residual retroperitoneal masses after chemotherapy and the presence of teratoma in those masses (Toner, 1990). It may therefore be advisable to recommend initial RPL rather than chemotherapy for these patients if they have a small volume of retroperitoneal disease as they will have a high risk of requiring surgery as a second treatment after chemotherapy.

We believe that all patients with a large tumor volume in the retroperitoneum (greater than 5 cm in diameter, or our Stage IIB) or with high marker levels (greater than 100) after allowing sufficient time for half-life decay to plateau, should undergo initial chemotherapy. Figure 17.1 is an algorithm for the expected course of 100 new, clinical Stage II patients based on what we know of their natural history and our experience with their management by RPL. If we accept that approximately two-thirds (67) will be of small volume, or clinical Stage IIA, 40 will have pathological small volume disease and 27 will be overstaged and therefore would need no treatment if staging procedures were more accurate. Of the remaining 40, 28 will be cured with surgery alone and the other 12 will need chemotherapy for relapse. The patients with more bulky disease or high markers (a total of 33) will receive initial chemotherapy, of whom up to 30%, or ten, will require surgery for a residual mass. In total, 77 RPLs will be performed and 45 patients will receive chemotherapy.

If initial or primary chemotherapy were given to all the patients, the burden of

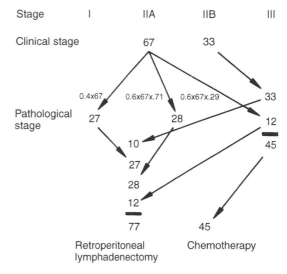

Fig. 17.1 An algorithm for the expected course of 100 new, clinical Stage II patients with non-seminomatous germ cell tumors, based on what we know of their natural history and our experience with their management by RPL.

treatment would be as summarized in Fig. 17.2. Again, if we accept that approximately two-thirds (or 67) will be of small volume, or clinical Stage IIA, 40 will have pathological small volume disease and 27 will be overstaged. Of the 40, all will receive chemotherapy (28 for retroperitoneal disease and 12 for more extensive metastatic disease). Eight of the former and four of the latter will require RPL for residual disease, based on a 30% surgery rate. Again, the patients with more bulky disease or high markers (a total of 33) will receive initial chemotherapy, of whom up to 30%, or ten, will require surgery for a residual mass. In total, 22 RPLs will be performed and 100 patients will receive chemotherapy for up to 400 cycles for an estimated greater burden of treatment.

It is our current belief that the policy of initial RPL for small volume defined as less that 5 cm in diameter, when markers are less than 100, results in equivalent survival with lower total morbidity.

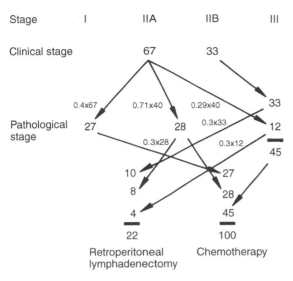

Fig. 17.2 An algorithm for the expected course of 100 new, clinical Stage II patients with non-seminomatous germ cell tumors, based on what we know of their natural history and management by initial or primary chemotherapy.

REFERENCES

Aass, N., Kaasa, S., Lund, E., Kaalhus, O., Heier, M.S. and Fosså, S.D. (1990) Long-term somatic side-effects and morbidity in testicular cancer patients. *Brit. J. Cancer*, **6**, 151–5.

Baniel, J., Foster, R.S., Rowland, R.G., Bihrle, R. and Donohue, J.P. (1994) Complications of primary retroperitoneal lymph node dissection. *J. Urol.*, **152**, 424–7.

Bokemeyer, C. and Schmoll, H.J. (1995) Treatment of testicular cancer and the development of secondary malignancies. *J. Clin. Oncol.*, **13**, 283–92.

Dieckmann, K.-P., Huland, H. and Gross, A.J. (1992) A test for the identification of relevant sympathetic nerve fibers during nerve sparing retroperitoneal lymphadenectomy. *J. Urol.*, **148**, 1450–2.

Donohue, J.P., Foster, R.S., Rowland, R.G., Bihrle, R., Jones, J. and Geier, G. (1990) Nerve sparing retroperitoneal lymphadenectomy with preservation of ejaculation. *J. Urol.*, **144**, 287–92.

Donohue, J.P., Maynard, B. and Zachary, M. (1982) The distribution of nodal metastases in the retroperitoneum from nonseminomatous testis cancer. *J. Urol.*, **128**, 315–20.

Donohue, J.P., Rowland, R.G., Kopecky, K. *et al.* (1987) Correlation of computerized tomographic changes and histological findings in 80 patients having radical retroperitoneal lymph node dissection after chemotherapy for testis cancer. *J. Urol.*, **137**, 1176–9.

Donohue, J.P., Thornhill, J.A., Foster, R.S., Bihrle, R., Rowland, R.G. and Einhorn, L.H. (1995) The role of retroperitoneal lymphadenectomy in clinical stage B testis cancer: the Indiana University experience (1965–1989). *J. Urol.*, **153**, 85–9.

Gerber, G.S., Bissada, N.K., Hulbert, J.C. *et al.* (1994) Laparoscopic retroperitoneal lymphadenectomy: Multi-institutional analysis. *J. Urol.*, **152**, 1188–91.

Hartlapp, J.H. (1987) Adjuvant chemotherapy in nonseminomatous testicular tumour stage II. *Int. J. Androl.*, **10**, 277–84.

Heritz, D.M. and Jewett, M.A.S. (1994) The evolving role for retroperitoneal lymphadenectomy. *Problems in Urology*, **8**, 118–26.

Horwich, A., Norman, A., Fisher, C., Hendry, W.F., Nicholls, J. and Dearnaley, D.P. (1994) Primary chemotherapy for stage II nonseminomatous germ cell tumors of the testis. *J. Urol.*, **151**, 72–8.

Jewett, M.A.S. (1990) Nerve-sparing technique for retroperitoneal lymphadenectomy in testicular cancer. *Urol. Cl. North Am.*, **17**, 449.

Jewett, M.A.S., Kong, Y.-S.P., Goldberg, S.D. *et al.* (1988) Retroperitoneal lymphadenectomy for testis tumor with nerve sparing for ejaculation. *J. Urol.*, **139**, 1220–4.

Klotz, L. (1994) Laparoscopic retroperitoneal lymphadenectomy for high-risk stage I nonseminomatous germ cell tumor: report of four cases. *Urol.*, **43**, 752–8.

Logothetis, C.J., Swanson, D.A., Dexeus, F. *et al.* (1987) Primary chemotherapy for clinical stage II nonseminomatous germ cell tumors of the testis: a follow-up of 50 patients. *J. Clin. Oncol.*, **5**, 906–11.

Pizzocaro, G., Nicolai, N., Salvioni, R. *et al.* (1992) Comparison between clinical and pathological staging in low stage nonseminomatous germ cell testicular tumors. *J. Urol.*, **148**, 76.

Pizzocaro, G. and Piva, L. (1984) Adjuvant chemotherapy in resected stage-II nonseminomatous testicular cancer. *Eur. Urol.*, **10**, 151.

Ray, B., Hajdu, S.I. and Whitmore, W.F.J. (1974) Lymph node metastases in testicular germinal tumors. *Cancer*, **33**, 340–8.

Recker, F. and Tscholl, R. (1993) Monitoring of emission as direct intraoperative control for nerve sparing retroperitoneal lymphadenectomy. *J. Urol.*, **150**, 1360–9.

Richie, J.P. and Kantoff, P.W. (1991) Is adjuvant chemotherapy necessary for patients with stage B1 testicular cancer? *J. Clin. Oncol.*, **9**, 1393–6.

Rørth, M., Jacobsen, G.K., von der Maase, H. *et al.* (1991) Surveillance alone versus radiotherapy after orchidectomy for clinical stage I nonseminomatous testicular cancer. *J. Clin. Oncol.*, **9**, 1543–8.

Sternberg, C.N. (1993) Role of primary chemotherapy in stage I and low-volume stage II nonseminomatous germ-cell testis tumors. *Urol. Clin. North Am.*, **20**, 93–116.

Sturgeon, J.F.G., Jewett, M.A.S., Alison, R.E. *et al.* (1992) Surveillance after orchidectomy for patients with clinical stage I nonseminomatous testis tumour. *J. Clin. Oncol.*, **10**, 564–8.

Toner, G.C., Panicek, D.M., Heelan, R.T. *et al.* (1990) Adjunctive surgery after chemotherapy for non-seminomatous germ cell tumors: recommendations for patient selection. *J. Clin. Oncol.*, **8**, 1983–94.

Travis, L.B., Curtis, R.E. and Hankey, B.F. (1995) Second malignancies after testicular cancer. *J. Clin. Oncol.*, **13**, 533–4.

Weissbach, L., Boedefeld, E.A. and the Group for the TTS (1987) Localization of solitary and multiple metastases in stage II nonseminomatous testis tumor as basis for a modified staging lymph node dissection in stage I. *J. Urol.*, **138**, 77–82.

Williams, S.D., Stablein, D.M., Eingorn, L.H. *et al.* (1987) Immediate adjuvant chemotherapy versus observation with treatment at relapse in pathological stage II testicular cancer. *N. Engl. J. Med.*, **317**, 1433–8.

Wischnow, K.I., Johnson, D.E. and Tenney, D. (1984) Are lymphangiograms necessary before placing patients with non-seminomatous testicular tumors on surveillance? *J. Urol.*, **141**, 1133–5.

PRIMARY CHEMOTHERAPY FOR STAGE II NON-SEMINOMA   18

A. Horwich

18.1 INTRODUCTION

As discussed in Chapter 17 the common practice in North America and certain European countries is to perform a retroperitoneal lymph node dissection in a patient with suspected small volume metastatic retroperitoneal lymphadenopathy, a procedure having both diagnostic and therapeutic value. In the United Kingdom the approach to clinical Stage II non-seminoma during the last 15 years has been with primary combination chemotherapy following orchidectomy, and lymphadenectomy has been reserved for patients with residual lymphadenopathy following chemotherapy. Since many patients avoid retroperitoneal lymphnode dissection the approach is perceived as less toxic; however, this judgement must be tempered by the fact that a somewhat greater proportion of patients receive chemotherapy, and unless assessment methodology is meticulous some patients may be treated with chemotherapy whose abdominal nodes were free from metastases.

18.2 THE ROYAL MARSDEN HOSPITAL SERIES

An analysis of the approach, which might be called primary chemotherapy, was undertaken on all 122 patients presenting to the Royal Marsden Hospital between 1979 and 1989 with metastatic testicular non-seminoma confined to the retroperitoneal nodes and measuring <5 cm in maximum transverse diameter (Horwich *et al.*, 1994a). Staging included histology review, CT scan of thorax, abdomen and pelvis, with lymphography reserved for equivocal abnormal nodes in patients with normal serum markers. A total of 26 patients did not have rising serum alpha-fetoprotein (AFP) or human chorionic gonadotrophin (HCG), and in the total series 64 patients had metastatic disease measuring <2 cm in diameter. All patients were treated with four cycles of platinum-based combination chemotherapy, and following completion of chemotherapy patients were selected for either follow-up observation or lymphadenectomy on the basis of a further CT scan. Lymphadenectomy was performed on those with a persistent postchemotherapy mass measuring at least 1 cm in diameter occurring at the site of previous lymphadenopathy. The dissection was confined to involved lymph nodes only. Of patients presenting with disease <2 cm in diameter, postchemotherapy lymphadenectomy was unilateral in nine and bilateral in one. Among those presenting with disease 2 to 5 cm in diameter, postchemotherapy lymphadenectomy was unilateral in 18 and bilateral in seven patients. Of the 35 patients who had lymphadenectomy

Testicular Cancer: Investigation and management. Second edition. Edited by Professor A. Horwich.
Published in 1996 by Chapman & Hall. ISBN 0 412 61210 0.

Table 18.1 Survival of patients with clinical Stage IIA and IIB non-seminomatous tumors (RMH 1979–1989)

Number of patients	122
Median yrs follow-up (range)	5.5 (2–11)
% 5-yr survival:	
Progression-free	92
Overall	97
Cause specific	98.5

Table 18.2 Overall toxicity of primary chemotherapy in 122 patients with clinical Stage II non-seminoma (RMH 1979–1989)

Toxicity	
Acute toxicities	
White blood count less than 1.5 × 109 l^{-1}	15 (12)
Platelets less than 50 × 109 l^{-1}	14 (11)
Haemoglobin less than 10 gm dl^{-1}	37 (30)
Neutropenic fever	5 (4)
Septicemia	2 (2)
Neuropathy	14 (11)
Dermatitis	23 (19)
Pneumonitis	6 (5)
Long-term toxicities	
% mean glomerular filtration rate decrease (range)	14 (0–46)
No. with Raynaud's phenomenon	14
No. with ejaculatory failure	5
No. with second malignancies (acoustic neuromas at 3 yrs)	1
No. undergoing surgical resection:	
Bowel	1
Kidney	1

because of residual lymphadenopathy after primary chemotherapy, the histology of the resected nodes was a mature teratoma in 29 patients, necrosis in only five patients and embryonal carcinoma in one patient.

The overall efficacy of this approach is shown in Table 18.1, in which it can be seen the overall 5-year survival was 97%. The four deaths were caused by progressive germ cell tumor in two patients, bleomycin pneumonitis in one patient and coincidental disease in one patient.

A total of ten patients demonstrated some evidence of progression after primary chemotherapy; however, in five of these progression was demonstrated to be due entirely to mature teratoma and was treated with surgery alone. In four of these five there had been a previous lymphadenectomy for mature teratoma. One of these suffered a secondary recurrence associated with raised AFP and was treated with further chemotherapy and radiation, and is currently well. Thus a total of six patients developed evidence of progressive undifferentiated tumor following their primary chemotherapy, of whom four have been successfully salvaged and two have died.

18.3   RMH SERIES – TOXICITY

The spectrum of toxicities identified in this series of 122 patients is listed in Table 18.2. The acute toxicities are typical of standard germ cell tumor chemotherapy and the long-term toxicities similarly relate to choice of chemotherapeutic agent and the need for post-chemotherapy lymphadenectomy. All five patients in this series who suffered ejaculatory failure were amongst those requiring lymphadenectomy. All those suffering from Raynaud's phenomenon following chemotherapy had been treated with at least 300 units of bleomycin and, as discussed in Chapter 20, consideration could be given to the reduction or deletion of the use of this drug in these particularly good prognosis presentations.

An important aspect of toxicity in young men is impairment of fertility, which could be due either to ejaculatory failure in those treated by node dissection or to impaired spermatogenesis in those treated with chemotherapy. In this series we found that of 36 patients with spermatogenesis prior to chemotherapy there was recovery of spermatogenesis in 32. A recent analysis of spermatogenesis after germ cell tumor chemotherapy was based on 178 patients treated with a variety of regimens. It was found that recovery of spermatogenesis to at least 1 million per milliliter occurred in 72% of patients with spermatogenesis prior to chemotherapy; recovery to 10 million per milliliter occurred in 49% of patients with spermatogenesis prior to chemotherapy. On multivariate analysis the significant factors predicting recovery were: higher prechemotherapy sperm count, reduced number of chemotherapy cycles and the use of carboplatin rather than cisplatin (Horwich *et al.*, 1995), however, randomized comparisons of carboplatin and cisplatin suggest that cisplatin is the more effective anticancer agent and should be retained in standard combination chemotherapy (Bajorin, Mazumdar and Vlamis, 1993; Horwich, *et al.* 1994).

18.4 MEDICAL RESEARCH COUNCIL SERIES

An analysis of prognosis in Stage II testicular non-seminoma was also performed in patients registered in the Medical Research Council Database (Horwich and Stenning, 1994). These comprised a subset of patients analyzed in a retrospective review of 795 men treated with chemotherapy for metastatic non-seminoma (Mead *et al.*, 1992). Patients had been treated with a range of different combination chemotherapy regimens following staging assessment. The analysis of Stage II non-seminoma was based on 287 patients, including 47 with node masses <2 cm in diameter (IIA), 175 with nodal metastases between 2 and 5 cm in diameter (IIB) and 65 with node metastases >5 cm in diameter (IIC). The number of patients with rising tumor markers postorchidectomy was 35 in Stage IIA, 115 in Stage IIB and 53 in Stage IIC. Table 18.3 shows the response to primary chemotherapy according to initial disease stage, and Table 18.4 illustrates the histology at postchemotherapy lymphadenectomy. In these tables complete response implied the absence of the residual mass measuring >1 cm in diameter, and it can been seen that it was unusual in patients presenting with node masses >5 cm in diameter. A total of 43 of the 222 patients who presented with node masses <5 cm in diameter had

Table 18.3 Chemotherapy response according to disease stage

Stage	n	CR (Ch)	CR (Ch + S)	NE (RM)
IIA	47	41	43	3
IIB	175	117	157*	18
IIC	65	16	53†	12

CR (Ch), Complete response to chemotherapy; CR (Ch + S), complete response to chemotherapy plus surgery; NE (RM), nonevaluable residual mass.
* Including eight patients with completely undifferentiated cancer.
† Including nine patients with completely resected undifferentiated cancer.
Data from the MRC analysis (Horwich and Stenning, 1994).

Table 18.4 Histology at postchemotherapy lymphadenectomy

Stage	n	Necrosis only	Mature teratoma	Carcinoma
IIA	3	0	3	0
IIB	40	13	19	8
IIC	37*	5	22	9

* In one case the histology was unknown.
Data from the MRC analysis (Horwich and Stenning, 1994).

postchemotherapy lymphadenectomy and in eight of these there was evidence of residual undifferentiated cancer, with a median follow-up of 6.5 years. The 3-year survival in patients presenting with Stage IIA disease was 98% (95% confidence intervals, 96–100%). In patients with Stage IIB disease the 3-year survival was 96% (95% confidence intervals, 93–9%).

18.5 DISCUSSION

Logothetis *et al.* (1987) have also reported from the M.D. Anderson Hospital on primary chemotherapy following orchidectomy in Stage I marker positive, and Stage II non-seminoma, including 11 patients with Stage IIA disease, 19 with IIB and nine with IIC. Eight of these 39 patients had postchemotherapy node dissection. The overall survival was excellent, with only one patient dying of progressive malignant disease.

If results from Chapters 17 and 18 are compared, it can be seen that, in patients presenting with Stage II small volume metastases from testicular non-seminoma, either primary retroperitoneal lymph node dissection or primary chemotherapy following orchidectomy appear to be equally successful in curing the great majority of patients. Since the clinical context is the young male patient with a high probability of cure, considerations of toxicity should be an important determinant of the treatment policy. The major problem of extensive bilateral lymph node dissection is dry ejaculation (Pizzocaro, 1987). However, this complication can clearly be mitigated by the use of nerve-sparing techniques in those with a limited extent of metastatic disease, as discussed in Chapter 16. The approach based on primary chemotherapy must confer a risk of chemotherapy-related toxicities as fully documented by Horwich *et al.*, (1994a) and summarized in Table 18.2. This toxicity was derived from a range of chemotherapy regimens; however, as discussed in Chapters 19 and 20, increased experience of chemotherapy has allowed the definition of low toxicity approaches such as the reduction of total number of chemotherapy cycles to only three (Einhorn *et al.*, 1989). In this context the risk of iatrogenic carcinogenesis is extremely low (Pedersen-Bjergaard *et al.*, 1991 Bokemeyer and Schmoll, 1993).

In the absence of a prospective comparative assessment of surgery or primary chemotherapy for Stage II small volume non-seminoma, the management decision should depend upon the expertise and resources available within the treatment center and should follow a full discussion with the patient of the advantages and disadvantages of these alternative approaches. The discussion should be guided by the importance of ejaculatory function to the long-term well-being of the patient (Rieker, Edbril and Garnick, 1985)

REFERENCES

Bajorin, D.F., Sarosdy, M.F., Bosl, G.J. and Mazumdar, M. (1992) Good risk germ cell tumour (GCT): a randomized trial of etoposide + carboplatin (EC) vs etoposide + cisplatin (EP). *Proc. Am. Soc. Clin. Oncol.*, **11**, 203.

Bokemeyer, C. and Schmoll, H.-J. (1993) Secondary neoplasms following treatment of malignant germ cell tumors. *J. Clin. Oncol.*, **11**(9), 1703–9.

Einhorn, L.H., Williams, S.D., Loehrer, P.J. *et al.* (1989) Evaluation of optimal duration of chemotherapy in favorable-prognosis disseminated germ cell tumors: A Southeastern Cancer Study Group protocol. *J. Clin. Oncol.*, **7**(3), 387–91.

Horwich, A., Lampe, H., Norman, A. *et al.* (1995) Fertility after chemotherapy for metastatic germ cell tumours. *Proc. Am. Soc. Clin. Oncol.*, **14**, 236.

Horwich, A., Norman, A., Fisher, C *et al.* (1994a). Primary chemotherapy for stage II non seminomatous germ cell tumors of the testis. *J. Urol.*, **151**, 72–8.

Horwich, A., Sleifer, D., Fosså, S. *et al.* (1994b) A trial of carboplatin-based combination chemotherapy in good prognosis metastatic testicular non-seminoma. *Proc. Am. Soc. Clin. Oncol.*, **13**, 231.

Horwich, A. and Stenning, S. (1994) Initial chemotherapy for stage II testicular non-seminoma. *World J. Urol.*, **12**(3), 148–50.

Logothetis, C.J., Swanson, D.A., Dexeus, F. *et al.* (1987) Primary chemotherapy for clinical stage II nonseminomatous germ cell tumors of the testis: A follow-up of 50 patients. *J. Clin. Oncol.*, **5**(6), 906–11.

Mead, G.M., Stenning, S.P., Parkinson, M.C. *et al.* (1992) The second Medical Research Council Study of prognostic factors in nonseminomatous germ cell tumours. *J. Clin. Oncol.*, **10**(1), 85–94.

Pedersen-Bjergaard, J., Daugaard, G., Hansen, S.W. *et al.* (1991) Increased risk of myelodysplasia and leukaemia after etoposide, cisplatin, and bleomycin for germ-cell tumours. *Lancet*, **338**, 359–63.

Pizzocaro, G. (1987) Retroperitoneal lymph node dissection in clinical stage IIA and IIB non-seminomatous germ cell tumours of the testis. *Int. J. Androl.*, **10**, 269–75.

Rieker, P.P., Edbril, S.D. and Garnick, M.B. (1985) Curative testis cancer therapy: psychosocial sequelae. *J. Clin. Oncol.*, **3**(8), 1117–26.

CHEMOTHERAPY FOR METASTATIC NON-SEMINOMA

C.R. Nichols and B.J. Roth

19.1 INTRODUCTION

Since the earliest attempts to use systemic cytotoxic agents in human neoplastic disease, and throughout the three-decade development of active chemotherapeutic regimens, germ cell tumors of the testis have demonstrated a unique sensitivity to a broad range of antineoplastic agents. In fact, virtually every agent tested has demonstrated some response in previously untreated patients.

Early recognition of this extraordinary chemosensitivity resulted in a long list of drugs with single agent activity, and the early use of combination regimens fueled the rapid progress of therapy for metastatic disease. Such improvement in metastatic chemotherapy is primarily responsible for the marked increase in survival rate for this disease over the past 20 years. Certainly, the extensive proliferative capacity of this malignancy contributed to sensitivity in early trials to cycle specific agents. However, kinetics alone is not a sufficient explanation for the unparalleled response rate to an agent such as cisplatin.

The response rates of testicular cancer to a number of single agents are summarized in Table 19.1. The review of such data over a 30-year period requires several caveats. (1) The early introduction of combination regimens resulted in a relative paucity of single agent data, even for the most active compounds. By today's standards, we would consider the majority of these early agents inadequately tested for consideration of incorporation into combination regimens. Such concerns failed to arise in view of the marked successes achieved with early combination regimens. (2) The information in Table 19.1 represents cumulative data from a variable number of trials, with a variety of dosages and schedules present for the more extensively tested compounds. (3) Response criteria varied over this interval, with stricter criteria predominating since the early 1970s. (4) Patients in these trials represent a heterogeneous group with respect to what are now well-defined prognostic variables, as well as the extent of prior therapy. The small number of active agents identified after 1975 is a reflection not of an altered natural history of the disease, but rather of the extent of prior chemotherapy. The curative potential of cisplatin-based therapy has resulted in the use of investigational agents only after patients' exposure to six to eight other cytotoxic drugs. While such a strategy is a clinical necessity in a potentially curable disease, it also markedly reduces the chance of discovering new agents with significant activity.

19.2 EARLY SINGLE AGENT ACTIVITY

In the first report of the use of systemic therapy in this disease, Friedgood, Danza and Bocca-

Testicular Cancer: Investigation and management. Second edition. Edited by Professor A. Horwich.
Published in 1996 by Chapman & Hall. ISBN 0 412 61210 0.

Table 19.1 Single agent activity in germ cell tumors

Agent	Year first reported	Number of patients	Number of responses	Number of complete responses	Reference
Nitrofurazone	1952	6	6 (100%)	1 (17%)	Friedgood, Danza and Boccabella (1952), Wildermuth (1955), Szczukowski, Daywitt and Elrick (1958)
Sarcolysin	1958	32	24 (75%)	11 (34%)	Blokhin et al. (1958)
Methotrexate	1958	15	4 (27%)	4 (27%)	Li, Hertz and Bergenstal (1958), Wyatt and McAninch (1961, 1967)
6-Mercaptopurine	1958	5	0	–	Li, Hertz and Bergenstal (1958)
5-Fluorouracil	1960	10	3 (30%)	0	Wilson (1960), Allaire et al. (1961), Hyman, Ultmann and Habif (1962)
Mithramycin	1960	305	113 (37%)	33 (11%)	Curreri and Ansfield (1960), Parker, Wiltsie and Jackson (1960), Kofman and Eisenstein (1963), Kofman, Medrek and Alexander (1964), Brown and Kenndey (1965), Kennedy, Griffen and Lober (1965), Koons, Sensenbrenner and Owens (1966), Ream et al. (1968), Ansfield (1969), Kennedy (1970)
Vinblastine	1961	30	13 (43%)	4 (13%)	Warwick, Alison and Dart (1961), Samuels and Howe (1970)
Vincristine	1962	6	4 (67%)	0	Costa, Hreshchyshyn and Holland (1962), Whitelaw et al. (1963), Shaw and Bruner (1964)
Chlorambucil	1966	8	4 (50%)	2 (25%)	MacKensie (1966)
Actinomycin-D	1966	22	8 (36%)	4 (18%)	MacKensie (1966)
Bleomycin	1970	45	14 (31%)	3 (7%)	Bonadonna et al. (1972), Blum, Carter and Agre (1973), Clinical Screening Co-operative Group of the EORTC (1970)
Cisplatin	1972	12	6 (50%)	3 (25%)	Rossof, Slayton and Perlia (1972), Higby et al. (1973, 1974)
Ifosfamide	1976	248	126 (51%)	55 (22%)	Bruhl et al. (1976), Schmoll, Rhomberg and Diehl (1978), Boutis, Stergion-Travantzis and Mourantidou (1982), Weibach and Kochs (1982), Niederle et al. (1983), Scheulen et al. (1983), Wheeler et al. (1986)
Etoposide (VP-16)	1977	96	24 (25%)	3 (3%)	Newlands and Bagshawe (1977), Cavalli et al. (1977, 1981), Fitzharris et al. (1980)
Vindesine	1979	19	3 (16%)	0	Reynolds et al. (1979)
m-AMSA	1981	22	0	–	de Jager et al. (1981), Williams, Duncan and Einhorn (1983)
Mitoxantrone	1985	11	0	–	Williams et al. (1985)
Iproplatin	1986	34	1 (3%)	0	Clavel et al. (1986), Drasga et al. (1987)
Carboplatin	1987	44	3 (7%)	1 (2%)	Motzer et al. (1987), Trump et al. (1987)
Epirubicin	1987	20	3 (15%)	0	Schultz et al. (1987)

bella (1952) used nitrofurans (a group of topical antiseptics known to result in testicular degeneration in rodents when used internally), and reported that all four seminoma patients treated demonstrated 'marked degeneration of the tumor cells, increased fibrosis and decreased cellularity of the tumor'. The activity of these agents was subsequently confirmed by others (Wildermuth, 1955; Szczukowski, Daywitt and Elrick, 1958).

Blokhin *et al.* (1958) reported on the Soviet experience with the alkylating agent sarcolysin (DL-*p*-di(2-chloroethyl) amino-phenylalanine hydrochloride) in 200 patients, including 32 with testicular cancer, and documented 24 responses, with 11 achieving complete remission. All 11 complete remissions were in patients with pure seminoma, a pattern often repeated in these early trials. Small numbers of patients were later treated with a number of other alkylating agents, including thiotepa, melphalan and cyclophosphamide. All of these agents yielded roughly similar results in seminoma, but were devoid of activity in non-seminomatous disease. Because of the disparity of response based on histology, and the availability of an alternative curative therapy in early stage seminoma (i.e. radiotherapy), interest in clinical trials with these agents dissipated rapidly.

Multidisease trials with several antimetabolites also appeared in the late 1950s and early 1960s. Methotrexate was shown to be a very active agent in female choriocarcinoma, but again significantly less so in male non-seminomatous disease (Li, Hertz and Bergenstal, 1958; Wyatt and McAninch, 1961, 1967), and no responses were observed with the purine antagonist 6-mercaptopurine (Li, Hertz and Bergenstal, 1958). Similar trials demonstrated modest activity of 5-fluorouracil (Wilson, 1960; Allaire, Thieme and Korst, 1961; Hyman, Ultmann and Habif, 1962).

The naturally occurring plant alkaloids, vinblastine and vincristine, first demonstrated activity in lymphomas and Hodgkin's disease, but were subsequently used in patients with testicular cancer (Warwick, Alison and Darte, 1961; Costa, Hreshchyshyn and Holland, 1962; Whitelaw *et al.*, 1963; Shaw and Brunner, 1964; Samuels and Howe, 1970). Particularly in the case of vinblastine, the induction of several complete remissions of short duration provided a useful tool in (and the impetus for) the development of subsequent combination regimens.

Several antibiotics derived from the fermentation of *Streptomyces* were found to have antitumor activity, including actinomycin-D and mithramycin. Remarkably few single agent trials of actinomycin-D were performed prior to its incorporation into early combination regimens, although MacKensie (1966) reported eight responders in 22 patients, including four complete remissions. On the other hand, mithramycin was extensively tested in testicular cancer patients, and provided a response rate of 30%, with nearly 30% of responders achieving complete remission (Curreri and Ansfield, 1960; Parker, Wiltsie and Jackson, 1960; Kofman and Eisenstein, 1963; Kofman, Medreck and Alexander, 1964; Brown and Kennedy, 1965; Kennedy, Griffen and Lober, 1965; Koons, Sensenbrenner and Owens, 1966; Ream *et al.*, 1968; Ansfield, 1969; Kennedy, 1970). Unfortunately, most responses were of short duration, and patients experienced significant hepatic, renal and bone marrow toxicity, prompting discontinuation of clinical trials.

19.3 EARLY COMBINATION CHEMOTHERAPY REGIMENS

The single agent data in testicular cancer in the late 1950s were both promising and disappointing. Despite the reproducible response rates using alkylating agents, antimetabolites or antitumor antibiotics, most responses were of short duration, with only anecdotal reports of 3-year survivors.

Li, Hertz and Bergenstal (1960) reported the results of a number of combination regimens using members of each of these three

Table 19.2 Early combination chemotherapy regimens

Regimen	Number of patients	Number of responses	Complete responses	Reference
Actinomycin-D/chlorambucil/	23	12 (52%)	7 (30%)	Li *et al.* (1960)
methotrexate	90	38 (42%)	10 (11%)	MacKensie (1966)
	11	5 (45%)	1 (9%)	Moore (1968)
	21	14 (67%)	4 (13%)	Ansfield *et al.* (1969)
	29	11 (38%)	0	Astrakan and Monul (1976)
	174	80 (46%)	22 (13%)	
Actinomycin-D/chlorambucil	9	2 (22%)	1 (11%)	Li *et al.* (1960)
	31	14 (45%)	5 (16%)	MacKensie (1966)
	40	16 (40%)	6 (15%)	
Actinomycin-D/nitrogen mustard	14	4 (29%)	1 (7%)	Jacobs, Johnson and Wood (1966)
Actinomycin-D/vincristine/ cyclophosphamide	10	5 (50%)	1 (10%)	Jacobs (1970)
Actinomycin-D/vincristine/ cyclophosphamide mithramycin	7	5 (71%)	3 (43%)	Jacobs (1970)
Methotrexate/nitrogen mustard	15	5 (33%)	2 (13%)	Jacobs *et al.* (1966)
Vincristine/methotrexate/melphalan	12	9 (75%)	1 (8%)	Steinfeld *et al.* (1966)
Vincristine/methotrexate/melphalan or cyclophosphamide	12	4 (33%)	0	Jacobs *et al.* (1966)
6MP/DON	8	1 (13%)	0	Li *et al.* (1960)
Chlorambucil/DON	2	0	–	Li *et al.* (1960)
Vincristine/methotrexate/ cyclophosphamide/5-FU	17	7 (41%)	5 (29%)	Mendelson and Serpick (1970)

6MP, 6-mercaptopurine. DON, 6-diazo-5-oxo-levo-norleucine. 5-FU, 5-fluorouracil.

classes of drugs in 36 patients with testicular tumors. Twenty-three patients were treated with a dose-intensive 25-day regimen consisting of methotrexate (5 mg, PO for 16 to 25 days), actinomycin-D (0.5 mg IV days 3–7) and chlorambucil (10 mg PO daily). Twelve of the 23 (52%) demonstrated an objective response and, significantly, seven of the 12 achieved complete remission. At the time of the report, five patients were disease free at 9–39 months. This particular three-drug regimen was popular throughout the 1960s, and the data from published trials are summarized in Table 19.2. These studies established the response rate with this regimen to be close to 50%, with almost a third of responses being complete responses, but long-term survivors were much less common. A number of other two- to four-drug regimens were developed in the 1960s (Table 19.2), but none

demonstrated significant improvement over the results of Li *et al.* A model for true cyclic chemotherapy in this disease was initially reported by Mendelson and Serpick (1970), and involved the bolus injections of four drugs over a 5-day course, with the interval between courses based on toxicity. In this regimen, vincristine (0.025 mg kg^{-1}), methotrexate (0.75 mg kg^{-1}) and cyclophosphamide (7.5 mg kg^{-1}) were given on days 1 and 4, while 5-fluorouracil (7.5 mg kg^{-1}) was administered daily for 5 days. Seven of 17 patients (41%) responded, with five of seven responses being complete.

It was clear that combination regimens of this era provided some improvement in therapy when compared with single agents, with 50–70% of all patients responding, and 10–20% achieving complete remission. The percentage of patients achieving durable complete remissions, however, was only slightly better than for single agents, and the combination regimens were clearly more toxic. While the concept of combination therapy became accepted, further advances awaited the development of new active agents.

19.4 BLEOMYCIN

The discovery and isolation of a third antitumor antibiotic, from *Streptomyces verticullus*, by Umezawa *et al.* (1966a, b; 1971) was the key to the development of modern combination regimens. The first report of single agent activity in testicular cancer came in 1970, when the Clinical Screening Cooperative Group of the EORTC (1970) noted four responses in six patients, including two complete responses. Other clinical trials revealed a unique, dose-related pulmonary toxicity of interstitial fibrosis that was dose limiting. The lack of hematological toxicity provided an excellent opportunity for use of this drug in full dose as part of a combination regimen.

While preclinical studies failed to reveal a clear mechanism of action of the drug, they did demonstrate a relative cell cycle specificity. Barranco and Humphrey (1971) showed that Chinese hamster ovary cells were the most sensitive to the cytotoxic effects of the drug during mitosis, but also in the G_2 phase of the cell cycle. With this high degree of cycle specificity, there was added impetus for the use of this drug in a rapidly proliferative malignancy such as testicular cancer.

19.5 VINBLASTINE/BLEOMYCIN

The next major advance in the development of effective therapy, as reported by Samuels from the M.D. Anderson Hospital, involved the use of vinblastine and bleomycin in combination, based on their single agent activities and the presence of nonoverlapping toxicities. Additionally, there was a reasonable anticipation of synergism on kinetic grounds, as vinblastine was capable of arresting cells in

mitosis, and bleomycin appeared to have its greatest cytotoxic potential during the mitotic phase of the cell cycle.

Samuels, Johnson and Holoye (1973, 1975, 1976) began treating patients with these two drugs in combination. The regimen (termed VB-1) consisted of vinblastine administered by IV push at a dosage of 0.4–0.6 mg kg^{-1} (split dosage on days 1 and 2), and bleomycin 30 units given IM twice weekly for ten doses. These treatments were given every 4–6 weeks based on toxicity, for a total of four to six cycles. Of the initial 50 patients treated with this regimen, 35 (70%) demonstrated an objective response, with 17 of 35 responding patients attaining complete remissions, and four of the 17 complete responders (CR) (24%) subsequently relapsing. These data were subsequently updated on 70 treated patients, with 53 (76%) responders, and 22 complete responders. Maximum response was related to histology (44% CR for teratocarcinoma versus 26% for pure embryonal carcinoma), extent of prior therapy and volume of disease (CR in ten out of 17 with minimal pulmonary involvement versus four of 21 with advanced pulmonary disease). However, because of a relatively poor response rate in patients with embryonal carcinoma, several changes were made in an attempt to improve the response rate.

Subsequent protocols altered the schedule of administration of bleomycin to a continuous infusion, based on the drug's short half-life and its cell cycle specificity. Additionally, there were preclinical data suggesting that continuous exposure resulted in increased cell kill (Drewinko, Novak and Barranco, 1972). The first attempt at this (VB-2) consisted of a 5-day continuous infusion of bleomycin (30 units day^{-1}) followed by vinblastine, again in split dosage on days 5 and 6. Only three patients were treated with this protocol before it was abandoned because of prolonged hematological toxicity.

The next protocol (VB-3) changed the order of administration, with vinblastine being ad-

Table 19.3 Vinblastine plus bleomycin combination regimens

Regimen	Number of patients	Number of responses	Complete responses	Reference
VB–1 V: 0.4–0.6 mg kg^{-1} IV divided days 1, 2 B: 30 U IM × 2/week × 10 doses	50	35 (70%)	17 (33%)	Samuels, Johnson and Holoye (1973, 1975, 1976)
VB–3 V: 0.4–0.6 mg kg^{-1} IV divided days 1, 2 B: 30 U d^{-1} × 5 days continuous infusion	91	86 (95%)	59 (65%)	Samuels *et al.* (1975, 1977, 1979)
V: 0.4 mg kg^{-1} IV divided days 1, 2 B: 15 U m^{-2} IV × 2/week to 400 mg	11	9 (82%)	5 (45%)	Spigel and Coltman (1974)
V: 15 mg m^{-2} IV divided days 1, 2 B: 15 U m^{-2} IV 2 ×/week to 230 U m^{-2}	48	31 (65%)	21 (44%)	Spigel *et al.* (1978)
V: 0.2 mg kg^{-1} IV B: 30 U IV × 2/week	25	18 (76%)	16 (64%)	Stoter, Struyvenberg and Vendrik (1978)

V, vinblastine. B, bleomycin.

ministered on days 1 and 2, followed by a 5-day continuous infusion of bleomycin. This protocol was initiated in 1973, and results were ultimately reported on 91 evaluable patients (Samuels *et al.*, 1975, 1977, 1979). The overall response rate was 95%, with 65% of patients achieving a complete remission, and virtually identical response rates for those with teratocarcinoma or embryonal carcinoma. These responses appeared to be durable, as the mean survival was 142 weeks for those with embryonal carcinoma, and 117 weeks for patients with teratocarcinoma.

Myelosuppression and pulmonary interstitial fibrosis were the dose-limiting toxicities observed with VB-3 (Samuels *et al.*, 1979). Seventeen patients experienced culture-positive septicemia, with one septic death. The incidence of sepsis was directly related to vin-

blastine dosage, and was seen in only 2.3% of patients receiving ≤0.45 mg kg^{-1} compared with a 9.2% incidence in those getting ≥0.5 mg kg^{-1}. The mean cumulative bleomycin dosage was 700 mg, and the corresponding incidence of pulmonary fibrosis was 7%, with half of those patients dying from this side-effect of therapy.

These excellent therapeutic results have been duplicated by other investigators and are summarized in Table 19.3. Thus, the combination of vinblastine and bleomycin represented a significant therapeutic advance in the early 1970s. However, the toxicity data from these trials made it clear that further improvements would not be possible with dose escalations of these two drugs, and instead would rely on the introduction of another active agent, cisplatin.

19.6 CISPLATIN

Few serendipitous findings have had an impact on clinical oncology as has the discovery by Rosenberg, Van Camp and Krigas (1965) of the ability of platinum coordination compounds to inhibit bacterial cell growth. Subsequent investigations of several of these compounds led to the discovery of significant antitumor activity for *cis*-diamminedichloroplatinum (II) (Drobnik, 1983). Early clinical studies revealed that cisplatin was the most active agent yet known in non-seminomatous germ cell tumors with single agent response rates of 70% and an impressive 50% complete remission rate (Rosoff, Slayton and Perlia, 1972; Higby, Wallace and Holland, 1973; Higby *et al.*, 1974). Although cisplatin produced severe nausea and a degree of renal dysfunction, its relative lack of myelosuppression encouraged its incorporation into combination regimens. Such cisplatin-containing regimens were subsequently developed at Memorial Sloan-Kettering Cancer Center and Indiana University.

19.7 VINBLASTINE/ACTINOMYCIN-D/ BLEOMYCIN REGIMENS 1–6

In an attempt to improve on the response rates seen in the vinblastine/bleomycin (VB) regimens, investigators at Memorial Hospital treated 50 patients with actinomycin-D added to vinblastine and bleomycin (VAB-1) (Wittes *et al.*, 1976). The overall response rate was 34%, including 15% complete responses, and clearly did not represent an improvement over the VB regimens. Actinomycin-D thus appears not to add significantly to modern chemotherapeutic regimens.

From 1974 to 1976, 50 patients were treated on the first VAB regimen to contain cisplatin, termed VAB-2 (Cheng *et al.*, 1978). During the induction phase of this regimen, patients received vinblastine (0.6 mg kg^{-1}) and actinomycin-D (0.02 mg kg^{-1}) on day 1, bleomycin (0.25–0.5 mg kg^{-1}) by continuous infusion days 1–7, and cisplatin 1.2 mg kg^{-1} on day 8. During the first maintenance phase, vinblastine, actinomycin-D and bleomycin were given weekly, with cisplatin replacing actinomycin-D every third week for 4 months. After a second course of induction therapy at 4 months, a second maintenance phase was started, and included daily oral chlorambucil, vinblastine and actinomycin-D every 3 weeks for 2–3 years. Overall 42 of 50 patients (84%) responded, with a complete response rate of 50%. At the time of the report, the median survival had not yet been reached, and 11 of the complete responders were free of disease at 16–33 months. Although 15% experienced leukopenia, there were no episodes of sepsis, and one patient died secondary to bleomycin-induced pulmonary fibrosis. The relapse rate from complete remission was 56%.

From 1975 to 1977, 74 evaluable patients were treated with the next generation regimen, VAB-3 (Reynolds *et al.*, 1981). This complicated regimen used a five-drug induction regimen, including cyclophosphamide (600 mg m^{-2}). Following induction, six 3-week cycles of maintenance were given, which included chlorambucil (4 mg m^{-2} d^{-1}, days 1–14), vinblastine (4 mg m^{-2} day 1) and a third drug rotated with each cycle of therapy, either doxorubicin (30 mg m^{-2} day 1), actinomycin-D (1 mg m^{-2} day 1), or cisplatin (50 mg m^{-2} day 1). Reinduction was undertaken at 5 months, followed by further maintenance for a total of 24–30 months of therapy. The response rate was 81%, including a complete response rate of 61%. At the time of the report, the median follow-up was 27.5 months and the median survival had not yet been reached. Forty-five per cent of those treated were alive and disease free, and the relapse rate from complete remission had fallen to 31%.

Between 1976 and 1978, the VAB-4 program was used to treat 41 evaluable patients (Vugrin *et al.*, 1981). This protocol differed from the previous one only in the schedule of administration of drugs in an attempt to decrease the early relapses seen with VAB-3 (within 8 months). These changes included a bleomycin bolus followed by a 6-day infusion during induction, omission of bleomycin at the 4-month reinduction, but the addition of a full reinduction period at 8 months. The overall response rate was 85%, with 61% achieving complete remission with chemotherapy alone, and an additional 15% who attained complete remission after resection of residual disease. With a median follow-up of 27 months, 68% were alive and disease free, with three complete responders (12%) relapsing at 8, 14 and 26 months.

VAB-5 represented an intensive variant of VAB-4 developed for use in poor prognosis patients, and accrued 38 evaluable patients from 1977 to 1979 (Vugrin, Whitmore and Golbey, 1983a). Those poor prognostic factors identified included the presence of metastases >5 cm, palpable retroperitoneal disease, brain or liver metastases, involvement of two or more parenchymal organs, pure choriocarcinoma, human chorionic gonadotrophin (HCG) or alpha-fetoprotein (AFP) >1000 IU l^{-1}, lactate dehydrogenase IU l^{-1} >400 IU l^{-1}, and failure on prior chemotherapy. In this regimen, the dose of vinblastine was doubled, the dose of actinomycin-D was increased by 50%, and cyclophosphamide, doxorubicin and cisplatin were added on day 28. With this regimen, 18 of 38 patients (47%) achieved complete remission (11 with chemotherapy alone, seven after resection of residual disease). Not surprisingly, toxicity was significant, as 82% experienced granulocytopenic fevers, 29% had rises in serum creatinine >2 mg dl^{-1} (including two patients requiring hemodialysis), and mucositis was severe. Thirty per cent of treated patients refused to complete the planned treatment regimen.

VAB-6 was started in 1980, and the results in 34 evaluable patients have been reported (Vugrin *et al.*, 1981; Vugrin, Whitmore and Golbey, 1983b). Alterations of the VAB-4 regimen to achieve VAB-6 were based on

an increased emphasis on the importance of induction therapy, decreased emphasis on the need for maintenance therapy, and the need for additional chemotherapy if viable carcinoma was present in the postchemotherapy resected specimen. Thus, induction cycles were shortened (from 7 to 4 days), given at 3–4-week intervals (compared with every 4 months in VAB-4), and patients with malignant elements in resected specimens received two additional cycles of chemotherapy. Maintenance therapy with vinblastine and actinomycin-D was given every 3 weeks for a total of 1 year of therapy. Thirty-one of 34 patients (91%) achieved complete remission, and 28 of those were still disease free with a median follow-up of >24 months. This regimen eliminated the mucositis, renal insufficiency and pulmonary fibrosis seen with prior regimens. Myelosuppression remained the dose-limiting toxicity, with 18% experiencing a granulocytopenic fever.

19.8 TRIALS AT INDIANA UNIVERSITY

In 1974, maturing results from several clinical trials laid the framework for development of cisplatin-based chemotherapy in germinal neoplasms. The synergistic combination of vinblastine plus bleomycin was showing major activity in testicular cancer (Table 19.3). In addition to producing complete response rates of 30–50%, a proportion of patients maintained durable, complete remissions suggesting the possibility of cure. Concurrently, *cis*-diamminedichloroplatinum, one of a group of platinum coordination complexes, was shown to have remarkable single agent activity in patients with refractory testicular cancer and was nearly devoid of significant myelosuppression (Rossof, Slayton and Perlia, 1972; Higby, Wallace and Holland, 1973; Higby *et al.*, 1974). The serial clinical trials performed at Indiana University are representative of the development and refinement of cisplatin-based chemotherapy in testicular cancer.

By integrating cisplatin into the regimen of vinblastine plus bleomycin, Einhorn and Donohue (1977) were able to develop a regimen that combined full doses of agents with excellent single agent activity since none of the agents had overlapping toxicity. The original cisplatin/vinblastine/bleomycin (PVB) schedule at Indiana University incorporated cisplatin in full doses (20 mg m^{-2} d^{-1} × 5) in combination with vinblastine (0.4 mg kg^{-1}) every 3 weeks. Bleomycin (30 units) was given weekly for 12 weeks. Maintenance vinblastine and BCG immunotherapy were also employed in an attempt to maintain remissions.

The results obtained with this treatment protocol represented a major breakthrough in the treatment of testicular cancer. Fifty patients with disseminated testicular cancer were entered. Three patients were deemed inevaluable owing to death within 2 weeks of initiation of therapy. Clinical remissions were achieved with chemotherapy alone in 33 of the 47 patients (74%). Fourteen patients obtained partial remissions and five of these partial remittors were converted to disease-free status by complete surgical resection of teratoma (three patients) or residual viable cancer (two patients). There were four therapy-related deaths, two related to septicemia, one to pulmonary fibrosis, and one to bowel obstruction. Seven patients relapsed from complete remission. Overall, 27 (57%) patients were long-term disease-free survivors.

The acute toxicity of this regimen was formidable, but manageable. Nausea and vomiting of a moderate to severe nature were uniformly encountered. Bleomycin cutaneous toxicity along with fever and chills at the time of administration were common. Vinblastine produced myalgias in half of the patients. Significant anemia and thrombocytopenia were rarely seen. The most fearsome complication was severe leukopenia with subsequent infection. Eighteen patients required hospitalization for presumed sepsis associated with granulocytopenia. Seven had documented

sepsis and infection contributed to the death of two patients. An important negative finding was that significant cisplatin-induced, renal insufficiency could be all but eliminated with the simple expedient of continuous saline hydration without mannitol or other diuretics.

Rather than the usual incremental advances seen in therapy of most malignant disorders, this trial represented an astonishing leap forward. Of all evaluable patients, 85% obtained a disease-free status with over half of all patients with widely disseminated germ cell cancer being long-term survivors. This trial also demonstrated that chemotherapy could significantly alter the course of the disease, even without producing complete remissions. The regimen seemed capable of converting inoperable patients to operable status, often with the findings of residual benign teratoma. These findings found confirmation in clinical trails conducted at other institutions in the USA and Europe (Einhorn and Donohue, 1977; Ginsberg *et al.*, 1977; Krikorian *et al.*, 1978; Garnick *et al.*, 1979; Stoter *et al.*, 1979; Wilkinson *et al.*, 1979; Bosl *et al.*, 1980; Ramsey *et al.*, 1980).

Thus the concept of multimodal management of disseminated testicular cancer became firmly entrenched and the goal of therapy in all patients became inducing complete remissions. An additional observation in this study was that, as expected, volume of metastatic disease was a useful discriminant of outcome. Despite these remarkable therapeutic accomplishments, the severe toxicity of myalgias and leukopenic sepsis remained troublesome and outcome in patients with far advanced metastatic disease was still unsatisfactory. The next generation of studies at Indiana University was designed to address these issues.

In an effort to minimize toxicity while maintaining therapeutic effect, a trial was designed and conducted at Indiana University comparing standard PVB (vinblastine, 0.4 mg kg^{-1}) with PVB (vinblastine 0.3 mg kg^{-1}) (Einhorn and Williams, 1980). A third arm had an even lower dose of vinblastine (0.2 mg kg^{-1}) but added a fourth drug, Adriamycin (Adria Laboratories, Columbus, Ohio) (doxorubicin hydrochloride). Between 1976 and 1978, 78 patients were entered on trial. Fifty-three patients (68%) obtained complete remission with chemotherapy alone. An additional 11 patients (14%) were rendered disease free by postchemotherapy surgery for an overall complete remission rate of 82%. There was no difference in outcome among the three treatment arms. Thus, the therapeutic promise of the initial PVB study was maintained, with 78% of patients entering the trial becoming disease free. An equally important observation was that these results could be obtained with lower (and less toxic) doses of vinblastine.

While there was no difference with respect to therapeutic outcome among the different treatment arms, the incidence of leukopenic sepsis was markedly different. In the high dose vinblastine arms (0.4 mg kg^{-1}), there was a 35% incidence of granulocytopenic fever, with a 12% incidence of documented sepsis. With PVB (vinblastine 0.2 mg kg^{-1}) plus Adriamycin, 24%, patients had granulocytopenic fever, with 4% incidence of documented sepsis. With PVB (vinblastine 0.3 mg kg^{-1}) without Adriamycin, 15% had fever and no patient had documented sepsis.

Throughout the early trials at Indiana University and other institutions, maintenance therapy was employed in an effort to induce and maintain remissions. Several observations called the use of routine maintenance therapy into question. First, the use of regular maintenance therapy rarely improved the remission status obtained with primary induction therapy. Second, those patients who did relapse while on maintenance therapy developed recurrent disease soon after the completion of induction therapy, implying that primary therapy had been ineffective.

With these questions in mind, maintenance therapy became the next focus for refining treatment of testicular cancer. Indiana University and the Southeastern Cancer Study Group (SECSG) performed a trial comparing PVB to PVB plus the addition of Adriamycin to validate the previous small trial at Indiana University (Einhorn *et al.*, 1981). A second randomization allocated patients obtaining a complete remission to receive maintenance vinblastine or to be observed without further therapy. There were no differences in the induction arms with 132 out of 171 eligible patients (80%) obtaining a complete remission. Thirteen of 132 patients obtaining complete remission did so after complete resection of carcinoma and were given postoperative cisplatin-based therapy. Six other patients obtained complete responses only after late resolution of radiographic abnormalities. Thus, 113 patients were entered into the second randomization, 58 patients received vinblastine maintenance (0.3 mg kg^{-1} per month for 20 months) and 55 patients were observed without further therapy. There were five relapses (9%) in the group receiving the vinblastine maintenance and four relapses (7%) in the group receiving no further therapy.

The therapeutic outcomes in this trial resulted in a major shift in the chemotherapy approach to testicular cancer. With the lack of additional benefit of prolonged low-dose treatment after cisplatin-based induction therapy, the framework for the modern day regimens was established. Intense brief induction therapy without maintenance treatments eliminated the morbidity of such treatments and allowed rapid resumption of a normal lifestyle in these young patients. That prolonged therapy was unnecessary was confirmed independently by other investigators (Bosl *et al.*, 1980).

During the period of investigations prior to 1982, some patients who failed primary chemotherapy responded to etoposide (Cavalli *et al.*, 1977, 1981: Newlands and Bagshawe, 1977; Fitzharris *et al.*, 1980). Investigators at Indiana University evaluated this drug in combination with cisplatin alone or with other drugs in previously treated patients (Williams *et al.*, 1980). A small portion of these patients achieved durable complete remissions. Etoposide therapy, compared with vinblastine therapy, was nearly devoid of neuromuscular or other nonhematological toxicities. In addition, etoposide and cisplatin demonstrated synergy in animal tumor models (O'Dwyer *et al.*, 1985).

With the evidence of excellent single agent activity of etoposide and the potential for diminished toxicity relative to vinblastine, a trial was designed at Indiana University and the SECSG with a straightforward substitution of etoposide for vinblastine as primary therapy of testicular cancer (Williams *et al.*, 1987). Between 1982 and 1984, patients with disseminated germ cell cancer were randomly allocated to receive cisplatin 20 mg m^{-2} daily × 5, bleomycin 30 units weekly × 12, and either vinblastin 0.3 mg kg^{-1} (PVB) or etoposide 100 mg m^{-2} d^{-1} × 5 (BEP). Cycles were repeated every 3 weeks for four cycles.

A total of 261 patients from 24 institutions were entered on this trial. Three patients were ineligible by reason of pathological errors or lack of disseminated disease. Fourteen patients were inevaluable for response but were included in the overall survival analysis. Detailed analysis of this large patient population revealed that the two groups were well balanced with respect to primary site, tumor type and extent of disease.

Among 121 patients treated with PVB, 74 patients achieved complete remission with chemotherapy alone and an additional 15 patients became disease free after complete surgical resection of teratoma (ten patients) or carcinoma (five patients). Of 123 patients treated with BEP, 74 achieved complete response with chemotherapy alone and 28 patients were rendered disease free after resection of teratoma (22 patients) or residual cancer (six patients). Thus, 74% of patients receiving PVB and 83% of patients receiving BEP became disease free. There were 15 relapses (nine on PVB, six on BEP).

Both regimens were associated with substantial acute toxicity. Granulocytopenia was common, with 59% of all patients experiencing an absolute granulocyte count less than 500 cells per mm^3 at some time during therapy. Despite this, only six patients (2%) died of sepsis (four on PVB, two on BEP). While both regimens appeared equally myelotoxic, there was a substantial difference in nonhematological toxicity. Paresthesias occurred more commonly with PVB (38%) than with BEP (23%) ($p = 0.02$). Abdominal cramps occurred in 20% of patients receiving PVB and only 5% of patients receiving BEP ($p = 0.0008$) and myalgias occurred in 19% of patients receiving PVB and only one patient receiving BEP ($p = 0.0002$).

Results of this large multi-institutional randomized trial suggested that BEP was therapeutically equivalent to PVB but associated with substantially less nonhematological toxicity. Thus, at Indiana University, BEP became the preferred therapy. Therapeutic results obtained with BEP were with doses of etoposide of 100 mg m^{-2} d^{-1} for 5 days. The results may have been different if the dose employed by Royal Marsden Hospital (120 mg m^{-2} d^{-1} for 3 days) had been used (Peckham *et al.*, 1983).

Careful analysis of previous trials with PVB at Indiana University and the SECSG suggested that disease volume and extent were powerful predictors of outcome with chemotherapy. Birch *et al.* (1986), carefully analyzed these clinical features employed in the Indiana University classification system. This system is given in Table 7.3 (Section 7.3). The system was able to discriminate between a group of patients with minimal or moderate extent metastatic disease (98 and 92%, respectively, obtaining disease-free status) and those patients with advanced disease that had a relatively poor outcome with conventional chemotherapy (59% obtaining disease-free status). This classification schema was applied prospectively to a study of PVB versus BEP and found to be an excellent predictor of outcome. Among these three clinically defined prognostic groups in the Indiana classification system, 95, 81 and 50% of patients in the minimal, moderate and advanced disease categories, respectively, obtained long-term survival. It is interesting that 14 of the 37 patients (38%) with advanced disease who received PVB obtained disease-free status, whereas 22 of the 35 patients (63%) receiving BEP obtained disease-free status ($p = 0.06$). This finding of superior outcome in advanced disease supports the use of BEP as first line therapy in disseminated germ cell cancer.

The definition of prognostic factors for favorable outcome in disseminated germ cell tumors and the validation of these factors in a large clinical trial has allowed the development of therapeutic approaches with diverse goals. In a group of patients with a predicted cure rate of 50% or less, the therapeutic goal has not been achieved and subsequent advances will be in the addition of new agents and intensification of therapy. In a group of favorable patients with an 85–100% chance of cure, the therapeutic goal has been achieved and a reasonable focus for investigation seems to be in diminution of toxicity.

19.9 TREATMENT OF PATIENTS WITH 'GOOD RISK' DISSEMINATED DISEASE

Although there is debate regarding the relative importance of a number of potential prognostic factors, in general those patients with either serum marker elevation only, small volume infra- or supradiaphragmatic involvement (or both) without visceral involvement are highly curable and are categorized as good risk. This group of patients constitutes approximately 70% of patients presenting with disseminated disease.

Stratification by selected prognostic factors in a series of randomized clinical trials has confirmed their predictive value. In the mid 1980s, several clinical trials were designed specifically for this group of patients. Because virtually all of these patients achieve complete remission with standard chemotherapy, these trials addressed the possibility of reducing the amount of chemotherapy administered (thus decreasing acute and chronic toxicity) while maintaining the excellent cure rate. Several approaches to this reduction in therapy have been employed, including a shortening of the duration of therapy, use of chemotherapeutic agents with less single agent toxicity, and a reduction in the number of agents used.

The SECSG performed a trial in which patients with good risk disease were randomized to receive either four courses of cisplatin + VP-16 + bleomycin (then considered standard therapy) or three courses of the same three agents (Einhorn *et al.*, 1989). There was no difference in the percentage of patients achieving complete remission with either three (98%) or four (97%) courses of therapy, and 92% of patients on both arms were disease free with a median follow-up of 19 months. Based on the results of this study, three courses of BEP have become the standard therapy for patients with minimal and moderate disease at Indiana University.

Several trials attempted to reduce the toxicity of therapy further for small volume metastatic disease. The Eastern Cooperative Oncology Group has completed a trial randomizing patients with minimal or moderate disease to receive three courses of either BEP or cisplatin + VP-16 alone in an attempt to eliminate the inconvenience (and possible pulmonary toxicity) of weekly bleomycin (Loehrer *et al.*, 1991). A trial at Memorial Hospital randomized good risk patients to receive VP-16 combined with either cisplatin for four cycles (standard arm) or the platinum analogue carboplatin (Bajorin *et al.*, 1993). The advantages of carboplatin in this setting are its relative lack of nephrotoxicity and neurotoxicity, and the ability to administer this compound as an outpatient without aggressive prehydration. However, analysis of both of these trials and similar trials around the world attempting to reduce toxicity further by the elimination of bleomycin or the substitution of carboplatin for cisplatin has shown therapeutic inferiority for the experimental arm, with an increased number of patients relapsing from complete remissions. Accordingly, we believe the standard therapy for good risk germ cell tumor remains three cycles of BEP.

The current standard of therapy in this patient population has minimal acute and probably even less long-term toxicity, based on results with more aggressive therapy. Further reductions in the amount of therapy given are therefore unlikely to reduce toxicity significantly, but certainly have the potential to reduce the cure rate in this stage of disease.

19.10   TREATMENT OF PATIENTS WITH 'POOR RISK' DISSEMINATED DISEASE

Since the mid 1980s, the focus of clinical investigation in patients with poor risk features has been to improve the cure rate by intensifying therapy or adding new agents.

Rigid testing of the impact of high dose cisplatin therapy in disseminated germ cell cancer was accomplished in the successor trial of the SEGSG in advanced germ cell cancer (Nichols *et al.*, 1991). This trial enrolled only patients with advanced disease by the Indiana University classification system. Patients were assigned at random to receive standard doses of etoposide and bleomycin and either standard dose cisplatin (20 mg m^2 daily for 5 days) or high-dose cisplatin (40 mg m^2 daily for 5 days). Between 1984 and 1989, 159 patients with advanced disseminated germ cell cancer were enrolled, 153 were evaluable for toxicity and response. Among 76 patients assigned to high-dose therapy, 52 (68%) became disease free with chemotherapy alone or subsequent surgery. Among 77 patients on the standard dose arm, 56 (73%) became disease free with chemotherapy alone or surgical resection of residual disease. Eleven patients relapsed (three on high dose and eight on standard dose) from

disease free status. Overall, 74% of patients receiving the high-dose cisplatin are alive and 63% are continuously free of disease compared with 74% alive and 61% continuously free of disease on the standard-dose arm. In addition, the high dose arm was associated with significantly more ototoxicity, neurotoxicity, gastrointestinal toxicity and myelosuppression. This large randomized trial found no therapeutic benefit to dose escalation of cisplatin beyond standard doses.

In follow-up to the SEG trial of cisplatin dose intensity, the Eastern Cooperative Oncology Group conducted a trial testing the substitution of ifosfamide for bleomycin (Loehrer *et al.*, 1993). From 1987 to 1992, 304 patients with advanced stage disseminated germ cell cancer by the Indiana Classification system were entered on this trial which randomized patients to either four standard courses of BEP or to four courses of VIP with etoposide (75 mg m^{-2} d^{-1} × 5), ifosfamide (1.2 g m^{-2} d^{-1} × 5) and cisplatin (20 mg m^{-2} d^{-1} × 5). In the preliminary analysis, 278 patients were fully evaluable for survival and toxicity. Of 128 patients randomized to VIP, 69 (54%) became disease free compared with 61 of 125 (49%) patients randomized to BEP (P = NS). Sixty-two patients (48%) on VIP and 52 patients (42%) on BEP are continuously free of disease (p = NS). Grade-IV or greater toxicity, primarily hematological, was significantly greater on the VIP arm (p = 0.0001). There were five therapy-related deaths on each arm. This preliminary analysis failed to demonstrate benefit for the experimental arm, VIP, relative to standard therapy with BEP as treatment for poor risk germ cell tumor.

19.10.1   CURRENT STUDIES

Other ongoing trials in poor risk patients have incorporated high dose cisplatin therapy along with newer agents or high dose therapy with bone marrow transplantation. While preliminary results are encouraging, randomized comparisons of these new therapies to standard dose cisplatin-based therapy are needed to evaluate the role of these innovative approaches.

Several groups are investigating the addition of other active agents to the traditional three-drug regimen or modest dose escalation with the addition of growth factors or stem cells. At Indiana University, a pilot trial of the five-drug regimen VIP/VB (standard dose VIP plus vinblastine 0.18 mg kg^{-1} day 1 and bleomycin 30 units weekly plus G-CSF) (Blanke *et al.*, 1994). In this Phase II trial, 20 patients were entered. Toxicity was significant, but manageable. There was only one therapy-related death in a patient who died of bleomycin lung disease during postchemotherapy surgery. Twelve of the 18 patients evaluable for response obtained a complete remission and two additional patients obtained a marker negative partial remission with residual, but minimal radiogaphic abnormalities (4+, 10+ months). With minimum follow-up of 3 months, ten patients remain progression free.

The EORTC/MRC trial for poor risk germ cell cancer is comparing bleomycin, oncovin and cisplatin and etoposide, ifosfamide and cisplatin (BOP/VIP) with standard therapy with BEP. The French trial for poor risk disease compares BEP with the M.D. Anderson regimen of CISCA/VB. Accrual to both of these important trials is recently completed and analysis is pending.

Investigators in Hanover and other institutions in Germany have attempted to intensify therapy for poor risk patients by incorporating growth factors and peripheral blood progenitor cell support to give high-dose, repetitive chemotherapy cycles. In the most recent update of this Phase I/II trial, patients with poor risk disseminated germ cell tumors were given repetitive cycles of cisplatin 25–30 mg m^{-2} days 1–5, etoposide 100–250 mg m^{-2} days 1–5 and ifosfamide 2 g m^{-2} days 1–5 Q22 days for four cycles. At the highest dose levels, support with growth factors and peripheral

blood progenitor cells were required. With these supportive care techniques, this high-dose therapy was tolerated with no dose-limiting myelosuppression, mucositis, renal toxicity or neurotoxicity. Three of the 32 patients at the highest dose levels have died related to therapy. Of the 23 evaluable for response, 20 (83%) have obtained disease-free status and three patients have relapsed. Accrual to this important exploratory trial is ongoing.

Investigators at M.D. Anderson have incorporated some of the principles of alternating therapy and have attempted to intensify therapy by shortening the interval between cycles of individually effective therapies (Amato, Hutchinson and Striegel, 1994). In a small pilot trial, poor risk patients received rapidly alternating cycles of BOP (7 days' delay), CISCA (14 days), POMB (10 days), ACE (14 days). In 17 patients, remission was achieved after an average of 3.5 cycles. Of 11 patients evaluable for response, eight achieved a disease-free status (73%). Toxicity was substantial, with significant requirements for red blood cell and platelet transfusions. There were no therapy-related deaths. Accrual is continuing.

This series of Phase II trials suggests that more intensive, nonmyeloablative chemotherapy can be given safely. Therapeutic results are not obviously better than less-intense, standard therapy. The impact of such approaches will require randomized comparisons with standard treatment.

19.10.2   HIGH-DOSE CHEMOTHERAPY AS PRIMARY TREATMENT OF POOR RISK DISEASE

The randomized trial from the Institut Gustave Roussey has been reported wherein poor risk patients were randomized to receive conventional therapy with cisplatin, vinblastine, etoposide and bleomycin versus similar therapy followed by a single high dose cycle of cisplatin, etoposide and cyclophosphamide

(Droz *et al.*, 1992). Patients were randomized to receive either the double dose cisplatin, vinblastine, bleomycin and etoposide regimen described by Ozols and colleagues (1988) or a modified regimen with etoposide 100 mg m^{-2} days 1–5, vinblastine 0.2 mg kg^{-1} on day 1, cisplatin 40 mg m^{-2} days 1–5 and bleomycin 20 units continuous infusion on days 1–5 followed by bolus injections on days 8, 15 and 22 of each cycle. Two such cycles were given followed by high dose consolidation with cisplatin 40 mg m^{-2} on days 1–5, etoposide 350 mg m^{-2} on days 1–5 and cyclophosphamide 1.6 g m^{-2} on days 1–4 with autologous bone marrow support.

Between 1988 and 1991, 115 patients who were poor risk by the Institut Gustave Roussey prognostic model were enrolled. One patient was incorrectly determined to have poor risk features and was ineligible. Fifty-seven patients were randomized to each arm. In the conventional arm, six patients failed to complete treatment owing to progressive disease (4), refusal (1) and toxic death (1). In the high-dose arm, 16 patients did not complete treatment due to early death prior to transplant (6), refusal (3), toxic death (2) poor performance status (1) and HIV infection (1). In long-term follow-up, 40 out of 57 (70%) of patients are progression free on the standard therapy arm compared with 33/57 (58%) on the high dose arm.

This trial failed to demonstrate any advantage for the high dose arm. As with many emerging new treatments, however, the high dose arm of this trial would be considered substandard by modern criteria and different prognostic factors have emerged as important predictors of outcome. Accordingly, there is currently a large scale trial being conducted in very poor risk patients that will compare standard therapy (BEP) with brief conventional therapy followed by two cycles of very high dose carboplatin, etoposide and cyclophosphamide. This trial is being conducted jointly by Memorial Sloan-Kettering, the Southwest Oncology Group, and the Eastern Cooperative Oncology Group. It is hoped that this trial will answer definitively the role of high dose chemotherapy as primary therapy of poor risk disease. This trial concept is based on the preliminary experience of high-dose chemotherapy as primary treatment from Memorial Sloan-Kettering where patients with poor predicted CR rates (<0.5) by the MSKCC classification system were treated with VAB-6 and, for those patients exhibiting marker decline consistent with a prolonged half-life (>7 days' AFP, >3 days' HCG), high dose chemotherapy with carboplatin, etoposide and cyclophosphamide was added (Motzer, Mazumdar and Gulati, 1993). Twenty-eight patients were entered and 22 patients proceeded to two cycles of high dose carboplatin, etoposide and cyclophosphamide plus autologous bone marrow transplant (ABMT). Overall 12 of the 22 patients (55%) receiving high dose therapy and 15 of 27 (56%) achieved a disease-free status; two via resection of residual carcinoma. Eleven patients remain continuously free of disease with a median follow-up of 31 months.

19.11 LATE EFFECTS OF TREATMENT

Case reports and clinical alerts have suggested treatment with high dose etoposide can result in the development of a unique secondary leukemia (Pedersen-Bjergaard *et al.*, 1991). To estimate the risk for developing leukemia in the more common clinical setting of patients receiving conventional doses of etoposide along with cisplatin and bleomycin, we reviewed records of patients with germ cell cancer entering clinical protocols using etoposide at Indiana University (Nichols *et al.*, 1993). Between 1982 and 1991, 538 patients entered serial clinical trials with planned etoposide doses from 1500 mg m^2 to 2000 mg m^2 in combination with cisplatin plus either ifosfamide or bleomycin; 348 patients received an etoposide combination as initial chemotherapy and 190 patients received etoposide as part of salvage treatment. Currently 315 patients are alive and 337 patients have follow-up beyond 2 years. The median follow-up for patients still alive is 4.9 years. Two patients (0.37%) developed leukemia. One patient developed acute undifferentiated leukemia with a $t(4:11)(q21:q23)$ cytogenetic abnormality 2.3 years after starting etoposide-based therapy and one patient developed acute myelomonoblastic leukemia with normal chromosome studies 2.0 years after beginning chemotherapy. During this period, a number of patients were seen who did not enter clinical trials and we are aware of several hematological abnormalities seen in this group, including one patient with acute monoblastic leukemia with a $t(11:19)$ $(q13:p13)$ abnormality. Secondary leukemia after treatment with chemotherapy containing conventional dose etoposide does occur. However, this low incidence of secondary leukemia does not alter the risk:benefit ratio of etoposide-based chemotherapy in germ cell cancer.

Additional concern regarding the toxicity of treatment has been raised with respect to cardiovascular toxicity of combination chemotherapy for germ cell tumors. Several anecdotal reports of major cardiovascular events in young men receiving chemotherapy for testis cancer suggested a causal association between chemotherapy treatments and these events (Vogelzang, Frenning and Kennedy, 1980; Doll *et al.*, 1986; Cantwell *et al.*, 1988). To evaluate the true risk of acute vascular events in patients receiving cisplatin-based chemotherapy for testicular cancer, questionnaires to assess cardiovascular toxicity were distributed to all participants in the Testicular Cancer Intergroup Study and toxicity reviews from the chemotherapy flow sheets were conducted (Nichols *et al.*, 1990).

Patients with pathological Stage I testicular cancer were registered to the study and observed after retroperitoneal lymphadenectomy. Patients with pathological Stage II disease were randomized to receive two postoperative courses of adjuvant cisplatin-based

chemotherapy or observation. Any patient who recurred after observation or adjuvant therapy was given four cycles of cisplatin-based chemotherapy.

Review of toxicity of treatment for those patients receiving adjuvant chemotherapy ($n = 97$) or chemotherapy for recurrent disease ($n = 83$) revealed no cases of acute cardiovascular toxicity. When the median follow-up after study enrollment was 5.1 years, 459 questionnaires were mailed and 270 were returned. Percentage return was equal among the observed, adjuvant and recurrent groups (59%, 54%, 64%). There was a significant increase in the incidence of extremity paresthesias in the two groups receiving chemotherapy. Fatal myocardial infarction was reported in two patients in the observation group and one nonfatal infarct was reported in the adjuvant treatment group. No patient in any group reported stroke. Three patients in the observation group and one patient in the recurrent group experienced a thromboembolic event. Despite sporadic case reports suggesting a causal association between chemotherapy for testicular cancer and acute vascular events, this retrospective analysis provides no evidence of an increased risk for subsequent cardiovascular disease in this patient population.

19.12 STANDARD MANAGEMENT OF GERM CELL TUMORS AT INDIANA UNIVERSITY

In this rare subset of an uncommon illness for which significant therapeutic questions remain, all such patients should be referred for participation in clinical trials. Off protocol or in those patients too ill to travel, standard management should include prompt initiation of combination chemotherapy with standard BEP for a planned three cycles of treatment for patients with good risk features and four courses for those with more advanced disease. In some cases, serologic confirmation of suspected germ cell tumor is sufficient to initiate therapy for patients *in extremis* from massive tumor dissemination. Patients presenting with brain metastases should have modern, curative-intent radiotherapy administered along with chemotherapy.

Patients should receive chemotherapy on schedule with as few delays as possible. Concerns regarding myelosuppression at the scheduled time of the next cycle (day 22) are often overblown. Despite low white blood cell counts, almost all of these young healthy patients have evidence of incipient hematological recovery. Therapy should be initiated in these patients and only if no recovery is seen over the course of the 5-day treatment is the last day of etoposide held.

Patients should have tumor markers obtained with each cycle of therapy and compared with previous values. If markers are not falling consistently with the half-life (HCG = 18 hours and AFP = 5 days), considerations should be made for alternative salvage treatments. In this situation, one must, however, consider the possibility of occult disease at a sanctuary site (CNS and testis) and rule out involvement of these areas prior to labeling the program as a failure.

Depending on the stage at diagnosis, 20–50% of patients who undergo induction chemotherapy for disseminated germ cell tumor have significant residual radiographic abnormalities. It is common practice for patients facing extensive postchemotherapy resection to discontinue bleomycin after the tenth dose and not receive the eleventh and twelfth week of bleomycin. In this subset of patients, postchemotherapy resection of residual disease is often performed to remove residual teratoma or viable cancer. Several points bear emphasis in this setting. Firstly, consideration of postchemotherapy surgery should be made only if the serum AFP and HCG have normalized. Patients with persistantly elevated serum markers should be considered for salvage chemotherapy rather than surgical 'debulking'. Secondly, post-chemotherapy resection of residual abnor-malities is rarely urgent and sufficient time should be taken to allow the patient to recover from the effects of induction chemotherapy. Typically, patients are taken to surgery 6 weeks after the last course of chemotherapy. Thirdly, repeat imaging of the areas of abnormality should be performed prior to surgery. In some patients, continued involution of residual masses occurs after the completion of therapy and surgical resection is not necessary.

Patients with persistant retroperitoneal disease undergo resection using either a midline or thoracoabdominal approach. Resection of residual radiogaphic abnormalities after induction chemotherapy for disseminated non-seminomatous germ cell cancer has a surprisingly low rate of significant complications. The most common intraoperative complication is injury to the renal vessels, which can be repaired at the time of surgery in most cases. Significant postoperative complications include wound infections, ileus, prolonged atelectasis or pneumonia. Development of lymphoceles can occur and can be mistaken for recurrent disease on abdominal CT scan. Overall, significant morbidity is rare and operative mortality almost non-existant. However, the majority of patients undergoing bilateral radical retroperitoneal lymphadenectomy will be rendered infertile as a result of retrograde ejaculation. Recent developments in urological surgery have allowed for preservation of the sympathetic fibers that control ejaculation while maintaining the therapeutic template of the cancer surgery. Depending on the extent of residual disease, many patients can retain ejaculatory function after undergoing resection of residual disease after chemotherapy.

Patients with unilateral disease in the pulmonary parenchyma or mediastinum can have resection of this supradiaphragmatic disease through a thoracotomy incision. Patients with combined thoracic and abdominal disease frequently require a median sternotomy as well as a midline abdominal approach. Patients who have received bleomycin as part of induction chemotherapy require specialized management. These patients may have subtle restrictive pulmonary disease and diminished carbon monoxide diffusion capacity. Care should be taken during anesthesia to avoid overhydration and to use colloid fluid replacement rather than crystalloid. Of most importance, inspired O_2 concentration should not exceed 25% in either the intraoperative period or post-operative recovery.

The histopathological findings in postchemotherapy surgical specimens help define the need for further treatment. In earlier reports, about 40% of cases revealed teratoma, 40% had fibrous necrotic debris and 20% had residual viable germ cell cancer. Analysis of recent series suggests that the incidence of persistent cancer is decreasing. In the recent study of optimal duration of chemotherapy in minimal extent disseminated germ cell cancer, 14 of 107 patients were found to have residual teratoma in the post chemotherapy specimen and no patient was found to have viable carcinoma (Einhorn et al., 1989). In the same study, 19 of 77 patients with moderate volume disease were found to have teratoma while only six had residual cancer. In the recent study of 153 advanced disease patients, 30 patients were found to have residual teratoma and only six had persistent germ cell cancer (Nichols et al., 1991). This apparent decrease in the incidence of residual cancer has been reported by others and is, in part, due to better selection of patients for surgery and improvements in primary chemotherapy.

Those patients with persistent cancer identified and totally removed at postchemotherapy surgery require special management. If the surgical margins are free of tumor, all sites of known disease are removed and the serum tumor markers remain normal, patients should receive two post-operative cycles of cisplatin-based therapy similar to induction therapy. Those patients with unresectable disease, positive surgical margins or elevated

tumor markers should be considered for full salvage therapy using new agents and more prolonged courses of therapy. About two-thirds of patients receiving additional postoperative cisplatin-based chemotherapy after total resection of residual viable cancer will remain free of disease (Fox et al., 1993).

19.13   CONCLUSIONS

Although there is debate regarding the relative importance of a number of potential prognostic factors, in general those patients with either serum marker elevation only, small volume infra- or supradiaphragmatic involvement (or both) without visceral involvement are highly curable and are categorized as good risk. This group of patients constitutes approximately 70% of patients presenting with disseminated disease. The current standard of therapy in this patient population has minimal acute and probably even less long-term toxicity, based on results with more aggressive therapy. Further reductions in the amount of therapy given are therefore unlikely to significantly reduce toxicity, but certainly have the potential to reduce the cure rate in this stage of disease.

Depending on what system of classification is used, only about one-half of all patients with poor risk disseminated germ cell tumors survive their illness. Standard therapy in this setting is four timely cycles of cisplatin, etoposide and bleomycin coupled, when necessary, with aggressive and complete resection of residual radiographic abnormalities. The foci of clinical investigations in this area are twofold. First is the exploration of more intensive scheduling or dosing of existing active agents and the recently begun randomized intergroup trial of BEP compared with abbreviated BEP plus high dose carboplatin, etoposide, and cyclophosphamide will serve to validate or refute the role of very high dose chemotherapy in the management of patients with very poor risk germ cell cancer. Second, ongoing efforts to define new agents with activity in this disease are critical to developing alternative regimens. Perhaps most important will be enhanced biological understanding of these unique malignancies, which will serve to discriminate between clinically identical, but biologically diverse, presentations as well as yield new targets for rationally designed therapeutics.

REFERENCES

Allaire, F.J., Thieme, E.T. and Korst, D.R. (1961) Cancer chemotherapy with 5-fluorouracil alone and in combination with X-ray therapy. *Can. Chemother. Rep.*, **14**, 59–75.

Amato, R., Hutchinson, L. and Striegel, A. (1994) Modulation of dose intensity (DI) by reducing chemotherapy (CHT) intervals in patients (pts) with high volume non-seminomatous germ cell tumors (HV-GCT). *Proc. Am. Soc. Clin. Oncol.*, **13**, 253.

Ansfield, F.J. (1969) Clinical studies with mithramycin. *Oncology*, **23** 283–8.

Ansfield, F.J., Korbitz, B.C., Davis, H.L. and Ramirez, G. (1969) Triple drug therapy in testicular tumors. *Cancer*, **24**, 442–6.

Astrakhan, V. and Monul, F. (1976) Combined chemotherapy of testicular tumors resistant to sarcolysin. *Vopr. Onkol.*, **13**, 87–90.

Bajorin, D., Sarosdy, M., Pfister, D. *et al.* (1993) A randomized trial of etoposide + cisplatin *vs.* etoposide and carboplatin in patients with good-risk germ cell tumors: A multiinstitutional study. *J. Clin. Oncol.*, **11**, 598–606.

Barranco, S.C. and Humphrey, R.M. (1971) The effects of bleomycin on survival and cell progression in Chinese hamster cells *in vitro*. *Can. Res.*, **31**, 1218–23.

Birch, R., Williams, S., Cone, A. *et al.* (1986) Prognostic factors for favorable outcome in disseminated germ cell tumors. *J. Clin. Oncol.*, **4**, 400–7.

Blanke, C., Loehrer, P., Einhorn, L. and Nichols, C. (1994) A phase II trial of VP-16 plus ifosfamide plus cisplatin plus vinblastine plus bleomycin (VIP/VB) with filgrastim for advanced stage testicular cancer. *Proc. Am. Soc. Clin. Oncol.*, **13**, 234.

Blokhin, N., Larinov, L., Perevodchikova, N. *et al.* (1958) Clinical experiences with sarcolysin in neoplastic diseases. *Ann. N.Y. Acad. Sci.*, **68**, 1128–32.

Blum, R.H., Carter, S.K. and Agre, K. (1973) A clinical review of bleomycin – a new antineoplastic agent. *Cancer*, **31**, 903–14.

Bonadonna, G., De Lena, M., Monfardini, S. *et al.* (1972) Clinical trials with bleomycin in lymphomas and in solid tumors. *Eur. J. Can.*, **8**, 205–15.

Bosl, G.J. *et al.* (1980) Vinblastine, bleomycin and *cis*diammine-dichloroplatinum in the treatment of advanced testicular carcinoma: Possible importance of larger induction and shorter maintenance schedules. *Am. J. Med.*, **68**, 492–6.

Boutis, L.L., Stergion-Travantzis, J. and Mourantidou, D. (1982) Ifosfamide chemotherapy of disseminated non-seminomatous testicular tumors, in *Proceedings of the Thirteenth International Cancer Congress, Seattle*, (Abstract 1017).

Brown, J.H. and Kennedy, B.J. (1965) Mithramycin in the treatment of disseminated testicular neoplasms. *N. Engl. J. Med.*, **272**, 111–8.

Bruhl, P., Gunther, U., Hoefer-Janker, H. *et al.* (1976) Results obtained with fractionated ifosfamide massive-dose treatment in generalized malignant tumours. *Int. J. Clin. Pharmacol. Ther. Toxicol*, **14**, 29–39.

Cantwell, B., Mannix, K., Roberts, J., Ghani, S. and Harris, A. (1988) Thromboembolic events during combination chemotherapy for germ cell malignancy. *Lancet* ii, 1086–7.

Cavalli, F., Klepp, O., Renard, J. *et al.* (1981) A phase II study of oral VP16–213 in nonseminomatous testicular cancer. *Eur. J. Cancer*, **17**, 245–9.

Cavalli, F., Sonntag, R.W. and Brunner, K.W. (1977) Epipodophyllotoxin derivative (VP16–213) in treatment of solid tumors. *Lancet*, ii, 362.

Cheng, E., Cvitkovic, E., Wittes, R.E. and Golbey, R.B. (1978) Germ cell tumors (II): VAB II in metastatic testicular cancer. *Cancer*, **42**, 2162–8.

Clavel, M., Monfardini, S., Siegenthalen, P. *et al.* (1986) Phase II trial of CHIP in previously treated disseminated testicular cancer. *Proc. Am. Soc. Clin. Oncol.*, **5**, 108.

Clinical Screening Co-operative Group of the EORTC (1970) Study of the clinical efficiency of bleomycin in human cancer. *BMJ*, **2**, 643–5.

Costa, G., Hreshchyshyn, M.M. and Holland, J.F. (1962) Initial clinical studies with vincristine. *Cancer Chemother. Rep.*, **24**, 39–44.

Curreri, A.R. and Ansfield, F.J. (1960) Mithramycin–human toxicology and preliminary therapeutic investigation. *Cancer Chemother. Rep.*, **8**, 18–22.

Doll, D., List, A., Greco, F., Hainsworth, J.,

Hande, K. and Johnson, D. (1986) Acute vascular ischemic events after cisplatin-based combination chemotherapy for germ-cell tumors of the testis. *Ann. Intern. Med.*, **105**, 48–51.

Drasga, R.E., Williams, S.D., Einhorn, L.H. and Birch, R. (1987) Phase II evaluation of iproplatin in refractory germ cell tumors: a Southeastern Cancer Study Group trial. *Cancer Treat. Rep.*, **71**, 863–4.

Drewinko, B., Novak, J. and Barranco, S.C. (1972) The response of human lymphoma cells *in vitro* to bleomycin and 1,3-*cis*-(chloroethyl)-nitrosourea. *Cancer Res.*, **32**, 1206–8.

Drobnik, J. (1983) Antitumor activity of platinum complexes. *Cancer Chemother. Pharmacol.*, **10**, 145–9.

Droz, J., Pico, J., Biron, P. *et al.* (1992) No evidence of a benefit of early intensified chemotherapy (HDCT) with autologous bone marrow transplantation (ABMT) in first line treatment of poor risk non seminomatous germ cell tumors. *Proc. Am. Soc. Clin. Oncol.*, **11**, 197.

Einhorn, L.H. and Donohue, J.D. (1977) Cis-diamminedichloroplatinum, vinblastine, and bleomycin combination chemotherapy in disseminated testicular cancer. *Ann. Intern. Med.*, **87**, 293–8.

Einhorn, L.H. and Williams, S.D. (1980) Chemotherapy of disseminated testicular cancer. A random prospective study. *Cancer*, **46**, 1337–44.

Einhorn, L.H., Williams, S.D., Loehrer, P.J. *et al.* (1989) Evaluation of optimal duration of chemotherapy in favorable-prognosis disseminated germ cell tumors: A Southeastern Cancer Study Group protocol. *J. Clin. Oncol.*, **7**(3), 387–91.

Einhorn, L.H., Williams, S.D., Troner, M. *et al.* (1981) Role of maintenance therapy in disseminated testicular cancer. A Southeastern Cancer Study Group evaluation. *N. Engl. J. Med.*, **305**, 727–31.

Fitzharris, B.M., Kaye, S.B., Saverymuttu, S. *et al.* (1980) VP16–213 as a single agent in advanced testicular tumors. *Eur. J. Can.*, **16**, 1193–7.

Fox, E., Weathers, T., Williams, S. *et al.* (1993) Outcome analysis for patients with persistent germ cell carcinoma in post chemotherapy retroperitoneal lymph node dissections. *J. Clin. Oncol.*, **11**, 1294–9.

Friedgood, C.E., Danza, A.L. and Boccabella, A. (1952) The effects of nitrofurans on the normal testis and on testicular tumors (seminoma). *Can. Res.*, **12**, 262–4.

Garnick, M.B. *et al.* (1979) Sequential combination chemotherapy and surgery for disseminated testicular cancer: Cis-diamminedichloroplatinum (II), vinblastine, and bleomycin remission induction followed by cyclophosphamide and Adriamycin. *Cancer Treat. Rep.*, **63**, 1681–6.

Ginsberg, S.J. *et al.* (1977) Vinblastine and inappropriate ADH secretion. *N. Engl. J. Med.*, **296**, 941.

Higby, D.J., Wallace H.J., Albert, D.J. and Holland, J.F. (1974) Diamminedichloroplatinum: a phase I study showing responses in testicular and other tumors. *Cancer*, **33**, 1219–25.

Higby, D.J., Wallace, H.J. and Holland, J.F. (1973) Cis-diamminedichloroplatinum (NSC-119875): a phase I study. *Cancer Chemother. Rep.*, **57**, 459–63.

Hyman, G.A., Ultmann, J.E. and Habif, D.V. (1962) Factors to be considered in the clinical evaluation of a new chemotherapeutic agent (5-fluorouracil). *Cancer Chemother. Rep.*, **16**, 397–9.

Jacobs, E.M. (1970) Combination chemotherapy of metastatic testicular germinal cell tumors and soft part sarcomas. *Cancer*, **25**, 324–32.

Jacobs, E.M., Johnson, F.D. and Wood, D.A. (1966) Stage III metastatic malignant testicular tumors: treatment with intermittent and combined chemotherapy. *Cancer*, **19**, 1697–704.

de Jager, R., Siegenthaler, P., Dombernowsky, P. *et al.* (1981) Phase II study of 4'-(9-acridinylamino)-methane sulfon-M-anisidide (*m*-AMSA, NSC 249992). *Proc. Am. Soc. Clin. Oncol.*, **22**, 367.

Kennedy, B.J. (1970) Mithramycin therapy in advanced testicular neoplasms. *Cancer*, **26**, 755–766.

Kennedy, B.J., Griffen, W.O. and Lober, P. (1965) Specific effect of mithramycin on embryonal carcinoma of the testis. *Cancer*, **18**, 1631–6.

Kofman, S. and Eisenstein, R. (1963) Mithramycin in the treatment of disseminated cancer. *Cancer Chemother. Rep.*, **32**, 77–96.

Kofman, S., Medrek, T.J. and Alexander, R.W. (1964) Mithramycin in the treatment of embryonal cancer. *Cancer*, **17**, 938–48.

Koons, C.R., Sensenbrenner, L.L. and Owens, A.H. (1966) Clinical studies of mithramycin in patients with embryonal cancer. *Bull. Hopkins, Hosp.*, **118**, 462–75.

Krikorian, J.G. *et al.* (1978) Variables for predicting serious toxicity (vinblastine dose, performance status, and prior therapeutic experience): Chemotherapy for metastatic testicular cancer with cis-dichlorodiammine platinum (II), vinblastine, and bleomycin. *Cancer Treat. Rep.*, **62**, 1455–63.

Li, M.C., Hertz, R. and Bergenstal, D.M. (1958) Therapy of choriocarcinoma and related trophoblastic tumors with folic acid and purine antagonists. *N. Engl. J. Med.*, **259**, 66–74.

Li, M.C., Whitmore, W.F., Golbey, R. and Grabstald, H. (1960) Effects of combined drug therapy on metastatic cancer of the testis. *JAMA*, **174**, 1291–9.

Loehrer, P., Einhorn, L., Elson, P. *et al.* (1993) Phase III study of cisplatin (p) plus etoposide (VP-16) with either bleomycin (B) or ifosfamide (I) in advanced stage germ cell tumors (GCT): An intergroup trial. *Proc. Am. Soc. Clin. Oncol.*, **12**, 261.

Loehrer, P.J., Elson, P., Johnson, D.H., Williams, S.D., Trump, D.L. and Einhorn, L.H. (1991) A randomized trial of cisplatin plus etoposide with or without bleomycin in favorable prognosis disseminated germ cell tumors. *Proc. Am. Soc. Clin. Oncol.*, **10**, 169.

MacKensie, A.R. (1966) Chemotherapy of metastatic testis cancer: results in 154 patients. *Cancer*, **19**, 1369–76.

Mendelson, D. and Serpick, A.A. (1970) Combination chemotherapy of testicular tumors. *J. Urol.*, **103**, 619–23.

Moore, C.A. (1968) Triple chemotherapy in the treatment of metastatic testicular neoplasms. *J. Urol.*, **100**, 527–9.

Motzer, R.J., Bosl, G.J., Tauer, K. and Golbey, R. (1987) Phase II trial of carboplatin in patients with advanced germ cell tumors refractory to cisplatin. *Cancer Treat. Rep.*, **71**, 197–8.

Motzer, R., Mazumdar, M. and Gulati, S. (1993) Phase II trial of high dose carboplatin and etoposide with autologous bone marrow transplantation in first line therapy for patients with poor-risk germ cell tumors. *J. Natl. Cancer Inst.*, **85**, 1828–35.

Newlands, E.S. and Bagshawe, K.D. (1977) Epipodophyllotoxin derivative (VP16–213) in malignant teratomas and choriocarcinomas. *Lancet*, **ii**, 87.

Nichols, C., Breeden, E., Loehrer, P., Williams, S. and Einhorn, L. (1993) Secondary leukemia associated with a conventional dose of etoposide: Review of serial germ cell tumor trials. *J. Natl. Cancer Inst.*, **85**, 36–40.

Nichols, C., Roth, B., Williams, S. *et al.* (1990) Cardiovascular complications of chemotherapy for testicular cancer. *Proc. Am. Soc. Clin. Oncol.*, **9**, 132.

Nichols, C., Williams, S., Loehrer, P. *et al.* (1991) Randomized study of cisplatin dose intensity in advanced germ cell tumors: A Southeastern Cancer Study Group and Southwest Oncology Group protocol. *J. Clin. Oncol.*, **9**, 1163–72.

Niederle, N., Scheulen, M.E., Cremer, M. *et al.* (1983) Ifosfamide in combination chemotherapy for sarcomas and testicular carcinomas. *Cancer Treat. Rev.*, **10** (Suppl. A), 129–35.

O'Dwyer, P.J. *et al* (1985) Etoposide (VP-16–213): Current status of an active anticancer drug. *N. Engl. J. Med.*, **312**, 692–700.

Ozols, R.F., Ihde, D.C., Linehan, W.M. *et al.* (1988) A randomized comparison of standard chemotherapy versus a high-dose chemotherapy regimen in the treatment of poor prognosis non-seminomatous germ cell tumors. *J. Clin. Oncol.*, **6**, 1031–40.

Parker, G.W., Wiltsie, D.S. and Jackson, C.B. (1960) The clinical evaluation of PA-144 (mithramycin) in solid tumors of adults. *Cancer Chemother. Rep.*, **8**, 23–6.

Peckham, M.J., Barrett, A., Liew, K. *et al.* (1983) The treatment of metastatic germ cell testicular tumors with bleomycin, etoposide and cisplatin (BEP). *Br. J. Cancer*, **47**, 613–19.

Pedersen-Bjergaard, J., Hansen, S., Larsen, S., Daugaard, G., Philip, P. and Rørth, M. (1991) Increased risk of myelodysplasia and leukaemia after etoposide, cisplatin and bleomycin for germ cell-tumours. *Lancet*, **338**, 359–63.

Ramsey, E.W. *et al.* (1980) The management of disseminated testicular cancer. *Br. J. Urol.*, **52**, 45–9.

Ream, N.W., Perlia, C.P., Wolter, J. and Taylor, S.G. (1968) Mithramycin therapy in disseminated germinal testicular cancer. *JAMA*, **204**, 96–102.

Reynolds, T.F., Vugrin, D., Cvitkovic, E. *et al.* (1979) Phase II trial of vindesine in patients with germ cell tumors. *Cancer Treat. Rep.*, **63**, 1399–401.

Reynolds, T.F., Vugrin, D., Cvitkovic, E. *et al.* (1981) VAB-3 combination chemotherapy of metastatic testicular cancer. *Cancer*, **48**, 888–98.

Rosenberg, B., Van Camp, L. and Krigas, T. (1965) Inhibition of cell division in *E. coli* by electrolysis products from a platinum electrode. *Nature*, **205**, 698–9.

Rossof, A.H., Slayton, R.E. and Perlia, C.P. (1972) Preliminary clinical experience with *cis*-diamminedichloroplatinum (*II*) (NSC 119875, CACP). *Cancer*, **30**, 1451–6.

Samuels, M.L., Holoye, P.Y. and Johnson, D.E. (1975) Bleomycin combination chemotherapy in the management of testicular neoplasia. *Cancer*, **36**, 318–26.

Samuels, M.L. and Howe, C.D. (1970) Vinblastine in the management of testicular cancer. *Cancer*, **25**, 1009–17.

Samuels, M.L., Johnson, D.E., Brown, B. *et al.* (1979) Velban plus continuous infusion bleomycin (VB–3) in stage III advanced testicular cancer: results in 99 patients with a note on high dose velban and sequential *cis*-platinum, in *Cancer of the Genitourinary Tract* (eds D.E. Johnson and M.L. Samuels), Raven Press, New York, pp. 159–72.

Samuels, M.L., Johnson, D.E. and Holoye, P.Y. (1973) The treatment of stage 3 metastatic germinal cell neoplasia of the testis with bleomycin combination chemotherapy. *Proc. Am. Assoc. Cancer Res.*, **42**, 23.

Samuels, M.L., Johnson, D.E. and Holoye, P.Y. (1975) Continuous intravenous bleomycin (NSC-125066) therapy with vinblastine (NSC-49842) in stage III testicular neoplasia. *Cancer; Chemother. Rep.*, **59** 563–70.

Samuels, M.L., Lanzotti, V.J., Holoye, P.Y., Johnson, D.E. *et al.* (1976) Combination chemotherapy in germinal cell tumors. *Cancer Treat. Rev.*, 3, 185–204.

Samuels, M.L., Lanzotti, V.J., Holoye, P.Y. and Howe, C.D. (1977) Stage III testicular cancer: complete response by substage to velban plus continuous bleomycin infusion (VB-3). *Proc. Am. Assoc. Cancer Res.*, **18**, 146.

Scheulen, M.E., Niederle, N., Bremer, K. *et al.* (1983) Efficacy of ifosfamide in refractory malignant diseases and uroprotection by mesna: results of a clinical phase II study with 151 patients. *Cancer Treat. Rev.*, **10** (Suppl. A), 93–101.

Schmoll, H., Rhomberg, W. and Diehl, V. (1978) Ifosfamide (NSC 109427): Activity in testicular cancer using mono- and combination therapy. *Procedures of the 10th International Congress on Chemotherapy (Zurich)*, **2**, 1089–91.

Schultz, S., Loehrer, P., Williams, S. and Einhorn, L. (1987) A phase II trial of epirubicin in the salvage therapy of germ cell tumors. *Proc. Am. Soc. Clin. Oncol.*, **6**, 99.

Shaw, R.K. and Bruner, J.A. (1964) Clinical evaluation of vincristine (NSC-67574). *Cancer Chemother. Rep.*, **42**, 45–8.

Spigel, S.C. and Coltman, C.A. (1974) Vinblastine (NSC-49842) and bleomycin (NSC-125066) therapy for disseminated testicular tumors. *Cancer Chemother, Rep.*, **58**, 213–16.

Spigel, S.C., Stephens, R.L., Haas, C.D. *et al.* (1978) Chemotherapy of disseminated germinal tumors of the testis – comparison of vinblastine and bleomycin with vincristine, bleomycin, and actinomycin D. *Cancer Treat. Rep.*, **62**, 129–30.

Steinfeld, J.L., Solomon, J. Marsh, A.A. *et al* (1966) Chemical therapy of patients with advanced metastatic germinal tumors. *J. Urol.*, **96**, 933–40.

Stoter, G., Struyvenberg, A. and Vendrik, C.P. (1978) Development of chemotherapy of metastatic testicular teratoma. *Med. Tijdschr. Geneeskd.*, **122**, 1427.

Stoter, G.J., Sleijfer, D.T., Vendrik, C.P. *et al.* (1979) Combination chemotherapy with *cis*-diamminedichloroplatinum, vinblastine, and bleomycin in advanced testicular non seminoma, *Lancet*, **i**, 941–5.

Szczukowski, M.J., Daywitt, A.L. and Elrick, H. (1958) Metastatic testicular tumor treated with nitrofurazone: report of a case *JAMA*, **152**, 1066–8

Trump, D.L., Elson, P., Brodovsky, H. and Vogl, S.E. (1987) Carboplatin in advanced refractory germ cell neoplasms: a phase II Eastern Cooperative Oncology Group study. *Cancer Treat. Rep.*, **71**, 989–90.

Umezawa, H. (1971) Natural and artificial bleomycins: chemistry and antitumor activities. *Pure Appl. Chem.*, **28**, 665–80.

Umezawa, H., Maeda, K., Takeuechi, T. and Okami, Y. (1966b) New antibiotics, bleomycin A and B. *J. Antib. Ser. A..*, **19**, 200–9.

Umezawa, H., Suhara, Y., Takita, T. and Maeda, K. (1966a) Purifications of bleomycins. *J. Antib ser. A..*, **19**, 210–15.

Vogelzang, N., Frenning, D. and Kennedy, B. (1980) Coronary artery disease after treatment with bleomycin and vinblastine. *Cancer Treat. Rep.*, **64**, 1159–60.

Vugrin, D., Cvitkovic, E., Whitmore, W.F. *et al*, (1981) VAB-4 combination chemotherapy in the treatment of metastatic testis tumors. *Cancer*, **47**, 833–9.

Vugrin, D., Herr, H.W., Whitmore, W.F. *et al* (1981) VAB-6 combination chemotherapy in disseminated cancer of the testis. *Ann. Intern. Med.*, **95**, 59–61

Vugrin, D., Whitmore, W.F. and Golbey, R.B. (1983a) VAB-5 combination chemotherapy in prognostically poor risk patients with germ cell tumors. *Cancer*, **51**, 1072–5.

Vugrin, D., Whitmore, W.F. and Golbey, R.B. (1983b) VAB-6 combination chemotherapy in treatment of disseminated cancer of the testis. *Cancer*, **51**, 211–15.

Warwick, O.H., Alison, R.E. and Darte, J.M.M. (1961) Clinical experience with vinblastine sulfate. *Can. Med. Assoc. J.*, **85**, 579–83.

Weissbach, L. and Kochs, R. (1982) Monotherapy with ifosfamide in the treatment of testicular tumours (non-seminomas). *Proceedings of the Thirteenth International Cancer Congress*, Seattle, (Abstract 3596).

Wheeler, B.M., Loehrer, P.J., Williams, S.D. and Einhorn, L.H. (1986) Ifosfamide in refractory male germ cell tumors. *J. Clin. Oncol.*, **4**, 28–34.

Whitelaw, D.M., Cowan, D.H. Cassidy, F.R. and Patterson, T.A. (1963) Clinical experience with vincristine. *Cancer Chemother, Rep.*, **30**, 13–20.

Wildermuth, O. (1955) Testicular cancer: management of metastases with report of a new chemotherapeutic agent, *Radiology*, **65**, 599–603.

Wilkinson, P. *et al.* (1979) Combination chemotherapy for metastatic malignant teratoma of testis. *Lancet*, **i**, 1185.

Williams, S.D., Birch, R., Einhorn, L.H. *et al.* (1987) Treatment of disseminated germ-cell tumors with cisplatin, bleomycin, and either vinblastine or etoposide. *N. Engl. J. Med.*, **316**, 1435–40.

Williams, S.D., Birch, R., Gams, R. and Irwin, L. (1985) Phase II trial of mitoxantrone in refractory germ cell tumors: a trial of the Southeastern Cancer Study Group. *Cancer Treat. Rep.*, **69**, 1455–6.

Williams, S.D., Duncan, P. and Einhorn, L.H. (1983) Phase II study of AMSA in refractory testicular cancer. *Cancer Treat. Rep.*, **67**, 309–10.

Williams, S.D., Einhorn, L.H., Greco, F.A. *et al.* (1980) VP-16-213 salvage therapy for refractory germinal neoplasms. *Cancer*, **46**, 2154–8.

Wilson, W.L. (1960) Chemotherapy of human solid tumors with 5-fluorouracil. *Cancer*, **13**, 1230–9.

Wittes, R.E., Yagoda, A., Silvay, O. *et al.* (1976) Chemotherapy of germ cell tumors of the testis: I. Induction of remissions with vinblastine, actinomycin D, and bleomycin. *Cancer*, **37**. 637–45.

Wyatt, J.K. and McAninch, L.N. (1961) Experiences with antimetabolites in the treatment of genitourinary carcinoma. *Can. Med. Assoc. J.*, **84**, 309–11.

Wyatt, J.K. and McAninch, L.N. (1967) A chemotherapeutic approach to advanced testicular carcinoma. *Can. J. Surg.*, **10**, 421–6.

MANAGEMENT OF METASTATIC GERM CELL TUMORS: TOXICITY REDUCTION AND THE USE OF BLEOMYCIN

G.J. Bosl

20.1 INTRODUCTION

The treatment of metastatic germ cell tumors has been one of the success stories in the management of solid tumors in the last 20 years. The introduction of cisplatin-based chemotherapy in the mid 1970s radically changed the expectations of oncologists toward this and other solid neoplasms (Einhorn and Donohue, 1977; Reynolds *et al.*, 1981). Modifications of these early programs led to the deletion of maintenance chemotherapy (Einhorn *et al.*, 1981; Vugrin, Whitmore and Golbey, 1983), the deletion of doxorubicin (Einhorn, 1981) and the expectation that 70–80% of patients with metastatic disease would be cured. With the recognition that most patients would be cured came the initial detailed studies of prognostic variables to attempt to identify those patients most likely to be rendered free of disease (Bosl *et al.*, 1983). By 1983, etoposide had been established as an essential component of salvage chemotherapy (Williams *et al.*, 1980; Bosl *et al.*, 1985), and clinical trials were designed to incorporate etoposide into first line therapy.

These successes in initial and salvage chemotherapy led to the widespread recognition that there were two groups of previously untreated patients with germ cell tumors:

(1) those who were highly likely to achieve complete remission (CR), and (2) those who were not. The goals of therapy for these two groups are different. For those most likely to achieve CR, treatment programs had to be designed to reduce toxicity. For those who are unlikely to achieve CR, programs had to be designed with efficacy in mind and with toxicity as only a secondary element. Thus the stage was set for good and poor risk studies.

During the evolution of these successful combined modality treatment programs, the toxicity of therapy was being evaluated. The acute toxicities of myelosuppression and bleomycin pneumonitis were widely known, and occasionally patients died as a consequence of such therapy (Williams *et al.*, 1987). In addition to acute bleomycin pneumonitis, about 20% of patients receiving bleomycin also had reduction in the vital capacity and/or diffusion capacity of carbon monoxide as subclinical evidence of bleomycin lung damage (Bosl *et al.*, 1986). In 1981, a high frequency of Raynaud's phenomenon was reported from the University of Minnesota in 37% of patients treated with vinblastine plus bleomycin with or without cisplatin (Vogelzang *et al.*, 1981). This early report was confirmed by the Dana Farber (Cancer Institute in 13% of their patients

Testicular Cancer: Investigation and management. Second edition. Edited by Professor A. Horwich.
Published in 1996 by Chapman & Hall. ISBN 0 412 61210 0.

(Garnick, Canellos and Richie, 1983), and eventually in a randomized trial conducted by the Southeastern Cancer Study Group (SECSG) in 6–7% of patients (Williams *et al.*, 1987). The early reports were accompanied by case studies of germ cell tumor patients who had experienced other vascular events, including myocardial infarction (Vogelzang, Frenning and Kennedy, 1980) and malignant hypertension (Harrell, Sibley and Vogelzang, 1982). A review was published by Vogelzang (1984).

The role of bleomycin in the management of germ cell tumors had never been carefully studied. It was initially incorporated into germ cell tumors regimens prior to the introduction of cisplatin. Bleomycin was added to actinomycin-D and vinblastine at Memorial Sloan-Kettering Cancer Center (MSKCC) in an attempt to improve upon the single agent activity of actinomycin-D (Mackenzie, 1966) and vinblastine (Samuels and Howe, 1970). This three-drug combination ('VAB-1') had a 24% CR rate in previously untreated patients and a 11% cure rate, not obviously different from that of actinomycin-D as a single agent (Wittes *et al.*, 1976). At the M.D. Anderson Tumour Institute, Samuels *et al.* (1976) first added a bolus and later continuous infusion bleomycin to high doses of vinblastine. The use of vinblastine plus continuous infusion bleomycin had a 49% CR rate. At MSKCC, bleomycin by continuous infusion was added to a subsequent regimen with relatively low doses of cisplatin (60 mg m^{-2}), with an improvement of the CR rate to 50% (Cheng *et al.*, 1978). However, it was not until the addition of high doses of cisplatin ($\geq$100 mg m^{-2}), that the high CR rates expected today were first observed (Einhorn and Donohue, 1977; Reynolds *et al.*, 1981). Thus the role of bleomycin has never been proven.

Because of the high cure rate, the apparent ability to distinguish between good and poor risk patients, and the acute and chronic toxicities which could at least be partly attributed to bleomycin, clinical trials were designed to evaluate the role of bleomycin.

20.2 TOXICITY REDUCTION IN GOOD RISK PATIENTS

The first clinical trial without bleomycin was a report of etoposide/cisplatin (EP) in 'low volume' patients from the Royal Marsden Hospital (Table 20.1) (Peckham *et al.*, 1985). In this study, 12/16 (75%) patients achieved CR; this was less than the 16/18 (89%) CR which was reported with EP plus bleomycin (PEB) (Peckham *et al.*, 1983) (Table 20.2). However, the total etoposide dose was only 360 mg m^{-2}. This is lower than the 500 mg m^{-2} administered in other trials (Table 20.1). This factor along with the scheduling and the small numbers render the results of this trial difficult to interpret.

The initial randomized trial intended to evaluate the role of bleomycin was begun at MSKCC and was designed to compare a five-drug treatment program with cisplatin/ continuous infusion bleomycin/cyclophosphamide/vinblastine/actinomycin-D (VAB-6) with a two-drug treatment program with etoposide/cisplatin (EP) (Tables 20.1 and 20.2). Good risk patients defined by MSKCC criteria (Bosl *et al.*, 1983, 1988) were randomly allocated to receive either VAB-6 or EP in the setting of standard combined modality therapy including postchemotherapy surgical resection of apparent residual disease. One hundred and sixty-four eligible and fully evaluable patients were treated, with 96% of patients receiving VAB-6 and 93% of patients receiving EP achieving a CR. The study completed accrual in 1986 and was fully reported in 1988 (Bosl *et al.*, 1988). The relapse-free, total and event-free survivals were equal in the two arms. There were nine relapses from CR in patients treated with VAB-6 and nine relapses from CR in patients treated with EP. This study showed that the two-drug treatment program had less quantitative emesis, myelosuppression, mucositis and magnesium wasting. No patient in either arm experienced treatment mortality, but 16% of patients on the VAB-6 arm had bleomycin

Table 20.1   Treatment programs investigating the value of bleomycin

---

Royal Marsden Hospital

Etoposide 120 mg m^{-2} IV days 1, 2 and 3   Four cycles administered at 3-week intervals
Cisplatin 20 mg m^{-2} IV days 1–5

Memorial Sloan-Kettering Cancer Center (Bosl *et al.*, 1986, 1988)

VAB–6
Cyclophosphamide 600 mg m^{-2} IV day 1   Three cycles administered at 4-week intervals
Vinblastine 4 mg m^{-2} IV day 1   No bleomycin in cycle three
Bleomycin 30 units IV push day 1
Bleomycin 20 units m^{-2} days 1–3 by continuous
    infusion
Cisplatin 120 mg m^{-2} IV day 4 with mannitol
    diuresis

EP
Etoposide 100 mg m^{-2} IV days 1–5   Four cycles administered at 3–4 week intervals
Cisplatin 20 mg m^{-2} IV days 1–5

European Organization for the Research and Treatment of Cancer (Stoter and Denis, 1985)

PEB
Cisplatin 20 mg m^{-2} IV days 1–5
Etoposide 120 mg m^{-2} days 1, 3 and 5
Bleomycin 30 units IV days 2, 9 and 16

EP
Cisplatin 20 mg m^{-2} IV days 1–5
Etoposide 120 mg m^{-2} days 1, 3 and 5

Eastern Cooperative Oncology Group (Einhorn *et al.*, 1989)

PEB
Cisplatin 20 mg m^{-2} IV days 1–5   Three cycles every 21 days compared to four
Etoposide 100 mg m^{-2} IV days 1–5   cycles every 21 days
Bleomycin 30 units IV days 2, 9, 16

Australasian Germ Cell Neoplasm Trial Group (Levi *et al.*, 1993)

PVB
Cisplatin 100 mg m^{-2} IV day 1   Four cycles administered at 3-week intervals
Bleomycin 30 units IV days 2, 9 and 16
Vinblastine 6 mg m^{-2} IV days 1 and 2

PV
Cisplatin 100 mg m^{-2} IV days 1–5   Four cycles administered at 3-week intervals
Vinblastine 6 mg m^{-2} IV day 1 and 2

Southwest Oncology Group

PVB
Cisplatin 120 mg m^{-2} IV day 3   Four cycles administered at 3-week intervals
Vinblastine 12 mg m^{-2} IV day 1   Bleomycin deleted after 200 units m^{-2}
Bleomycin 15 units m^{-2} twice weekly

VPVe
Cisplatin 120 mg m^{-2} IV day 3   Four cycles administered at 3-week intervals
Vinblastine 8 mg m^{-2} IV day 1
Etoposide 50 mg m^{-2} days 2–5

Table 20.2   Results of studies on deletion of bleomycin from chemotherapy regimens

Reference	Regimen	Number of patients	Complete responses	Number of relapses
Bosl *et al.* (1986, 1988)	VAB-6	82	79 (96%)	9 (12%)
	EP	82	76 (93%)	9 (12%)
Peckham *et al.* (1985)	EP	16	12 (75%)	0 (–)
Levi *et al.* (1993)	PVB	110	96 (87%)	5 (5%)
	PV	108	88 (82%)	8 (7%)
Samson *et al.* (1989)	PVB	77	59 (77%)	5
	VPVe	83	61 (73%)	7
Stoter and Denis (1985)	PEB	67	64 (96%)	1 (2%)
	EP	62	59 (95%)	2 (3%)
Stoter and van Oosterom (1990)*	BEP	144	137 (95%)	5 (3.5%)
	EP	134	122 (91%)	3 (2.5%)
Einhorn (1990)†	BEP (×3)	82		15% unfavorable response‡
	EP (×3)	82		32% unfavorable response

NS, not stated. VAB-6, vinblastine/actinomycin-D/bleomycin/cisplatin/cyclophosphamide. EP, etoposide/cisplatin. PVB, cisplatin/vinblastine/bleomycin. VPVe, vinblastine/cisplatin/etoposide. PEB, cisplatin/etoposide/bleomycin.
* Update by personal communication of the EORTC study reported by Stoter and Denis (1985). (Analysis Feb 1990. Presented at UICC congress, Hamburg.)
† Personal communication. L.H. Einhorn 1990.
‡ Unfavorable response = relapse, non remission or positive biopsy after chemotherapy.

eliminated after the first cycle of therapy because of a ≥20% reduction in the vital capacity and/or diffusion capacity of carbon monoxide. As of October 1990, no further patients had relapsed or died with a median follow-up of 61 months. This study showed that a treatment program without bleomycin can achieve a high cure rate with less toxicity. However, it does not directly address the question of the need for bleomycin. In a subsequent randomized trial comparing EP with etoposide plus carboplatin, 121 out of 134 (90%) of patients randomized to EP achieved CR, with only four relapses (3%), attesting to the validity of the first randomized trial (Bajorin *et al.*, 1993).

Two ongoing studies were designed to answer this question, but neither has been reported yet in other than abstract form. The larger of these two was conducted by the European Organization for Research in the Treatment of Cancer (EORTC). In this study, etoposide/bleomycin/cisplatin (PEB) is directly compared with EP in patients deemed to be good risk by the criteria of the EORTC (Stoter and Denis, 1985; Stoter *et al.*, 1987) (Tables 20.1 and 20.2). With 278 patients entered into the study, 95% of the evaluable patients receiving PEB and 91% of patients receiving EP had achieved CR. Of the complete responders, two receiving EP and one receiving PEB relapsed. Unfortunately, this study also uses a lower etoposide dose (Table 20.1). Patient accrual is closed, but follow-up continues in order to be certain that a small difference in response proportion and/or survival does not exist between the two arms, and a recent analysis is also presented in Table 20.2 (personal communication A. Van Oosterom).

The Australasian Germ Cell Neoplasm Trial Group randomly allocated patients to receive either cisplatin/vinblastine/bleomycin (PVB) or cisplatin/vinblastine (PV) (Tables 20.1 and 20.2). With 218 patients entered, 82% of the patients receiving PV and 87% of patients receiving PVB had achieved CR (Levi *et al.*, 1993). However, only 71% of patients receiving PV were continuously disease free, com-

Table 20.3 Myelosuppression in trials comparing chemotherapy with and without bleomycin in germ cell tumor patients

Reference	Parameter	Bleomycin	No bleomycin	P
Bosl *et al.* (1988)	WBC (median)	1 850	2 200	0.06
	Platelets (median)	95 000	117 000	0.01
Levi *et al.* (1993)	WBC (<2000)	50%	40%	0.04
	Platelets <100 000	16%	8%	0.04
Stoter and Denis (1985)	WBC (<2000)	45%	25%	–
	Platelets (<75 000)	29%	18%	–

WBC, white blood cells. CBC, complete blood count. NS, not stated. GR 3–4, World Health Organisation Toxicity Grade 3–4.

pared with 84% of patients receiving PVB. Cumulative survival probability between the two treatment arms was similar ($p = 0.70$). Tumor deaths were more frequent in the PV arm ($p = 0.02$), while treatment deaths were more frequent in the PVB arm ($p = 0.06$). These data suggest that, in regimens based on vinblastine, bleomycin may be important but is associated with greater treatment mortality. One additional randomized trial, conducted by the Southwest Oncology Group (SWOG), compared PVB with a combination of vinblastine/cisplatin/etoposide (VPVe) (Tables 20.1 and 20.2). In this study, 59 of 77 patients (77%) receiving PVB and 61 of 83 (73%) receiving VPVe achieved CR (Samson *et al.*, 1989). The toxicity experienced in the treatment arms without bleomycin was less than that observed in the bleomycin-containing arms in each of these studies.

The Eastern Cooperative Oncology Group (ECOG) performed a comparison of EP × three cycles and BEP × three cycles. The trial has been terminated after an interim analysis suggested less favorable responses with EP (Table 20.2).

Pneumonitis is the most feared of bleomycin side-effects. However, one unexpected outcome of the above randomized trials is that the myelosuppression of the bleomycin-containing arm was greater than that observed in the arm without bleomycin (Table 20.3). Bleomycin is not generally recognized as a myelosuppressive agent, and its effect on

blood counts has not been widely studied. However, the results reported in the above trials show that the use of bleomycin decreases nadir blood counts to some degree, thereby increasing the likelihood of septicemia at a time of granulocytopenia. This unrecognized effect may have contributed to the 4% mortality with PEB and 6% mortality with PVB noted in the SECSG study.

20.3 DISCUSSION AND RECOMMENDATIONS

The deletion of bleomycin from treatment programs for patients with metastatic germ cell tumors continues to be studied. Treatment regimens based on EP appear to be as efficacious as those containing bleomycin when combined with standard postchemotherapy and surgical excision of residual disease. The data from the SECSG study most clearly define the likelihood of lethal toxicity. Of 244 patients treated, five treated with either PVB or PEB died as a result of bleomycin pneumonitis. An additional six died as a consequence of septicemia. The incidence of Raynaud's phenomenon was equal in both arms (6% and 7%, respectively) (Williams *et al.*, 1987). Thus the substitution of etoposide for vinblastine did not eliminate this side-effect. However, in both the MSKCC and EORTC studies, no Raynaud's phenomenon has been reported in the EP arms. Thus, it is likely that the bolus administration of bleomycin is responsible for the Raynaud's phenomenon.

Whether bleomycin should be eliminated in community practice remains somewhat controversial. Three cycles of PEB were as effective as four cycles of PEB (Einhorn *et al.*, 1989) with only one treatment death in patients deemed to be good risk by the criteria of Indiana University (Birch *et al.*, 1986). Thus 4 months of EP or 3 months of PEB appear to be equivalent therapy.

It must be emphasized that the studies deleting bleomycin have been exclusively performed in patients deemed to be 'good risk' by a set of criteria. Although there is substantial debate over the value of such criteria in identifying 'poor risk' patients, the criteria of MSKCC (Bosl *et al.*, 1983), Indiana University (Birch *et al.*, 1986) and the EORTC (Stoter and Denis, 1985) all identify good risk patients with a very high proportion of CR (Bajorin *et al.*, 1988). Two-drug therapy is not appropriate in poor risk patients. Thus, the community use of two-drug treatment programs that delete bleomycin should be limited to 'good risk' patients using one of the established criteria.

If bleomycin is used, strict criteria should be used to interrupt its use based upon changes in pulmonary function. The standard criteria at MSKCC are conservative and have resulted in an absence of lethal bleomycin pulmonary toxicity in all of its reports; no deaths have been reported in >300 patients receiving VAB-6. In patients receiving bleomycin, a 20% reduction from a pretreatment baseline in either the vital capacity or the diffusion capacity of carbon monoxide is sufficient evidence to delete bleomycin from the treatment program. Bleomycin pneumonitis may not be completely abrogated by routine pulmonary function testing, but the risk will be reduced as awareness is increased. Given the doubtful benefit of bleomycin in good risk patients, the continued use of bleomycin in the presence of subclinical but definite evidence of pulmonary dysfunction is unwarranted. The presence of cough, dyspnoea or interstitial pulmonary infiltrates is nearly always too late in the course of the disease and usually results in a lethal outcome.

Bleomycin was an important element of early treatment programs for germ cell tumors. Given the extraordinary efficacy of etoposide and cisplatin, its role is doubtful. Standard therapy for good risk patients can be either four cycles of EP or three cycles of PEB.

ACKNOWLEDGEMENTS

Supported in part by grant CA05826 and contract CM-57732 from the National Cancer Institute.

REFERENCES

Bajorin, D., Katz, A., Chan, E. *et al.* (1988) Comparison of criteria for assigning germ cell tumor patients to 'good risk' and 'poor risk' studies. *J. Clin. Oncol.*, **6**, 786–92.

Bajorin, D.F., Sarosdy, M.F., Pfister, D.G. *et al.* (1993) Randomized trial of etoposide and cisplatin versus etoposide and carboplatin patients with good-risk germ cell tumors: A multiinstitutional study. *J. Clin. Oncol.*, **11**, 598–606.

Birch, T., Williams, S., Cone, A. *et al.* (1986) Prognostic factors for favorable outcome in disseminated germ cell tumors. *J. Clin. Oncol.*, **4**, 400–7.

Bosl, G.J., Geller, N.L., Cirrincione, C.C. *et al.* (1983) Multivariate analysis of prognostic variables in patients with metastatic testicular cancer. *Cancer Res.*, **43**, 3403–7.

Bosl, G.J., Yagoda, A., Golbey, R.B. *et al.* (1985) Role of etoposide-based chemotherapy in the treatment of patients with refractory or relapsing germ cell tumor. *Am. J. Med.*, **78**, 423–8.

Bosl, G.J., Gluckman, R., Geller, N. *et al.* (1986) VAB-6: an effective chemotherapy regimen for patients with germ cell tumor. *J. Clin. Oncol.*, **4**, 1493–9.

Bosl, G.J., Geller, N.L., Bajorin, D. *et al.* (1988) A randomized trial of etoposide + cisplatin versus VAB-6 (vinblastine + bleomycin + cisplatin + cyclophosphamide + actinomycin D) in patients with good prognosis germ cell tumor. *J. Clin. Oncol.*, **6**, 1231–8.

Cheng, E., Cvitkovic, E., Wittes, R.E. and Golbey, R.B. (1978) Germ cell tumors (II). VABII in metastatic testicular cancer. *Cancer*, **42**, 2162–8.

Einhorn, L.H. (1981) Testicular cancer as a model for a curable neoplasm. The Richard and Hinda Rosenthal Foundation Award Lecture. *Cancer Res.*, **41**, 3275–80.

Einhorn, L.H. and Donohue, J.P. (1977) *Cis*-diamminedichloroplatinum, vinblastine, and bleomycin combination chemotherapy in disseminated testicular cancer. *Ann. Intern. Med.*, **87**, 293–8.

Einhorn, L.H., Williams, S.O. Loehrer P.L. *et al.* (1989) Evaluation of optimal duration of chemotherapy in favorable-prognosis disseminated germ cell tumors: A Southeastern Cancer Study Group protocol. *J. Clin. Oncol.*, **7**, 387–91.

Einhorn, L.H., Williams, S.D., Troner, M. *et al.* (1981) The role of maintenance chemotherapy in disseminated testicular cancer. *N. Engl. J. Med.*, **305**, 727–31.

Garnick, M.B., Canellos, G.P., Richie, J.P. (1983) Treatment and surgical staging of testicular and primary extragonadal cell tumors. *JAMA*, **250**, 49, 1733–41.

Harrell, R.M., Sibley, R.J. and Vogelzang, N.J. (1982) Renal vascular lesions after chemotherapy with vinblastine, bleomycin, and cisplatin. *Am. J. Med.*, **73**, 429–34.

Levi, J., Raghavan, D., Harvey, V. *et al.* (1993) The importance of bleomycin in combination chemotherapy for good-prognosis germ cell carcinoma. *J. Clin. Oncol.*, **11**, 1300–5.

Mackenzie, A.R. (1966) Chemotherapy of metastatic testis cancer. Results in 154 patients. *Cancer*, **19**, 1369–76.

Peckham, M.J., Barret, A., Lieu, K.H. *et al.* (1983) The treatment of metastatic germ cell testis tumors with bleomycin, etoposide, and cisplatin *Br. J. Cancer*, **47**, 613–19.

Peckham, M.J., Horwich, A., Blackmore, C. and Hendry, W.F. (1985) Etoposide and cisplatin with or without bleomycin as first-line chemotherapy for patients with small-volume metastases of testicular nonseminoma. *Cancer Treat. Rep.*, **69**, 483–8.

Reynolds, T.F., Vugrin, D., Cvitkovic, E. *et al.* (1981) VAB-3 combination chemotherapy of metastatic testicular cancer. *Cancer*, **48**, 888–91.

Samson, M.K., Crawford, E.D., Natale, R. *et al.* (1989) A randomized trial of cisplatin (P), vinblastine (VLB) plus either bleomycin (PVB) or VP-16 (VPV) in patients with advanced testicular cancer. *Proc. Am. Soc. Clin. Oncol.*, **8**, 134 (Abstract 522).

Samuels, M.L. and Howe, C.D. (1970) Vinblastine in the management of testicular cancer. *Cancer*, **25**, 1009–17.

Samuels, M.L., Lanzoti, V.J., Holoye, P.Y. *et al.* (1976) Combination chemotherapy in germinal cell tumors. *Cancer Treat. Rev.*, **3**, 185–204.

Stoter, G. and Denis, L. (1985) The chemotherapy of disseminated testicular nonseminomatous germ cell tumors and the clinical research of the EORTC Genitourinary Group. *Acta Urol. Belg.*, **53**, 428–35.

Stoter, G., Kaye, S., Jones, W. *et al.* (1987) Cisplatin (P) and VP16 (E) +/− bleomycin (BEP vs. EP) in good risk patients with disseminated non-seminomatous testicular cancer; a randomized EORTC GU group study. *Proc. Am. Soc. Clin. Oncol.*, **6**, 110 (Abstract 432).

Vogelzang, N.J. (1984) Vascular and other complications of chemotherapy for testicular cancer. *Wld J. Urol.*, **2**, 32–7.

Vogelzang, N.J., Bosl, G.J., Johnson, K. *et al.* (1981) Raynaud's phenomenon: A common toxicity after combination chemotherapy for testicular cancer. *Ann. Intern. Med.*, **95**, 288–92.

Vogelzang, N.J., Frenning, D.H. and Kennedy, B.J. (1980) Coronary artery disease after treatment with bleomycin and vinblastine. *Cancer Treat. Rep.*, **64**, 1159–60.

Vugrin, D., Whitmore, W. and Golbey, R. (1983) VAB-6 combination chemotherapy without maintenance in treatment of disseminated cancer of the testis. *Cancer*, **51**, 211–15.

Williams, S.D., Birch, R., Einhorn, L.H. *et al.* (1987) Treatment of disseminated germ cell tumors with cisplatin, bleomycin and either vinblastine or etoposide. *N. Engl. J. Med.*, **316**, 1435–40.

Williams, S.D., Einhorn, L.H., Greco, F.A. *et al.* (1980) VP-16–213 salvage therapy for refractory germinal neoplasms. *Cancer*, **46**, 2154–8.

Wittes, R.E., Yagoda, A., Silvay, O. *et al.* (1976) I. Induction of remission with vinblastine, actinomycin-D, and bleomycin. *Cancer*, **37**, 637–45.

DOSE ESCALATION OF CISPLATIN IN THE CHEMOTHERAPY OF POOR RISK GERM CELL TUMOR PATIENTS

M. Rørth

21.1 INTRODUCTION

Achievement of long-term survival of most patients with metastatic germ cell tumors is one of the most impressive results of modern medical oncology. The earliest results by Einhorn and Donohue (1977) were rapidly confirmed by many groups all over the world. Subsequently, the standard chemotherapy of the late 1970s (the cisplatin/vinblastine/bleomycin (PVB) regimen) has been improved, i.e. toxicity has been reduced by replacing vinblastine with etoposide (PEB) (Peckham *et al.*, 1983) and lately by decreasing the necessary number of chemotherapy cycles in the management of subsets of patients with good prognosis. Concomitant with a reduction in

toxicity and without increasing the aggressiveness of the treatment, the therapeutic results have continuously improved over time. This evolution reflects a more or less systematic improvement of regimens and probably also a better overall handling of patients with germ cell tumors including an improvement in the handling and prevention of toxicity problems (Einhorn, 1986).

In the Indiana University/Southeastern Cancer Study Group (SECSG) series (Nichols *et al.*, 1991), it has been shown that in subsets of patients with poor prognosis the PEB regimen gives better therapeutic results than the PVB regimen (Table 21.1). It is important to realize that these results are with standard, relatively nontoxic chemotherapy, and form a

Table 21.1 Treatment of high risk patients with 'standard' chemotherapy using cisplatin, 20 mg m^{-2} daily for 5 days

Other drugs used in combination with cisplatin	Time between cycles (weeks)	Dose (mg m^{-2}) every 3 weeks	Number of patients	No evidence of disease	Reference
Vinblastine/bleomycin	3	100	36	12 (33%)	Einhorn (1986)
Vinblastine/bleomycin	3	100	18	6 (33%)	Ozols *et al.* (1988)
Etoposide/bleomycin	3	100	40	34 (85%)	Pizzocaro *et al.* (1985)
Etoposide/bleomycin	3	100	14	12 (86%)	Peckham *et al.* (1983)
Vinblastine/bleomycin	3	100	25	4 (16%)	Daugaard *et al.* (1987a)

Testicular Cancer: Investigation and management. Second edition. Edited by Professor A. Horwich.
Published in 1996 by Chapman & Hall. ISBN 0 412 61210 0.

baseline for comparison with more aggressive approaches. It is, however, agreed that there are still subsets of patients with poor prognosis, i.e. patients where aggressive therapy is justified and necessary if long-lasting remission is to be obtained.

Improvement of therapeutic results in young patients with aggressive, heterogenous tumors can conceivably be achieved by adding new drugs to the current regimens or by increasing the efficacy of the drugs already in use. New and old drugs such as ifosfamide (Loehrer, Einhorn and Williams, 1986), epirubicin, vincristine, cyclophosphamide and carboplatin (Marangolo *et al.*, 1989, Nichols *et al.*, 1992) are currently being investigated in different protocols for patients with poor prognosis. The present review deals in more detail with the second type of strategy, i.e. attempts to increase the efficacy of the supposedly most important drug in the treatment schedules, cisplatin.

21.2 RATIONALE FOR, AND FEASIBILITY OF, DOSE ESCALATION

From *in vitro* experiments (Durand *et al.*, 1987) and early clinical trials (Hayes *et al.*, 1977; Samson *et al.*, 1984) we know that a certain dose–effect relationship exists for the action of cisplatin on germ cell tumors. This effect has not been studied systematically in the clinical setting and only the amount of drug per cycle has been looked at, not the total amount of drug delivered over a period of time. In the dose range 40–150 mg cisplatin per cycle, dose dependence was shown in germ cell patients by Hayes *et al.* (1977). Such a relationship has not been conclusively demonstrated for higher dose ranges in clinical trials. In the early days of the cisplatin era, increasing the dose of cisplatin above approximately 100 mg m^{-2} per cycle was hampered by renal toxicity. By the proper use of hydration with isotonic saline and diuretics like mannitol it has been shown, however, that the reduction in renal function as measured by glomerular filtration rate (GFR) estimate (e.g. Cr-EDTA clearance) is very small and not clinically important. Application of higher doses of cisplatin have thus become feasible and other types of toxicity are experienced as clinically important, in particular neurotoxicity.

Indirect evidence for a dose–response relationship has been produced in small series of patients previously treated with cisplatin or progressing while on standard dose chemotherapy (Table 21.2). Some, although admittedly few, of these patients achieved lasting remission with high dose cisplatin, i.e. 40 mg m^{-2} daily × 5. In germ cell cancers, as well as in several other aggressive, chemosensitive tumors, it is generally agreed that the battle against the disease should be won at the very start of the treatment. In other words, aggressive therapy should be used as a first line treatment in those patients who, by standard regimens, have a relatively poor prognosis, e.g. a predicted chance of obtaining disease-free survival (or no evidence of disease, NED) of less than 50%. The first step in defining the overall strategy thus becomes the identification of prognostic factors and definition of poor risk groups.

21.3 SELECTION OF POOR RISK PATIENTS

Vogelzang (1987) has compiled an overview of the existing information on prognostic factors based on a standardized inquiry to 18 clinical centers. In order to derive useful information for the subsequent identification of patients eligible for aggressive therapy, special emphasis was given to the results of multivariate analysis of possible prognostic factors in patients treated with standard dose cisplatin-based chemotherapy. The series analyzed are not directly comparable because of minor or major differences in treatment schedules and in differences in patient selection and referral. In contrast to most other analyses of similar problems in other cancers, the performance status of patients is not an

Table 21.2 High dose cisplatin regimens in previously treated patients using cisplatin, 40 mg m^{-2} daily for five days

Other drugs used in combination	Time between cycles (weeks)	Number of patients	Evaluable	Complete response*	Deaths from toxicity	No evidence of disease (NED)	Median observation time for NED (months)	Reference
Etoposide/bleomycin	3	7	7	5	0	4 (57%)	22	Daugaard et al. (1987a)
Etoposide/ifosfamide	4	33	29	8	3	3 (9%)	19	Droz et al. (1989a)
Etoposide/ifosfamide + ABMT	?	8	8	3	0	6 (75%)	15.5	Biron et al. (1989)
Etoposide/vinblastine/ bleomycin + ABMT	3	5	5	0	?	0	–	Ozols et al. (1988) (crossover from PVB in randomized trial)
Etoposide	4	12	12	5		1	–	Trump and Hortvet (1985)

* Includes complete responses after secondary surgery.
ABMT, autologous bone marrow transplantation.

important variable, simply because the vast majority of germ cell tumor patients is in very good performance status even with very advanced disease. Tumor volume is, however, as in other diseases, definitely of importance. For germ cell tumors, tumor markers are of special importance because the markers human chorionic gonadotrophin (HCG) and alpha-fetoprotein (AFP) fulfil most of the demands for ideal tumor markers. Likewise, histological subtypes are reasonably well defined and the presence or absence of certain components in the primary tumor could conceivably be of importance. Finally, specific sites of metastases in germ cell cancers were considered in several series.

Direct measurements of total tumor volume related to prognosis (and to marker levels) were attempted by Horwich *et al.* (1987). Using total body computed tomography scans, an estimate of tumor volume in cubic centimeters was made. It was not, however, possible to include pulmonary metastases in the measurements, a fact that of course limits the overall applicability of the approach. Total tumor volume was found to correlate clearly with prognosis. In an analysis of 171 patients at the Memorial Sloan-Kettering Cancer Center (Bosl *et al.*, 1983), tumor volume entered the prognostic formula in terms of number of sites of metastases. In the EORTC study (Stoter *et al.*, 1987) comprising 214 patients, the size and number of lung metastases were of significance. The disparity in criteria to define the adverse group is obvious (Birch *et al.*, 1986; Einhorn, 1986; Daugaard *et al.*, 1987a; Schmoll *et al.*, 1987; Ozols *et al.*, 1988; Kaye *et al.*, 1989) and therefore comparison between results is difficult and sometimes even meaningless. A consensus should be sought, preferably with the use of easily standardized and objective measures, i.e. number and size (diameter) of metastases.

In nearly all analyses, the levels of tumor markers, especially HCG, achieved significant prognostic importance (Chapter 7). Most groups ascribe a prognostic significance to

the HCG and/or the AFP levels *per se*, but the cut-off levels differ considerably. For HCG, levels of 6000 IU l^{-1} (Droz *et al.*, 1988), 10 000 IU l^{-1} (Ozols *et al.*, 1988), 50 000 IU l^{-1} (Pizzocaro *et al.*, 1985) and 100 000 IU l^{-1} (Daugaard *et al.*, 1987a) have been used. The cut off level of AFP when used has been 1000 μg l^{-1} in most groups (Pizzocaro *et al.*, 1985; Stoter *et al.*, 1987; Droz *et al.*, 1988; Ozols *et al.*, 1988). For both these markers, a standardization of assays, interlaboratory control, and analysis of assay variations are mandatory if certain cut-off levels are to be universally accepted. The level of lactate dehydrogenase (LDH) in serum may be useful as a prognostic factor (Bosl *et al.*, 1983), but relatively few groups have used levels of this enzyme systematically in the classification of patients. Lactate dehydrogenase is obviously not a tumor marker in the strict sense, but the level in serum could reflect tumor mass or high levels could reflect high metabolic activity and/or cell turnover. It is thus obvious that also in the area of tumor markers a consensus is needed with regard to the use of the cut-off limits.

Few studies deal with the prognostic significance of histology in patients with advanced disease. Prognostic significance has been ascribed to the presence of choriocarcinoma in the primary tumor (Stoter *et al.*, 1987; Ozols *et al.*, 1988).

Retrospective analysis of different series have indicated that patients with liver, bone or CNS metastases (Birch *et al.* 1986; Daugaard *et al.*, 1987a; Schmoll *et al.*, 1987; Ozols *et al.*, 1988), should automatically be considered as having very advanced disease. In most studies, however, a systematical search for bone, liver or CNS metastases has not been carried out prior to the initiation of therapy. The proper influence of metastases to these sites thus awaits a prospective analysis.

In recent years, an international collaborative effort (including EORTC, MRC and several other European and American centers) has succeeded in defining three groups of patients with germ cell cancer: good, intermediate and poor risk patients. Based on data from approximately 6000 patients treated with *cis*-platinum-containing regimens for germ cell cancer the cut-off limits were defined (Mead and Stenning, 1993). Poor risk is defined as NSGCT with liver, bone or brain metastases, or mediastinal primary, or one poor 'marker' i.e. LDH > ten × normal value, HCG > 50 000 IU l^{-1} or AFP > 10 000 μg l^{-1}. This classification will hopefully form the basis for future randomized trials.

21.4 RESULTS OF TRIALS EMPLOYING HIGH CISPLATIN DOSES

The dose of cisplatin in most standard regimens has been 20 mg m^{-2} daily for 5 days combined with bleomycin 15 mg m^{-2} weekly and vinblastine or etoposide. In most series, the treatment is repeated after 3–4 weeks. Examples are given in Table 21.1 of treatment results with standard regimens given to patients with poor prognosis. The results vary, but it is evident that improvements have been experienced over time and that PEB is superior to PVB in this group of patients (Einhorn, 1986). The impressive results obtained by Pizzocaro *et al.* (1985) were obtained by using five courses of PEB and with early aggressive surgery in 25 of the 40 patients after the first three series. One of the 34 NED patients was salvaged with additional surgery and chemotherapy. The criteria used for selection of high risk patients were similar to other groups. The results of this 'moderate' strategy needs to be confirmed in other series. In the series of Peckham *et al.* (1983) the group of high risk patients included patients with retroperitoneal metastases >5 cm (Stage IIC), a cut-off limit considerably lower than that used by other groups, a fact that could explain the very high NED figure.

Increase in the intensity of cisplatin treatment can be achieved by increasing the single dose, by giving cisplatin in the same doses for more days in each cycle or by giving cisplatin with shorter intervals. The basic assumption made here is that dose intensity of cisplatin during the treatment period is a crucial variable for therapeutic outcome. In Table 21.3 a compilation has been made of reported series, including more than 15 patients and with dose intensity of cisplatin exceeding 100 mg m^{-2} per 3 weeks. Comparison of results is hampered by the above-mentioned very significant differences in criteria for patient selection. It is evident from the table that many of the applied regimens differ from the standard PEB not only in terms of high cisplatin dose, but also by including other drugs such as ifosfamide, vincristine and cyclophosphamide (Wandl *et al.*, 1989; Ghosn *et al.*, 1988). Also, the doses of etoposide used differ considerably, ranging from 300 mg m^{-2} per cycle (Kaye *et al.*, 1989) to 1000 mg m^{-2} per cycle (Daugaard *et al.*, 1987a). Finally, autologous bone marrow transplantation (ABMT) has been used in some patients. Given these premises it is hazardous to draw firm conclusions based on this compilation.

Close to 100% of the patients do respond to the intensive treatment, i.e. *a priori* complete clinical resistance to high dose cisplatin chemotherapy is seldom if ever seen in patients with germ cell cancer. It is, furthermore, evident that high rates (>70%) of lasting NED are achievable even in the group of patients with the most heavy combination of poor prognostic features (e.g. Daugaard *et al.*, 1987a). It is also clear that toxic deaths do occur in a significant number of patients who are receiving intensive first line treatment. In the series from the Finsen Institute (Daugaard *et al.*, 1987a) toxic deaths due to heavy myelosuppression (etoposide) have been observed. Improvement in handling of infectious complications, the proper use of ABMT and maybe in particular the use of colony-stimulating factors such as GM-CSF or G-CSF could conceivably abolish this serious drawback.

Table 21.3 High dose cisplatin regimens in previously untreated patients

Cisplatin dose	Other drugs	Dose intensity of cisplatin (mg m^{-2} every 3 weeks)	Time between cycles	Number of patients	Number evaluable	Complete response*	Deaths from toxicity	No evidence of disease (NED)	Median observation time for NED (months)	Comments	Reference
40 mg m^{-2} daily × 5	EVB	200	3 weeks	34	34	30	2	23 (68%)	30	9% alive with disease†	Ozols et al. (1988)
40 mg m^{-2} daily × 5	EB	200	3 weeks	33	32	28	4	24 (72%)	18.5	–	Daugaard et al. (1987a)
35 mg m^{-2} daily × 5	EB	175	3 weeks	116	98	62	8	58 (59%)	26	14% alive with disease†	Schmoll et al. (1987)
1) 50 mg m^{-2} daily × 2	BO	210	10 days	56	39	23	0	23 (59%)	14	15% alive with disease†	Kaye et al. (1989)
2) 20 mg m^{-2} daily × 5	EIFX	100	3 weeks								
1) 20 mg m^{-2} daily × 5 + 1 mg kg^{-1}	BO	210	10 days	29	27	20	2	22 (85%)	24	–	Horwich et al. (1989)
2) 20 mg m^{-2} daily × 5	E(B)	100	3 weeks								

* Includes complete responses after secondary surgery.
† Unresected residual disease, marker negative.
E, etoposide. B, bleomycin. v, vinblastine. IFX, ifosfamide. O, vincristine. ABMT, autologous bone marrow transplantation. NED, no evidence of disease.

Table 21.4 Cisplatin dose escalation in chemotherapy of NSGCT randomized study of Southeastern Cancer Study Group and Southwest Oncology Group

Regimen	Cisplatin dose	Patients	CR/NED*	Relapse	CDFS	S
BEP	100 mg m^{-2}	77	72%	8%	61%	74%
BEP	200 mg m^{-2}	76	68%	7%	63%	74%

* Including results after secondary surgery.
CDFS, Continuous disease-free survival. S, Survival.
From Nichols *et al.*, 1991.

back. In the context of toxicity, the principle applied by Kaye *et al.* (1989) and Horwich *et al.* (1989) may be of special interest. They have achieved a high dose intensity of cisplatin by decreasing the time interval between cisplatin treatments and not by increasing the single dose (see Chapter 22). The high dose intensity is sustained for a relatively short period of time, i.e. the high dose intensity does not necessarily lead to a high cumulative dose. Furthermore, the myelosuppression experienced is modest.

A randomized trial comparing standard PEB with standard EB + high dose cisplatin (40 mg m^{-2} daily $\times$ 5) in poor risk patients according to the Indiana University Staging Classification has been performed (Nichols *et al.*, 1991). No significant difference with regard to overall survival was found between the two arms in that study (Table 21.4). Thus, even though confirmative trials would have been nice, the available evidence indicates that standard doses of cisplatinum (100 mg m^{-2} for 3 weeks) is as effective as the achievable higher doses of cisplatinum (up to 200 mg m^{-2} for 3 weeks). The only other published randomized trial is that of Ozols *et al.* (1988) from NCI, USA. They compared the classical PVB with high dose cisplatin plus vinblastine + etoposide (100 mg m^{-2} daily $\times$ 5) + bleomycin. A significant better survival was found for the high dose regimen. The high dose regimen differs from the standard PVB, not only by using a higher dose of cisplatin, but also by replacement of vinblastine with etoposide – a difference which the Indiana University/Southeastern Cancer Study Group

has shown to influence the survival results significantly (Nichols *et al.*, 1991). Thus, as also stated by the authors, the improved survival in the high dose arm cannot at present be attributed to the high dose cisplatin alone.

With the advent of growth factors and bone marrow or peripheral stem cell support much higher doses of myelosuppressive drugs are achievable. With regard to platinum compounds this has led to the use of very high doses of carboplatinum in several successful phase II trials (Nichols *et al.*, 1992; Barnett *et al.*, 1993; Motzer *et al.*, 1993; Siegert *et al.*, 1994). Whether or not these aggressive regimens are superior to standard PEB still awaits the execution of well-designed randomized trials. Most of the experience existing today is based on the treatment of relapsing patients.

21.5 TOXICITY

21.5.1 MYELOSUPPRESSION

Cisplatin is not myelosuppressive to a high degree but thrombocytopenia is known to occur with high cumulative doses. This complication is, however, seldom life threatening. The addition of myelosuppressive drugs, in particular etoposide, in the high dose regimens leads to significant leukopenia with a concomitant risk of sepsis and toxic death. Toxic deaths due to sepsis have been reported in Danish (Daugaard *et al.*, 1987a), German (Schmoll *et al.*, 1987), and French studies (Droz *et al.*, 1989b). Improvements in the application of antibiotic strategies, colony-stimulating factors and ABMT can conceivably diminish this problem.

21.5.2   RENAL TOXICITY

As stated earlier, renal toxicity can be reduced by the use of high volumes of isotonic saline. Ozols *et al.* (1988) recommend, apart from intensive isotonic hydration, the use of 3% saline with the cisplatin infusion since animal experiments have indicated that renal function is protected with this high NaCl concentration. Ozols *et al.* (1988) claim that no renal dysfunction was experienced; others have reported the same experience. Most of the clinical results are, however, based on serum creatinine measurements and such measurements are more or less useless in the context of high dose cisplatin treatment. By using Cr-EDTA clearance measurements, Daugaard, Rossing and Rørth (1988) showed that GFR was significantly reduced (by approximately 30%) in patients who were treated with high dose cisplatin (three series, cumulative dose 600 mg m^{-2}). The reduction was more than twice that seen in patients who received standard dose cisplatin when comparing renal toxicity after the same cumulative dose of cisplatin. Even though a 30–50% reduction of GFR can be tolerated without immediate clinical problems, it is possible that patients treated with high dose cisplatin have an increased risk of renal hypertension or renal insufficiency later in life. Long-term follow-up investigations are needed. Protective methods might be improved by using protective drugs or in particular by avoiding other nephrotoxic drugs such as aminoglycosides.

21.5.3   HYPOMAGNESEMIA

All patients who are treated with high dose cisplatin experience a negative magnesium balance with hypomagnesemia to various degrees. Severe hypomagnesemia is nearly always followed by hypocalcemia and hypokalemia. It is important to realize that these latter electrolyte disturbances are not manageable unless magnesium substitution is carried out. Thus, nearly all patients on high dose cisplatin treatment need magnesium supplements in the form of intravenous magnesium. Long-term follow-up of the magnesium balance in these patients is necessary and it has still not been clarified to what extent and for how long hypomagnesemia prevails after cisplatin treatment.

21.5.4   NEUROPATHY

Peripheral neuropathy is a major side-effect in nearly all patients treated with high dose cisplatin. The subjective complaints are typically tingling, numbness and pain in hands and feet leading to functional problems including gait disturbances, and inability to feel and to identify things. Objective measurements have indicated a clear deterioration of the sensory nerves, but also deterioration at the level of the synapses in medulla spinalis (Daugaard *et al.*, 1987b; Krarup-Hansen *et al.*, 1993). The peripheral neuropathy is related to the cumulative dose of cisplatin with typical distinct progression of symptoms after a total dose of 600 mg m^{-2}. Peripheral neuropathy is also related to age, so that elderly patients experience a higher degree and a longer duration of peripheral neuropathy. This side-effect has a definitive influence on the quality of life of the patients (Ostchega *et al.*, 1988). Peripheral neuropathy is at least partly reversible. Longer follow-up studies are needed and more studies with objective investigations should be done.

21.5.5   OTOTOXICITY

Loss of hearing at high frequencies is invariably found in patients who are treated with cisplatin. This loss is irreversible and some patients need permanent hearing aids. Tinnitus is a very distressing side-effect in some patients. The reversibility of this has not been evaluated in detail.

Both with regard to neuropathy and oto-toxicity, protective methods are very much needed, but there is no clear indication as to what type of protective methods would be effective.

21.5.6 LUNG TOXICITY

Cisplatin is not directly lung toxic, but several groups have reported that problems of bleomycin-induced lung toxicity are becoming more serious with the use of high dose cisplatin. This could be due to an influence of cisplatin on the excretion of bleomycin in the kidney. Scrutinized use of lung function measurements, in particular carbon monoxide diffusion capacity, is recommended. The carbon monoxide diffusion capacity is very dependent on hemoglobin concentration in the blood and it is therefore recommended that measurements are carried out at normalized hemoglobin levels. Several of the toxic deaths reported and cited in Table 21.3 were related to pulmonary toxicity.

21.5.7 VASCULAR TOXICITY

Raynaud's disease is present in more than 50% of germ cell cancer patients treated with cisplatin-based chemotherapy (Hansen and Olsen, 1989). The relative influence of the different drugs (cisplatin, bleomycin, vinblastine, etoposide) in the regimens has not been defined. The influence of high dose cisplatin has not been thoroughly investigated, but such studies are on their way.

Long-term toxicity problems related to psychosocial factors (Chapter 31), fertility and the risk of secondary cancer need further studies with larger groups of patients and long-term follow-up.

21.5.8. SECONDARY LEUKEMIA

A new type of secondary leukemia has been described in patients treated with inhibitors of the enzyme topoisomerase II (Pedersen-

Bjergaard J *et al.*, 1991). Etoposide is such a drug, and now several cases of secondary leukemia have been described in PEB-treated patients. It is not clear whether or not the risk of leukemia is dependent on the dose of platinum used, but a definite influence of dose of etoposide has been found.

21.6 FUTURE ASPECTS

In view of the impressive results of treatment of patients with advanced germ cell tumor, it is obviously important to concentrate efforts on improvement of therapy of those patients who still today face a poor prognosis. An analysis of the existing data makes it painfully clear that standardization of patient selection, i.e. clear definition of poor risk patients, is a very important task. Randomized trials are clearly needed to provide answers to many of the clinical problems. One of the most pertinent problems for the moment is to define the optimal dose intensity of platin treatment. In view of its favorable toxicity profile, it is likely that carboplatin and not cisplatin will be the major platinum compound in forthcoming, high dose regimens. Growth factors, bone marrow transplantation and peripheral stem cells have effectively reduced the problems of myelosuppression. However, as carboplatinum might show less antineoplastic efficacy compared with cisplatinum, it could be prudent to include both *cis*-platinum and carboplatinum in the intensive schedules. It is to be hoped that the established lines of collaboration and the achieved agreement on prognostic factors can form the basis of the necessary randomized trials of intensive chemotherapy versus standard PEB in high-risk patients. Protective methods that can diminish toxicity, especially neurotoxicity, should be looked for, and finally the study of long-term toxicity is becoming increasingly important for the evaluation of the overall effect of an aggressive and toxic chemotherapeutic approach to young patients with potentially curable disease.

REFERENCES

Barnett, M.J., Coppin, C.M.L., Murray, N. *et al.* (1993) High-dose chemotherapy and autologous bone marrow transplantation for patients with poor prognosis nonseminomatous germ cell tumours. *Br. J. Cancer*, **68**, 594–8.

Birch, R., Williams, S., Cone, A. *et al.* (1986) Prognostic factors for favorable outcome in disseminated germ cell tumors. *J. Clin. Oncol.*, **4**, 400–7.

Biron, P., Brunat-Montigny, M., Bayle, J.Y. *et al.* (1989) Cisplatinum-VP16 and ifosfamide (VIC) + autologous bone marrow transplantation (ABMT) in poor prognostic non seminomatous germ cell tumors (NSGCT). *Proc. Am. Soc. Clin. Oncol.*, **8**, 576, 148.

Bosl, G.J. Geller, N., Cirricione, C. *et al.* (1983) Multivariate analysis of prognostic variables in patients with metastatic testicular cancer. *Cancer Res.*, **43**, 3403–7.

Daugaard, G. *et al.* (1987a) Management of advanced metastatic germ cell tumours. *Int. J. Androl.*, **10**, 319–24.

Daugaard, G. *et al.* (1987b) Electrophysiological study of the peripheral and central neurotoxic effect of cis-platin. *Acta Neurol. Scand.*, **76**, 86–93.

Daugaard, G., Rossing, N. and Rørth, M. (1988) Effects of cisplatin on different measures of glomerular function in the human kidney with special emphasis on high-dose. *Cancer Chemother. Pharmacol.*, **21**, 163–7.

Droz, J.P. *et al.* (1988) Prognostic factors in advanced nonseminomatous testicular cancer. A multivariate logistic regression analysis. *Cancer*, **62**, 564–8.

Droz, J. P., *et al.* (1989a) Phase II trial with etoposide (VP16) plus ifosfamide plus high-dose cisplatin (VIhP regimen) in refractory germ cell tumors, in *Therapeutic Progress in Urological Cancers* (eds G.P. Murphy and S. Khoury), Alan R. Liss Inc., New York, pp. 739–47.

Droz, J.P., Pico, J.L., Ghosn, M. *et al.* (1989b) High complete remission (CR) and survival rates in poor prognosis (PP) non seminomatous germ cell tumors (NSGCT) with high dose chemotherapy (HDCT) and autologous bone marrow transplantation (ABMT). *Proc. Am. Soc. Clin. Oncol.*, **8**, 505, 130.

Durand, R.E. *et al.* (1987) Interaction of etoposide and cisplatin in an *in vitro* tumor model. *Cancer Treat. Rep.*, **71**, 673–9.

Einhorn, L.H. (1986) Have new aggressive chemotherapy regimens improved results in advanced germ cell tumors? *Eur. J. Cancer Clin Oncol.*, **22**, 1289–93.

Einhorn, L.H. and Donohue, J.P. (1977) Cis-diammine-dichloroplatinum, vinblastine and bleomycin combination chemotherapy in disseminated testicular cancer. *Ann. Intern. Med.*, **87**, 292–8.

Ghosn, M. *et al.* (1988) Salvage chemotherapy in refractory germ cell tumors with etoposide (VP16) plus ifosfamide plus high-dose cisplatin. A VIhP regimen. *Cancer*, **62**, 24–7.

Hansen, S.W. and Olsen, N. (1989) Raynaud's phenomenon in patients treated with cisplatin, vinblastin and bleomycin for germ cell cancer: Measurement of vasoconstrictor response to cold. *J. Clin. Oncol.*, 7, 940–3.

Hayes, D.M. *et al.* (1977) High dose cisplatinum diammine dichloride. Amelioration of renal toxicity by mannitol diuresis. *Cancer*, **39**, 1372–81.

Horwich, A., Brada, M., Nicholls, J. *et al.* (1989) Intensive induction chemotherapy for poor risk non-seminomatous germ cell tumours. *Eur. J. Cancer Clin. Oncol.*, **25**, 177–84.

Horwich, A., Easton, D., Nicholls, J. *et al.* (1987) Prognosis following chemotherapy for metastatic malignant teratoma. *Br. J. Urol.*, **59**, 578–83.

Kaye, S., Harding, M., Stoter, G. *et al.* (1989) 'BOP/VAP' – a new intensive regime for poor prognosis germ cell tumours. *Proc. Am. Soc. Clin. Oncol.*, **8**, 136.

Krarup-Hansen, A., Fuglholm, K., Helweg-Larsen, S. *et al.* (1993) Examination of distal involvement in cisplatin induced neuropathy in man. *Brain*, **116**, 1017–41.

Loehrer, P.J., Einhorn, L.J. and Williams, S.D. (1986) VP-16 plus ifosfamide plus cisplatin as salvage therapy in refractory germ cell cancer. *J. Clin. Oncol.*, **4**, 528–36.

Marangolo, M., Rosti, G., Leoni, M. *et al.* (1989) Very high-dose carboplatin (JM8) + etoposide (VP16) and ABMT in refractory germinal-cell tumor. A pilot study. *Proc. Am. Soc. Clin. Oncol.*, **8**, 142.

Mead, G.M., Stenning, S.P. on behalf of the IGCCCG (1994) Prognostic factors for metastatic germ cell cancers treated with platinum-based chemotherapy: The international germ cell cancer collaborative group (IGCCCG) project to standardise risk criteria. *Proc. Am. Soc. Clin. Oncol.*, **13**, 790.

Motzer, R.J., Mazumdar, M., Gulati, S.C. *et al.* (1993) Phase II trial of high-dose carboplatin and etoposide with autologous bone marrow transplantation in first-line therapy for patients with poor-risk germ cell tumors. *J. Natl. Cancer Inst.,* **85**, 1828–35.

Mulder, P.O.M., DeVries, E., Koops, H. *et al.* (1988) Chemotherapy with maximally tolerable doses of VP 16–213 and cyclophosphamide followed by autologous bone marrow transplantation for the treatment of relapsed or refractory germ cell tumors. *Eur. J. Cancer Clin. Oncol.,* **24**, 675–7.

Nichols, C.R., Andersen, J., Lazarus, H.M. *et al.* (1992) High-dose carboplatin and etoposide with autologous bone marrow transplantation in refractory germ cell cancer: An Eastern Cooperative Oncology Group Protocol. *J. Clin. Oncol.,* **10**, 558–63.

Nichols, C.R., Williams, S.D., Loehrer, P.J. *et al.* (1991) Randomized study of cisplatin dose intensity in poor-risk germ cell tumors: A Southeastern Cancer Study Group and Southwest Oncology Group Protocol. *J. Clin. Oncol.,* **9**, 1163–72.

Ostchega, Y. *et al.* (1988) High-dose cisplatin-related peripheral neuropathy. *Cancer Nursing,* **11**, 23–32.

Ozols, R., Ihode, D.C., Linchan, W. *et al.* (1988) A randomized trial of standard chemotherapy *vs* a high-dose chemotherapy regimen in the treatment of poor prognosis nonseminomatous germ-cell tumors. *J. Clin. Oncol.,* **6**, 1031–40.

Peckham, M.J., Barrett, A., Liew, K. *et al.* (1983) The treatment of metastatic germ-cell testicular tumours with bleomycin, etoposide and cisplatin (BEP). *Br. J. Cancer,* **47**, 613–19.

Pedersen-Bjergaard, J., Daugaard, G., Hansen, S.W. *et al.* (1991) Increased risk of myelodysplasia and leukaemia after etoposide, cisplatin, and bleomycin for germ-cell tumours. *Lancet,* **338**, 359–63.

Pizzocaro, G., Piva, L., Salvioni, R. *et al.* (1985) Cisplatin, etoposide, bleomycin first-line therapy and early resection of residual tumor in far-advanced germinal testis cancer. *Cancer,* **56**, 2411–15.

Samson, M.K., Rivkin, S.E., Jones, S.E. *et al.* (1984) Dose-response and dose-survival advantage for high versus low-dose cisplatin combined with vinblastine and bleomycin in disseminated testicular cancer. *Cancer,* **53**, 1029–35.

Schmoll, H.J., Schubert, I., Arnold, H. *et al.* (1987) Disseminated testicular cancer with bulky disease: results of a phase-II study with cisplatin ultra high dose/VP-16/bleomycin. *Int. J. Androl.* **10**, 311–17.

Siegert, W., Beyer, J., Strohscheer, I. *et al.* (1994) High-dose treatment with carboplatin, etoposide, and ifosfamide followed by autologous stem-cell transplantation in relapsed or refractory germ cell cancer: A phase I/II study. *J. Clin. Oncol.,* **12**, 1223–31.

Stoter, G., Sylvester, R., Sleijifer, D.T. *et al.* (1987) Multivariate analysis of prognostic factors in patients with disseminated nonseminomatous testicular cancer: Results from a European Organization for Research on Treatment of Cancer multi-institutional phase III study. *Cancer. Res.,* **47**, 2714–18.

Trump, D.L. and Hortvet L. (1985) Etoposide and very high dose cisplatin: salvage therapy for patients with advanced germ cell neoplasms. *Cancer Treat. Rep.,* **69**, 259–61.

Vogelzang, N.J. (1987) Prognostic factors in metastatic testicular cancer. *Int. J. Androl.,* **10**, 225–37.

Wandl, U. *et al.* (1989) Treatment of high risk nonseminomatous testicular cancer (NSTC) with cisplatin, ifosfamide and bleomycin (PIB). *Proc. Am. Soc. Clin. Oncol.,* **8**, 147.

INTENSIVE INDUCTION CHEMOTHERAPY FOR POOR RISK TUMORS

22

D.P. Dearnaley

22.1 INTRODUCTION

The improvement in survival for patients with testicular teratoma has been impressive and gratifying since the introduction of platinum-containing regimens some 15 years ago (Einhorn and Donohue, 1977). However, there remains a subgroup of 10–20% of men presenting with metastases who die from their disease (Horwich, 1989). Prognostic factor analyses have been used to identify the patients at highest risk (Bosl *et al.*, 1983; Medical Research Council Working Party on Testicular Tumours, 1985; Birch *et al.*, 1986b; Logothetis *et al.*, 1986; Stoter *et al.*, 1987; Hitchins *et al.*, 1989; Mead, 1995) and there is general agreement that measures of tumor volume and extent of disease together with serum levels of the beta subunit of human chorionic gondatrophin, alpha-fetoprotein and lactate dehydrogenase (BHCG, AFP, LDH) can predict outcome. Using these systems, groups of patients can be identified with a 50% or more chance of relapsing (Chapter 7). For these men, strategies for increasing the efficacy of chemotherapy are required.

There are four main methods for modifying standard chemotherapy schedules: (a) the introduction of new chemotherapy agents, (b) the use of alternating drug combinations (Chapter 23), (c) high dose chemotherapy schedules (Chapter 2) and (d) chemotherapy schedules using drugs at increased frequency – intensive induction chemotherapy. This chapter will discuss the rationale of treatment with drugs at an increased frequency, describe our results using intensive induction chemotherapy in a high risk group of patients, and where possible compare this approach with other methods of treatment modification.

22.2 RATIONALE FOR INTENSIVE INDUCTION CHEMOTHERAPY

The growth rate of teratoma metastases may be rapid. Malaise *et al.* (1974) found the mean volume-doubling time of lung metastases from embryonal tumors to be 19.5 days as measured from serial chest X-ray examinations, which is significantly lower than for other carcinomas and sarcomas (range 29.5–90.4 days). Volume-doubling time is largely influenced by cell loss, which ranges from 29 to 97% (mean 77%) for a range of human tumors, and potential doubling times may be considerably faster at between 3 and 23 days (Steel, 1977). The proliferation rate of primary non-seminomatous germ cell tumors has been measured by Fosså *et al.* (1985) using

Testicular Cancer: Investigation and management. Second edition. Edited by Professor A. Horwich.
Published in 1996 by Chapman & Hall. ISBN 0 412 61210 0.

Table 22.1   Repopulation during 3-weekly chemotherapy schedule

	Increase in cell number compared with no proliferation						
Doubling time (d)	21	10.5	7	5	4	3	2
Two courses chemotherapy	2	4	8	18.4	38.1	128	1448
Four courses chemotherapy	8	64	512	6208	5.5×10^4	2.1×10^6	3.0×10^9

DNA flow cytometry and the S phase fraction estimated at between 22 and 51% – two to four times higher than generally shown in human cancers. Similar indications of high proliferative rate have been found by incubating or infusing primary tumors with tritiated thymidine and measuring the [^{3}H]thymidine labelling index. In 46 embryonal carcinomas the mean labelling index was 42% (range 1.6–77.3%) (Silvestrini *et al.*, 1985), and Rabes (1987) found labelling indexes of 80% with a calculated potentional doubling time as low as 0.6 days in areas of maximal proliferation. The Indiana University group (Sledge *et al.*, 1988) have found that a high proliferative index measured from DNA histograms from archived material of primary tumors shows a highly significant correlation with survival when tested in multivariate analysis. The Royal Marsden group (Price *et al.*, 1988) have studied tumor marker production (TMP) doubling times calculated from serial estimations of serum BHCG or AFP levels taken after orchidectomy but prior to the start of chemotherapy. This method gives an estimate of the growth of metastases and marker production doubling times ranging from 0.5 to >80 days (median 8 days for HCG and 13 days for AFP), with 14 out of 51 (29%) patients showing TMPs of less than 4 days. Short TMPs occurred more frequently in advanced presentations and correlated with relapse following chemotherapy (Price *et al.*, 1988, 1990). A further complicating factor is the accelerated proliferation of tumor cells that can occur after the start of treatment. This phenomenon is well documented for radiation therapy (Tubiana, 1982; Fowler, 1989; Mead, 1995), when doubling times may shorten by a factor of 2.5–5, and new accelerated fractionation schedules that reduce the overall treatment time are under study to determine whether this approach can lead to improved tumor control (Horwich *et al.*, 1988; Saunders *et al.*, 1989).

Chemotherapy for testicular cancer has conventionally been given on 3-weekly cycles to allow for adequate recovery from marrow suppression. On the basis of results achieved with the BEP regimens (bleomycin, etoposide, cisplatin) (Einhorn, 1986; Williams *et al.*, 1987b), we can estimate the level of tumor cell kill that must be achieved in order to obtain the observed responses. Patients with a minimal or moderate volume of disease according to the Indiana staging system (Einhorn, 1986) (up to perhaps 100 g and containing around 10^{11} teratoma cells) are controlled by three courses of chemotherapy (Einhorn, 1986). Each course must therefore reduce the fraction of surviving tumor cells by at least 2×10^{-4}. Microscopic disease (containing perhaps 10^9 teratoma cells) is controlled by two courses of chemotherapy (Williams *et al.*, 1987b), which implies a surviving fraction of approximately 3×10^{-5} per course of treatment. The surviving fraction of tumor cells at the end of each course of chemotherapy will be determined both by the proportion of cells killed by chemotherapy and by the capacity of the residual tumor to proliferate. Table 22.1 indicates the proliferation that will occur during either adjuvant (two courses) or a standard four courses of chemotherapy. When doubling

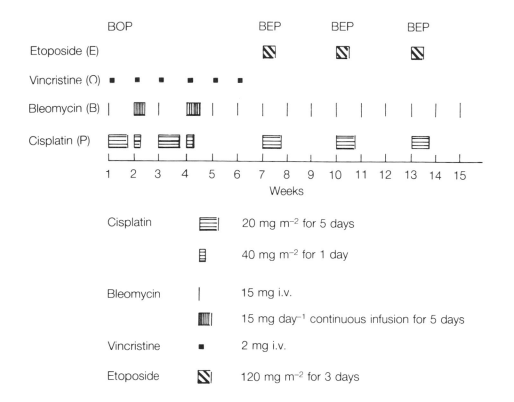

Fig. 22.1 Intensive induction regimen of platinum, vincristine, bleomycin and etoposide (BOP–BEP). In the C–BOP regimen, carboplatin is additionally given at a dose calculated to give an AUC of 3 on weeks 2 and 4 and etoposide is at 100 mg m^{-2} for 5 days.

times fall to the order of five days or less, the repopulation factor increases very steeply. For example if repopulation occurs with a tumor-doubling time of 3 days then cell numbers will increase by a factor of over 100 during each 3-weekly cycle of treatment. Over a standard four-cycle course of chemotherapy repopulation could increase cell numbers by a factor of about 2×10^6 (Table 22.1) – an effect that might at best require an additional two courses of chemotherapy to compensate, but which might also permit the development of drug-resistant clones. Tumor regrowth between courses of chemotherapy might therefore explain failure of conventional treatment in patients (Tubiana, 1982).

22.3 DESIGN OF INTENSIVE INDUCTION CHEMOTHERAPY SCHEDULE

To overcome rapid tumor proliferation as a potential cause for treatment failure in patients with poor risk non-seminomatous germ cell tumors, we have used an accelerated program of initial treatment. The intensive induction regimen (Horwich *et al.*, 1989) was based on that of Wettlaufer and colleagues (Wettlaufer *et al.*, 1984) using platinum, vincristine and bleomycin on a weekly schedule (Fig. 22.1). However, vincristine was substituted for vinblastine (Einhorn and Donohue, 1977) or etoposide (Peckham *et al.*, 1983; Williams *et al.*, 1987a) so as to avoid dose-limiting myelosuppression. Vincristine alone may have little antimitotic effect in germ cell tumors (Costa and Hreshchyshyn, 1962; Shaw and Bruner, 1964) but may show synergism when used in combination with bleomycin and cisplatin; clinically favorable results have been found by a number of groups (Merrin, 1980; Newlands *et al.*, 1983; Wettlaufer *et al.*, 1984). Samuels and associates (Samuels *et al.*, 1975) found that 5 days of continuous bleomycin was the most effective of the bleomycin combination programs against large volume tumors, and we used continuous infusions of bleomycin during weeks 2 and 4 of treatment (Fig. 22.1). After the first six courses of weekly chemotherapy a further three cycles of BEP chemotherapy (bleomycin, etoposide, platinum) (Peckham *et al.*, 1983) was given and the overall treatment time was 13 weeks.

22.4 PATIENTS AND METHODS

Eighty-two patients were treated with high intensity induction chemotherapy between January 1985 and January 1992. For the purpose of survival analysis, entry to the study was the first day of chemotherapy. Patients' ages ranged from 15 to 52 years (median 26 years). The diagnosis was established by initial orchidectomy in 61 cases, biopsy of an abdominal mass in two, and of mediastinal tumors in five cases. The remaining 14 patients were treated with their primary disease *in situ* (seven cases), presented with an occult primary (four cases) or with a mediastinal primary (three cases). All of these 14 patients had significantly raised BHCG or AFP serum levels and the diagnosis of non-seminomatous germ cell tumors was accepted on clinical grounds. Histological specimens were reviewed in the Royal Marsden Hospital Department of Histopathology. Thirteen patients had malignant teratoma trophoblastic (MTT) (choriocarcinoma pure or with other cell types), 33 patients had malignant teratoma undifferentiated (MTU) (embryonal carcinoma), 17 cases had malig-

nant teratoma intermediate (MTI) (teratocarcinoma), one patient had differentiated teratoma (TD), Stage IVC, L3 with brain metastases and HCG of 184 600 IU l^{-1}), and three cases had seminoma (one Stage IVC with bone metastases, HCG 14 000 IU l^{-1}; one stage IV with liver and lung metastases (>20) and one mediastinal tumor HCG > 16 000 IU l^{-1}). An additional nine patients had seminomatous elements seen in the primary tumor: one combined with MTT, five with MTU and three with MTI.

Staging investigations included full physical examination, assay of serum AFP and BHCG, chest X-ray and computerized tomography (CT) of the thorax and abdomen. Patients with multiple lung metastases (L3) or high serum HCG concentrations (>50 000 IU l^{-1}) or liver involvement (based on CT evidence) had central nervous system staging by CT of brain and by CSF marker analysis and cytology. Patients were then classified on the Royal Marsden Hospital staging system and the eligible 'high risk' subgroup was defined by extent of disease and serum marker concentration (Stage IIC with AFP > 500 kU l^{-1} or HCG > 1000 IU l^{-1}, Stage IV L3, liver, bone or brain metastases, mediastinal primary, HCG $\geqslant$ 10 000 IU l^{-1}, AFP $\geqslant$ 5000 kU l^{-1}.

Details of the initial extents of disease are given in Table 22.2. Of the 82 patients, 83% had Stage IV disease, 44% advanced lung disease (>20 lung metastases), 16% bulky (>10 cm) abdominal disease and 37% visceral metastases. Serum HCG levels were elevated >1000 IU l^{-1} in 51% and AFP > 1000 IU l^{-1} in 33% of patients respectively.

The intensive induction chemotherapy regimen (Fig. 22.1) consisted of cisplatin 20 mg m^{-2} d^{-1}, days 1–5 (total 100 mg m^{-2}), vincristine 2 mg IV on day 1 and bleomycin 15 units IV on day 1 for weeks 1 and 3. For weeks 2 and 4, cisplatin 40 mg m^{-2} with vincristine 2 mg was given on day 1, with a continuous 5-day infusion of bleomycin 15 units per 24 h on days 1 to 5 (total 75 units).

Table 22.2   Initial extent of disease in 82 patients

		Number of patients		
		BOP–BEP	C–BOP–BEP	%
Stage	IIB/C	3	2	6
	IIIC	1	1	2
	IV	54	14	83
Primary mediastinum		3	4	9
Lung metastases >20		27	9	44
Abdominal disease >10 cm		10	3	16
Visceral metastases	Liver	14	3	21
	Bone	7	3	10
	Brain	8	1	10
	Other*	7	1	10
Tumor markers	AFP >1000	20	7	33
	HCG >1000	34	8	51

* Skin × 2, bladder, kidney, intracardiac, extensive pleural.
AFP, alpha-fetoprotein.
HCG, human chorionic gonadotrophin.

Cisplatin was given with hydration (1 liter of 1 mol l^{-1} saline plus 20 mmol l^{-1} KCl every 6 hours) and 200 ml of 10% mannitol for 30 min prior to cisplatin. Magnesium supplementation (20 mM MgCl L^{-1}) was prescribed during infusion chemotherapy and hydrocortisone 100 mg IV was given 12-hourly during bleomycin infusions. Vincristine 2 mg and bleomycin 15 units IV were given on weeks 5 and 6, to be followed by three 21-day cycles of BEP chemotherapy (Peckham *et al.*, 1983), which commenced on week 7. Patients entered into the protocol between January 1985 and April 1986 received 30-unit rather than 15-unit doses of bleomycin in their induction therapy; the incidence of bleomycin lung was substantial (see below) and subsequently 15-unit doses were used in both the induction and subsequent phase of treatment with BEP. From August 1988, 12 patients with either trophoblastic tumors and multiple lung metastases or brain metastases received additional treatment with high dose methotrexate. A dose of 1 g m^{-2} was given 24 hours prior to cisplatin during weeks 2 and 4 of treatment, followed by folinic acid rescue

(15 mg 4-hourly × 6 or as determined by serum methotrexate levels) with additional intrathecal methotrexate (10 mg) during weeks 1, 3, 5 and 6. We have subsequently treated 21 patients between August 1989 and January 1992 adding carboplatin during weeks 2 and 4 of the intensive induction schedule (Horwich *et al.*, 1993, 1994). The initial 13 patients were given doses calculated to achieve an AUC (area under the serum concentration/time curve) of 2 mg ml × minutes and in the remaining eight patients 3 mg ml^{-1} × minutes according to the dose calculations of Calvert and colleagues (Calvert *et al.*, 1989). The etoposide dose has also been increased to give 100 mg m^{-2} for 5 days during the three cycles of BEP.

Patients with brain metastases received whole brain irradiation to a dose of 40 Gy in 20 fractions, with a further 10 Gy boost to solitary lesions. Radiotherapy was commenced during weeks 5 and 6 of chemotherapy, but interrupted during subsequent courses of chemotherapy, which were given at the usual time. Residual masses were resected whenever possible in patients with normal serum markers after completion of chemotherapy.

22.5 RESULTS

Fifty-seven of the 61 patients treated with BOP–BEP schedule are evaluable for response. Two patients died from overwhelming sepsis during the first month of chemotherapy (see below); postmortem examination showed extensive necrosis with no viable tumor in either case. An additional two patients treated with the higher initial doses of bleomycin developed fatal lung toxicity 12 and 14 weeks after commencement of treatment, whilst in complete marker remission and with regressing tumor masses. All cases were included in the cause-related survival analysis. Two patients dying from intercurrent illness (suicide in an AIDS patient and pulmonary infection in a cystic fibrosis patient, both 16 months post-treatment) were censured at the time of death. Response to chemotherapy was judged both radiologically and by tumor marker assay. Nineteen patients (32%) had a complete remission with chemotherapy alone and a further 20 (34%) after resection of residual masses. Thirteen patients had persistent masses with negative tumor markers. Overall 54 out of 61 (89%) cases became marker negative. Only two recurrences (5%) have occurred in the 39 patients entering complete remission, with or without surgery, with a total of eight recurrences (15%) out of the 54 patients having complete tumor marker remission. Seven out of these eight recurrences occurred 6–8 months after the commencement of chemotherapy; the remaining one occurred at 18 months in a patient who was found to have sarcomatous change in an expanding pulmonary lesion, partially removed at thoracotomy. None of the five patients who failed to achieve marker remission has been salvaged, but two out of eight patients who recurred after entering marker remission have been rendered disease free with combined modality treatment using high dose carboplatin/etoposide or *cis*-platinum/ifosfamide chemotherapy, surgical resections of liver and lung

masses and radiotherapy to recurrent cerebral and pulmonary disease. These two patients remain without active disease 12 and 26 months respectively after recurrence. Overall, 43 patients (71%) are alive and disease free, 11 (18%) have died from recurrent teratoma, 5 (8%) from chemotherapy-related toxicity and 2 (3%) from intercurrent illness. The actuarial 2-year cause-related survival is 67% (Fig. 22.2).

Of the 21 patients treated with intensified C–BOP schedule, 18 remain continuously free from progressive disease. One patient who had had carboplatin-based chemotherapy (GFR at presentation 81 ml min^{-1}) died from neutropenic sepsis during week 12 of treatment. No viable tumor was found at postmortem. A further patient developed progressive disease and declined further treatment. He died 12 months after completing chemotherapy. The third patient remained with multiple large cystic masses postchemotherapy but, despite a marker relapse, has been disease free for 2 years after salvage radiotherapy and extensive surgery to remove all demonstrable disease. The overall survival of these patients is shown in Fig. 22.3, 2-year overall survival rates being 90% and failure-free survival 86%.

22.6 TOXICITY OF TREATMENT (TABLE 22.3)

The intensive induction phase of treatment was generally well tolerated. Most patients experienced a degree of nausea and vomiting during the first 24 hours of cisplatin infusions, but symptoms were substantially controlled with high dose dexamethasone, maxolon and lorazepam. The major hematological toxicity was of myelosuppression, which was maximal in weeks 6 or 9 of treatment. Of the 49 patients treated with the BOP–BEP regimen, 28% had a nadir total white cell count (WBC) <1.0 at some time during treatment; 18% had neutropenic fevers with two (5%) septic deaths. The

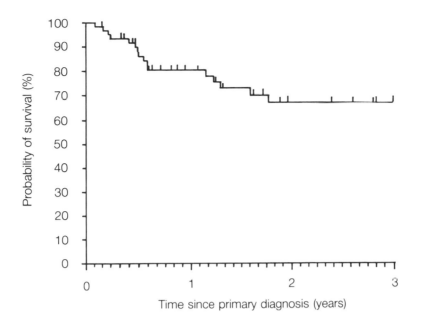

Fig. 22.2 Cause-related survival of patients with high risk NSGCT treated with BOP–BEP chemotherapy.

addition of high dose methotrexate in 12 patients increased toxicity, 45% of patients having a nadir WBC < 1.0, and 27% had neutropenic fever with one septic death. Two of the infective deaths occurred in patients who presented in a moribund condition having neglected febrile episodes whilst outside hospital, and the third man developed an overwhelming pneumococcal and candidal respiratory infection during his third week of chemotherapy, which failed to response to appropriate antibiotics. The C–BOP schedule also increased myelotoxicity. Seven patients (33%) had episodes of neutropenic sepsis and there was one septic death.

Mucositis was infrequent and mild using the BOP regimen but Grade 2 toxicity was noted in seven and Grade 3 toxicity in two of the 12 patients treated with additional methotrexate. Bleomycin lung toxicity was seen in six out of 16 (38%) patients treated with the higher 30-unit doses (total dose 450 units) of bleomycin, and was fatal in two cases. A further patient recovered following treatment

with high doses of corticosteroids and the remaining three patients had radiological evidence of pneumonitis but remained asymptomatic. Of the 65 patients treated using 15-unit doses (total dose 345 units) only two had symptomatic pneumonitis; radiological changes were present in a further two cases, but there were no fatalities.

Kidney function was assessed using clearance of chromium-51 labelled ethylenediamine tetra-acetic acid (Cr-51-EDTA). The mean initial clearance pretreatment was 143 ml min^{-1} (range 41–200 ml min^{-1}) and fell to 83 ml min^{-1} (range 26–147 ml min^{-1}), representing a mean fall to 58% of pretreatment values. Overall 21% of patients had a >50% reduction of clearance and 16% had a final Cr-51-EDTA clearance of <60 ml min^{-1}. In 16 patients carboplatin was substituted for cisplatin owing to falls in renal clearance.

Severe peripheral neuropathy developed in four patients, with slow recovery following completion of chemotherapy, and one patient developed transient steatorrhea and mal-

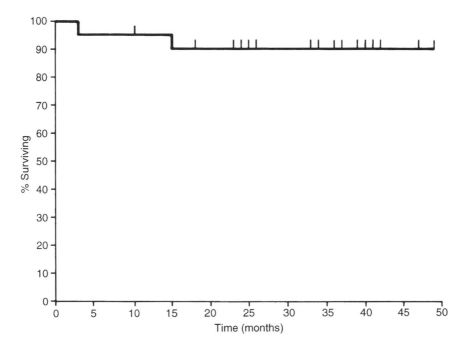

Fig. 22.3   Overall survival of patients with high risk NSGCT treated with C–BOP–BEP chemotherapy. (Reproduced from Horwich *et al.* (1994) Accelerated chemotherapy for poor prognosis germ cell tumors, *Eur. J. Cancer*, **30A** (11) 1607–11, with kind permission from Elsevier Science Ltd, The Boulevard, Langford Lane, Kidlington OX5 1GB, UK.)

absorption that rapidly resolved after treatment.

22.7   DISCUSSION

Intensive induction chemotherapy using platinum, vincristine and bleomycin was first described by Wettlaufer *et al.* (1984), who reported a 93% complete response rate in 29 patients with 'high risk' disease (advanced abdominal Stage B₃ or Stage C). Surgical resection of residual masses was undertaken after seven weekly cycles of treatment followed by consolidation chemotherapy using three courses of cisplatin, actinomycin-D and vincristine in most patients; an 83% overall survival was found with a median follow-up of 31 months. Favorable results have subsequently been reported in single arm studies using similar intensive weekly treatment

regimens in both poor risk as well as more favorable cases. Murray *et al.* (1987) found an 85% survival rate in 16 patients with advanced disease defined by the Indiana staging system (Table 7.3, p. 91) and Daniels *et al.* (1987) reported a 90% control rate in 45 unselected patients using six weekly courses of platinum, etoposide, vincristine and bleomycin. Our own approach (Horwich *et al.* 1989) has been to modify the original Wettlaufer regimen, adding three courses of BEP chemotherapy (Peckham *et al.*, 1983) after the intensive induction period. Patients have been selected on the basis of risk factors identified by the Medical Research Council (MRC) (Medical Research Council Working Party on Testicular Tumours, 1985; Mead *et al.*, 1992). Our results show an overall disease-free survival of 71% (2-year actuarial survival 67%), with 18% of deaths from

Table 22.3   Toxicity of intensive BOP induction chemotherapy

		No. of patients	WHO grade (maximum) %					Infective episodes %	Infective deaths %
			0	*1*	*2*	*3*	*4*		
1. Hematological									
BOP	WBC	49	2	20	40	24	28	18	5
	Plat	49	62	4	10	14	10		
BOP–MTX	WBC	12	0	9	18	27	45	27	8
	Plat	12	27	9	18	18	27		
C–BOP	WBC	21	0	24	24	29	24	33	5
	Plat	21	0	29	29	29	14		

2. Renal

Initial EDTA clearance (mean)	143 ml min^{-1} (41–200)
Final EDTA clearance (mean)	83 ml min^{-1} (26–147)
Final EDTA clearance <50% of pretreatment	21%
Final EDTA clearance <60 ml min^{-1}	16%

3. Pulmonary

	No. treated	Total	Bleomycin lung symptomatic	Fatal
Bleomycin dose 450 units (30 unit-doses)	16	6	4	2
Bleomycin dose 345 units (15 unit-doses)	66	4	2	0

disease, 8% from treatment-related complications and 3% from intercurrent illness, following the BOP schedule. The further intensification using C–BOP has given an 86% failure-free and 90% overall survival (Horwich *et al.*, 1994). These results are better than those previously achieved with BEP chemotherapy at the Royal Marsden Hospital, particularly for patients in the high risk MRC category (very large volume disease plus high markers) (Medical Research Council Working Party on Testicular Tumours, 1985) who had a 27% survival (Dearnaley *et al.*, 1988). Our patients have also been evaluated using prognostic criteria developed by other groups. Fifty-seven out of 61 cases treated with BOP fell into the Indiana high risk group (Birch *et al.*, 1986b) with a 67% survival. Nineteen out of 21 cases treated with C–BOP were in the Indiana University advanced disease category and 17 (89%) remain disease free 2 years after treatment. The majority of patients (61–97%) fell into the high risk categories as defined by other groups (Pizzocaro *et al.*, 1985; Daugaard

and Rørth, 1986; Newlands *et al.*, 1986; Schmoll *et al.*, 1987; Ozols *et al.*, 1988) but these classifications failed to stratify our patients further into high or low risk categories.

It has been proposed that chemotherapy dose and dose intensity are of major importance in determining the outcome of chemotherapy treatment (Frei and Canellos, 1980). The most detailed studies have been undertaken by Hryniuk and colleagues (Hryniuk and Bush, 1984; Levin and Hryniuk, 1987) who have retrospectively analyzed the chemotherapy given to patients with breast and ovarian cancers and in Hodgkin's disease (Carde *et al.*, 1983). Response rates correlated well with dose intensity, calculated by measuring the quantity of drugs administered per unit time compared with those given in standard regimens. The importance of dose–time factors in chemotherapy has been discussed by Dembo (1987). Increases in dose intensity of treatment can be achieved either by increasing the dosage per course and keeping the interval between treatment constant or by increasing the frequency of courses and keeping the doses constant. If there is a very steep dose–response curve then the former approach is attractive. However, if failure results from significant tumor proliferation during the period of treatment and the dose–response curve is shallow then smaller frequent doses may provide a better strategy. There is relatively little information available concerning dose and dose intensity for germ cell tumors. In a randomized study, Samson *et al.* (1984) demonstrated that, in combination with vinblastine and bleomycin, increasing the dose of cisplatin from 75 mg m^{-2} to 120 mg m^{-2} improved survival from 59% to 83%. Further dose escalations of platinum have been made possible by the reduction of cisplatin renal toxicity by hydration with hypertonic saline. However, a randomized study by the SWOG (Nichols *et al.*, 1991) comparing standard BEP with the same regimen utilizing double dose cisplatin (200 mg m^{-2} per course) failed to show any benefit in response rate or survival and was associated with greater toxicity. It therefore appears that dose escalation of cisplatin above 100–120 mg m^{-2} appears unrewarding using 3-week treatment schedules. Retrospective reviews have shown that dose reductions of vinblastine and bleomycin in the PVB regimen (Einhorn and Donohue, 1977) owing to myelosuppression or lung toxicity have no detrimental effect on survival (Levi *et al.*, 1989) and, similarly, modifications in the dosage of vincristine, bleomycin, actinomycin-D and cyclophosphamide have no effect on survival using the Charing Cross POMB/ACE regimen (Crawford *et al.*, 1989). However, this group suggested that reductions in the dosage of cisplatin, etoposide and methotrexate were associated with an increased risk of treatment failure. The Royal Marsden Hospital BEP regimen uses etoposide at a dose of 120 mg m^{-2} or 3 days. Although highly successful in the MRC low and intermediate risk categories, with 95% and 75% long-term survivals respectively (Peckham

et al., 1983, 1988; Dearnaley *et al.*, 1988), there was a suggestion that, in the highest risk group, the 27% survival is less satisfactory than that achieved with a dosage of 100 mg m^{-2} for 5 days as reported by other groups (Pizzocaro *et al.* 1985; Williams *et al.*, 1987a). In the randomized study of PVB versus BEP (Williams *et al.*, 1987a) prolongation of treatment intervals of >7 days was associated with a significantly higher risk of disease recurrence and reduced survival (Birch *et al.*, 1986a), thus giving support to the idea that dose frequency as well as total dose is important in determining treatment efficacy.

The total dose and dose intensity of cisplatin, etoposide and bleomycin for regimens used in high risk disease are shown in Table 22.4. Compared with BEP, the intensive induction weekly schedules can achieve a 40–100% increase in platinum dose delivered during the first month of therapy. This is at the expense of substituting the nonmyelosuppressive vinca alkaloid vincristine for etoposide. Although weekly treatment with etoposide in addition to cisplatin, vincristine and bleomycin has been studied (HIPE regimen) (Murray *et al.*, 1987), the increase in bone marrow toxicity prevented any increase in dose intensity compared with standard BEP (Table 22.4). Overall bone marrow toxicity from the BOP–BEP schedule is quite similar to that from BEP with 28% of patients having nadir leukocyte counts <1000 mm^{-3} compared with 20%, and neutropenic fever occurring in 20% and 15% respectively. Similarly, thromboctyopenia (platelets <50 000 mm^{-3}) occurred slightly more often with the BOP–BEP regimen (24% versus 14%), although only 10% of patients had platelets <25 000 at any time. The alternative method of increasing dose intensity is by escalating chemotherapy dose (Daugaard and Rørth, 1986; Schmoll *et al.*, 1987; Ozols *et al.*, 1988) and keeping intervals between treatment constant (Chapter 21). A direct comparison with the more complex altern-

Table 22.4 Chemotherapy regimens for high risk NSGCT: dose and dose intensity

Regimen	Duration	Total dose in 12 wks CP mg m⁻²	VP16 mg m⁻²	BLE units	Mean dose/wk, wk 1–4 CP mg m⁻²	VP16 mg m⁻²	BLE units	Overall mean dose/wk CP mg m⁻²	VP16 mg m⁻²	BLE mg	Reference
BEP[46,63]	10	400	2000	360	50	250	30	40	200	30	Pizzocaro et al., 1985; Williams et al., 1987b
Intensive Induction											
BOP BEP	13	540	1080	345	70	0	45	42	83	25	Horwich et al., 1989
CBOP–BEP	13	666*	1500	345	100*	0	45	51*	115	25	Horwich et al., 1993, 1994
BOP	7	440	0	480	80	0	90	63	0	69	Wettlaufer et al., 1984
HIPE	9	486	1314	210	54	146	23	54	146	23	Murray et al., 1987
Alternating											
POMB ACE	13+	480	1500	120	60	0	15	37	115	9	Newlands et al., 1983
CISCA VB	13+	360	1000°	300	30	250°	38	28	77°	23	Logothetis et al., 1986
BOP VIP	12	600	900	90	75	0	18	50	75	8	Kaye et al., 1995
PVB BEP	10	400	1720	360	50	225	30	40	172	30	Stoter et al., 1986
VAB–6 EP	20	600	2100°	450	44	150°	30	33	75°	23	Bosl et al., 1987
High Dose											
PEB	7	600	3000	270	100	500	38	86	428	30	Daugaard & Rørth, 1986
PEB	10	700	2400	360	88	300	38	70	240	30	Schmoll et al., 1987
PVeBV	7	600	2490°	270	100	415°	38	86	355°	30	Ozols et al., 1988
Growth factors + stem cell support											
IPE (Standard)	10	400	1500	24*	50	188	3*	40	150	2.4*	Nichols et al., 1995
IPE (GSF)	10	600	4000	32*	75	500	4*	60	400	3.2	Bokemeyer et al., 1994
IPE (stem cells + GCSF)	10	600	5000	40*	75	625	5*	60	500	4	Bokemeyer et al., 1995

* Approximate equivalence taking carboplatin AUC 3 as similar to cisplatin 60 mg m⁻².

° Approximate equivalence taking 0.15 mg kg⁻¹. Vinblastine Days 1–2 as similar to 100 mg m⁻². VP16 Days 1–5.

Additional drugs. Total/mean weekly doses m⁻²: (* total doses). BOP-BEP. VCR 12 mg/1 mg*: BOP VCR 14 mg/2 mg*: HIPE VCR 7 mg/0.8 mg: POMB ACE VCR 4 mg/MTX1200 mg/160 mg. Act D 2.25 mg/0.18 mg*, CY 1500 mg/125 mg: CISCA VB Adr 240 mg/20 mg. BOP VIP VCR 6 mg/0.5 mg. IF 15 g/1.25 mg: VA: Act D 3.0 mg/0.15 mg, CY 1800 mg/90 mg.

Abbreviations: CP = cisplatin, BLE = bleomycin, VCR = vincristine, MTX = methotrexate, Act D = actinomycin, CY = cyclophosphamide, Adr = adriamycin, IF = ifosfamide.

ating multiagent chemotherapy programs (Chapter 23) is difficult. Those using 3- or 4-weekly schedules (BEP–PVB, VAB–6–EP, Table 22.4) at standard intensity found similar myelotoxicity as BEP and have shown no increase in response rates when compared with standard regimens (Stoter *et al.*, 1986; Bosl *et al.*, 1987). The other alternating schedules (POMB–ACE, CISCA–VB, BOP–VIP) not only introduce additional chemotherapy agents but also have more frequent programs of drug administration. However, the Charing Cross (POMB–ACE) (Newlands *et al.*, 1986; Hitchins *et al.*, 1989) and M.D. Anderson (CISCA–VB) (Logothetis *et al.*, 1986) groups have reported impressive results with 82% and 83% long-term survival for patients with high risk disease. The contribution to the success of these regimens from case selection, increased frequency of drug administration, alternation of drug schedules or the individual chemotherapy agents remains uncertain. The preliminary results of the MRC/EORTC trial comparing BEP with BOP–VIP, which included 380 patients, has shown no advantage for the hybrid regimen. Complete response was seen in 59% and 58% of patients treated with BEP and BOP–VIP respectively and, with a median follow-up of 1.5 years, 26% and 33% of patients respectively had developed disease progression (Kaye *et al.*, 1995). In this study the incidence of treatment modification, granulocytopenic fever and toxic death were significantly reduced by the use of G-CSF (Filgrastim) (Fosså *et al.*, 1995).

There are major limitations to comparing the results of different chemotherapy series because of the differences in criteria for patient selection (Bajorin *et al.*, 1988), as well as the variable lengths of follow-up between different series and the different methods used for reporting survival results (Chapter 7). During the last decade, improved treatment results have been obtained in successive cohorts of patients of similar clinical stage and marker level using the same chemotherapy drug combinations. This improvement of prognosis has been ascribed to more appropriate use of chemotherapy and postchemotherapy surgery (Merrin, 1980; Einhorn, 1986), but further restricts the value of comparison between nonrandomized series. The survival results do not convincingly demonstrate an advantage for regimens using drugs at increased total dose or dose intensity, nor for the use of additional agents in alternating schedules over the 'standard' BEP regimen (Williams *et al.*, 1987a). Although there are sound biological reasons for believing that the rapid proliferation rate of some testicular teratomas may be an important contributory factor leading to failure of control following standard cytotoxic chemotherapy, approaches modifying both the total dose and dose intensity of active agents need to be carefully evaluated in additional prospective randomized studies.

Further escalation of dose intensity will require use of hematopoetic growth factors or bone marrow/peripheral stem cell support to avoid excessive drug-induced myelosuppression. Although the addition of ifosfamide to cisplatin and etoposide (IPE) in first line treatment has shown no advantage compared with BEP (Nichols *et al.*, 1995), the German Testicular Cancer Study Group has shown that dose intensity of this three-drug regimen may be increased by a factor of 1.4 using growth factor support. Dose-limiting toxicity was severe mucositis/enteritis and prolonged thrombocytopenia (Bokemeyer *et al.*, 1994). Further studies of G-CSF in conjunction with peripheral blood stem cell rescue have been made and in a careful ongoing Phase I/II dose escalation protocol, which has now included 118 patients, etoposide dose per course has reached 1250 mg m^{-2} and ifosfamide dose per course of 10 g m^{-2}. Overall 2-year survival and event-free survival rates of 72% and 68% have been reported with acceptable morbidity in patients with poor risk presentations (Bokemeyer *et al.*, 1995).

Such treatment intensification programs have not yet been proven to improve survival in patients with adverse presentations from germ cell tumors. However, these new approaches do appear promising, but need to be carefully evaluated in prospective randomized studies so as to be able to balance the risks from increased treatment morbidity against any improvements in tumor control.

REFERENCES

Bajorin, D., Katz, A. *et al.* (1988) Comparison of criteria for assigning germ cell tumour patients to 'good risk' and 'poor risk' studies. *J. Clin. Oncol.*, **6**(5), 786–92.

Birch, R., Loehrer, P., *et al.* (1986a) The effect of delay of therapy on response to cisplatin chemotherapy in disseminated germ cell tumors. The Southeastern Cancer Group (SEG) experience (abstract). *Proc. ASCO*, **5**, 409.

Birch, R., Williams, S., *et al.* (1986b) Prognostic factors for favorable outcome in disseminated germ cell tumors. *J. Clin. Oncol.*, **4**(3), 400–7.

Bokemeyer, C., Harstrick, A., *et al.* (1994) The role of granulocyte-macrophage colony-stimulating factor in the treatment of germ cell tumors. *Sem. Oncol.*, **21**(6) (Suppl. 16)), 57–63.

Bokemeyer, C., Harstrick, A., *et al.* (1995) Sequential treatment with high-dose VIP-chemotherapy plus peripheral blood stem cell (PBSC) support in advanced germ cell cancer. *Proc. ASCO*, **14**, 230.

Bosl, G.J., Geller, N.L., *et al.* (1983) Multivariate analysis of prognostic variables in patients with metastatic testicular cancer. *Cancer Res.*, **43**, 3403–7.

Bosl, G.J., Geller, N.L., *et al.* (1987) Alternating cycles of etoposide plus cisplatin and VAB-6 in the treatment of poor-risk patients with germ cell tumors. *J. Clin. Oncol.*, **5**(3), 436–40.

Calvert, A.H., Newell, D.R., *et al.* (1989) Carboplatin dosage: Prospective evaluation of a simple formula based on renal function. *J. Clin. Oncol.*, **7**, 1748–56.

Carde, P., Mackintosh, F.R., *et al.* (1983) A dose and time response analysis of the treatment of Hodkin's disease with MOPP chemotherapy. *J. Clin. Oncol.*, **1**, 146–53.

Costa, G. and Hreshchyshyn, M.M., (1962) Initial clinical studies with vincristine. *Cancer Chemother. Rep.*, **42**, 45–8.

Crawford, S.M., Newlands, E.S., *et al.* (1989) The effect of intensity of administered treatment on the outcome of germ cell tumours treated with POMB/ACE chemotherapy. *Bri. J. Cancer*, **59**, 243–26.

Daniels, J.R., Russell, C., *et al.* (1987) Malignant germinal neoplasms: Intensive weekly chemotherapy with cisplatin, vincristine, bleomycin and etoposide (abstract). *Proc. ASCO*, **6**, 104.

Daugaard, G. and Rørth, M., (1986) High-dose cisplatin and VP-16 with bleomycin, in the management of advanced metastatic germ cell tumors. *Eur. J. Cancer Clin. Oncol.*, **22**, 477–85.

Dearnaley, D.P., Nicholls, J., *et al.* (1988) BEP chemotherapy for metastatic teratoma: Royal Marsden Hospital experience 1979–1986 (abstract). *Br. J. Cancer*, **58**, 526.

Dembo, A.J. (1987) Time-dose factors in chemotherapy: expanding the concept of dose-intensity. *J. Clin. Oncol.*, **5**, 694–6.

Einhorn, L.H. (1986) Have new aggressive chemotherapy regimes improved results in advanced germ cell tumours? *Eur. J. Cancer*, **22**, 1289–93.

Einhorn, L.H. and Donohue, J.P., (1977) Cis-diamminedicholoroplatinum, vinblastine and bleomycin chemotherapy for disseminated testicular cancer. *Ann. Intern. Med.*, **87**, 293–8.

Fosså, S., Kaye, S.B., *et al.* (1995) An MRC/EORTC randomised trial in poor prognosis metastatic teratoma comparing treatment with/without filgrastim (G-CSF) (abstract). *Proc. ASCO*, **14**, 245.

Fosså, S.D., Pettersen, E.O., *et al.* (1985) DNA flow cytometry in human testicular cancer. *Cancer Lett.*, **28**, 55–60.

Fowler, J.F. (1989). Fractionation and therapeutic gain, in *Biological Basis of Radiotherapy*, 2nd edn, (eds G.G. Steel, G.E. Adams and A. Horwich), Elsevier Science Publishers, Amsterdam, pp. 181–207.

Frei, E. and Canellos, G.P., (1980) Dose: A critical factor in cancer chemotherapy. *Am. J. Med.*, **69**, 585–94.

Hitchins, R.N., Newlands, E.S., *et al.* (1989) Long-term outcome in patients with germ cell tumours treated with POMB/ACE chemotherapy: comparison of commonly used classification systems of good and poor prognosis. *Br. J. Cancer*, **59**, 236–42.

Horwich, A. (1989) Germ cell tumour chemotherapy. *Br. J. Cancer*, **59**(2), 156–9.

Horwich, A., Brada, M., *et al.* (1989) Intensive induction chemotherapy for poor risk non-seminomatous germ cell tumours. *Eur. J. Cancer*, **25**(2), 177–84.

Horwich, A., Dearnaley, D.P., *et al.* (1994) Accelerated chemotherapy for poor prognosis germ cell tumours. *Eur. J. Cancer*, **30A**(11), 1607–11.

Horwich, A., Duchesne, G., *et al.* (1988) Accelerated fractionation (AF) for bladder cancer (abstract). *Br. J. Cancer*, **58**, 526.

Horwich, A., Wilson, C., *et al.* (1993) Increasing the dose intensity of chemotherapy in poor-prognosis metastatic non-seminoma. *Eur. Urol.*, **23**(1), 219–22.

Hryniuk, W. and Bush, H., (1984) The importance of dose intensity in chemotherapy of metastatic breast cancer. *J. Clin. Oncol.*, **2**, 1281–8.

Kaye, S.B., Mead, G.M., *et al.* (1995) An MRC/EORTC randomised trial in poor prognosis metastatic teratoma comparing BEP with BOP-VIP (abstract). *Proc. ASCO*, **14**, 246.

Levi, J.A., Thomson, D., *et al.* (1989) Dose intensity and outcome with combination chemotherapy for germ cell carcinoma. *Eur. J. Cancer Clin. Oncol.*, **25**, 1073–7.

Levin, L. and Hryniuk, W.M., (1987) Dose intensity analysis of chemotherapy regimens in ovarina carcinoma. *J. Clin. Oncol.*, **5**, 756–7.

Logothetis, C.J., Samuels, M.L., *et al.* (1986) Cyclic chemotherapy with cyclophosphamide, doxorubicin and cisplatin plus vinblastine and bleomycin in advanced germinal tumors. *Am. J. Med.*, **81**, 219–28.

Malaise, E.P., Chavaudra, N., *et al.* (1974) Relationship between the growth rate of human metastases, survival and pathological type. *Eur. J. Cancer*, **10**, 451–9.

Mead, G.M. on behalf of the IGCCCG (1995) International consensus prognostic classification for metastatic germ cell tumours treated with platinum based chemotherapy; final report of the International Germ Cell Cancer Collaborative Group (IGCCCG) (abstract). *Proc. ASCO*, **14**, 235.

Mead, G.M., Stenning, S.P., *et al.* (1992) The second Medical Research Council study of prognostic factors in nonseminomatous germ cell tumours. *J. Clin. Oncol.*, **10**(1), 85–94.

Medical Research Council Working Party on Testicular Tumours (1985) Prognostic factors in advanced non-seminomatous germ-cell testicular tumours: results of a multicentre study. *Lancet*, **i**, 8–11.

Merrin, C. (1980) Combined chemotherapy and cytoreductive surgery for the treatment of advanced testes tumors: 6 years follow-up in 77 patients. (abstract). *Proc. ASCO*, **21**, 400.

Murray, P.O.M., De Vries, E.G.E., *et al.* (1987)

Weekly high intensity cisplatin etoposide (HIPE) for far advanced germ cell cancer (GCC) (abstract). *Proc. ASCO*, **6**, 101.

Newlands, E.S., Bagshawe, K.D., *et al.* (1986) Current optimum mangement of anaplastic germ cell tumors of the testis and other sites. *Br. J. Urol.*, **58**(3), 307–14.

Newlands, E.S., Begent, R.H., *et al.* (1983) Further advances in the management of malignant teratomas of the testis and other sites. *Lancet*, **I**, 948–51.

Nichols, C., Loehrer, P.J., *et al.* (1995) Phase III Study of cisplatin, etoposide and bleomycin (PVP16B) or etoposide, ifosfamide and cisplatin (VIP) in advanced stage germ cell tumors: An intergroup trial. *Proc. ASCO*, **14**, 239.

Nichols, C.R., Williams, S.D., *et al.* (1991) Randomized study of cisplatin dose intensity of advanced germ cell tumors. *J. Clin. Oncol.*, **9**, 1163–72.

Ozols, R.F., Ihde, D.C., *et al.* (1988) A randomized trial of standard chemotherapy v. a high-dose chemotherapy regimen in the treatment of poor prognosis nonseminomatous germ-cell tumors. *J. Clin. Oncol.*, **6**, 1031–40.

Peckham, M.J., Barrett, A., *et al.* (1983) The treatment of metastatic germ-cell testicular tumours with bleomycin, etoposide and cisplatin (BEP). *Br. J. Cancer*, **47** 613–19.

Peckham, M.J., Horwich, A., *et al.* (1988) The management of advanced testicular teratoma. *Br. J. Urol.*, **62**(1), 63–8.

Pizzocaro, G., Piva, L., *et al.* (1985) Cisplatin, etoposide, bleomycin first-line therapy and early resection of residual tumor in far-advanced germinal testis cancer. *Cancer*, **56**, 2411–15.

Price, P., Hogan, S.J., *et al.* (1990) The growth factor of metastatic nonseminomatous germ cell testicular tumours measured by marker production doubling time – II. Prognostic significance in patients treated by chemotherapy. *Eur. J. Cancer*, **26**(4), 453–7.

Price, P., Hogan, S.J., *et al.* (1988) Tumour proliferation rate as a predictive factor in testicular teratomas. *Br. J. Cancer*, **59**, 525–6.

Rabes, H.M. (1987) Proliferation of human testicular tumours. *Int. J. Androl.*, **10**, 127–37.

Samson, M.K., Rivkin, S.E., *et al.* (1984) Dose–response and dose–survival advantaged for high versus low-dose cisplatin combined with vinblastine and bleomycin in disseminated testicular cancer. A Southwest Oncology Group study. *Cancer*, **53**(5), 1029–35.

Samuels, M.L., Holoye, P.Y., *et al.* (1975) Bleomycin combination chemotherapy in the management of testicular neoplasia. *Cancer*, **36**, 318–26.

Saunders, M.I., Dische, S., *et al.* (1989) Continuous hyperfractionated accelerated radiotherapy in locally advanced carcinoma of the head and neck region. *Int. J. Rad. Oncol., Biol., Phys.*, **17**(6), 1287–93.

Schmoll, H.J., Schubert, I., *et al.* (1987) Disseminated testicular cancer with bulky disease: Results of a phase II study with cisplatin ultra high dose/VP-16/bleomycin. *Int. J. Androl.*, **10**, 311–17.

Shaw, R.K. and Bruner, J.A., (1964) Clinical evaluation of vincristine (NSC-67574). *Cancer Chemother. Rep.*, **42**, 45–8.

Silvestrini, R., Costa, A., *et al.* (1985) Cell kinetics in human germ cell tumors of the testis, in *Testicular Cancer and Other Tumors of the Genitourinary Tract*, (eds M. Pavone–Macaluss, P.H. Smith and M.A. Bagshaw), Plenum Publishing Corp, New York and London, 55–62.

Sledge, G.W., Eble, J.N., *et al.* (1988) Relation of proliferative activity to survival in patients with advanced germ cell cancer. *Cancer Res.*, **48**, 3864–8.

Steel, G.G. (1977). *The Growth Kinetics of Tumours*, Clarendon Press, Oxford.

Stoter, G., Kaye, S., *et al.* (1986) Preliminary results of BEP (bleomycin, etoposide, cisplatin) versus an alternating regimen of BEP and PVB (cisplatin, vinblastine, bleomycin) in high volume metastatic (HVM) testicular non-seminomas. An EORTC study (abstract). *Proc. ASCO*, **5**, 106.

Stoter, G., Sylvester, R., *et al.* (1987) Multivariate analysis of prognostic factors in patients with disseminated nonseminomatous testicular cancer: Results from a European Organization for Research on Treatment of Cancer multiinstitutional phase III study. *Cancer Res.*, **47**, 2714–18.

Tubiana, M. (1982), 'L.H. Gray Medal Lecture: Cell kinetics and radiation oncology. *Int. J. Rad. Oncol., Biol., Phys.*, **8**, 1471–89.

Wettlaufer, J.N., Feiner, A.S., *et al.* (1984) Vincristine, cisplatin and bleomycin with surgery in the management of advanced metastatic non-seminomatous testis tumors. *Cancer*, **53**, 203–9.

Williams, S.D., Birch, R., *et al.* (1987a) Treatment of disseminated germ-cell tumors with cisplatin, bleomycin and either vinblastine or etoposide. *N. Engl. J. Med.*, **316**(23), 1435–40.

Williams, S.D., Stablein, D.M., *et al.* (1987b) Immediate adjuvant chemotherapy versus observation with treatment at relapse in pathological stage II testicular cancer. *N. Engl. J. Med.*, **317**(23), 1433–8.

ALTERNATING REGIMENS TO OVERCOME DRUG RESISTANCE IN POOR RISK GERM CELL TUMOR PATIENTS

R. de Wit and G. Stoter

23.1 INTRODUCTION

The rationale for alternating administration of different chemotherapy combinations is based on the theoretical consideration that a given tumor mass contains cell populations which are sensitive to one combination, but resistant to the other, and vice versa. Such drug resistance can either exist before any antitumor pharmacotherapy (natural resistance), or develop during systemic therapy (acquired resistance) as a result of biochemical modulation or genetic mutation (Zijlstra, de Vries and Mulder, 1987; Bosl *et al.*, 1989).

Until 15 years ago, metastatic germ cell tumors were mostly incurable, despite the initial sensitivity of this type of cancer to a wide variety of drugs (Anderson, 1979). The introduction of cisplatin in 1974 has changed this situation completely. The mere addition of cisplatin to the combination of vinblastine and bleomycin – the most effective combination in the early seventies – has rendered germ cell cancer into a potentially curable disease. This three-drug combination yields disease-free 10-year survival rates of 60–70% Williams *et al.*, 1987; Stoter *et al.*, 1989). It has become clear that patients who do not

respond to any form of (salvage) therapy, and die of progressive disease, usually have extensive disease, i.e. a large volume of metastatic tumor (Rodenburg and Stoter, 1988). It has recently been shown that the substitution of VP-16–213 (a podophyllotoxin) for vinblastine is more effective, particularly in poor prognosis patients with extensive tumor burden (Williams *et al.*, 1987).

The relationship between tumor burden and drug resistance can be explained by a mathematical model developed by Goldie and colleagues (Goldie, Coldman and Gudauskas, 1982; Goldie and Coldman, 1984). They have demonstrated that the graphical depiction of the development of drug resistance takes a sigmoid form, in which the tumor turns from completely sensitive to almost completely resistant in a relatively small margin of proliferation. The absolute time to the development of complete drug resistance is thus dependent on the mutation rate, which appears to be approximately $1:10^6$ cells (K. Nooter, personal communication). The theory of Goldie and Coldman has formed the basis for the application of noncross-resistant chemotherapy regimens. In the face of present

Testicular Cancer: Investigation and management. Second edition. Edited by Professor A. Horwich.
Published in 1996 by Chapman & Hall. ISBN 0 412 61210 0.

knowledge about the multiple aspects of drug resistance mechanisms, this theory is bound to be a simplification of the reality (Schabel *et al.*, 1980). Increased efflux of drugs from the tumor cell (Pastan and Gottesman, 1987), defects in transmembrane influx (Zijlstra, de Vries and Mulder, 1987), accelerated metabolism and detoxification (de Graeff, Slebos and Rodenhuis, 1988), increased DNA repair and decreased DNA binding (Fichtinger-Schepman *et al.*, 1987; de Graeff, Slebos and Rodenhuis, 1988), as well as intrinsic genetic abnormalities (Bosl *et al.*, 1989) may be involved in various combinations. To overcome these problems, different treatment strategies should be investigated including increased doses of chemotherapeutic drugs (Peckham, 1988), the use of competitive compounds to block membrane molecules responsible for drug efflux (Pastan and Gottesman, 1987; Nooter *et al.*, 1988), addition of new drugs to conventional treatment schemes, and alternating chemotherapy regimens (Peckham, 1988).

In the case of germ cell cancer no clear insight exists to explain the cause(s) of eventual drug resistance. It is likely that natural resistance is the main factor since this type of cancer is rapidly proliferating and the duration of chemotherapy is short, i.e. 3–4 months (Williams *et al.*, 1987; Stoter *et al.*, 1989). These considerations favor the approach with alternating chemotherapy with different combinations. A summary of clinical studies using this strategy are described below.

23.2 PHASE II STUDIES

Drug combinations in sequence have been explored at the Charing Cross Hospital with POMB/ACE chemotherapy (Newlands *et al.*, 1983). The chemotherapy schedules used are summarized in Table 23.1. Recently, an updated analysis concerning 206 patients treated between 1977 and 1988, was published (Hitchins *et al.*, 1989). One hundred and six out of 193 fully evaluable patients had large volume

Table 23.1 POMB/ACE regimen

POMB
Day 1: vincristine 1 mg m^{-2} IV; methotrexate 300 mg m^{-2} as a 12-h infusion
Day 2: bleomycin 15 mg given as a 24-h infusion; folinic acid rescue started 24 h after the start of methotrexate, 15 mg 12-hourly for four doses
Day 3: bleomycin 15 mg as a 24-h infusion
Day 4: cisplatin 120 mg m^{-2} as a 12-h infusion, given together with hydration and 3 g magnesium sulphate supplementation

ACE
Etoposide 100 mg m^{-2} days 1–5
Actinomycin-D 0.5 mg IV days 3, 4 and 5
Cyclophosphamide 500 mg m^{-2} IV day 5

OMB
Day 1: vincristine 1 mg m^{-2} IV; methotrexate 300 mg m^{-2} as a 12-h infusion
Day 2: bleomycin 15 mg as a 24-h infusion; folinic acid rescue starts 24-h (after the start of methotrexate) 15 mg 12-hourly for four doses
Day 3: bleomycin 15 mg as a 24-h infusion

Treatment
Two courses of POMB are followed by ACE, then POMB is alternated with ACE until patients are in biochemical remission as measured by serum HCG and AFP levels. The usual number of courses of POMB has been 3–5. Following biochemical remission, ACE is alternated with OMB until the remission has been maintained for 12 weeks. The intervals between each course of chemotherapy has been kept to a minimum; usually 9–11 days.

---

metastatic disease (according to the Royal Marsden Hospital staging classification), i.e. Stage IIC (lymph node metastases >5 cm) or L3 (lung metastases >2 cm). These 106 patients with advanced disease had an overall survival of almost 80% (Hitchins *et al.*, 1989).

The efficacy of the POMB/ACE regimens was confirmed in a series of 60 patients with large or very large volume metastases (according to the Royal Marsden Hospital staging classification), resulting in a 5-year survival rate of about 70% (Cullen *et al.*, 1988). Toxicity included severe myelosuppression, resulting in septicemia in five cases, leading to death in one case. Overall, three patients died as a direct result of treatment. Troublesome mucositis, cisplatin-associated auditory problems and peripheral neuropathy (severe enough to stop treatment in two cases) were observed as well.

In 1985, Logothetis *et al.* reported 48 patients with advanced disease (according to M.D. Anderson criteria) treated with a combination of cyclophosphamide, doxorubicin and cisplatin (CISCA), and a combination of vinblastine and bleomycin (VB) (Table 23.2).

Forty-four patients (92%) achieved a complete response (CR). Similarly, an 85% durable CR rate was achieved in a series of 100 patients, as published 1 year later (Logothetis *et al.*, 1986). Although the toxicity (stomatitis,

Table 23.2 CISCA/VB regimen

CISCA
Cyclophosphamide 500 mg m^{-2} IV day 1+2
Doxorubicin (Adriamycin) 40 to 45 mg m^{-2} IV day 1+2
Cisplatin 100 to 120 mg m^{-2} as a 2-h infusion on day 3

VB
Vinblastine 3 mg m^{-2} IV days 1–5, continuously for 24 h
Bleomycin 30 mg IV days 1–5 simultaneously
VB is given after recovery from myelosuppression
(>2 × 10^9 l^{-1} granulocytes, >100 × 10^9 l^{-1} platelets)

Patients receive two courses of chemotherapy beyond a marker negative status

paralytic ileus, leukopenic fever) of this cyclic chemotherapy was formidable, only one of the 100 patients died as a result of the treatment. Bleomycin pulmonary toxicity (with a drop in vital capacity of more than 10%) was observed in only one case. According to the authors, this low incidence of pulmonary toxicity was based on the continuous infusion of bleomycin.

Bosl *et al.* (1987) reported a 6-month schedule of alternating cycles of etoposide plus cisplatin and VAB-6 (cyclophosphamide, vinblastine, actinomycin-D, bleomycin, cisplatin) in 41 poor risk patients (Table 23.3). All patients

Table 23.3 VAB-6 EP regimen

EP	
Etoposide 100 mg m^{-2} IV days 1–5	
Cisplatin 20 mg m^{-2} IV days 1–5	months 1, 3, 5
VAB-6	
Vinblastine 4 mg m^{-2} IV day 1	
Cyclophosphamide 600 mg m^{-2} IV day 1	
Actinomycin-D 1 mg m^{-2} IV day 1	months 2, 4, 6; no bleomycin in month 6
Bleomycin 30 mg IV day 1 – push	
Bleomycin 20 mg m^{-2} IV days 1–3 continuously	
Cisplatin 120 mg m^{-2} IV day 4 with forced diuresis	

Cycles are repeated every 4 weeks. Six alternating cycles of EP and VAB—6 are administered, starting with EP.

were considered to be poor risk using the criteria: (1) extragonadal non-seminomatous germ cell tumor or (2) testicular cancer with a probability of CR of < 0.5. The method for calculating the probability of CR is based on lactate dehydrogenase (LDH) and human chorionic gonadotrophin (HCG) levels and the number of metastatic sites. The durable overall CR rate was 37%. There were no treatment-related deaths in these 41 evaluable patients.

The response and survival of these patients were found to be identical to the results of 29 historical controls with poor risk germ cell tumors treated with VAB-6 alone at Memorial Sloan-Kettering Cancer Center. Thus, the 6-month schedule of VAB-6/EP was not superior over 3 months of VAB-6 alone, and was not recommended by the authors.

23.3 PHASE III STUDIES

In 1982, the EORTC embarked on a randomized study comparing four cycles of bleomycin/etoposide/cisplatin (BEP) versus an alternating regime of cisplatin/vinblastine/bleomycin (PVB) and BEP for a total of four cycles for patients with 'high volume' metastases (defined as lymph node metastases >5 cm or lung metastases >2 cm in diameter) (Stoter *et al.*, 1986) (Table 23.4).

Thirty-five out of 45 (78%) patients achieved CR to BEP and 33/43 (77%) to PVB/BEP. The PVB/BEP regimen proved to be more toxic with respect to bone marrow function and

neuromuscular symptoms. It was concluded that the alternating regimen of PVB/BEP did not yield a better CR rate than BEP (Stoter *et al.*, 1986).

In an updated analysis as of April 1994, 208 patients were fully evaluable (de Wit *et al.*, 1995). Of these, 76 out of 108 (72%) achieved CR to BEP and 78 out of 103 (76%) to PVB/BEP. Also the relapse rates were similar for both treatment groups: after an average follow-up of 6 years the relapse rates from CR were 16% on BEP and 12% on PVB/BEP. There were no significant differences in duration of survival between the two treatment groups. Bone marrow suppression proved to be more severe in the PVB/BEP arm. Leukocytopenia Grade IV was observed in 28% of the patients on PVB/BEP, whereas only 5% of the patients on BEP, had Grade IV leukocytopenia ($p < 0.001$). Similarly, thrombocytopenia Grade IV was observed in 10% following PVB/BEP and in 1% of the patients following BEP. In addition, granulocytopenic fever was noticed in 16% of the patients on the alternating arm, compared with 5% of the patients on BEP. Finally, there proved to be a higher incidence of neuropathy ($p < 0.001$) in the patients on the alternating regimen; 47% versus 25%, respectively. In conclusion, this study showed that an alternating regimen of PVB/BEP is not superior to BEP and that it was more myelo- and neurotoxic. In 1990, the MRC/EORTC initiated a randomized trial comparing standard therapy with six cycles of bleomycin 30 mg weekly × 12, etoposide 100 mg m^{-2} days 1 to 5 and cisplatin 20 mg m^{-2} days 1 to 5 (BEP) given 3-weekly, against three cycles of bleomycin 30 mg, vincristine 2 mg and cisplatin 50 mg m^{-2} days 1 and 2 (BOP) given every 10 days, followed by three cycles of etoposide 100 mg m^{-2} days 1, 3 and 5, ifosfamide 1 g m^{-2} days 1 to 5 and cisplatin 20 mg m^{-2} days 1 to 5 (VIP) given 3-weekly (Table 23.5). The BOP/VIP schedule incorporates rapid induction followed by potentially noncross-resistant chemotherapy, and had previously been tested in a pilot

Table 23.4 PVB/BEP regimen

PVB

Cisplatin 20 mg m^{-2} IV days 1–5
Vinblastine 0.15 mg kg^{-1} IV days 1+2 } at 3-week intervals
Bleomycin 30 mg IV days 2, 9, 16

BEP

Cisplatin 20 mg m^{-2} IV days 1–5
Etoposide 120 mg m^{-2} IV days 1, 3, 5 } at 3-week intervals
Bleomycin 30 mg IV days 2, 9, 16

Table 23.5 BOP/VIP regimen

BOP

Bleomycin 30 mg
Vincristine 2 mg } every 10 days
Cisplatin 50 mg m^{-2} days 1 + 2

VIP

Etoposide 100 mg m^{-2} days 1, 3, 5
Ifosfamide 1 g m^{-2} days 1–5 } at 3-week intervals
Cisplatin 20 mg m^{-2} days 1–5

study in 91 cases (Lewis *et al.*, 1991). Between January 1990 and June 1994 a total of 380 cases were randomized (Kaye *et al.*, 1995). Eligible patients had one or more of the following: liver/bone or brain metastases; BHCG $\geq$ 10 000 IU l^{-1} or AFP $\geq$ 1000 ku l^{-1}; lung metastases $\geq$ 20; lymph node mass $\geq$ 10 cm maximum diameter below or $\geq$ 5 cm above the diaphragm. Following chemotherapy, patients in CR had to have normal tumor markers, a normal CT scan or no evidence of viable tumor in any post-treatment resected specimens. At the present time (May 1995), 228 of the 229 patients (150 on BEP, 149 on BOP/VIP) for whom data are available are evaluable for response. Of these, 68 of 116 (59%) on BEP and 65 of 112 (58%) on BOP/VIP achieved CR. With a median follow-up of almost 1.5 years, 46 of 175 (26%) on BEP and 57 of 173 (33%) on BOP/VIP have progressed or died (HR = 1.33; p = 0.15). Among the patients who achieved CR, 10 of 68 (15%) on BEP and seven of 65 (11%) on BOP/VIP have progressed or died (HR = 0.84, p = 0.73). There were a total of 14 deaths attributed to toxicity, six on BEP and eight on BOP/VIP. This preliminary analysis suggests no advantage to the more intensive schedule, although longer follow-up is required.

23.4 DISCUSSION

It is unlikely that the concept of alternating administration of different chemotherapy combinations would be the prime solution to the problem of drug resistance, since drug resistance is probably a multifactorial issue. For instance, the multidrug resistance phenotype impacts in the efficacy of anthracyclines, vinca alkaloids, dactinomycin and epipodophyllotoxins, while a tumor may become unresponsive to cisplatin because of at least five different mechanisms (de Graeff, Slebos and Rodenhuis, 1988), like increased glutathione transferase activity and increased DNA repair. As a result, one can doubt whether noncross-resistant regimens do exist. To date, alternating sequential chemotherapy has not been proven to be superior to one particular combination. For instance, in breast cancer cyclophosphamide/methotrexate/5-fluorouracil (CMF) compared with CMF and Adriamycin (doxorubicin hydrochloride)/vincristine in alternating courses did not yield improvement of response rate and median survival (Hellman *et al.*, 1982). In addition, alternating drug regimens in small cell lung cancer give comparable results to conventional regimens (Spiro, 1985; Roth *et al.*, 1992). Also in Hodgkin's disease alternating therapy of mechlorethamine/vincristine/procarbazine/prednisone and doxorubicin/bleomycin/vinblastine/dacarbazine (MOPP/ABVD) has not found to be superior to either MOPP or ABVD (Canellos *et al.*, 1992).

At present, there is no indication that alternating sequential chemotherapy is superior to standard chemotherapy (i.e. four cycles of BEP) in poor risk germ cell cancer. However, with the exception of the randomized EORTC and MRC/EORTC studies, it is difficult to assess the outcomes of the studies addressing the issue of alternating sequential chemotherapy since each group of investigators uses their own set of prognostic criteria (Vogelzang, 1987; Bajorin *et al.*, 1988). Thus, the possibility exists that some regimens may yield excellent results because of inclusion of good prognosis patients. In other words the results of a (Phase II) trial may be influenced significantly by the eligibility criteria.

Therefore, it seems justified to state that

only a prospective randomized study can substantiate whether alternating sequential chemotherapy is superior to standard regimens. However, we are of the opinion that only with the introduction of drugs with modes of action different from the present cytostatics, efficacious noncross-resistant regimens may be developed.

ACKNOWLEDGEMENTS

The authors express their thanks to Dr J. Verweij for advice and criticism, and to Ms I. Dijkstra and Mrs A. Sugiarsi for secretarial assistance.

REFERENCES

Anderson, T. (1979) Testicular germ cell neoplasms: recent advances in diagnosis and therapy. *Ann. Intern. Med.*, **90**, 373–85.

Bajorin, D., Katz, A., Chan, E. *et al.* (1988) Comparison of criteria for assigning germ cell tumor patients to 'Good Risk' and 'Poor Risk' studies. *J. Clin. Oncol.*, **6**, 786–92.

Bosl, G.J., Dmitrovsky, E., Reuter, V. *et al.* (1989) A specific karyotypic abnormality in germ cell tumors (GCT). *Proc. Am. Soc. Clin. Oncol.*, **8**, 131.

Bosl, G.J., Geller, N.L., Vogelzang, N.J. *et al.* (1987) Alternating cycles of Etoposide plus Cisplatin and VAB-6 in the treatment of poor-risk patients with germ cell tumors. *J. Clin. Oncol.*, **5**, 436–40.

Canellos, G.P., Anderson, I.R., Propert, K.J. *et al.* (1992) Chemotherapy of advanced Hodgkin's disease with MOPP, ABVD, or MOPP alternating with ABVD. *N. Engl. J. Med.*, **327**, 1478–84.

Cullen, M.H., Harper, P.G., Woodroffe, C.M. *et al.* (1988) Chemotherapy for poor risk germ cell tumours. An independent evaluation of the POMB/ACE regime. *Br. J. Urol.*, **62**, 454–60.

Fichtinger-Schepman, A.M.J., van Oosterom, A.T., Lohman, P.H.M. and Berends, F. (1987) *cis*-Diamminedichloroplatinum (II)-induced DNA adducts in peripheral leukocytes from seven cancer patients: Quantitative immunochemical detection of the adduct induction and removal after a single dose of *cis*-Diamminedichloroplatinum (II). *Cancer Res.*, **47**, 3000–4.

Goldie, J.H. and Coldman, A.J. (1984) The genetic origin of drug resistance in neoplasms: implications for systemic therapy. *Cancer Res.*, **44**, 3643–53.

Goldie, J.H., Coldman, A.J. and Gudauskas, G.A. (1982) Rationale for the use of alternating noncross-resistant chemotherapy. *Cancer Treat. Rep.*, **66**, 439–49.

de Graeff, A., Slebos, R.J.C. and Rodenhuis, S. (1988) Resistance to cisplatin and analogues: mechanisms and potential clinical implications. *Cancer Chemother. Pharmacol.*, **22**, 325–32.

Hellman, S., Harris, J.R., Canellos, G.P. and Fisher, B. (1982) Cancer of the breast, in *Cancer*, (ed. V.T. de Vita), Lippincot Company, Philadelphia, pp. 914–70.

Hitchins, R.N., Newlands, E.S., Smith, D.B. *et al.* (1989) Long-term outcome in patients with germ cell tumours treated with POMB/ACE chemotherapy: comparison of commonly used classification systems of good and poor prognosis. *Br. J. Cancer*, **59**, 236–42.

Kaye, S.B., Fosså, S., Cullen, M. *et al.* (1995) An MRC/EORTC randomised trial in poor prognosis metastatic teratoma, comparing BEP with BOP-VIP. *Proc. Am. Soc. Clin. Oncol.*, **14**, 246, Abstract 657.

Lewis, C.R., Fosså, S.D., Bokkel Huinink ten, W. *et al.* (1991) BOP/VIP – a new platinum-intensive chemotherapy regimen for poor prognosis germ cell tumours. *Ann. Oncol.*, **2**, 203–11.

Logothetis, C.J., Samuels, M.L., Selig, D.E. *et al.* (1985) Improved survival with cyclic chemotherapy for non-seminomatous germ cell tumors of the testis. *J. Clin. Oncol.*, **3**, 326–35.

Logothetis, C.J., Samuels, M.L., Selig, D.E. *et al.* (1986) Cyclic chemotherapy with Cyclophosphamide, Doxorubicin, and Cisplatin plus Vinblastine and Bleomycin in advanced germinal tumors. Results with 100 patients. *Am. J. Med.*, **81**, 219–28.

Newlands, E.S., Rustin, G.J.S., Begent, R.H.J. *et al.* (1983) Further advances in the management of malignant teratomas of the testis and other sites. *Lancet*, **i**, 948–51.

Nooter, K., Oostrum, R., Janssen, A. *et al.* (1988) Detection and treatment of typical multidrug resistance in refractory ANLL patients. *Proc. Am. Ass. Cancer Res.*, **29**, 303.

Pastan, I. and Gottesman, M. (1987) Multiple drug resistance in human cancer. *N. Engl. J. Med.*, **22**, 1388–93.

Peckham, M. (1988) Testicular cancer. *Acta Oncol.*, **4**, 439–53.

Rodenburg, C.J. and Stoter, G. (1988) Salvage therapy in refractory and relapsing testicular cancer, in *Therapeutic Progress in Urological Cancers* (eds G.P. Murphy and S. Khoury), Alan R. Liss Inc., New York, pp. 763–9.

Roth, B.J., Johnson, D.H., Einhorn, L.H. *et al.* (1992) Randomized study of cyclophosphamide, doxorubicin and vincristine versus etoposide and cisplatin versus alteration of these two regimens in extensive small-cell lung cancer: a phase III trial of the Southeastern Cancer Study Group. *J. Chim. Oncol.*, **10**, 282–91.

Schabel, Jr, F.M., Skipper, H.E., Trader, M.W. *et al.* (1980) Concepts for controlling drug-resistant tumor cells, in *Breast Cancer – Experimental and Clinical Aspects* (eds H.T. Mouridson and T. Palshof), Pergamon Press, Oxford, pp. 199–211.

Spiro, G. (1985) Chemotherapy of small cell lung cancer, in *Small Cell Lung Cancer* (ed. G. Spiro), W.B. Saunders, London, pp. 105–20.

Stoter, G., Kaye, S., Sleyfer, D. *et al.* (1986) Preliminary results of BEP (Bleomycin, Etoposide, Cisplatin) versus an alternating regimen of BEP and PVB (Cisplatin, Vinblastine, Bleomycin) in high volume metastatic (HVM) testicular non-seminomas. An EORTC-study. *Proc. Am. Soc. Clin. Oncol.*, **5**, 106.

Stoter, G., Koopman, A., Vendrik, C.P.J. *et al.* (1989) Ten-year survival and late sequelae in testicular cancer patients treated with cisplatin, vinblastine, and bleomycin. *J. Clin. Oncol.*, **7**, 1099–104.

Vogelzang, N.J. (1987) Prognostic factors in metastatic testicular cancer. *Int. J. Androl.*, **10**, 225–37.

Williams, S.D., Birch, R., Einhorn, L.H. *et al.* (1987) Treatment of disseminated germ cell tumors with cisplatin, bleomycin, and either vinblastine or etoposide. *N. Engl. J. Med.*, **316**, 1435–40.

de Wit, R., Stoter, G., Sleijfer, D.Th. *et al.* (1995) Four cycles of BEP versus an alternating regimen of PVB and BEP in patients with poor prognosis metastatic testicular non-seminoma; a randomised study of the EORTC Genitourinary Tract Cancer Cooperative Group. *Br. J. Cancer*, **71**, 1311–14.

Zijlstra, J.G., de Vries, E.G.E. and Mulder, N.H. (1987) Mechanism and circumvention of drug resistance in tumor cells. *Neth. J. Med.*, **30**, 85–93.

THE ROLE OF HEMATOPOIETIC GROWTH FACTORS IN THE CHEMOTHERAPY OF GERM CELL TUMORS

24

H.-J. Schmoll and C. Bokemeyer

24.1 INTRODUCTION

Human recombinant hematopoietic growth factors (HGF) have entered the clinical setting and have dramatically altered treatment strategies in hematology and oncology. One of the most frequent clinical problems addressed with the use of HGF has been the improvement in chemotherapy-related granulocytopenia and associated infective complications. For a variety of human malignancies clinical studies have demonstrated that HGF can reduce the incidence of infections following chemotherapy and possibly also reduce the duration of hospitalization and the use of antibiotics for the treatment of granulocytopenic fever (Boogaerts, 1994). Currently two growth factors are available for clinical use: granulocyte colony stimulating factor (G-CSF) and granulocyte–macrophage colony stimulating factor (GM-CSF). Both growth factors have been studied in a large number of human malignancies, either to reduce the duration of granulocytopenia after standard dose chemotherapy, to allow dose intensification of chemotherapy regimens, or to generate peripheral blood stem cells (PBSC) as hemato-poietic support after megadose chemotherapy (Diaz-Rubio and Adrover, 1994). In addition to G- and GM-CSF, interleukin-3 (IL-3) and stem cells factor (SCF) are on the verge of clinical use. This chapter will discuss the currently available knowledge on the biological interaction between hematopoietic growth factors and the malignant germ cells, as well as the clinical role for growth factors during standard dose chemotherapy and the use of growth factors for dose-intensive experimental approaches to high risk patients with testicular cancer.

24.2 BIOLOGICAL INTERACTIONS BETWEEN HGF AND MALIGNANT GERM CELL TUMORS

A biological relationship between early hematopoietic stem cells and germ cells during embryonic development has been suspected. Therefore, hematopoietic growth factors acting on hematopoietic stem cells and on committed blood cell precursors might also be able to interact with normal human germ cells and possibly even with malignant cells in germ cell cancer. The clinical association

Testicular Cancer: Investigation and management. Second edition. Edited by Professor A. Horwich.
Published in 1996 by Chapman & Hall. ISBN 0 412 61210 0.

between mediastinal germ cell tumors and the development of leukemia, in which the leukemic blasts show a typical cytogenetic marker also found in germ cell tumors, the isochromosome 12p ($i(12p)$), has been observed (Nichols *et al.*, 1990). It has therefore been an important issue to investigate the potential of growth factors active during hematopoiesis to stimulate the growth of testicular cancer cells in patients.

A variety of nonhematopoietic tumor cell lines, e.g. non-small cell lung cancer, adenocarcinoma of the stomach, and osteosarcoma, have been demonstrated to express receptors for GM-CSF (Miyagawa *et al.*, 1990). Furthermore, GM-CSF concentrations that result in hematopoietic colony formation have been shown to be able to promote the growth of human ovarian cancer cell lines *in vitro* (Cimoli *et al.*, 1991). However, growth promotion of human testicular cancer cell lines by either G- or GM-CSF has not been demonstrated so far. Buzello *et al.* showed that the addition of G-CSF to testicular cancer cells *in vitro* neither promoted tumor growth, nor interacted with the cytostatic activity of cisplatin (Buzello, 1995). In a large study by Roach *et al.* using cell lines established from human teratomas neither GM-CSF, interleukin-1, -2 or -3, nor SCF were able to promote tumor growth *in vitro* (Roach *et al.*, 1993). Using the established panel of human testicular cancer cell lines derived from patients at Hannover University Medical School, we have been able to demonstrate that neither GM-CSF, G-CSF, nor SCF are produced by tumor cell lines H 12.1, H 32, and 1428A in detectable amounts. The addition of G-CSF or GM-CSF *in vitro* to medium containing 15% fetal calf serum did not result in enhanced tumor cell proliferation. Only a weak enhancement of proliferative activity of SCF could be detected when high concentrations of SCF were added to cell lines in serum free medium culture conditions (Dunn *et al.*, 1994). Only very weak expression of SCF-receptors on these non-seminomatous germ cell tumor lines was

found. Immunhistochemical investigations of testicular cancer specimens for the expression of SCF and *c-kit*, the gene coding for the SCF-receptor, demonstrate that both are expressed in a large number of pure seminomas, but are not found on non-seminomatous germ cell tumor specimens (Sehrt *et al.*, 1994). The detection of SCF and *c-kit* in normal testicular tissue and their absence in non-seminomatous germ cell tumors argue against an important role of these proteins for tumor progression. They may rather form an important functional regulatory system for normal spermatogenesis.

The *in vivo* effect of GM-CSF on heterotransplanted human testicular cancer cell lines H 12.1 and H 23.1 has been studied in nude mice (Bokemeyer *et al.*, 1993a). During 14 days of daily GM-CSF injections a slight but not significant, reduction in tumor growth was observed compared with untreated control mice. Preliminary results from the application of G-CSF, either alone or in combination with SCF using heterotransplanted tumor cell lines H 12.1 and H 32 in nude mice, also seem to exclude stimulatory effects on tumor growth *in vivo*.

In summary, the results from *in vitro* and *in vivo* animal studies indicate that the use of hematopoietic growth, particularly G- and GM-CSF, does not promote the growth of malignant germ cell cancer. The importance of the SCF and *c-kit* regulatory system for normal spermatogenesis and fertility requires further evaluation, but a clinically significant stimulation of malignant germ cells by SCF seems unlikely.

24.3 CLINICAL USE OF HGF IN STANDARD DOSE COMBINATION CHEMOTHERAPY

24.3.1 GOOD RISK PATIENTS

24.3.1.1 Risk of infection

Three cycles of the combination of cisplatin, etoposide and bleomycin (PEB) are con-

Table 24.1 Incidence of neutropenic fever and septic death in patients treated with standard dose regimens for testicular cancer

Author	No. pts	Regimen	No. pts with granulocytopenic fever	No. pts septic death
Williams *et al.*, 1987	104	PVB × 4	n.s.	4 (4%)
	111	PEB × 4	n.s.	2 (2%)
Wozniak *et al.*, 1991	77	PVB × 4	5 (6%)	–
	83	PEV × 4	2 (2%)	1 (1%)
Nichols *et al.*, 1991	77	PEB × 4	12 (16%)	–
	76	$P_{40}EB × 4$	38 (50%)	1 (1%)
Daugaard and Rørth, 1992	69	$P_{40}E_{200}B × 4$	62 (90%)	6 (9%)
Schmoll *et al.*, 1987	98	$P_{35}EB × 4$	34 (35%)	2 (2%)
Harstrick *et al.*, 1991	48	PEBOI × 4	10 (21%)	–
Husband and Green, 1992	53	POMB/ACE	16 (30%)	–
Bajorin* *et al.*, 1995	49	VIP	(35%)	1 (2%)
	55	VIP + GM-GSF	(18%)	–
Fosså *et al.*, 1995	116	PEB × 6 or BOP/VIP × 3	34 (29%)	9 (8%)
	114	PEB × 6 or BOP/VIP × 3 + G-CSF	20 (17%)	1 (1%)
Blanke *et al.*, 1994	20	VIP/VB × 4 + G-CSF	8 (40%)	–

n.s. = not stated.
* Data are given in percentage of cycles and refere only to cycle 1 and 2.

sidered standard therapy for patients with 'good risk' metastatic testicular cancer (Einhorn *et al.*, 1989). Between 85 and 98% of these patients will be rendered long-term tumor free by this treatment. The classification of 'good risk' for these patients is based on the number of metastatic sites, tumor volume, tumor marker evaluation and the type of organ involvement. In the Indiana University classification these patients are found in the groups of 'minimal' or 'moderate disease' patients. According to MSKCC criteria 'good risk' patients will have a chance of >50% of achieving complete remission after induction chemotherapy, and a 5-year survival of 85–90% (Bosl *et al.*, 1983). Only scanty information is available on the severity of myelosuppression and the frequency of granulocytopenic infections in 'good risk' patients treated with PEB chemotherapy. However, based on data from larger randomized trials, the incidence of granulocytopenic infections is estimated to be lower than 20% of patients, including 1–2% death due to septicemia.

24.3.1.2 Recommendations for use of HGF

No trials prospectively evaluating the use of recombinant hematopoietic growth factors in this subpopulation of 'good risk' testicular cancer patients are available. Based on the assumption that minor treatment delays due to myelotoxicity will not effect overall curability and that the total frequency of granulocytopenic infections is low in these patients, the routine use of hematopoietic growth factors after chemotherapy would not be recommended at present. However, the use of HGF should be considered for selected patients who may either have a generally increased risk for severe infections due to concomitant medical illnesses or who have had a severe granulocytopenic infection during their previous cycle of chemotherapy.

Of particular concern is the 1–2% septic death rate in some older randomized trials in patients with good prognostic criteria and a 5-year life expectancy of 95% (Table 24.1). In the light of the high cure rate, this rate of septic death could be considered unacceptably high. Furthermore, since many patients with good prognosis testicular cancer, including the early stages IIA and B, are treated outside of protocols in a less experienced oncological setting or in private practice, the true rate of lethal septic complications may be higher than documented in these prospective randomized trials. Therefore it could be argued that, in the light of the excellent cure rate, the prophylactic application of G-CSF after standard dose PEB therapy would be justified in all patients with 'good risk' metastatic germ cell cancer, as well as for adjuvant chemotherapy. This question needs to be seriously discussed in the scientific community with particular respect to the costs of health care in the curative setting and the quality of patient care. Unfortunately, randomized trials will not be able to answer this question.

24.3.2   POOR RISK PATIENTS

24.3.2.1   Risk of infection

Approximately 15–30% of patients with metastatic testicular cancer will be considered 'poor risk', and their chance of cure will reach only 50% with standard chemotherapy regimens. According to the Indiana University classification these patients are classified as 'advanced disease', and according to the MSKCC prognostic model their chance of achieving complete remission will be < 50% (Bosl *et al.*, 1983). Four cycles of PEB therapy are regarded as standard treatment for these patients (Williams *et al.*, 1987). Granulocytopenia is the major reported toxic side-effect of treatment and various incidences of leukocytopenia with < 1000 leukocytes μl^{-1}, ranging from 6 to 85%, have been reported after standard PEB treatment (Table 24.1). In most studies, single patients with toxic death during granulocytopenia had been observed (Nichols *et al.*, 1991; Williams *et al.*, 1987; Wozniak *et al.*, 1991).

The impact of close schedule adherence during standard therapy and the importance of dose intensity for effective treatment results in 'poor risk' testicular cancer patients has been demonstrated (Husband and Green, 1992; Murphy *et al.*, 1993). This has stimulated the investigation of regimens including or supplementing drugs in the standard PEB regimen. In general these investigative treatments have been associated with a considerably higher degree of myelotoxicity and infections. For example in the study by Nichols *et al.* (1991) comparing PEB standard dose therapy with a double-dose platinum/etoposide/bleomycin regimen, 38 of 76 patients (50%) developed granulocytopenic fever in the experimental arm, compared with only 16% in the standard PEB arm. The frequency of neutropenic fever in a Phase II trial using double dose platinum and double-dose etoposide with bleomycin ranged from 50 to 90% from treatment cycle 1 to 6 (Daugaard and Rørth, 1992). Two studies that have compared a regimen composed of platinum, etoposide and ifosfamide (PEI) with the standard PEB regimen clearly demonstrated that the substitution of ifosfamide for bleomycin is associated with an increased myelotoxicity and that 30–40% of patients have developed granulocytopenic fever (Loehrer *et al.*, 1993; Stoter *et al.*, 1993). As can be seen in Table 24.1, the incidence of granulocytopenic infections following investigational multidrug regimens such as POMB–ACE or PEBOI chemotherapy has also been associated with an increased rate of neutropenic infections (Harstrick *et al.*, 1991; Husband and Green, 1992).

24.3.2.2   G-CSF

Only preliminary data using G-CSF as hematopoietic support following multiple drug regimens of standard dose chemotherapy for 'poor risk' testicular cancer are available. Blanke *et al.* demonstrated that a five-drug regimen composed of platinum, etoposide, ifosfamide, and vinblastine and bleomycin could be applied for a total of four cycles without either large treatment delay or unexpected toxicity (Blanke *et al.*, 1994). The only randomized study concerning the use of hematopoietic growth factors in 'poor prognosis' testicular cancer has been conducted by the MRC and EORTC and a preliminary analysis of the results is available (Fosså *et al.*, 1995). Six cycles of standard PEB chemotherapy were compared with three cycles of platinum, vincristine and bleomycin (POB) followed by three cycles of platinum, etoposide and ifosfamide (POB/VIP). From 263 patients, 130 were randomized to receive no hematopoietic growth factor after chemotherapy and 133 patients to G-CSF after chemotherapy. The preliminary analysis demonstrated that dose reductions were necessary in 71 of 116 (61%) patients without G-CSF compared with only 30 of 114 patients (26%) with G-CSF. Granulocytopenic fever developed in 17% of G-CSF-treated patients compared with 29% of those without. Most importantly, there were 8% toxic deaths in the group without G-CSF compared with only 1% in the G-CSF-treated group. After a median follow-up of 1 year there was no difference in response or overall survival.

24.3.2.3 GM-CSF

For GM-CSF, effective stimulation of hematopoietic recovery after chemotherapy for testicular cancer has been demonstrated during an early Phase I/II study (Jost, Pichert and Stahel, 1990). In addition, GM-CSF has been used after combination chemotherapy with carboplatin, etoposide and bleomycin (CEB) in a Russian study (Tjulandin *et al.*, 1993). Most data on GM-CSF in testicular cancer are available from patients treated with PEI chemotherapy. A randomized trial of patients with relapsed testicular cancer receiving GM-CSF after conventional dose PEI salvage treatment demonstrated that the effect of GM-CSF on amelioration of granulocytopenia

and prevention of infections was observed only during the first cycle of chemotherapy, and that this reduced rate of granulocytopenia was not associated with a clinical benefit for the patients (Bajorin *et al.*, 1995). In addition, the side-effects observed during treatment with GM-CSF in testicular cancer patients, particularly local inflammation at the injection site, fever and, in rare cases, anaphylactoid type reactions, have hampered the further evaluation of GM-CSF after standard dose chemotherapy in this disease (Bokemeyer, Schmoll and Harstrick, 1993).

24.3.2.4 Recommendations for use of HGF

For patients with 'poor risk' germ cell cancer, the delivery of at least four cycles of myelotoxic chemotherapy with adequate schedule adherence and the maintenance of dose intensity appear to be important variables for therapeutic success. Based on the high incidence of granulocytopenic infections, particularly for the aggressive experimental standard dose treatment regimens, and the results achieved in Phase II and randomized phase III studies evaluating the use of G-CSF after chemotherapy for 'poor risk' patients, the use of this growth factor should be recommended. Although no influence of G-CSF on response to treatment and on overall survival has been clearly demonstrated so far, in a young patient population receiving aggressive combination chemotherapy with a curative intention, the use of G-CSF can be encouraged despite the lack of further convincing clinical data.

24.4 THE ROLE OF HGF FOR EXPERIMENTAL HIGH DOSE TREATMENT APPROACHES

24.4.1 HGF AND DOSE-INTENSIFIED CHEMOTHERAPY

While the intensification of cisplatin in standard regimens for the treatment of testicular cancer is associated with increased non-hematological toxicity, particularly nephro-, oto- and neurotoxicity, etoposide and ifosfamide have been considered as candidates for dose escalation because of predominant hematological toxicity. Phase II trials in patients with relapsed disease have demonstrated that both high dose ifosfamide and high dose etoposide followed by autologous bone marrow rescue can achieve responses in patients refractory to standard doses of these agents (Motzer *et al.*, 1992; Mandanas *et al.*, 1993). Since myelotoxicity is one of the main side-effects of etoposide and ifosfamide, hematopoietic growth factors have been introduced into dose-escalated regimens of these agents. The value of growth-factor-supported dose-intensified chemotherapy has been studied as first line therapy for patients with 'poor risk' testicular cancer. A study by the Australian Germ Cell Tumour Study Group demonstrated that G-CSF at 5 µg kg^{-1} SC allowed the escalation of a carboplatin, etoposide and ifosfamide regimen to a maximum of 125% (Levi and Toner, 1993). The German Testicular Cancer Study Group has used a regimen composed of cisplatin, etoposide and ifosfamide followed by GM-CSF in 'advanced' testicular cancer. With 74 available patients in this trial a 1.4-fold increase in dose intensity could be achieved (Bokemeyer *et al.*, 1993b). Both mucositis and thrombocytopenia were dose limiting for further escalation. Dose escalation trials with different chemotherapy regimens in various human malignancies such as non-Hodgkin's lymphoma, Hodgkin's lymphoma, bladder cancer and others have demonstrated that hematopoietic growth factors will allow an approximately 1.5-fold increase of dose compared with standard chemotherapy regimes. However, while the feasibility of this approach has been demonstrated, the clinical value of dose escalation, in the range of 1–1.5 fold compared with standard chemotherapy, has not been proven in randomized trials in testicular cancer so far. While HGF can reduce the incidence of neutro-

penia and subsequent infections in most Phase II studies, they are not able to overcome the dose-limiting thrombocytopenia. Therefore the achievement of further dose escalations by the use of myeloid growth factors alone is very unlikely.

24.4.2 HIGH DOSE CHEMOTHERAPY WITH AUTOLOGOUS STEM CELL SUPPORT AND HGF

The poor results of salvage chemotherapy for patients with relapsed testicular cancer, which will achieve a durable complete response rate in only 20% of patients, have led to the investigation of high dose chemotherapy regimens with autologous bone marrow or peripheral stem cell rescue. While initially high dose regimens with without platinum compounds have been explored, more recent Phase II studies of high dose chemotherapy have used carboplatin and etoposide – two drugs with myelosuppression as their main toxicity. Aggressive regimens using high dose carboplatin, etoposide and ifosfamide or cyclophosphamide have recently been studied in patients with relapsed testicular cancer (Linkesch, Krainer and Wagner 1992; Motzer and Bosl, 1992; Mandanas *et al.*, 1993; Siegert *et al.*, 1994). These treatment approaches were initially associated with considerable toxicity and 5–20% of treatment-related deaths, particularly due to septic infection in a range of 7–21% of patients. The introduction of G-CSF or GM-CSF following autologous marrow reinfusion after high dose chemotherapy has resulted in reduced numbers of septic infections and toxic deaths (Linkesch, Krainer and Wagner, 1992; Motzer *et al.*, 1993a). Although not clearly evaluated in randomized trials, most recently performed studies of high dose chemotherapy for testicular cancer have used hematopoietic growth factors, particularly G-CSF, after bone marrow rescue.

The widespread availability of techniques for peripheral blood stem cell separation has further boosted the investigation of high dose

Table 24.2 Comparison of hematopoietic recovery after high dose CEI therapy followed either by bone marrow (BM) or peripheral blood stem cell rescue (PBSC) and G-CSF (Beyer *et al.*, 1994)

	PBSC + G-CSF	BM + G-CSF	p-*value*
No. pts	20	23	
Days to leukocytes >1000 μl^{-1}	10 (7–16)	11.5 (10–29)	<0.01
Days to neutrophils >500 μl^{-1}	10 (7–15)	11.5 (9–27)	<0.01
Days to platelets >20 000 μl^{-1}	10.5 (8–62)	17 (9–42)	<0.01
Days until hospital discharge	18.5 (11–33)	20 (13–51)	0.16
Days with IV antibiotics	9 (0–22)	11 (6–49)	0.06

chemotherapy regimens in testicular cancer. It has been demonstrated that, with the use of G-CSF ± interleukin-3, sufficient numbers of peripheral blood stem cells (PBSC) can be separated after standard dose chemotherapy with platinum, etoposide and ifosfamide (Brugger *et al.*, 1992). In a Phase II study of the German Testicular Cancer Study Group using a high dose regimen composed of carboplatin, etoposide and ifosfamide in patients with relapsed testicular cancer, both autologous bone marrow rescue or PBSC support have been used (Siegert *et al.*, 1994). All 20 patients of this study, receiving PBSC rescue plus G-CSF, experienced a full hematological recovery, demonstrating that the use of PBSC for stem cell rescue after high dose chemotherapy for testicular cancer can be considered safe (Lynch *et al.*, 1994). Furthermore, patients receiving PBSC rescue after HD–CEI treatment had a significantly faster recovery of neutrophils and platelets in comparison with patients receiving autologous bone marrow rescue. This was accompanied by a trend for a reduced need for IV antibiotics and a shortened hospital stay (Table 24.2) (Beyer *et al.*, 1994). Owing to the rapid progress made with the techniques of stem cell separation and data demonstrating highly effective regeneration of hematopoiesis after PBSC retransfusion, this technique is currently rapidly replacing the use of autologous bone marrow transplantation in solid tumors (Nakagawa *et al.*, 1994).

The value of the additional use of hematopoietic growth factors following PBSC rescue after high dose treatment for testicular cancer cannot yet be clearly assessed. Most recently conducted studies have routinely used growth factors after PBSC reinfusion (Linkesch, Krainer and Wagner, 1992; Motzer *et al.*, 1993; Siegert *et al.*, 1994; Sobrevilla-Calvo *et al.*, 1994). In the above-mentioned study of the German Testicular Cancer Study Group, 45 of 74 patients received G-CSF after marrow rescue; with only one of 74 patients dying from treatment-related infections, it appears likely that this approach will remain standard practice (Siegert *et al.*, 1994). In a randomized study of the use of growth factors after PBSC reinfusion in patients with different tumors, an improved neutrophil recovery was observed for those patients receiving G-CSF or GM-CSF. However, the detected clinical benefit was only moderate when compared with patients receiving PBSC without additional HGF (Spitzer *et al.*, 1994).

Although high dose chemotherapy is currently evaluated in different Phase II studies in patients with testicular cancer, the true value of this approach has not been demonstrated in randomized trials. Many questions are still unanswered, such as: Which is the optimal high dose chemotherapy treatment regimen, which patients should be included for high-dose treatment and how many cycles of high dose chemotherapy should be performed? However, from the data available in patients with relapsed disease it appears that high dose chemotherapy may be more effective and better tolerated when used early in the course of disease (Motzer *et al.*, 1993b).

Table 24.3 Dose-escalated scheme of PEI therapy for patients with 'advanced disease' germ cell cancer used by the GTCSG. Cycles were repeated on day 22 for a total of four cycles. GM-CSF was given sc at each cycle in levels 2 and 3, G-CSF + PBSC at each cycle at levels 4 and 5 (Bokemeyer *et al.*, 1994)

		Dose level				
		1	2	3	4	5
Cisplatin (mg m^{-2})	d 1–5	25	30	30	30	30
Etoposide (mg m^{-2})	d 1–5	120	150	200	200	250
Ifosfamide (mg m^{-2})	d 1–5	1200	1600	1600	2000	2000
GM-CSF (5/10 µg kg^{-1})	d 6–15	–	+	+	–	–
PBSC + G-CSF (5 µg kg^{-1})	d 7/d 6–15	–	–	–	+	+

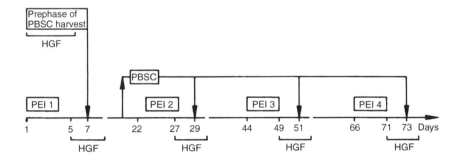

Fig. 24.1 Treatment strategy of sequential high dose PEI (cisplatin/etoposide/ifosfamide) chemotherapy and PBSC support in patients with advanced germ cell tumors.

This has led to the investigation of early intensification of chemotherapy in 'poor risk' patients not responding adequately during the first courses of standard dose induction chemotherapy, a strategy investigated at the Memorial Sloan-Kettering Cancer Center (Motzer *et al.*, 1993b). Based on the experience with dose intensified chemotherapy followed by GM-CSF in 'poor risk' patients, the German Testicular Cancer Study Group has used a treatment strategy of sequential 'high dose VIP' chemotherapy as first line treatment for this prognostically poor subgroup of patients (Bokemeyer *et al.*, 1995). Following PBSC harvest after stimulation with G-CSF alone during a 5-day prephase, patients will receive four sequential cycles of

intensified platinum, etoposide and ifosfamide, each cycle followed by retransfusion of PBSC and G-CSF application. This approach has allowed the application of four sequential cycles of therapy at the current dose level 5, as shown in Table 24.3. The treatment strategy is outlined in Fig. 24.1. The introduction of PBSC into this treatment concept has significantly reduced both the duration of granulocytopenia and thrombocytopenia, as could be demonstrated in patients at dose level 3 receiving either hematopoietic growth factors alone after chemotherapy or PBSC plus hematopoietic growth factors (Table 24.4) (Bokemeyer *et al.*, 1994). Currently 48 patients have been treated with sequential high dose VIP therapy followed by PBSC

Table 24.4 Hematopoietic recovery following four cycles of dose-intensive PEI chemotherapy at dose level 3 (see Table 24.3) supported either by GM-CSF alone or by PBSC plus HGF after each treatment cycle (Bokemeyer *et al.*, 1994)

	Cycle			
	1	*2*	*3*	*4*
Median no. of days with granulocytes <500 μ/l^{-1}				
GM-CSF alone (44 pts)	6	6.5	9.5	12*
PBSC + G-CSF (15 pts)	7	6	5	5*
Median no. of days with thrombocytes <20 000 μ/l^{-1}				
GM-CSF alone (44 pts)	2	4	7*	12*
PBSC + G-CSF (15 pts)	2.5	2.5	3.5*	3*

* Significant difference ($p <0.05$).

support, and with an overall survival >80% these initial results are promising. However, the true value of this concept needs to be addressed in a randomized trial (Bokemeyer, Beyer and Schmoll, 1994).

In conclusion, the availability of hematopoietic growth factors, particularly G-CSF, has substantially influenced the development of high dose chemotherapy regimens in patients with testicular cancer. It has been demonstrated that sufficient numbers of PBSC as hematopoietic support after high dose therapy can be gained either after stimulation with G- or GM-CSF alone or following the application of these factors after standard dose PEI treatment. With the use of hematopoietic growth factors and PBSC the treatment-associated morbidity of high dose chemotherapy has become acceptable. Therefore, HGF has allowed the investigation of the role of high dose chemotherapy in a large number of patients with testicular cancer and the introduction of high dose chemotherapy concepts earlier in the course of the disease.

REFERENCES

Bajorin, D.F., Nichols, C.R., Schmoll, H.-J., Kantoff, P.W., Bokemeyer, C., Demetri, G.D., Einhorn, L.H. and Bosl, G.J. (1995) Recombinant human granulocyte–macrophage colony-stimulating factor as an adjunct to conventional-dose ifosfamide-based chemotherapy for patients with advanced or relapsed germ cell tumors: A randomized trial. *J. Clin. Oncol.*, **13**, 79–86.

Beyer, J., Schwella, N., Strohscheer, I., Schwander, I., Zingsem, J., Serke, S., Huhn, D. and Siegert, W. (1994) Randomized comparison of hematopoietic rescue with stem/progenitor cells from bone marrow or peripheral blood after high-dose chemotherapy in germ cell tumors. *Bone Marrow Tranpl.*, **14**(1), 45.

Blanke, C., Loehrer, P.J., Einhorn, L.H. and Nichols, C. (1994) A phase II study of VP-16 plus ifosfamide plus cisplatin plus vinblastine plus bleomycin (VIP/VB) with filgrastim for advanced stage testicular cancer. *Proc. Am. Soc. Clin. Oncol.*, **13**, 723, (Abstract).

Bokemeyer, C., Beyer, J. and Schmoll, H.-J. (1994) The role of dose-intensified chemotherapy for the treatment of metastatic germ cell tumours. *Forum*, **4**, 671–80.

Bokemeyer, C., Harstrick, A., Rüther, U., Metzner, B., Arseniev, L., Kadar, J., Illiger, H.-J., Link, H., Raichele, A., Beyer, J., Hossfeld, D.K. and Schmoll, H.-J. (1995) Sequential treatment with high-dose VIP-chemotherapy plus peripheral blood stem cell (PBSC) support in advanced germ cell cancer. *Proc. Am. Soc. Clin. Oncol.*, **14**, 236.

Bokemeyer, C., Schmoll, H.-J., Arseniev, L., Metzner, B., Rüther, U., Illiger, H.-J., Link, H. and Poliwoda, H. (1994) Treatment of advanced testicular cancer with dose intensified chemotherapy plus GM-CSF alone or G-CSF and sequential harvesting and reinfusion of peripheral blood stem cells (PBSC). *Proc. Am. Soc. Clin. Oncol.*, **13**, 728, (Abstract).

Bokemeyer, C., Schmoll, H.-J., Casper, J., Kuczyk, M. and Poliwoda, H. (1993a) No growth stimulation of heterotransplanted human testicular cancer cell lines by recombinant human granulocyte-macrophage colony-stimulating factor (GM-CSF). *Int. J. Oncol.*, **3**, 77–80.

Bokemeyer, C., Schmoll, H.-J. and Harstrick, A. (1993) Side effects of GM-CSF in advanced testicular cancer. *Eur. J. Cancer*, **29A**, 924 (letter).

Bokemeyer, C., Schmoll, H.-J., Harstrick, A., Illiger, H.-J., Metzner, B., Räth, U., Hohnloser, J., Clemm, C., Berdel, W., Siegert, W., Rüther, U., Ostermann, H., Kneba, M., Hartlapp, J.H., Schröder, M. and Poliwoda, H. (1993b) A phase I/II study of a stepwise dose-escalated regimen of cisplatin, etoposide and ifosfamide plus granulocyte-macrophage colony-stimulating factor (GM-CSF) in patients with advanced germ cell tumours. *Eur. J. Cancer*, **29A**, 2225–31.

Boogaerts, M.A. (1994) Growth factors in hematology: Prophylactic versus interventional use. *Eur. J. Cancer*, **30A**, 238–43.

Bosl, G.J., Geller, N., Cirrincone, C. *et al.* (1983) Multivariate analysis of prognostic variables in patients with metastatic testicular cancer. *Cancer Res.*, **43**, 3403–7.

Brugger, W., Bross, K., Frisch, J. *et al.* (1992) Mobilization of peripheral blood progenitor cells by sequential administration of interleukin-3 and granulocyte-macrophage colony stimulating factor following polychemotherapy with etoposide, ifosfamide and cisplatin. *Blood*, **79**, 1193–200.

Buzello, H. (1995) Effect of granulocyte colony stimulating factor (G-CSF) on growth of testicular cancer cells in vitro, in *Hodentumoren – Testis Cancer*, (eds D. Schnorr, S.A. Loenig and L. Weißbach), Blackwell, Berlin.

Cimoli, G., Russo, P., Billi, G., Nariani, G.L., Rovini, E. and Venturini, M. (1991) Human granulocyte-macrophage colony-stimulating factor a growth factor active on human ovarian cancer cells. *Jap. J. Cancer Res.*, **82**, 1196–8.

Daugaard, G. and Rørth, M. (1992) Treatment of poor-risk germ-cell tumors with high-dose cisplatin and etoposide combined with bleomycin. *Ann. Oncol.*, **3**, 277–82.

Diaz-Rubio, E. and Adrover, E. (1994) Use of granulocyte growth factors in solid tumours. *Eur. J. Cancer*, **30A**, 120–2.

Dunn, T., Bokemeyer, C., Hartmann, K., Rae, C. and Schmoll, H.-J. (1994) Effect of hematopoietic growth factors (HGF's) on the growth of human embryonic carcinoma cell lines in reduced or serum free culture. *Ann. Oncol.*, **5** (Suppl. 8) 9, 38.

Einhorn, L.H., Williams, S.D., Loehrer, P.J., Birch, R., Drasga, R., Omura, G. and Greco, F.A. (1989) Evaluation of optimal duration of chemotherapy in favorable-prognosis disseminated germ cell tumors: A Southeastern Cancer Study Group Protocol. *J. Clin. Oncol.*, **7**, 387–91.

Fosså, S., Kaye, S.B., Cullen, M., De Wit, R., Bodrogi, I., van Groeningen, C., Sylvester, R., Stenning, S., Kaye, S.B., Cullen, M., Lallemand, E. and Mead, G.M. (1995) An MRC/EORTC randomized trial in poor prognosis metastatic teratoma, a comparing treatment with/without filgrastim. *Proc. Am. Soc. Clin. Oncol.*, in press.

Harstrick, A., Schmoll, H.-J., Köhne-Wömpner, C.-H. *et al.* (1991) Cisplatin, etoposide, ifosfamide, vincristine and bleomycin combination chemotherapy for far advanced testicular carcinoma. *Ann. Oncol.*, **2**, 197–202.

Husband, D.J. and Green, J.A. (1992) POMB/ACE chemotherapy in nonseminomatous germ cell tumours: Outcome and importance of dose intensity. *Eur. J. Cancer*, **28**(1), 86–91.

Jost, L.M., Pichert, G. and Stahel, R.A. (1990) Placebo controlled phase I/II study of subcutaneous GM-CSF in patients with germ cell tumors undergoing chemotherapy. *Ann. Oncol.*, **1**, 439–42.

Levi, J.A. and Toner, G. (1993) Dose intensive chemotherapy for poor prognosis germ cell malignancies. (Abstract). International Germ Cell Tumour Conference, Leeds, England.

Linkesch, W., Krainer, M. and Wagner, A. (1992) Phase I/II trial of ultrahigh carboplatin, etoposide, cyclophosphamide with ABMT in refractory or relapsed non-seminomatous germ cell tumors (NSGCT). *Proc. Am. Soc. Clin. Oncol.*, **11**, 600, (Abstract).

Loehrer, P.J., Einhorn, L.H., Elson, P. *et al.* (1993) Phase III study of cisplatin plus etoposide (VP16) with either bleomycin (B) or ifosfamide (I) in advanced stage germ cell tumours (GCT): An Intergroup trial. *Proc. Am. Soc. Clin. Oncol.*, **12**, 831, (Abstract).

Lynch, J., Lee, R., Gross, M., Vellis, K., Hutchenson, C., Ayash, L, Weiner, R. and Moreb, J. (1994) Time to myeloid recovery is related to number of peripheral blood (PB) pregenitors infused after high dose chemotherapy. *Proc. Am. Soc. Clin. Oncol.*, **13**, 189.

Mandanas, R.A., Broun, E.R., Nichols, C.R.,

Salzman, D., Turns, M. and Einhorn, L.H. (1993) Phase I/II dose escalation study of carboplatin (CBDCA) and etoposide (VP-16) with autologous marrow support done in tandem for refractory germ cell tumors (GCT). *Proc. Am. Soc. Clin. Oncol.*, **12**, 747, (Abstract).

Miyagawa, K., Chiba, S., Shibuya, K. *et al.* (1990) Frequent expression of receptors for granulocyte-macrophage colony-stimulating factor on non hematopoietic tumour cell lines. *J. Cell. Physiol.*, **143**, 483–7.

Motzer, R.J. and Bosl, G.J. (1992) High-dose chemotherapy for resistant germ cell tumors: Recent advances and future directions. *J. Natl. Cancer Inst.*, **84**, 1703–9.

Motzer, R.J., Gulati, S.C., Crown, J.P., Weisen S., Doherty, M., Herr, H., Fair, W., Sheinfeld, J., Sogani, P., Russo, P., and Bosl, G.J. (1992) High-dose chemotherapy and autologous bone marrow rescue for patients with refractory germ cell tumors. *Cancer*, **69**, 550–6.

Motzer, R.J., Gulati, S.C., Mazumdar, M., Bajorin, D.F., Vlamis, V., Lyn, P. and Bosl, G.J. (1993a) Phase II trial of VAB-6 + high-dose carboplatin + etoposide (HD C+E) with autologous bone marrow transplantation (AUBMT) for poor risk germ cell tumor (GCT) patients (PTS). *Proc. Am. Soc. Clin. Oncol.*, **12**, 720, (Abstract).

Motzer, R.J., Mazumdar, M., Subhash, C.G., Bajorin, D.F., Lyn, P., Vlamis, V. and Bosl, G.J. (1993b) Phase II trial of high-dose carboplatin and etoposide with autologous bone marrow transplantation in first-line therapy for patients with poor-risk germ cell tumors. *J. Natl. Cancer Inst.*, **85**, 1828–35.

Murphy, B.A., Motzer, R.J., Mazumdar, M. *et al.* (1993) An analysis of the effect of dose intensity on response, event-free survival and overall survival in patients with germ cell tumours (GCT) receiving ifosfamide-based salvage therapy. *Proc. Am. Soc. Clin. Oncol.*, **12**, 721, (Abstract).

Nakagawa, S., Sugimoto, K., Mikamie, K., Watanabe, H., Sonoda, Y., Kuzuyama, Y., Abe, T. and Fuji, H. (1994) Successful collection of peripheral blood stem cells mobilized by high-dose etoposide for patients with chemotherapy-resistant and/or poor prognostic testicular cancer. *Nippon Hinyokika Gakkai Zasshi*, **85**, 571–8.

Nichols, C.R., Roth, B.J., Heerema, N., Griep, J. and Tricot, G. (1990) Hematologic neoplasia associated with primary mediastinal germ cell tumours. *N. Engl. J. Med.*, **322**, 1425–9.

Nichols, C.R., Williams, S.D., Loehrer, P.J. *et al.* (1991) Randomized study of cisplatin dose intensity in poor risk germ cell tumours: A Southeastern Cancer Study Group and Southwest Oncology Group protocol. *J. Clin. Oncol.*, **9**(7), 1163–72.

Roach, S., Cooper, S., Bennet, W. and Pera, M.F. (1993) Cultured cell lines from human teratomas: Windows into tumor growth and differentiation and early human development. *Eur. Urol.*, **23**, 82–8.

Schmoll, H.-J., Schubert, I., Arnold, H., Dölken, G., Hecht, T., Bergmann, L., Illiger, J., Fink, U., Preiss, J., Pfreundschuh, M., Kaulen, H., Bonfert, B., Ho, A.D., Manegold, C., Mayr, A., Hoffmann, L., Weiss, J. and Hecker, H. (1987) Disseminated testicular cancer with bulky disease: results of a phase-II study with cisplatin ultra high dose/VP-16/bleomycin. *Int. J. Androl.*, **10**, 311–17.

Sehrt, J., Pietsch, T., Schöffski, P., Bokemeyer. C. *et al.* (1994) A possible role for stem cell factor (SCF) and its receptor C-kit in malignant germ cell tumors. *Proc. Am. Ass. Cancer Res.*, **35**, 255.

Siegert, W., Beyer, J., Strohscheer, I., Baurmann, H., Oettle, H., Zingsem, J., Zimmermann, R., Bokemeyer, C., Schmoll, H.-J. and Huhn, D. (1994) High-dose treatment with carboplatin, etoposide and ifosfamide followed by autologous stem-cell transplantation in relapsed or refractory germ cell cancer: A phase I/II study. *J. Clin. Oncol.*, **12**, 1223–31.

Sobrevilla-Calvo, P., Zinser, J.W., Lara, F.U., Acosta-Barreda, A., Guarner-Lans, J., Miranda-Lopez, E. and Reynoso-Gomez, E. (1994) High dose ICE (ifosfamide (I), carboplatin (C) and etoposide (E)) regimen supported with autologous transplantation of refrigerated peripheral blood stem cells (PAPBSC, mobilized with G-CSF: Description of a standard method to give high-dose chemotherapy (CT). *Proc. Am. Soc. Clin. Oncol.*, **13**, 161.

Spitzer, G., Adkins, D.R., Spencer, V., Dunphy, F.R., Petruska, P.J., Velasquez, W.S., Bowers, C.E., Kronmueller, N., Niemeyer, R. and McIntyre, W. (1994) Randomized study of growth factors post-peripheral-blood stem-cell transplant: Neutrophil recovery is improved with modest clinical benefit. *J. Clin. Oncol.*, **12**, 661–70.

Stoter, G., Sleijfer, D.T., Schornagel, J.H., ten Bokkel-Huinink, W.W., Vermeijlen, K. and Sylvester, R. on behalf of the EORTC Genito-

Urinary Group. (1993) BEP versus VIP in intermediate risk patients with disseminated non-seminomatous testicular cancer (NSTC). *Proc. Am. Soc. Clin. Oncol.*, **12**, 714, (Abstract).

Tjulandin, S., Garin, A., Stenina, M. *et al.* (1993) Carboplatin (CBDA), etoposide (VP-16), bleomycin (B) and GM-CSF in patients (pts) with poor risk nonseminomatous germ cell tumours (NSGCT). *Proc. Am. Soc. Clin. Oncol.*, **12**, 769, (Abstract).

Williams, S.D., Birch, R., Einhorn, L.H., Irwin, L., Greco, F.A. and Loehrer, P.J. (1987) Treatment of disseminated germ-cell tumors with cisplatin, bleomycin and either vinblastine or etoposide. *N. Engl. J. Med.*, **316**, 1435–40.

Wozniak, A.J., Samson, M.K., Shah, N.T., Crawford, E.D., Ford, C.D., Altman, S.J., Stephens, R.L., Natale, R.B., Bouroncle, B.A., Blumenstein, B.A and Cummings, G.D. (1991) A randomized trial of cisplatin, vinblastine and bleomycin versus vinblastin, cisplatin and etoposide in the treatment of advanced germ cell tumors of the testis: A Southwest Oncology Group Study. *J. Clin. Oncol.*, **9**, 70–6.

SALVAGE THERAPY AND AUTOLOGOUS BONE MARROW TRANSPLANTATION

25

A. Sandler and P. Loehrer

25.1 INTRODUCTION

Cisplatin combination chemotherapy has dramatically impacted upon the prognosis of patients with disseminated testicular cancer. In the past 15 years, the cure rate for metastatic disease has improved from less than one in five to approximately 80% of treated patients (Einhorn, 1981). Unfortunately, despite these successes, some patients may become candidates for salvage chemotherapy. These include patients who fail to achieve complete remission (CR) with induction chemotherapy, as well as those few who relapse from complete remission following chemotherapy. This chapter will present some of the nuances of salvage chemotherapy in recurrent and refractory germ cell tumors and highlight our experience with high dosage chemotherapy with autologous bone marrow transplantation.

25.2 PITFALLS IN SALVAGE CHEMOTHERAPY

Although patients failing to be cured with first line chemotherapy will be candidates for salvage therapy, occasionally the roentographic or serologic appearance of 'progressive disease' may mislead physicians to initiate inappropriate salvage chemotherapy. For ex-

ample, if the serum markers, i.e. the beta subunit of human chorionic gonadotrophin (BHCG) and alpha-fetoprotein (AFP), are falling appropriately but progressive pulmonary disease is noted during cisplatin chemotherapy, one might suspect pseudoprogression from either bleomycin lung disease or progression of benign teratoma (Loehrer *et al.*, 1987). New subpleural nodules (especially in areas outside previously known disease) are frequently noted on computed tomography (CT) scans of the chest following several cycles of bleomycin-containing chemotherapy and should not be confused with development of new disease (Figure 25.1). In contrast, when slow progression of previously known roentgenographic disease is noted despite normalization of serum markers, one should suspect the possibility of a growing benign teratoma. Not infrequently, patients may have histology that contains immature teratoma with non-germ cell elements (Table 25.1) (Loehrer *et al.*, 1985). Patients with this variant of teratoma may exhibit signs of rapidly growing disease, mimicking that of carcinoma but with normal serum markers. None the less, despite the rapidity of growth in this latter situation, complete surgical excision of the teratoma remains the treatment of choice.

25

25

25

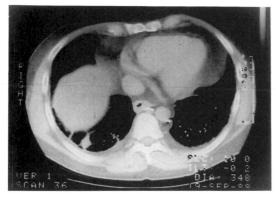

Fig. 25.1 Computed tomography scan of the chest following three courses of cisplatin, etoposide and bleomycin. The subpleural nodules secondary to bleomycin developed during therapy and mimic the appearance of pulmonary metastases.

Table 25.1 Non-germ cell elements in immature teratoma

Embryonal rhabdomyosarcoma
Myxoid liposarcoma
Epithelioid leiomyosarcoma
Adenosquamous carcinoma
Glioblastoma multiforme
Malignant giant cell tumor
Neuroblastoma
Nephroblastoma
Chondroblastoma
Cystosarcoma phylloides
Ganglioneuroma
Small cell carcinoma

False positive serum markers may occasionally occur. For BHCG, this may occur with cross-reactivity with luteinizing hormone (in states of relative hypogonadism), marijuana use and antibody formation (Phillips *et al.*, 1982; Loehrer *et al.*, 1987). Falsely elevated serum AFP may occur with hepatitis.

In patients undergoing treatment for metastatic disease, radiographic regression of cancer may be associated with serum marker elevation or plateau. Although an infrequent finding, a tumor sanctuary, e.g. occult testicular cancer or brain metastases, may be an explanation for those discordant results and

should be investigated by head CT scanning and/or testicular ultrasound. If progressive carcinoma is indeed documented, then salvage chemotherapy should be considered.

25.3 SALVAGE CHEMOTHERAPY

Following the successful combination of cisplatin with vinblastine and bleomycin (PVB), a new optimism sprang up for the treatment of patients with disseminated testicular cancer. Whereas 70% of all patients treated with PVB attained a CR, there was unfortunately a group of patients who either failed to achieve or relapsed from CR. The plight of these patients paralleled the dismal course of patients treated in the precisplatin era with a rapidly fatal disease. The dramatic impact that a single agent, cisplatin, made in the treatment of disseminated testicular cancer in early Phase II trials spurred hopes for similar stories for other newer agents tested in the refractory setting. Despite numerous trials with various agents, no drugs, with the exception of etoposide and ifosfamide, have emerged with a ⩾20% response rate in cisplatin-refractory disease.

Factors that adequately predict prognosis in patients with recurrent refractory germ cell tumors are difficult to discern because of the infrequent occurrence of resistant disease and the myriad of coexisting factors. In our experience, however, inability to achieve CR or quick relapse from a CR (⩽2 months) has been associated with few long-term survivors. In support of this, Bosl *et al.* (1985) reported only five partial remissions (PR) and no CR in 28 patients treated with cisplatin plus etoposide, all of whom had previous unresectable PR as their best response to previous cisplatin-based induction chemotherapy.

The term 'unresectable PR' includes two types of patients: those who demonstrate normalization of serum markers with persistent roentgenographic abnormalities that later progress, and those who fail to normalize their serum markers or progress during therapy. The prognosis in each setting may be different. Patients who exhibit concurrent roentgenographic and elevated serum marker progression following induction chemotherapy clearly have poor prognosis and should be targeted for innovative salvage chemotherapy (Wheeler *et al.*, 1986). However, those patients with residual disease and normal serum markers following induction chemotherapy have a variable clinical course. Although may of these latter patients will later relapse with progressive cancer manifested by rapidly growing disease and/or serum markers, many will show continued regression (implying necrotic tissue) or stable disease (implying benign teratoma). Slowly growing disease with persistently normal serum markers is almost pathognomic for recurrent benign teratoma and should be treated primarily with surgery.

An additional group of patients who are candidates for salvage therapy are those 9–10% of patients who relapse from CR following cisplatin induction chemotherapy. The majority of recurrences from CR occur during the first 1 to 2 years, with fewer than 5% of patients relapsing beyond 2 years (Einhorn, 1981; Roth *et al.*, 1988). Although it would appear likely that patients with late relapses might exhibit a broader range of sensitivity to chemotherapeutic agents, this, in fact, has not translated into an improved cure rate in our experience (Roth *et al.*, 1988).

25.3.1 THE ETOPOSIDE ERA

We believe that an important prognostic factor is the distinction between those who are cisplatin refractory (progressing during treatment) and those patients whose cancer recurs after cisplatin therapy. Prior to 1982, etoposide was the only drug to produce objective remissions in patients experiencing disease progression on cisplatin (Williams and Einhorn, 1982). Objective remissions were achieved in approximately one-third of

cisplatin refractory patients treated with single agent etoposide, but these remissions rarely lasted for longer than a few months.

Based on preclinical data of Schabel *et al.* (1979) demonstrating synergy of cisplatin plus etoposide, these two drugs were used in combination for patients with recurrent testicular cancer not refractory to cisplatin (the term 'refractory' being defined as a patient relapsing within 1 month of previous cisplatin) (Hainsworth *et al.*, 1985). In this setting, approximately 50% of patients achieved CR and 25% were cured with cisplatin/etoposide combination therapy, which represented a remarkable achievement and paved the way towards the successful evaluation of etoposide-containing regimens as initial therapy. Indeed, cisplatin/etoposide plus bleomycin (PVpB) not only demonstrated less toxicity but was more active and produced more cures than cisplatin/vinblastine/bleomycin (PVB) (Williams *et al.*, 1987). Most patients who currently present with recurrent or refractory germ cell tumors have been heavily pretreated and thus are generally considered for newer Phase II drugs.

As previously mentioned, only etoposide and ifosfamide have demonstrated response rates greater than 20% as single agents in cisplatin-refractory patients. The optimal schedule for etoposide is unclear. In a recent article by Slevin and his colleagues (1989), etoposide was administered to previously untreated patients with small cell carcinoma of the lung in two different dosage schedules (500 mg m^{-2} over 24 h versus 100 mg m^{-2} on days 1–5) in a protective randomized trial. Surprisingly, not only the response rate but also the overall survival rate was statistically significantly superior for the fractionated schedule. With the advent of an oral etoposide capsule, the opportunity to test schedule dependency further arose.

In a Phase II trial performed at Indiana University, etoposide was administered at a daily oral dose of 50 mg m^{-2} for 21 days in patients with recurrent or refractory germ cell tumor (Miller and Einhorn, 1990). This regimen has roughly the same total bioequivalency as seen in the intravenous schedule of 100 mg m^{-2} daily for 5 consecutive days. In 21 evaluable patients, three demonstrated partial remissions. Three additional patients had greater than 90% reduction in serum markers without roentgenographic change. The median length of treatment was 11.5 weeks (range 2–30 weeks) with a median white blood count nadir of $1.5 \times 10^9 \text{ l}^{-1}$ and a median platelet nadir of $184 \times 10^9 \text{ l}^{-1}$. Eight patients developed granulocytopenic fever, including two patients with pneumonia and one additional patient with bacteremia. The median survival time was 20.5 weeks (range 8–48 weeks) with the median time to progression being 13.8 weeks (range 5–38) weeks. The longest remission to date has been observed in a patient who relapsed following high dose carboplatin and VP-16 (etoposide) with bone marrow transplantation. How these data will be integrated into initial therapeutic regimens is uncertain. None the less, this study with daily oral etoposide is a reminder of the possible importance of drug scheduling as well as dosing in the treatment of malignant neoplasms.

Patients who relapse from CR or fail to achieve a CR have a poor prognosis. Given the activity of etoposide with prolonged daily oral administration in patients with relapsed or refractory germ cell tumors, researchers at Indiana University conducted a study evaluating the role of maintenance oral etoposide in patients who had achieved a disease-free status following salvage therapy (Cooper *et al.*, 1995). Patients who had achieved a partial remission were also included to determine whether oral etoposide could convert any of these patients into a CR.

Between July 1990 and December 1992, 37 patients with histologic evidence of germ cell tumor who had attained a CR or PR after salvage therapy (chemotherapy or surgery) were entered on the study. Three patients were not evaluable due to progression of disease prior to receiving oral etoposide. Oral

etoposide was administered in a dose of $50 \text{ mg m}^{-2} \text{ d}^{-1}$ for 21 consecutive days every 4 weeks for three cycles. Doses were rounded off to the nearest 25 mg. The toxicity of oral VP-16 was minor, with 25 of 34 patients (76%) completing all three courses. Only four patients received less than three courses because of toxicity (three with neutropenia, one with mucositis). Five patients progressed while receiving oral VP-16 and did not complete treatment.

At the time daily oral VP-16 was started, 23 patients were in CR and 11 patients were in PR. Seventeen of the 23 patients (74%) remain continuously disease free, with a median follow-up of 36 months (26–49 months). Three of 11 patients in PR were converted to CR during maintenance therapy. All three patients have since relapsed at 4, 7 and 18 months from initiation of maintenance oral VP-16 therapy.

It is expected that most, if not all, of the 17 patients who are continuously disease free are cured of their disease since the minimal follow-up time is 26 months. These results are encouraging given the fact that CRs obtained in the salvage setting are less durable than those achieved after first line therapy. The relapse rate from CR following salvage therapy, regardless of the clinical situation, is greater than 50%.

Given the excellent tolerability of oral maintenance VP-16 therapy and the encouraging results, the authors recommend maintenance daily oral VP-16 for patients who achieve a CR following any type of salvage therapy.

25.3.2 SINGLE AGENT IFOSFAMIDE

Ifosfamide is an oxazaphosphorine, which is a structural analogue of cyclophosphamide (Brock, 1983). Moving the chloroethyl group from the side chain to the ring structure produced differences in metabolism as well as an improved therapeutic index of ifosfamide over cyclophosphamide. The enhanced therapeutic index was largely achieved by the relative lack of myelosuppression of ifosfamide compared with its parent compound. The dose-limiting toxicity in early Phase I trials was hemorrhagic cystitis, which was thought to result from the production of acrolein and chloracetic acid (Morgan, Holdiness and Gillen, 1983; Brock *et al.*, 1984). This toxicity has been largely eliminated with the use of effective thiol compounds, such as *N*-acetylcysteine and mesna, which combine with the toxic metabolites to provide urothelial protection.

Early clinical trials proved ifosfamide to have a broad range of activity against both experimental and human tumors (Goldin, 1982; Hunter and Harrison, 1982). Indeed, numerous European studies demonstrated a high degree of activity for ifosfamide against testicular cancer although the majority of patients had minimal or no previous chemotherapy (Aiginger *et al.*, 1982; Schmoll, 1982). In heavily pretreated patients, ifosfamide produced lower response rates, but it had definite activity. For example, Scheulen *et al.* (1985) reported a 20% response rate with ifosfamide in refractory germ cell tumors.

From July 1982 to September 1983, 30 patients with recurrent or refractory germ cell tumors were entered into a trial at Indiana University to evaluate single agent ifosfamide (Wheeler *et al.*, 1986). Twenty-eight of the 30 patients had been treated with two or more cisplatin combination regimens, and 75% had progressed during or within 3 weeks of completion of a prior cisplatin combination regimen. Ifosfamide was administered at dosages of 1.5 to 2.0 g m^{-2} daily for 5 days with courses repeated every 3 weeks. Overall, one CR and six PR were observed, for an overall objective response rate of 23%. As was observed with single agent etoposide in a comparable patient population, the duration of remission and median survival time were limited. However, this activity in this heavily treated population provided the basis for

further evaluation of ifosfamide in a more favorable population.

25.3.3 IFOSFAMIDE COMBINATION THERAPY

Based on the demonstration of single agent activity of ifosfamide, as well as known preclinical synergy of oxazaphosphorines plus cisplatin (Goldin, 1982), a trial was initiated to evaluate etoposide/ifosfamide/cisplatin (VIP) and vinblastine/ifosfamide/cisplatin (VeIP) in patients with recurrent testicular cancer (Loehrer *et al.*, 1988). We felt that the optimal method for clarifying the impact of ifosfamide was to study patients with recurrent germ cell neoplasms who received ifosfamide as the only new drug in third line combination therapy or greater.

From April 1983 to July 1986, 57 eligible patients with progressive, recurrent germ cell neoplasms were entered into this trial. All patients had progressive recurrent disease and had received at least two previous cisplatin combination regimens (including prior exposure to both vinblastine and etoposide). Twenty-six (46%) of the patients had previously received three or more regimens and 22 patients had never achieved a CR with previous induction therapy. No patient, however, was excluded on the basis of performance status or metastatic site. With the exception of one female patient who had recurrent ovarian germ cell tumor, patients who demonstrated progressive disease within 3 weeks of receiving previous cisplatin combination chemotherapy, i.e. cisplatin-refractory patients, were not entered into this study but were referred for Phase II trials with other investigational drugs. The majority of patients had moderate or advanced disease according to the Indiana University staging system (Table 7.3, Section 7.3) (Birch *et al.*, 1986).

Patients on this VIP/VeIP trial were treated with cisplatin (20 mg m^{-2} days 1–5), ifosfamide (1.2 g m^{-2} days 1–5) and either etoposide (75 mg m^{-2} days 1–5) or vinblastine

(0.11 mg kg^{-1} days 1 and 2), respectively. Eligible patients were not randomly assigned to these regimens, but rather received vinblastine or etoposide depending on which drug was associated with previous best response, longest duration of remission, or least toxicity in prior induction therapies. From April 1983 to October 1984, N-acetylcysteine was administered as a uroepithelial protective agent. Since October 1984, mesna has been administered at an intravenous dosage of 120 mg m^{-2} given immediately before ifosfamide, followed by a continuous infusion (1200 mg m^{-2} daily for 5 consecutive days) with 0.9% normal saline. In those patients with prior chest or abdominal radiotherapy, the dosages of vinblastine or etoposide and ifosfamide were reduced by 25%. Courses were repeated every 21 days for a total of four cycles.

Fifty-six of 57 eligible patients were evaluable for response and survival. One patient who had incomplete resection of carcinoma with normal serum markers was evaluable for survival but not response. Overall 12 patients (21%) achieved a disease-free status after VIP or VeIP chemotherapy; an additional eight patients were free of disease following resection of teratoma (three patients) or carcinoma (five patients). Thus overall 20 patients (36%) achieved disease-free status (95% confidence intervals, 23.4–49.6%).

Various characteristics of the patients with respect to response rate are shown in Table 25.2. Fifteen of 32 patients (47%) achieved a favorable response to VIP compared with only five of 24 (21%) treated with VeIP. Although this difference was significant, other factors, including extent of disease and previous response, were also marginally significant. When a logistic regression analysis was performed and adjusted for extent of disease and previous best response, these differences in treatment regimens remained significant, with VIP yielding improved disease-free rates over VeIP. Yet, when these same factors were evaluated in terms of overall survival, the Cox proportional hazards model

revealed that only extent of disease was a statistically significant factor.

The median duration of CR in these 57 patients was 34 months (range 3–>42 months), including nine patients who remained continuously free of disease from 15 to over 42 months. Seven patients remained in continuous CR for 2 years or longer. Currently, 19 of 57 (33%) patients who are evaluable for survival remain alive from 16 to over 53 months. The median survival time for all patients was 12.7 months, and 15 of the 20 patients who achieved CR are still alive.

These data have provided the impetus to evaluate the role of ifosfamide in initial induction chemotherapy. An intergroup trial (ECOG, CALGB, SWOG) has evaluated cisplatin plus etoposide with either bleomycin (BEP) or ifosfamide (VIP) in patients with poor risk disseminated germ cell tumors, and found no obvious differences in survival (Nichols *et al.*, 1994).

Einhorn *et al.* (1992) have recently reported on an update of patients treated with vinblastine, ifosfamide and cisplatin (VeIP) as second line therapy after failing cisplatin, VP-16 and bleomycin (PEB). One hundred and twenty-four patients were treated with VeIP from July 1984 to August 1989. Minimal follow-up after initiation of VeIP was 27 months. Eighty-one patients had advanced disease (Indiana classification) at the start of PVP$_{16}$B and 59 patients at the initiation of VeIP. Thirty-one patients had extragonadal disease. Fifty-six (45%) patients achieved NED (no evidence of disease) status, including 15 (12%) NED teratoma and 7 (6%) NED with VeIP following resection of carcinoma. At the time of publication, 29 patients (23%) were continuously NED and 37 (30%) are currently NED. Median survival was 72 weeks (6–356 weeks). Seventy-seven (62%) patients never achieved an NED status with PVP$_{16}$B. Seventeen of these 77 patients achieved NED status with VeIP and 11 patients (14%) are continuously NED. Overall, 28 of 93 patients (30%) with refractory

Table 25.2 Prognostic factors following salvage chemotherapy with etoposide/ifosfamide/cisplatin (VIP) or vinblastine/ifosfamide/cisplatin (VeIP)

Characteristics	Favorable responses/ total number of patients	
Histological findings		
Embryonal cell carcinoma	5/13	(38%)
Teratoma plus embryonal carcinoma	1/9	(11%)
Choriocarcinoma	1/2	(50%)
Teratoma	1/1	(100%)
Seminoma	0/3	(0%)
Combination of above or other	12/18	(41%)
Primary site		
Testis	16/46	(34%)
Mediastinum	0/2	(0%)
Retroperitoneum	3/7	(43%)
Ovary	1/1	(100%)
Marker elevation		
Beta-human chorionic gonadotrophin (BHCG)	10/22	(45%)
Alpha-fetoprotein (AFP)	8/9	(42%)
Both BHCG and AFP	2/11	(18%)
None	0/4	(0%)
Disease extent		
Minimal	13/30	(43%)
Moderate	6/17	(35%)
Advanced	1/9	(11%)
Previous treatment		
Two previous chemotherapy regimens	10/31	(32%)
More than two previous chemotherapy regimens	10/15	(40%)
Previous best response to chemotherapy		
Complete (>2 months duration)	14/30	(47%)
Complete (≤2 months duration)	0/4	(0%)
Partial or no response	6/22	(27%)

testis cancer are continuously NED. Only six of 31 extragonadal patients attained an NED status and only one patient is continuously disease free.

The activity of ifosfamide-based combination chemotherapy in patients with germ cell tumors refractory to cisplatin-based chemotherapy has been confirmed by others. Motzer *et al.* (1992a) reported on 66 patients with germ cell tumors refractory to cisplatin plus etoposide or vinblastine-based chemotherapy subsequently treated with cisplatin, ifosfamide and vinblastine (VeIP)(16 patients) or eto-

poside (VIP)(50 patients). Sixty-two patients were evaluable for response. Complete response were seen in 21 patients (34%), 18 with chemotherapy alone and an additional three patients following surgery for carcinoma. At the time of publication six patients had relapsed, and 15 patients (24%) remain continuously NED with a median follow-up of 13 months (3+ to 41+ months).

Harstrick *et al.*, reported on 30 patients with refractory germ cell tumor who had failed to be cured by first line cisplatin-based chemotherapy (Harstrick *et al.*, 1991). Ten patients (33%) were disease free at the end of therapy, including four patients requiring surgery (two with teratoma, two with carcinoma). Six patients (20%) had normalization of tumor markers but persistent, unresectable disease. Of the ten patients with CR, nine (90%) patients have relapsed again (eight with carcinoma, one with teratoma). At the time of publication, seven of 30 patients were alive, and five were NED (17%).

Ifosfamide-based salvage chemotherapy has curative potential in refractory testis cancer but, with durable complete remissions in only about 25–30% of cases, other treatment modalities are being studied.

25.4   BONE MARROW TRANSPLANTATION

High dose chemotherapy with autologous bone marrow rescue appears to be an attractive concept in patients with relapsed testis cancer for several reasons: (1) Patients with testis cancer are generally young and without other significant medical problems. (2) Testicular cancer is an extremely chemosensitive tumor in which one might expect to find a dose–response relationship to chemotherapy. (3) Testicular cancer rarely metastasizes to bone marrow, making reinfusion of harvested marrow with contaminated tumor cells unlikely.

Initial attempts at high dose chemotherapy with autologous bone marrow transplantation have produced occasional complete responses that were typically of short duration (Table 25.3). The bulk of the experience utilized high dose etoposide without cisplatin. Pico and

his associates (1986) underscored the clinical importance of the platinum-compound–etoposide synergy that Schabel and colleagues (1979) demonstrated. Among 16 patients with recurrent testicular cancer (details regarding prior treatment not given) treated with high dose etoposide, cyclophosphamide and cisplatin in that series, five (31%) remain in continuous CR.

Carboplatin is an analogue of cisplatin that is virtually devoid of the severe dose-limiting nephrotoxicity and neurotoxicity observed with its parent compound. Myelosuppression is the dose-limiting toxicity of carboplatin. Like cisplatin, carboplatin has definite activity in patients with germ cell tumors (albeit low when used at conventional dosages in cisplatin-refractory patients; Motzer *et al.*, 1987; Trump *et al.*, 1987. As such, the incorporation of carboplatin and etoposide are ideal drugs to evaluate in testicular cancer in the light of their single activities and relatively mild nonhematological toxicity.

From September 1986 to June 1989 40 consecutive patients with refractory germ cell tumors were treated at Indiana University with high dose carboplatin (900 to 2000 mg m^{-2}) and etoposide (1200 mg m^{-2}) over 3 days (Nichols *et al.*, 1989; Broun *et al.*, 1992) (Fig. 25.2). Three patients also received ifosfamide (10 g m^{-2}). All patients had autologous bone marrow rescue. All eligible patients had extensive prior chemotherapy including 70% of patients exhibiting progressive disease within 4 weeks of completing cisplatin-based chemotherapy. Nineteen

Table 25.3 High dosage chemotherapy with autologous bone marrow transplantation in refractory testicular cancer

Reference	Number of patients	Chemotherapy regimen	Number of complete responses
Wolff *et al.* (1984)	11	VP-16	2 (20%)
Blijham *et al.* (1981)	13	Cy/VP-16	4 (30%)
Mulder *et al.* (1988)	11	Cy/VP-16	2
Corringham *et al.* (1983)	1	L-PAM	0

Cy, cyclophosphamide. VP-16, etoposide. L-PAM, melphalan.

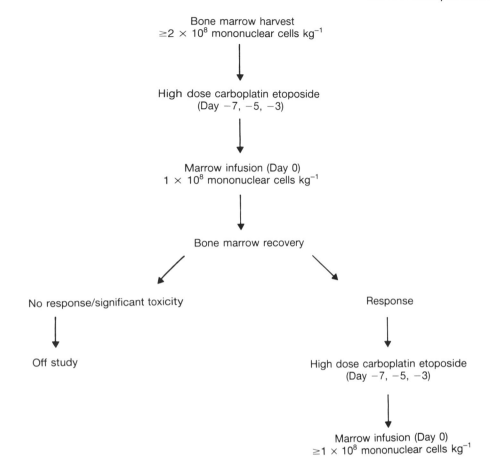

Fig. 25.2 A schematic diagram showing repetitive high dose chemotherapy with autologous bone marrow transplantation for refractory germ cell tumors.

patients (55%) had received three or more prior chemotherapy regimens. Two-thirds of the patients received a second course of chemotherapy at the same dosage. Of the 40 study patients 26 (65%) responded to treatment; 12 (30%) achieved a complete response. Of the 12 CRs, five patients have relapsed and one patient died of a treatment-related acute leukemia 27.5 months after treatment without evidence of germ cell cancer. Six of the original 40 patients (15%), of whom three were considered to be cisplatin refractory, remained NED after at least 2 years of follow-up. Seven patients (18%) died of treatment-related causes, including sepsis (four patients), veno-occlusive disease (one patient), and hemorrhage (two patients). Eight of the 40 patients had primary mediastinal germ cell tumors, of which no patient achieved a complete response.

This study demonstrates that a dose-intensive regimen is capable of overcoming cisplatin resistance in some cases, albeit with significant toxicity. A logical extension of these data is to incorporate high dose regimens earlier in the treatment planning of poor risk patients and not merely wait until these patients reach the end stages of their disease. As such, the Eastern Cooperative Oncology Group evaluated a protocol consisting of two induction cycles of VeIP followed by one single course of high dose carboplatin plus etoposide with autologous bone marrow rescue (ABMR) (Nichols *et al.*, 1992). From July 1988 to September 1989, 40 patients were entered on the study, of which 38 patients were deemed eligible, two were ineligible owing to incorrect histology and insufficient prior therapy. All patients either failed initial chemotherapy and a salvage combination regimen containing cisplatin and ifosfamide, or had progressive disease while receiving optimal cisplatin combination therapy or within 1 month of the last cisplatin dose. Nineteen patients (48%) were considered cisplatin refractory and 28 patients (70%) had received only one or two prior chemotherapy regimens. Treatment consisted of carboplatin (1500 mg m^{-2}) and etoposide (1200 mg m^{-2}) over 3 days followed by autologous bone marrow rescue. Patients who achieved a complete or partial response with the first cycle of therapy received a second identical cycle of chemotherapy and ABMR. Objective responses were seen in 17 of the 38 patients (45%), with nine patients achieving a CR. At the time of publication, five patients (13%) remain in continuous NED with a minimum follow-up of 1 year. Toxicity was principally hematological, with five patients (13%) dying of treatment-related complications including sepsis (one patient), bleeding (two patients), veno-occlusive disease (one patient) and liver failure secondary to disease progression and chemotherapy.

Broun and colleagues at Indiana University and Case Western-Reserve University reported on a trial involving high dose chemotherapy and ABMT for patients with relapsed germ cell tumors as second line therapy (Broun *et al.*, 1994). This trial excluded patients with extragonadal germ cell tumors. Twenty-three patients were treated with two cycles of induction chemotherapy (VeIP or PVB (cisplatin, vinblastine, and bleomycin) followed by carboplatin (1500–2100 mg m^{-2}) and etoposide (1200–2250 mg m^{-2}) over 3 days followed by ABMR. Eighteen of 23 patients com-

pleted therapy. Five patients did not receive high dose therapy due to: patient refusal (one); active infection (one), CNS metastasis (one), death during induction therapy (one), insurance refusal (one). Results from high dose therapy included 15 out of 18 response, with nine patients achieving a CR. There was only one patient treatment-related death, this occurred during the induction phase. There were no transplant-related deaths. At the time of publication, seven of the 18 patients (39%) completing high dose therapy were alive NED with a median follow-up of 26 months. Motzer and colleagues (Motzer *et al.*, 1992b) reported similar experiences with the use of high dose chemotherapy and ABMR in patients with relapsed germ cell tumor as initial salvage therapy.

To test further the hypothesis that early intervention with high dose chemotherapy may be superior to current standard therapy, the Eastern Cooperative Oncology Group will be conducting a trial comparing standard BEP versus high dose chemotherapy in previously untreated poor risk germ cell tumors. Eligible patients will be randomized to either four cycles of BEP or two cycles of BEP followed by carboplatin (1800 mg m^{-2}), etoposide (1800 mg m^{-2}) and cyclophosphamide (150 mg kg^{-1}), each divided over 3 days, followed by ABMR or stem cell reinfusion. Responding patients in the latter arm will also receive a second identical cycle of high dose chemotherapy followed by ABMR or stem cell reinfusion.

25.5 CONCLUSIONS

Testicular cancer is indeed a rare neoplasm but remains an important disease for clinical study, not only because of its unique biological aspects and its highly curable nature by surgery (in local disease) and chemotherapy (in metastatic disease), but also because it has served as a successful link between preclinical and clinical models of drug development. Many of the observations from trials of salvage therapy that have been successfully incorporated into first line therapy have broad implications in the treatment of other malignancies. Thus, testicular cancer remains a fertile testing ground for future drug development and remains a disease in which cautious optimism may remain for patients even in the salvage setting.

REFERENCES

Aiginger, P., Schwartz, H.P., Juzmits, R. *et al.* (1982) Ifosfamide and cisplatin in testicular tumor patients resistant to vinblastine, bleomycin, cisplatinum. *Proc. 13th Int. Cancer Congress 13*, **180**, (Abstract).

Birch, R., Williams, S.D., Cone, A. *et al.* (1986) Prognostic factors for favorable outcome in disseminated germ cell tumors. *J. Clin. Oncol.*, **4**, 400–7.

Blijham, G., Spitzer, G., Litam, J. *et al.* (1981) The treatment of advanced testicular carcinoma with high dose chemotherapy and autologous marrow support. *Eur. J. Cancer*, **17**, 433–41.

Bosl, G.J., Yagoda, A., Golbey, R.B. *et al.* (1985) Role of etoposide-based chemotherapy with refractory or relapsed germ cell tumors. *Am. J. Med.*, **78**, 423–38.

Brock, N. (1983) The oxazaphosphorines. *Cancer Treat. Rev.*, **10**, 3–15 (Suppl. A).

Brock, N., Hilgard, P., Pohl, J. *et al.* (1984) Pharmacokinetics and mechanism of action of detoxifying low-molecular-weight thiols. *J. Cancer Res. Clin. Oncol.*, **108**, 87–97.

Broun, E.R., Nichols, C.R., Kneebone, P. *et al.* (1992) Long-term outcome of patients with relapsed and refractory germ cell tumors treated with high-dose chemotherapy and autologous bone marrow rescue. *Ann. Intern. Med.*, **117**, 124–8.

Broun, E.R., Nichols, C.R., Turns, M. *et al.* (1994) Early salvage therapy for germ cell cancer using high dose chemotherapy with autologous bone marrow support. *Cancer*, **73**, 1716–20.

Cooper, M.A., and Einhorn, L.H. (1995) Maintenance Chemotherapy with daily oral etoposide following salvage therapy in patients with germ cell tumors. *J. Clin. Oncol.*, **13**, 1167–9.

Corringham, R., Gilmore, M., Prentice, H.G. *et al.* (1983) High dose melphalan with autologous bone marrow transplant. *Cancer*, **52**, 1783–8.

Einhorn, L.H. (1981) Testicular cancer as a model for curable neoplasm: The Richard and Hinda Rosenthal Foundation Award Lecture. *Cancer Res*, **41**, 3275–80.

Einhorn, L.H., Weathers, T., Loehrer, P. *et al.* (1992) Second line chemotherapy with vinblastine, ifosfamide, and cisplatin after initial chemotherapy with cisplatin, VP-16 and bleomycin (PVP$_{16}$B) in disseminated germ cell tumors. *Proc. Am. Soc. Clin. Oncol.*, **11**, 196.

Goldin, A. (1982) Ifosfamide in experimental tumor systems. *Sem. Oncol.*, **9**, 14–23.

Hainsworth, J.D., Williams, S.D., Einhorn, L.H. *et al.* (1985) Successful treatment of resistant germinal neoplasms with VP-16 and cisplatin: Results of a Southeastern Cancer Study Group Trial. *J. Clin. Oncol.*, **3**, 666–71.

Harstrick, A., Schmoll, H.J., Wilke, H. *et al.* (1991) Cisplatin, etoposide, and ifosfamide salvage therapy for refractory or relapsing germ cell carcinoma. *J. Clin. Oncol.*, **9**, 1549–55.

Hunter, H.L. and Harrison, E.F. (1982) The anticancer spectrum of ifosfamide. *Sem. Oncol.*, **9**, 96–100 (Suppl. 1).

Loehrer, P.J., Eisenhut, C., Sample, M. *et al.* (1987) How to cope with antibodies to HCG in laboratory testing. *J. Clin. Ligand Assay Soc.*, **10**, 58 (Abstract).

Loehrer, P.J., Lauer, P., Roth, B.J. *et al.*. (1988) Salvage therapy in recurrent germ cell cancer: Ifosfamide and cisplatin plus either vinblastine or etoposide. *Ann. Intern. Med.* **7**, 540–6.

Loehrer, P.J., Mandelbaum, I., Hui, S. *et al.* (1985) Resection of thoracic and abdominal teratoma in patients after cisplatin-based chemotherapy for germ cell tumors. Late results. *J. Thorac. Cardiovasc. Surg.*, **92**, 676–83.

Miller, J.C. and Einhorn, L.H. (1990) Phase II study of daily oral VP-16 in refractory germ cell tumors. *Sem. Oncol.*, **17**, 36–9.

Morgan, L.R., Holdiness, M.R. and Gillen, L.E. (1983) N-Acetylcysteine: Its bioavailability and interaction with ifosfamide metabolites. *Sem. Oncol.*, **10**, 56–61 (Suppl. 1).

Motzer, R.J., Bajorin, D.F., Vlamis, V. *et al.* (1992a) Ifosfamide-based chemotherapy for patients with resistant germ cell tumors: The Memorial Sloan Kettering Cancer Center Experience. *Sem. Oncol.*, **19**, 8–12 (Suppl. 12).

Motzer, R.J., Bosl, G.J., Taver, K. *et al.* (1987) Phase II trial of carboplatin in patients with advanced germ cell tumors refractory to cisplatin. *Cancer Treat. Rep.*, **71**, 197–8.

Motzer, R.J., Gulati, S.C., Crown, J.P. *et al.*

(1992b) High-dose chemotherapy and autologous bone marrow rescue for patients with refractory germ cell tumors. *Cancer*, **69**, 550–6.

Mulder, P.O.M,, DeVries, E.G.E., Koops, H.S. *et al.* (1988) Chemotherapy with maximally tolerable doses of VP-16-213 and cyclophosphamide followed by autologous bone marrow transplantation for the treatment of relapsed or refractory germ cell tumors. *Eur. J. Cancer Clin. Oncol.*, **24**, 674–9.

Nichols, C.R., Andersen, J., Lazarus, H.M. *et al.* (1992) High-dose carboplatin and etoposide with autologous bone marrow transplantation in refractory germ cell cancer: An Eastern Cooperative Oncology Group Protocol. *J. Clin. Oncol.*, **10**, 558–63.

Nichols, C.R., Loehrer, P.J., Einhorn, L.H. *et al.* (1994) Phase III study of cisplatin, etoposide and bleomycin or etoposide, ifosfamide and cisplatin in advanced stage germ cell tumors. An intergroup trial. *Proc. Am. Soc. Clin. Oncol.*, **14**, 239.

Nichols, C.R., Tricot, G., Williams, S.D. *et al.* (1989) Dose-intensive chemotherapy in refractory germ cell cancer – a phase I/II trial of high dose carboplatin and etoposide with autologous bone marrow transplantation. *J. Clin. Oncol.*, **7**, 937–9.

Phillips, M.I., Weiner, R., MacLaren, N. *et al.* (1982) Test of false positive testicular cancer marker by suppressing luteinizing hormone with testosterone. *Lancet*, **ii**, 928.

Pico, J.L., Droz, J.P., Gouyette, A. *et al.* (1986) 25 high dose chemotherapy regimens (HDCR) followed by autologous bone marrow transplantation (ABMT) in refractory or relapsed non-seminomatous germ cell tumor (NSGCT). *Proc. Am. Soc. Clin. Oncol.*, **5**, 111.

Roth, B.J., Greist, A., Kublili, P.S. *et al.* (1988) Cisplatin-based combination chemotherapy for disseminated germ cell tumors: Long term follow-up. *J. Clin. Oncol.*, **6**, 1239–47.

Schabel, F.M, Jr, Trader, M.W., Laster, W.R. Jr *et al.* (1979) *Cis*-dichlorodiammineplatinum (II): Combination chemotherapy and cross resistance studies with tumors of mice. *Cancer Treat. Rep.*, **63**, 1459–73.

Scheulen, M.E., Niederle, N., Hoffken, K. *et al.* (1985) Ifosfamide/mesna alone or in combination with etoposide: Salvage therapy for patients with metastasized non-seminomatous testicular cancer. *Proc. Am. Soc. Clin. Oncol.*, **4**, 97 (Abstract).

Schmoll, H.J. (1982) The role of ifosfamide in testicular cancer. *Proc. 13th Int. Cancer Congress.*, **13**, 1981 (Abstract).

Slevin, M.L., Clark, P.I., Joel, S.P. *et al.* (1989) A randomized trial to evaluate the effect of schedule on the activity of etoposide in small-cell lung cancer. *J. Clin. Oncol.*, **7**, 1333–40.

Trump, D.L., Elson, P., Brodovsky, H. *et al.* (1987) Carboplatin in advanced, refractory germ cell neoplasms: A Phase II Eastern Cooperative Oncology Group study. *Cancer Treat. Rep.*, **71**, 989–90.

Wheeler, B.M., Loehrer, P.J., Williams, S.D. *et al.* (1986) Ifosfamide in refractory male germ cell tumors. *J. Clin. Oncol.*, **4**, 28–34.

Williams, S.D., Birch, R., Einhorn, L.H. *et al.* (1987) Disseminated germ cell tumors: Chemotherapy with cisplatin plus bleomycin plus either vinblastine or etoposide. A trial of the Southeastern Cancer Study Group. *N. Engl. J. Med.*, **316**, 1435–40.

Williams, S.D. and Einhorn, L.H. (1982) Etoposide salvage therapy for refractory germ cell tumors: An update. *Cancer. Treat. Rev.*, **9**, 67–71 (Suppl.).

Wolff, S.N., Johnson, D.H., Hainsworth, J.D. *et al.* (1984) High dose VP-16-213 monotherapy for refractory germinal malignancies: A phase II study. *J. Clin. Oncol.*, **2**, 271–4.

ABDOMINAL SURGERY POSTCHEMOTHERAPY IN METASTATIC NON-SEMINOMA

W.F. Hendry

26.1 INTRODUCTION

After completion of chemotherapy, a residual mass is left behind in almost one-quarter of cases (Tait *et al.*, 1984). Ever since the introduction of effective chemotherapy in 1976, these masses have been the subject of intense interest in our Testicular Tumour Unit (Hendry *et al.*, 1977; Boyd *et al.*, 1978; Husband *et al.*, 1979), and we have demonstrated that computed tomography (CT) scanning is more than 95% accurate in defining their site, size and extent (Kennedy *et al.*, 1985). Initially it was hoped that radiotherapy would eliminate any active tumor remaining after chemotherapy. However, comparative studies showed that there was still residual undifferentiated tumor in 20% of cases after planned chemotherapy and radiotherapy, compared with 24% after chemotherapy alone (Hendry *et al.*, 1981). Furthermore, side-effects after radiotherapy following chemotherapy were not inconsiderable, and so this treatment modality was abandoned at our center, although it is still used by others (Read, Johnson and Wilkinson, 1986). It became our policy to recommend excision of all substantial residual masses 1 month or so after completion of chemotherapy. Since the likelihood of residual active tumor was shown to be related to the size of the mass (Hendry *et al.*, 1981), we set a lower limit of 2 cm transverse diameter; only rarely has active tumor been found in nodes smaller than this (Dexeus *et al.*, 1989).

It should be appreciated that the persistence of a mass on CT scanning was never regarded as a failure of chemotherapy. It was always made clear to patients with metastatic disease, before commencing chemotherapy, that surgical excision might be necessary for any bits of cancer that did not disappear. As a result, patients coming to the Joint Testicular Tumour Clinic for assessment for surgery arrive with minds well prepared, with no sense of disappointment or feeling that all has not gone as well as expected. This positive approach makes the surgeon's job much easier than it is with patients referred in from some other units, when an air of despondency surrounds the discussion of the forthcoming operation. It is generally only necessary to explain to our patients that the lump has to be removed (a) to get rid of it, and (b) to make sure that the chemotherapy has completely eliminated the cancer. Most testicular tumor patients are young and adapt well psychologically to their disease, provided it is explained adequately (Cassileth and Steinfeld, 1987), although inevitably a

Testicular Cancer: Investigation and management. Second edition. Edited by Professor A. Horwich.
Published in 1996 by Chapman & Hall. ISBN 0 412 61210 0.

few have long-term psychosocial problems if treatment results in alteration in sexual function (Tamburini *et al.*, 1989).

Preparation for excision of residual masses therefore commences at presentation, and by the time chemotherapy is completed it is fairly clear which patients are likely to require surgery. An appointment is made at this time for joint consultation with surgeon and oncologist. All relevant recent radiographs and scans are made available, up-to-date marker results are obtained, and the patient is told the purpose of the meeting. Close relatives are welcome to attend.

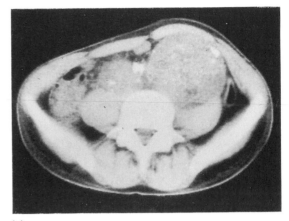

(a)

26.2 PLANNING AND PREPARATION

The surgeon needs to know exactly where the masses are, and their size. Adjacent structures may be at risk of damage, or may have to be removed along with the mass, and this can only be assessed by careful reference to the scans. Not only is this essential for the surgeon to plan the operative approach, but the patient and his relatives **must** be advised of the likely extent of the surgery, and be warned of any likely effect on other organs. In particular, failure to warn the patient of potential loss of a major organ such as a kidney, or interference with ejaculation, could be interpreted as negligence. None the less, a positive matter-of-fact approach should be taken, and whilst potential risks should not be ignored or glossed over, they need not be dwelt upon.

In 70% of cases, the residual masses are in the para-aortic lymph nodes in the retroperitoneum, in 18% they are in the chest, and in 12% they are above and below the diaphragm. In the latter group the thoracic surgeon and the urologist should meet to discuss whether it is possible to remove all the tumors at once, through a thoracoabdominal incision, or whether a staged approach is preferable. In general, we have found that it is better not to be overambitious, hoping to remove everything in one operation, since access and hence safety may be compromised. Our approach is

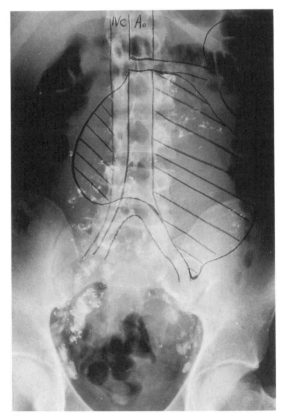

(b)

Fig. 26.1 (a) A computed tomography scan, and (b) a 'scanogram' showing extent of residual mass and its relation to the great vessels. Since the tumor lies below the renal vessels, an anterior approach provides adequate access.

Table 26.1   Incisions used to remove masses in 140 patients (Royal Marsden Hospital data, 1976–1984)

| | | Sites of residual masses | | | |
| | | Para-aortic | | | |
Incision	Number	Unilateral	Bilateral	Mediastinum	Lung
Midline	109	69	40		
Thoracoabdominal	29	17	12	9	13
Nagamatsu	2	2			
Total	140	88	52	9	13

that masses above the diaphragm are always best dealt with by a thoracic surgeon (Chapter 27), while those in the neck may require a separate operation by a third surgical specialist.

In planning the surgical approach to retroperitoneal or other abdominal masses, it is very helpful indeed to have a 'scanogram' – this is a freehand drawing of the tumor showing its relation to the great vessels, and in particular to the renal vessels and kidneys (Fig. 26.1b). The first decision that must be made is whether an anterior, long midline incision will provide adequate access. Analysis of 140 para-aortic lymphadenectomies at the Royal Marsden Hospital over a 10-year period (Hendry *et al.*, 1987, 1988) indicated that this incision was used in over three-quarters of cases (Table 26.1). It has the great advantage that it provides excellent direct access to the great vessels, with equally good exposure on either side: as a result even very large masses can be completely excised, provided they are below the renal vessels (Fig. 26.2). Occasionally the vena cava itself may be involved (Hendry *et al.*, 1980; Maeda *et al.*, 1986; Ahlering and Skinner, 1989; Jacqmin *et al.*, 1989) (Fig. 26.3); this should be recognized in advance so that adequate arrangements can be made for blood transfusion, and a vascular surgeon may be invited to the operation. Similarly, if a liver metastasis is present it may be sensible to involve a surgeon who is experienced at hepatic resection. Particular attention must be paid to the kidneys: the metastatic tumor commonly causes

ureteric obstruction, and although some renal function may return after chemotherapy there may be significant postobstructive atrophy of one or even both kidneys. The residual mass may be inseparably stuck on to the kidney, its vessels or the ureter, and in our experience nephrectomy had to be done in 11% of cases; obviously it was essential in these cases to make sure that contralateral kidney function was adequate.

A thoracoabdominal approach is essential if simultaneous excision of supradiaphragmatic masses is to be carried out (Chapter 27). Excellent access is provided to retrocrural nodes (Fig. 26.4), and this incision may be chosen for massive tumors that are predominantly on one side (Fig. 26.5).

Decisions on optimum approach, possible involvement of adjacent organs, the need for additional surgical expertise, transfusion requirements and any postchemotherapy lung function defects that might lead to anesthetic difficulties should all be addressed at the planning visit in the outpatient clinic, in a calm considered atmosphere and not left to the last moment before surgery. Many of these masses are large – 23% being over 10 cm in diameter in our experience – and they may present a formidable appearance. Perhaps the most difficult decision is to know when the case is inoperable. Tumors below the renal vessels can be excised (Fig. 26.2), and most nodal deposits above this level, but occasionally a case is encountered in which tumor encases the coeliac axis and superior mesenteric vessels, extending into the small

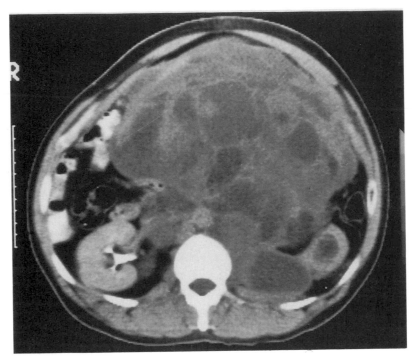

Fig. 26.2   Huge mass resembling full-term pregnancy. All of it was situated below the renal vessels and removed completely through an anterior approach.

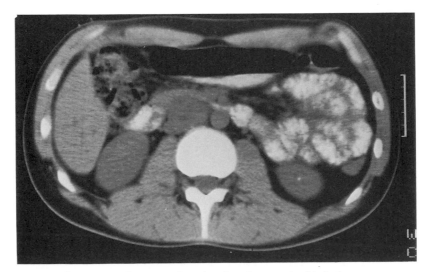

Fig. 26.3   A computed tomography scan showing involvement of inferior vena cava.

bowel mesentery (Fig. 26.6). Surgery has little to offer such cases, and these patients should not be subjected to the additional suf-fering associated with unnecessary laparot-omy.

Finally, tumor may be present in an undes-

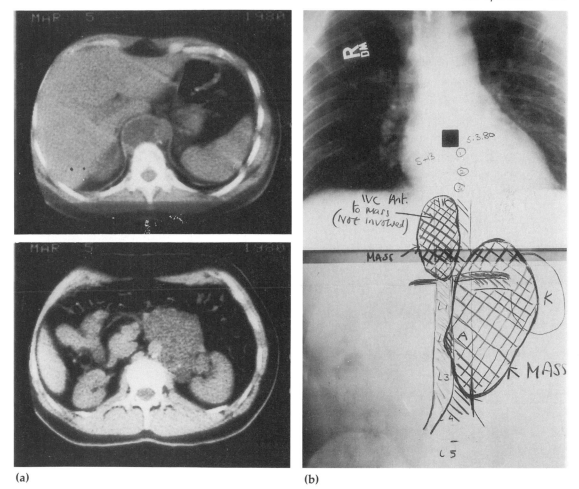

Fig. 26.4 (a) A computed tomography scan, and (b) a scanogram showing a large mass displacing the left kidney and a right retrocrural node. These residual masses were removed completely through a left thoracoabdominal incision.

cended, abdominal testis (Fig. 26.7). Following chemotherapy, it is usually suprisingly easy to remove the affected testicle.

26.3 THE OPERATION

This is usually scheduled to take place 4–6 weeks after completion of chemotherapy (Fig. 26.8). The patient is admitted 48 h prior to operation, to allow preoperative blood tests, chest X-ray, cross-matching, bowel preparation and physiotherapy to be arranged.

Prophylactic broad-spectrum antibiotics are started preoperatively.

26.3.1 ANTERIOR APPROACH

The patient lies supine and the abdomen is opened in the midline from xiphisternum to symphysis pubis. After checking the liver and abdominal cavity for metastases, the transverse colon is placed on the chest between moist packs and the small bowel is packed away to the right. The classical technique of

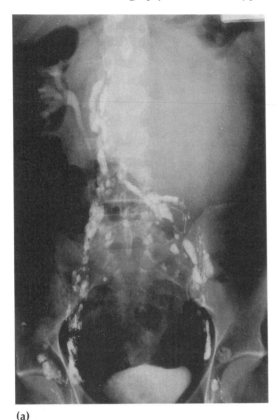

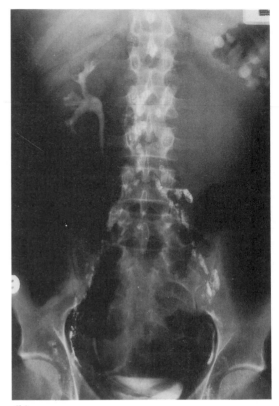

(a)

(b)

Fig. 26.5 Intravenous urograms (a) before and (b) after chemotherapy. This residual mass was removed with the left kidney through a left thoracoabdominal incision.

para-aortic lymphadenectomy has been well described elsewhere (Mallis and Patton, 1958; Staubitz *et al.*, 1969), and the basic principles remain the same in excision of residual masses in this region. The posterior peritoneum is incised from the bifurcation of the right common iliac artery up between the aorta and vena cava, between the duodenum and the inferior mesenteric vein until the splenic vein is reached (Fig. 26.9). The entire ascending colon can be mobilized by extending the peritoneal incision around the cecum and up the lateral paracolic gutter as far as the foramen of Winslow, thus gaining access to the vena cava, right kidney and suprahilar space (Donohue, 1977). Alternatively, the descending colon can be mobilized to identify the left ureter and left iliac vessels below

the tumor mass – these can be traced up and safely separated from the mass at a later stage.

Care must be taken in separating the back of the duodenum from the front of the tumor mass, and the third and fourth parts of the duodenum are packed away to the right, exposing the right ureter. The inferior mesenteric artery can be preserved with right-sided masses, but is often surrounded by or adherent to left-sided tumors, and should be divided electively at its origin from the aorta, to gain access to the left side of the aorta. Care should be taken not to disturb the tissues around the aorta below this level unnecessarily, in particular below the bifurcation of the aorta where the hypogastric plexus lies, so as to minimize the possibility of interference with ejaculation (Jewett *et al.*,

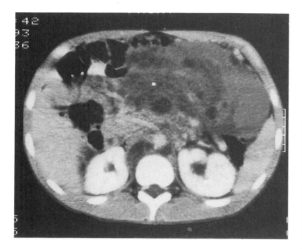

Fig. 26.6 A CT scan. This mass involved the celiac axis and superior mesenteric artery with invasion of the small bowel mesentery and was therefore inoperable.

1988; Sherlag, O'Brien and Graham, 1989). The left ureter is identified below the mass and dissected off its lateral aspect by mobilizing the descending colon, and after dividing the left testicular vessels.

Once the boundaries of the residual mass have been defined and freed from surrounding normal tissues, work can commence on patiently and delicately dissecting the mass from the great vessels (Fig. 26.10). It is generally best to free it from the vena cava first, and then the aorta. If the vena cava is damaged it can be repaired by oversewing, or even ligated above and below the site of injury with no ill effect (Skinner, 1976). Extensive injury to the aorta is more serious and may require grafting. Some tumors seem to induce softening of the aortic wall, perhaps by myxoid degeneration, and the surgeon should be prepared to control the aorta above the renal vessels while inserting an aortic graft. The renal vessels may be surrounded by tumor, and great care must be exercised in approaching the origin of the renal arteries. The left kidney is not uncommonly inseparable from the tumor mass, and provided contralateral renal function is

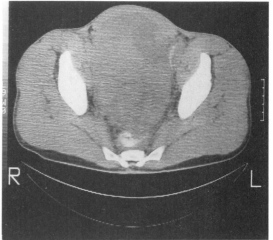

(a)

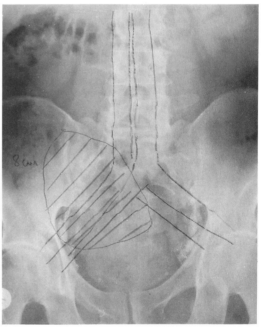

(b)

Fig. 26.7 (a) A computed tomography scan, and (b) a scanogram of a tumor in the abdominal testis. After chemotherapy the testis was easily removed.

adequate, it should be removed with the mass rather than risk leaving tumor behind in the renal hilum.

Once hemostasis has been achieved, the wound is closed in layers without drainage

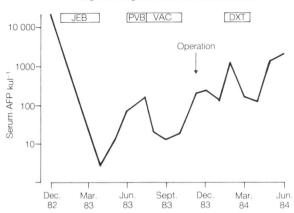

Fig. 26.8 Serum alpha-fetoprotein levels in a patient initially treated with carboplatin/etoposide/bleomycin (JEB). A residual mass was not removed in April 1983 because of pneumonitis and there was subsequent inexorable disease progression despite salvage chemotherapy with a platinum combination of cisplatin/vinblastine/bleomycin (PVB) and vincristine/Adriamycin/cyclophosphamide (VAC), surgery and radiotherapy (DXT).

using continuous deep nylon sutures to the muscle layer and linea alba. A bladder catheter is inserted for a few days.

26.3.2 THORACOABDOMINAL APPROACH

If the mass extends above the renal vessels, or if it is massive and predominantly unilateral, the patient should be positioned with supports below the shoulder and buttock on the side of the tumor mass, and a thoracoabdominal incision made (Merrill, 1977; Skinner, 1977). The incision is made along the most prominent rib over the middle of the lymph node mass (usually the 8th, 9th or 10th) and extends from the midaxillary line to the midline, and then down the midline as far as necessary. The chest may be entered above the rib, or after excising it, and the abdomen opened widely in the same line; the diaphragm is incised as necessary. The colon is mobilized, with or without the spleen on the left, or the duodenum on the right, and the lateral and upper margins of the tumor mass are defined. The colon is allowed to fall back into place while the great vessels are exposed and dissected out as described above. It is essential that the tumor mass is freed from the great vessels, including dissection and division of the lumbar vessels if necessary, before mobilization of the main tumor mass is attempted. Ipsilateral nephrectomy may be required, and involvement of the vena cava may occasionally be encountered. Once the mass has been excised, the wound is closed with a water-sealed chest drain.

26.4 POSTOPERATIVE CARE

The patient is nursed in an intensive care or high dependency unit for the first 48 hours. Blood replacement and fluid losses are monitored by arterial and central venous monitoring. Urine output is carefully recorded. Early active physiotherapy encourages chest expansion and limb movement. Paralytic ileus is common, and intravenous fluids and nasogastric suction are required for a few days. Antibiotics are discontinued as soon as the patient is mobile and arterial and venous lines, and urinary catheter are-removed.

Most patients go home 10–14 days after operation, and are advised to limit their physical activity for a month.

26.5 RESULTS AND PROGNOSTIC FACTORS

Amongst 231 consecutive patients undergoing para-aortic lymphadenectomy after chemotherapy at the Royal Marsden Hospital between 1976 and 1990, there was residual undifferentiated teratoma (MTU) in 48 (21%), differentiated teratoma (TD) in 131 (57%) and only fibrosis/necrosis in 52 cases (22%) (Hendry *et al.*, 1993). The incidence of residual MTU in this series is similar to that reported from other centres (Table 26.2) (Bracken *et al.*, 1983; Harding *et al.*, 1989; Staehler *et al.*, 1989; Mulders

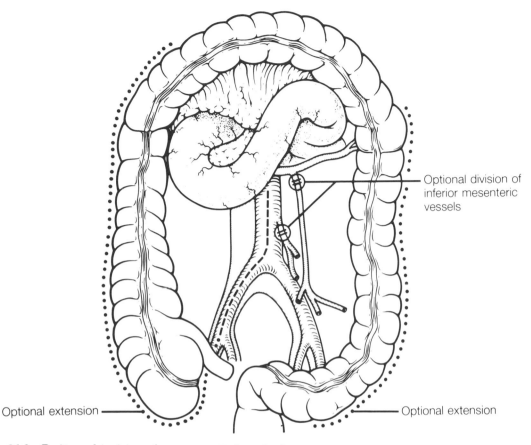

Fig. 26.9 Peritoneal incisions for para-aortic lymphadenectomy.

et al., 1990; Herr *et al.*, 1991; Kulkarni *et al.*, 1991). The histological findings had a profound effect on prognosis, as did completeness of surgical excision (Figs 26.11 and 26.12). Multivariate analysis was performed, and completeness of excision, pathology of the excised mass, elective versus salvage surgery and year of treatment (before or after 1984) were found to be independent prognostic variables, whereas serum markers at the time of surgery, and size were not found to be of any additional prognostic value once pathology and completeness of excision were taken into account. Since it is impossible to distinguish radiologically those patients with MTU from the rest, we recommend excision of all substantial residual masses 1 month or so after completion of chemotherapy.

What size of residual mass is substantial enough to merit excision? We have excised all masses greater than 2 cm diameter, and although MTU was found in only 13% of masses less than 3 cm diameter in our series, it has been recorded in a mass only 1.7 cm in diameter (Dexeus *et al.*, 1989). We therefore examined carefully all masses 1–2 cm diameter and selected those for surgery that did not continue to shrink with time. Donohue (Donohue *et al.*, 1987) has observed that those who have greater than 90% reduction of measured tumor volume in metastases from MTU all had necrosis/fibrosis in their resected specimens; however, it remains to be seen whether this will become established as such a good prognostic feature that surgical excision can be omitted (Sheinfeld and Bajorin, 1993).

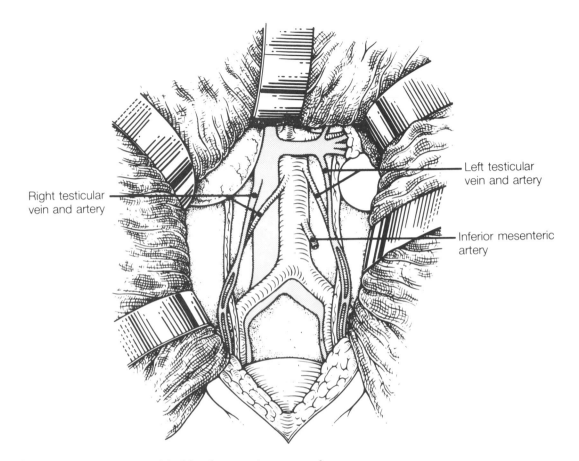

Fig. 26.10 Exposure provided by the anterior approach.

Table 26.2 Comparison of histological findings in excised residual masses following chemotherapy

| | | Histology of residual mass | | |
| | | Fibrosis necrosis | | |
Authors	No.	(%)	TD (%)	MTU (%)
Bracken *et al.* (1983)	60	25 (42)	14 (23)	17 (28)
Staehler *et al.* (1989)	65	23 (35)	25 (39)	17 (26)
Harding *et al.* (1989)	42	15 (36)	14 (33)	9 (21)
Williams *et al.* (1989)	25	13 (52)	9 (36)	3 (12)
Mulders *et al.* (1990)	55	31 (56)	12 (22)	12 (22)
Herr *et al.* (1991)	122	57 (47)	48 (39)	17 (14)
Kulkarni *et al.* (1991)	67	18 (27)	29 (47)	20 (30)
Donohue and Foster (1994)	557	150 (27)	273 (49)	134 (24)
Hendry *et al.* (1993)	231	52 (22)	131 (57)	48 (21)

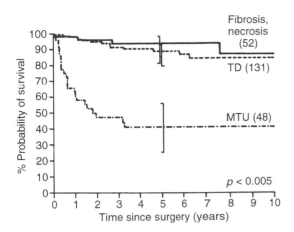

Fig. 26.11 Comparison of survival by pathology of excised tissue. (Reproduced by permission of the *British Journal of Urology*.)

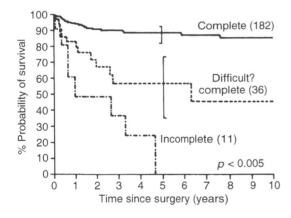

Fig. 26.12 Survival related to completeness of surgical excision. (Reproduced by permission of the *British Journal of Urology*.)

Heading the list of factors associated with poor prognosis are incomplete excision of the residual mass, and presence of undifferentiated tumor. These two factors are related, since tissue with persistent active malignancy is undoubtedly more difficult to remove; however, complete clearance of residual masses that do turn out to contain active disease is clearly of therapeutic benefit, as shown by the results of the multivariate analysis, which indicated that these two factors were independently significant. The presence of sarcoma in the excised tissue is recognized as a particularly bad sign, but surgical excision is potentially curative (Little *et al.*, 1994). There was residual undifferentiated teratoma in 14% of our patients with normal serum markers after chemotherapy, and so neither this finding nor the mere size of the mass should lull the oncologist into believing that surgery is unnecessary. On the other hand, raised serum markers at the time of surgery was highly predictive of the presence of undifferentiated tumor in the residual mass, and of subsequent relapse and death. Nevertheless, it can be seen that 50% of such patients were long-term survivors after excision of the residual masses with follow-on chemotherapy, when otherwise their prognosis would have been poor. Survival was significantly worse after salvage, compared with elective surgery after primary chemotherapy, probably reflecting the lower complete remission rate after salvage chemotherapy.

26.6 COMPLICATIONS

There is a cost that must be paid for such major surgery. Operative mortality within 1 month of surgery in our series was 0.9% (Hendry *et al.*, 1993), similar to that recorded by Donohue (Baniel *et al.*, 1995). One patient developed severe respiratory failure 2–3 days after thoracolaparotomy and died, possibly related to bleomycin lung toxicity; this complication has been observed by others (Donohue and Rowland, 1981) and emphasizes the need for careful preoperative lung function studies. One died of renal failure a year after injury to a renal artery, when the contralateral kidney had postobstructive atrophy, despite dialysis and kidney transplantation. Impairment of renal function, and severe hypertension, have been observed by others (Beck and Stutzman, 1979), and underline the need for obsessively careful technique when dissecting around the renal pedicles. The third patient died of secondary hemorrhage 10 days after excision of a huge necrotic mass which was involving the femoral nerve roots. Hemorrhage, primary or secondary, is the greatest risk in this operation. The aorta or iliac artery was resected or grafted in 4%, and the vena cava was resected or tied off without ill effect in 3%. Sometimes what appears to be a simple little node can be inextricably adherent to the aorta, defying all attempts at removal without doing damage; in others, a large mass may have such a well-developed plane of cleavage round it that removal is child's play. It is, therefore, imperative that adequate exposure is obtained in all cases, to allow proximal control of repair or grafting of major vessels if necessary.

The ipsilateral kidney was removed with the lymph node mass in 12.5% of our patients. It is better to remove such a kidney than to risk leaving tumor behind (Skinner, 1976). Chylous ascites or chylothorax has been recorded (Jacqmin *et al.*, 1989), but has not been seen in this series possibly because drains were not used. Lymphocele has been seen occasionally, and has been noted by others (Messing, Love and Kvols, 1986). Wound infection was not a problem, perhaps because we did not do incidental appendicectomy (Sago, Ball and Novicki, 1979).

Loss of ejaculation occurred significantly more often after bilateral (46%) compared with unilateral (14%) lymphadenectomy, and was related to the size of the excised mass (<4 cm 4%; 4–8 cm 19%; >8 cm 60%); a nerve-sparing operative technique led to a significant reduction in ejaculatory dysfunction, from 37% to 19% in our experience of 186 patients (Jones *et al.*, 1993). Loss of ejaculation is caused by division of the sympathetic nerves on both sides of the great vessels (Leiter and Brendler, 1967), or removal of the hypogastric plexus, which lies just below the bifurcation of the aorta (Fig. 26.13). Attempts to modify para-aortic lymphadenectomy to reduce the incidence of this

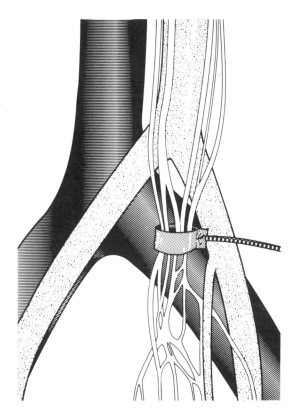

Fig. 26.13 Sympathetic nerves controlling ejaculation shown here with hypogastric plexus stimulator *in situ* used to obtain semen from paraplegic men. (Reproduced from Brindley, Sauerwein and Hendry, 1989, by courtesy of the *British Journal of Urology*.)

complication have met with limited success (Fosså *et al.*, 1985, Fritz and Weissbach, 1985; Jewett *et al.*, 1988; Sherlag, O'Brien and Graham, 1989). Despite optimistic reports of return of ejaculation with the use of drugs such as ephedrine (Lynch and Maxted, 1983) or imipramine (Nijman *et al.*, 1982, 1987) we have had no success with treating this complication, which should probably be regarded as permanent. However, success has been reported in these cases with electroejaculation (Ohl, 1993). It is most important to recognize patients at high risk of loss of ejaculation early in the course of their treatment so that seminal analysis and cryopreservation of semen can be arranged in suitable cases (Hendry *et al.*, 1983). Increasingly successful therapy, a more open society and legal precedent all now demand that reproductive function and future fertility are kept in mind, and fully discussed with both patient and relatives before, during and after treatment (Hendry, 1995).

26.7 CONCLUSIONS

With the passage of time since the introduction of effective chemotherapy for metastatic testicular teratoma, the number of reports of late relapse in the retroperitoneum is steadily growing (Carr, Gilchrist and Carbone, 1981; Geier *et al.*, 1983; Gelderman *et al.*, 1989; Maatman, Bukowski and Montie, 1984; Chan, Ford and Sikora, 1985; Kuzmits and Ludwig, 1986). The unstable nature of teratomatous metastases, even those composed of apparently adult tissue, was recognized by Logothetis *et al.* (1982); furthermore Dexeus *et al.* (1989) have recorded carcinoma in a residual para-aortic mass as small as 1.7 cm in diameter. The difficulties inherent in treating patients with established relapse (Chapter 25) make prevention a preferable alternative. Routine excision of residual masses allows early recognition of adverse prognostic features, and elimination of unstable or frankly malignant tissue. We are not alone (Donohue, 1989; Staehler *et al.*, 1989) in believing that this policy is preferable to the 'wait-and-see' approach recommended by others (Levitt *et al.*, 1985, Read *et al*, 1986). Nevertheless, the surgery is difficult and can be dangerous and it should be done in specialist cancer centers.

REFERENCES

Ahlering, T.E. and Skinner, D.G. (1989) Vena caval resection in bulky metastatic germ cell tumours. *J. Urol.*, **142**, 1497–9.

Baniel, J., Foster, R.S., Rowland, R.G., Bihrle, R. and Donohue, J.P. (1995) Complications of post-chemotherapy retroperitoneal lymph node dissection. *J. Urol.*, **153**, 976–80.

Beck, P.H. and Stutzman, R.E. (1979) Complications of retroperitoneal lymphadenectomy for nonseminomatous tumours of the testis. *Urology*, **13**, 244–7.

Boyd, P.J.R., Husband, J.E., Peckham, M.J. *et al.* (1978) CT scanning and the surgery of metastatic teratoma of the testis: a preliminary report. *Br. J. Urol.*, **50**, 609–11.

Bracken, B.R., Johnsen, D.E., Frazier, O.H., Logothetis, C.J., Trindade, A. and Samuels, M.L. (1983) The role of surgery following chemotherapy in Stage III germ cell neoplasms. *J. Urol.*, **129**, 39–43.

Brindley, G.S., Sauerwein, D. and Hendry, W.F. (1989) Hypogastric plexus stimulators for obtaining semen from paraplegic men. *Br. J. Urol.*, **64**, 72–7.

Carr, B.I., Gilchrist, K.W. and Carbone, P.P. (1981) The variable transformation in metastases from testicular germ cell tumours: the need for selective biopsy. *J. Urol.*, **126**, 52–4.

Cassileth, B.R. and Steinfeld. A.D. (1987) Psychological preparation of the patient and family. *Cancer*, **60**, 547–52.

Chan, S.Y.T., Ford, G. and Sikora, K. (1985) Late relapse in testicular teratoma after chemotherapy. *Lancet*, **ii**, 773–4.

Dexeus, F.H., Shirkhoda, A., Logothetis, C.J. *et al.* (1989) Clinical and radiological correlation of retroperitoneal metastasis from nonseminomatous testicular cancer treated with chemotherapy. *Eur. J. Cancer Clin. Oncol.*, **25**, 35–43.

Donohue, J.P. (1977) Retroperitoneal lymphadenectomy. *Urol. Clin. North Am.*, **4**, 509–21.

Donohue, J.P. (1989) The case for retroperitoneal lymphadenectomy after chemotherapy for selected patients with nonseminomatous tumours of the testis, in *Controversies in Urology* (ed. C.E. Carlton), Year Book Publishers Chicago, pp. 225–9.

Donohue, J.P. and Foster, F.S. (1994) Management of retroperitoneal recurrence: seminoma and non-seminoma. *Urol. Clin. North Am.*, **21**, 761–72.

Donohue, J.P. and Rowland, R.G. (1981) Complications of retroperitoneal lymph node dissection. *J. Urol.*, **125**, 338–40.

Donohue, J.P., Rowland, R.G., Kopecky, K., Steidle, C.P., Geier, G., Ney, K.G., Einhorn, L., Williams, S. and Loehrer, P. (1987) Correlation of computerized tomographic changes and histological findings in 80 patients having radical retroperitoneal lymph node dissection after chemotherapy for testis cancer. *J. Urol.*, **137**, 1176–9.

Fosså, S.D., Ous, S., Abyholm, T. *et al.* (1985) Post treatment fertility in patients with testicular cancer I. Influence of retroperitoneal lymph node dissection on ejaculatory potency. *Br. J. Urol.*, **57**, 204–9.

Fritz, K. and Weissbach, L. (1985) Sperm parameters and ejaculation before and after operative treatment of patients with germ cell testicular cancer. *Fertil. Steril.*, **43**, 451–4.

Geier, L.J., Volk, S.A., Weldon, E. *et al.* (1983) Late relapse in testicular cancer after chemotherapy. *Lancet*, **i**, 1049.

Gelderman, W.A., Oosterhuis, J.W., Koops, H.S. *et al.* (1989) Late recurrence of mature teratoma in nonseminomatous testicular tumours after PVB chemotherapy and surgery. *Urology*, **33**, 10–14.

Harding, M.J., Brown, I.L., Macpherson, S.G., Turner, M.A. and Kaye, S.B. (1989) Excision of residual masses after platinum based chemotherapy for nonseminomatous germ cell tumours. *Eur. J. Cancer Clin. Oncol.*, **25**, 1689–94.

Hendry, W.F. (1995) Cancer therapy and fertility, in *Oncology – A Multidisciplinary Textbook*. (ed. A. Horwich), Chapman & Hall, London, pp. 213–21.

Hendry, W.F., A'Hern, R.P., Hetherington, J.W., Peckham, M.J., Dearnaley, D.P. and Horwich, A. (1993) Para-aortic lymphadenectomy after chemotheraphy for metastatic non-seminomatous germ cell tumours: prognostic value and therapeutic benefit. *Br. J. Urol.*, **71**, 208–13.

Hendry, W.F., Barrett, A., McElwain, J.J. *et al.* (1980) The role of surgery in the combined management of metastases from malignant teratomas of testis. *Br. J. Urol.*, **52**, 38–44.

Hendry, W.F., Goldstraw, P., Horwich, A. *et al.* (1988) Paraaortic lymphadenectomy after chemotherapy for testicular tumour. *Br. J. Urol.*, **62**, 470–1.

Hendry, W.F., Goldstraw, P., Husband, J.E. *et al.* (1981) Elective delayed excision of bulky para-aortic lymph node metastases in advanced nonseminomatous germ cell tumour of testis. *Br. J. Urol.*, **53**, 648–53.

Hendry, W.F., Goldstraw, P. and Peckham, M.J. (1987) The role of surgery in the combined management of metastases from malignant teratomas of testis. *Br. J. Urol.*, **59**, 358.

Hendry, W.F., Stedronska, J., Jones, C.R., Blackmore, C.A., Barrett, A. and Peckham, M.J. (1983) Semen analysis in testicular cancer and Hodgkin's disease: pre- and post-treatment findings and implications for cryopreservation. *Br. J. Urol.*, **55**, 769–73.

Hendry, W.F., Tyrrell, C.J., Macdonald, J.S. *et al.* (1977) The detection and localisation of abdominal lymph node metastases from testicular teratomas. *Br. J. Urol.*, **49**, 739–45.

Herr, H.W., Toner, G.C., Geller, N.L. and Bosl, G.J. (1991) Patient selection for retroperitoneal lymph node dissection after chemotherapy for non-seminomatous germ cell tumours. *Eur. Urol.*, **19**, 1–5.

Husband, J.E., Peckham, M.J., Macdonald, J.S. and Hendry, W.F. (1979) The role of computed tomography in the management of testicular teratoma. *Clin. Radiol.*, **30**, 243–52.

Jacqmin, D., Bertrand, P., Ansieau, J.P. *et al.* (1989) Involvement of the caval vein lumen by a metastasis of a nonseminomatous testicular tumour. *Eur. Urol.*, **16**, 233–4.

Jewett, M.A.S., Kong, Y-S.P., Goldbert, S.D. *et al.*, (1988) Retroperitoneal lymphadenectomy for testis tumour with nerve sparing for ejaculation. *J. Urol.*, **139**, 1220–4.

Jones, D.R., Norman, A.R., Horwich, A. and Hendry, W.F. (1993) Ejaculatory dysfunction after retroperitoneal lymphadenectomy. *Eur. Urol.*, **23**, 169–71.

Kennedy, C.L., Husband, J.E., Bellamy, E.A. *et al.* (1985) The accuracy of CT scanning prior to paraaortic lymphadenectomy in patients with bulky metastases from testicular teratoma. *Br. J. Urol.*, **57**, 755–8.

Kulkarni, R.P., Reynolds, K.W., Newlands, E.S., Dawson, P.M., Makey, A.R., Theodorov, N.A., Bradley, J., Begent, R.H.J., Rustin, G.J.S. and Bagshawe, R.D. (1991) Cytoreductive surgery n disseminated nonseminomatous germ cell tumours of testis. *Br. J. Surg.*, **78**, 226–9.

Kuzmits, R. and Ludwig, H. (1986) Late relapse in testicular cancer from a residual tumour. *Lancet*, **i**, 1207–8.

Leiter, E. and Brendler, H. (1967) Loss of ejaculation following bilateral retroperitoneal lymphadenectomy. *J. Urol.*, **98**, 375–8.

Levitt, M.D., Reynolds, P.M., Sheiner, J.H. *et al.* (1985) Nonseminomatous germ cell testicular tumours – masses after chemotherapy. *Br. J. Surg.*, **72**, 19–21.

Little, J.S., Foster, R.S., Ulbright, T.M. and Donohue,

J.P. (1994) Unusual neoplasms detected in testis cancer patients undergoing post-chemotherapy retroperitoneal lymphadenectomy. *J. Urol.*, **152**, 1144–9.

Logothetis, C.J., Samuels, M.L., Trindale, A. *et al.* (1982) The growing teratoma syndrome. *Cancer*, **50**, 1629–35.

Lynch, J.H. and Maxted, W.C. (1983) Use of ephedrine in post-lymphadenectomy ejaculatory failure: a case report. *J. Urol.*, **129**, 379.

Maatman, T., Bukowski, R.M. and Montie, J.E. (1984) Retroperitoneal malignancies several years after initial treatment of germ cell cancer of the testis. *Cancer*, **54**, 1962–5.

Maeda, O., Yokokawa, K., Oka, T. *et al.* (1986) Inferior vena cava thrombus after retroperitoneal lymphadenectomy for testicular tumour. *Urol. Int.*, **41**, 318–20.

Mallis, N. and Patton, J.F. (1958) Transperitoneal bilateral lymphadenectomy in testis tumour. *J. Urol.*, **80**, 501–3.

Merrill, D.C. (1977) Modified thoracoabdominal approach to the kidney and retroperitoneal tissue. *J. Urol.*, **117**, 15–18.

Messing, E.M., Love, R.R. and Kvols, L.K. (1986) Lymphocele after retroperitoneal node dissection for testis tumour. *Cancer*, **57**, 871–4.

Mulders, P.F.A., Oosterhof, G.O.N., Boestes, C., De Mulder, P.H.M., Theeuwes, A.G.M. and Debruyne, F.M.J. (1990) The importance of prognostic factors in the individual treatment of patients with disseminated germ cell tumours. *Br. J. Urol.*, **66**, 425–9.

Nijman, J.M., Jager, S., Boer, P.W. *et al.* (1982) The treatment of ejaculation disorders after retroperitoneal lymph node dissection. *Cancer*, **50**, 2967–71.

Nijman, J.M., Koops, H.S., Oldhoff, J. *et al.* (1987) Sexual function after bilateral retroperitoneal lymph node dissection for nonseminomatous testicular cancer. *Arch. Androl.*, **18**, 255–67.

Ohl, D.A. (1993) Electroejaculation. *Urol. Clin. North Am.*, **20**, 181–8.

Read, G., Johnson, R.J. and Wilkinson, P.M. (1986) The role of radiotherapy after chemotherapy in the management of persistent para-aortic nodal disease in nonseminomatous germ cell tumours. *Br. J. Cancer*, **53**, 623–8.

Sago, A.L., Ball, T.P. and Novicki, D.E. (1979) Complications of retroperitoneal lymphadenectomy. *Urology*, **13**, 241–3.

Sheinfeld, J. and Bajorin, D. (1993) Management of the postchemotherapy residual mass. *Urol. Clin. North Amer.*, **20**, 133–43.

Sherlag, A.P., O'Brien, D.P. and Graham, S.D. (1989) Use of limited retroperitoneal lymphadenectomy in nonseminomatous germ cell tumours. *Urology*, **33**, 355–7.

Skinner, D.G. (1976) Complications of lymph node dissection, in *Complications of Urologic Surgery: Prevention and Management*. (eds R.B. Smith and D.G. Skinner), W.B. Saunders, Philadelphia, pp. 422–35.

Skinner, D.G. (1977) Surgical management of advanced nonseminomatous tumours of the testis. *Urol. Clin. North Am.*, **4**, 465–76.

Staehler, G., Wiesel, M., Clemm, C., Gokel, J.M. and Marchner, M. (1989) Significance of salvage lymphadenectomy in the therapeutic concept of advanced nonseminomatous germ cell tumours. *Urol. Int.*, **44**, 84–6.

Staubitz, W.J., Magoss, I.V., Grace, J.T. *et al.* (1969) Surgical management of testis tumours. *J. Urol.*, **101**, 350–5.

Tait, D., Peckham, M.J., Hendry, W.F. *et al.* (1984) Post chemotherapy surgery in advanced nonseminomatous germ cell testicular tumours: the significance of histology with particular reference to differentiated (mature) teratoma. *Br. J. Cancer*, **50**, 601–9.

Tamburini, M., Filiberti, A., Barbieri, A. *et al.* (1989) Psychological aspects of testis cancer therapy: a prospective study. *J. Urol.*, **142**, 1487–90.

Williams, S.N., Jenkins, B.J., Baithun, S.I. *et al.* (1989) Radical retroperitoneal node dissection after chemotherapy for testicular tumours. *Br. J. Urol.*, **63**, 641–3.

THORACOTOMY POSTCHEMOTHERAPY IN NON-SEMINOMA PATIENTS

P. Goldstraw

27.1 INTRODUCTION

The previously dismal prognosis for young men with disseminated non-seminomatous germ cell tumors has been dramatically improved with the development of effective chemotherapy (Einhorn and Donohue, 1977; Peckham *et al.*, 1983; Vugrin, Whitmore and Golbey, 1983), and the diagnosis and monitoring of such cases have been further aided by the development of the serum tumor markers, alpha-fetoprotein (AFP) and the beta fraction of human chorionic gonadotrophin (BHCG) (Lehrman, 1979). The initial treatment of Stage III and IV cases [Royal Marsden Hospital staging categories (Peckham *et al.*, 1977)] is now chemotherapy, and primary surgery has been abandoned (Javadpour *et al.*, 1982). Yet surgery, principally the excision of retroperitoneal lymph node masses (Hendry *et al.*, 1981), still has an important role in approximately 25% of patients with advanced disease: those in whom bulky residual disease remains following normalization of tumor markers with chemotherapy. It has been estimated that prior to treatment pulmonary metastases are present in 50% of patients with retroperitoneal node involvement and in up to 10% of those without such extension (Pizzocaro,

1989). Bulky disease remains in the chest in up to 50% of such cases (Pizzocaro, 1986) and the excision of these deposits, mediastinal nodes and/or pulmonary metastases may involve the thoracic surgeon. Of 211 patients presenting to the Testicular Tumour Group at the Royal Marsden Hospital in London with lung or mediastinal disease, 125 had residual intrathoracic disease after chemotherapy, of whom 39 were referred for surgery. Additionally, a residual mass is almost always present after chemotherapy for a mediastinal primary germ cell tumor, and surgery should be planned routinely for all those without widespread metastases.

The surgical excision of bulky residual disease is justified on the following grounds:

1. Following the completion of chemotherapy for advanced disease, prognosis is influenced by the histology of residual masses (Tait *et al.*, 1984). Residual malignancy may persist in 22–35% of patients (Vugrin *et al.*, 1981, Donohue and Rowland, 1984; Tait *et al.*, 1984). This group have not been cured and require additional chemotherapy, whilst the other patients may be spared such treatment. Marker normalization does not reliably exclude residual malignancy (Hendry *et*

Testicular Cancer: Investigation and management. Second edition. Edited by Professor A. Horwich.
Published in 1996 by Chapman & Hall. ISBN 0 412 61210 0.

al., 1981), and if one waits for relapse to identify this group, chemotherapy is then less likely to produce cure (see Chapter 25). Given the additional advantages of surgery, a 'wait-and-see' policy is untenable. There is evidence that the complete excision of residual malignancy contributes to cure (Hendry, Goldstraw and Peckham, 1987).

2. Residual deposits will consist of cystic and fully differentiated tumor in 22–44% of cases (Vugrin *et al.*, 1981, Donohue and Rowland, 1984; Tait *et al.*, 1984). Whilst such deposits appear benign histologically, we, and others (Logothetis *et al.*, 1982; Schrafford Koops *et al.*, 1986), have observed relapse after several years of stability, and now consider such deposits unstable and best excised.

3. Cystic deposits may persist, and even enlarge, following chemotherapy, causing pressure symptoms. Mediastinal deposits may cause pain by bone erosion or nerve entrapment, dyspnea if compressing the airway, and on one occasion we have seen an intracardiac deposit cause inflow obstruction (Pillai *et al.*, 1986). The excision of such symptomatic deposits may be thus justified on palliative grounds.

27.2 PERSONAL EXPERIENCE

Between January 1980 and December 1988 we performed 70 thoracic operations on 53 patients to excise residual deposits after treatment for non-seminomatous germ cell tumors. All were male, with a mean age of 32 years ($\pm$ 8.35 SD). The primary site was testis in all but one patient who had a retroperitoneal primary. Initial treatment in all patients included chemotherapy, and thoracotomy was only considered once tumor markers had normalized. The extent of residual disease was documented using computed tomography (CT) of the chest and abdomen. Contiguous cuts were obtained through the whole of both lung fields. Intravenous contrast was used to enhance the vessels, greatly aiding the interpretation of the mediastinum. The scans were reviewed by the thoracic surgeon, paying particular attention to the apices and costodiaphragmatic fringes where deposits may easily be overlooked. A urological colleague similarly assessed the abdomen. If residual deposits remained on both sides of the diaphragm, a combined approach was considered in all cases. Whilst such a combined approach was possible in 12 patients, for the majority, separate abdominal and thoracic operations have been preferred for the improved access such an approach affords.

Patient fitness was assessed and set against the scale of proposed surgery. Evaluation for surgery was delayed for several weeks following the completion of chemotherapy to assess the full response by clinical, radiological and tumor marker criteria. By this time any toxicity related to chemotherapy had stabilized. Hematological effects had largely recovered, although a slight anemia was common. Renal impairment, by chemotherapy and previous abdominal surgery, could often be demonstrated if glomerular filtration rate was measured but serum creatinine was normal. Pulmonary toxicity, related to bleomycin, was usually evidenced on the CT scan of the lung fields. Whilst this possibility was taken into consideration by our anesthetists (see below) it was not severe enough to show on crude assessment of global lung function. Lung function was assessed by spirometric testing, measuring forced expiratory volume (FEV_1) and forced vital capacity (FVC). In our wider experience of pulmonary metastasectomy (Goldstraw, 1987; Venn, Sarin and Goldstraw, 1989) an FEV_1 of 1 litre and FEV_1 : VC ratio in excess of 50% has proved sufficient to allow safe surgery on one lung, ensuring an active lifestyle postoperatively. In practice, in this young population patient fitness has not proved a limitation. We have in the last 10 years refused surgery in only one patient, and that on the grounds that extensive

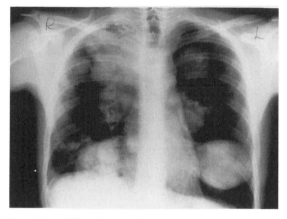

Fig. 27.1 The chest radiograph of a young man with bulky residual deposits in both lungs and widespread mediastinal deposits following chemotherapy. The excision of the pulmonary deposits was judged to require lobectomy on each side and considerable damage to the remaining lobes. He was judged to be inoperable.

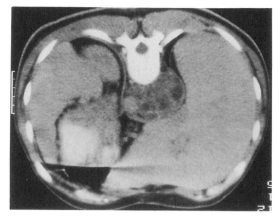

Fig. 27.2 A CT scan showing a residual node deposit behind the right crus of the diaphragm. Having tried a number of surgical approaches we would now advise a right thoracolaparotomy incision to excise deposits in this location.

pulmonary deposits would have required the resection of a crippling amount of lung tissue (Fig. 27.1).

27.2.1 INCISIONS

The incision to be used was decided upon once the extent of disease had been documented, and if abdominal disease was found, following discussion with our urological colleagues. The left or right thoracolaparotomy incision allows good access to the ipsilateral lung, ipsilateral part of the posterior mediastinum and the upper abdomen. Access to the superior mediastinum from such an incision is not good, and a high lateral thoracotomy is to be preferred if disease has to be excised from above the aortic arch. Our urologist would prefer a separate laparotomy if a difficult abdominal or pelvic dissection is anticipated. On two occasions we have found it possible to resect favorably sited, contralateral pulmonary deposits through a lateral thoracolaparotomy incision, by dissection across the mediastinum. The right thoraco-

laparotomy incision has been found to give good exposure to those inaccessible deposits behind the crurae of the diaphragm (Fig. 27.2). A midline thoracolaparotomy provides excellent access to the anterior mediastinum, reasonable access in selected cases to both lungs, and limited exposure to the upper abdomen. The use of this incision is thus somewhat limited, and it has been used on only two occasions. When dealing only with intrathoracic disease we have used a median sternotomy approach selectively to deal with bilateral pulmonary deposits. Of 13 patients with bilateral pulmonary metastases, six underwent synchronous combined resection of deposits from both lungs using a sternotomy incision. The other seven patients were operated upon through staged, lateral thoracotomy incisions for one or more of the following reasons:

1. Concurrent pulmonary and posterior mediastinal deposits.
2. Large pulmonary deposits where excision was judged difficult from an anterior approach.
3. If deposits lay close to hilar structures, such that the improved exposure afforded

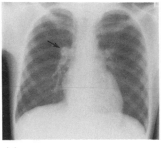

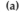

(a)

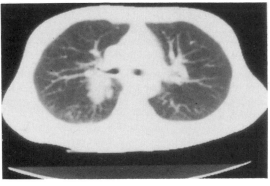

(b)

Fig. 27.3 (a) A chest radiograph, and (b) CT scan showing a right pulmonary metastasis (arrow) lying close to the hilar structures. There was also a deposit in the left lung. We elected to undertake staged lateral thoracotomy incisions. The right-sided lesion was excised with the posterior segment of the upper lobe, a difficult procedure through a sternotomy incision. The left-sided deposit was subsequently excised by wedge excision through a left thoracotomy.

by lateral thoracotomy would render conservative resection more feasible, or make segmentectomy or lobectomy safer (Fig. 27.3).

4. If large deposits lay in the posterior aspects of the lungs, especially the basal segments of the lower lobes. We undoubtedly find access to these areas superior through a lateral thoracotomy incision (Fig. 27.4).

Thus our 53 patients underwent 60 initial operations. Forty (75%) with unilateral disease underwent thoracotomy or thoraco-laparotomy, and, of the 13 (25%) with bilateral disease, six underwent median sternotomy and seven staged lateral thoracotomy or thoracolaparotomy.

27.2.2 FURTHER SURGERY

At relapse further chemotherapy was given. If further residual disease remained, further surgery was undertaken. Eight of our patients underwent a second round of surgery, and in one patient third line surgery was performed.

27.2.3 EXCISIONS

All patients underwent bronchoscopy prior to resection to exclude endobronchial extension and to determine bronchial anatomy. The anesthetist inserts a double lumen endobronchial tube so that each lung in turn can be palpated, aerated and collapsed. We have found this of considerable advantage as subpleural deposits are more easily palpated with the lung aerated, whilst deeply sited deposits are best appreciated with the lung collapsed. There is some debate as to the deleterious effects of high inspired oxygen concentration on lungs previously damaged by chemotherapy, and it is the routine of our anesthetists to keep this as low as possible during surgery, consistent with adequate arterial oxygenation (Gothard and Macrae, 1987). Arterial blood gases are carefully monitored during surgery. Whilst an inspired oxygen concentration of 40% is usually sufficient when both lungs are being ventilated, it is usually necessary to increase this once single lung ventilation is required.

Having carefully checked the preoperative prediction each deposit is then tagged with a suture. The excision is conservative and we aim to remove the deposit with as little damage as possible. Mediastinal deposits may be adherent to adjacent structures, and care is necessary to avoid key structures such as the recurrent laryngeal nerve or thoracic

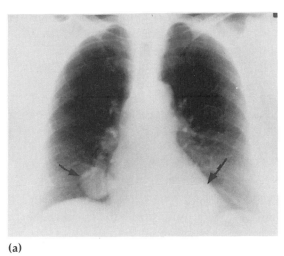

(a)

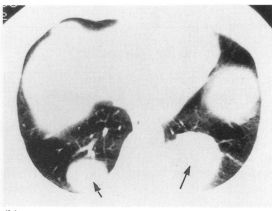

(b)

Fig. 27.4 (a) A chest radiograph, and (b) CT scan showing large pulmonary metastases at each lung base (arrows). We have in our earlier experience resected such lesions via a sternotomy incision. Having found excision difficult and, in the light of subsequent events, sometimes incomplete, we would now recommend a staged approach through lateral thoracotomy incisions.

duct. Posterior mediastinal deposits usually lie along the vertebral bodies, and we strive not to damage intercostal arteries that may be important in spinal perfusion. Particular care is necessary in the lower mediastinum, as the artery of Adamkiewicz, an important vessel in spinal perfusion, may arise from any of the lower intercostal arteries (Smith, Stallone and Yee, 1979). Paraplegia can result from the

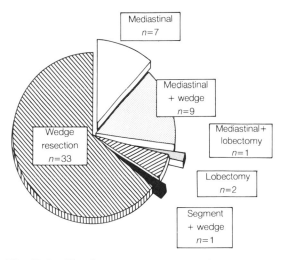

Fig. 27.5 The thoracic resections performed in 53 patients at initial surgery.

transection of this vessel, a devastating complication, which we have so far escaped. Each pulmonary metastasis is excised with a thin rim of surrounding lung tissue. If very large, the removal of a deposit may leave the segment or lobe irretrievably damaged, or if deposits lie close to hilar structures resection may damage adjacent segments or the lobe. In such circumstances more formal resection is necessary. The resections necessary in our series are shown in Fig. 27.5. In our series all pulmonary metastases were excised by one or more local wedge excisions, except in four patients, three of whom required lobectomy and one segmentectomy. The number of pulmonary metastases excised at each operation ranged from 1 to 18 with a mean of 3.5 ($\pm$ 3.3).

27.2.4 ACCURACY OF COMPUTED TOMOGRAPHY SCANS

In 52 patients the original CT scan was available to check its prediction against the operative findings and histological report. The number of deposits was correctly predicted in 77% of scans. In 3.8% of scans the report overestimated the number of pulmonary metastases, and in a fifth of cases (19.2%) the scan underestimated the number of metastases found at surgery. The error was usually only one or two deposits and it was rare for the discrepancy to undermine the rationale of surgery. This accuracy was similar for other cell types coming to metastasectomy (Goldstraw, 1987; Venn, Sarin and Goldstraw, 1989).

27.2.5 HISTOLOGY

The histology of resected deposits was described as showing residual malignancy in 12 patients (23%), fully differentiated, mature teratoma in 18 patients (34%), and only necrosis or fibrosis in 23 patients (43%). These figures differ only slightly from those in our other series (Tait *et al.*, 1984), with the percentage containing residual malignancy being the same but with greater numbers showing mature teratoma versus necrosis/fibrosis. This may reflect statistical problems with the smaller number or the relative ease with which residual abnormalities are seen on thoracic CT scans.

27.2.6 MORBIDITY AND MORTALITY

Early in our experience we encountered considerable problems with wound infection. One patient developed severe, fulminating wound infection within 2 days of surgery. Our immunologists have identified a wide range of defects in cellular immunity, which persist for 12 to 24 months following chemotherapy. This problem has been overcome with the routine use of perioperative prophylactic antibiotics, and it has not been a problem since. Overall wound infection occurred in three patients (4%), proving troublesome in two, one of whom was grossly obese and developed an incisional hernia, and one requiring the removal of sternal wires. One patient developed a chylothorax which required re-exploration and ligation of the thoracic duct, a surprisingly rare complication given the proximity of the duct to posterior mediastinal node deposits. One patient died with adult respiratory distress syndrome (ARDS) following thoracolaparotomy and excision of mediastinal and retroperitoneal deposits, a mortality of 1.8% per patient (0.4–6.8%, 70% confidence limits), and 1.4% per operation (0.3–5.2%, 70% confidence limits).

27.2.7 SURVIVAL

Detailed follow-up was available in 50 patients (95%), the other three being lost to follow-up. The mean period of follow-up was 40 months from surgery ($\pm$ 30·4 SD), the longest period being 98 months. The actuarial survival for all 53 patients is shown in Fig. 27.6. The 5-year survival was 75.8% ($\pm$ 7.3). This figure is very similar to the survival in larger series dominated by abdominal disease (Einhorn *et al.*, 1981; Tait *et al.*, 1984; Pizzocaro, 1986; Hendry, Goldstraw and Peckham, 1987). Figure 27.7 shows survival of those patients who only had pulmonary deposits, set against that for patients who also had mediastinal node deposits. The 5-year actuarial survival for the former was 84% ($\pm$ 7.5) and for the latter 60% ($\pm$ 14.4). Whilst this difference appears large and the two curves are diverging, the difference does not reach statistical significance ($p < 0.10$). The numbers are too small to analyze separately the influence of histology on this observation. The actuarial survival is shown in Fig. 27.8 set against the histology of the resected deposits. Those patients whose deposits showed necrosis and/or fibrosis did best, with a 5-year survival of 93.1% ($\pm$ 6.6), compared with 71.2% ($\pm$ 12.6) for those showing mature teratoma and 61.8% ($\pm$ 15.3) for those with active malignancy. There was statistical significance between the best and worst groups ($p < 0.05$), and the latter fared better than has been reported following abdominal clearance (Tait *et al.*, 1984; Schrafford Koops *et al.*, 1986).

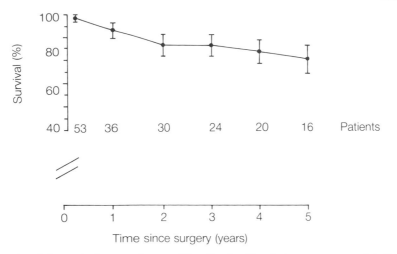

Fig. 27.6 The actuarial survival curve for our 53 patients. The data are expressed ± the standard error of the mean. The number entering the analysis each year is shown above the horizontal axis.

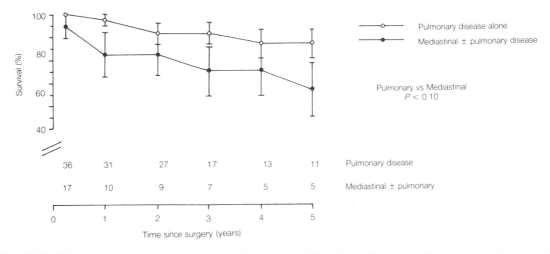

Fig. 27.7 The actuarial survival curves of patients with only pulmonary disease, and those with coexisting mediastinal deposits. The data are shown ± the standard error of the mean. The number entering the analysis each year is shown above the horizontal axis.

27.3 CONCLUSIONS

Following chemotherapy and marker normalization, thoracotomy and excision of bulky residual disease in the chest, pulmonary metastases and mediastinal node deposits, may be undertaken with low mortality and minimal morbidity. The histology of resected deposits gives valuable information on pro-gnosis and identifies those patients who will benefit from additional chemotherapy, allowing such treatment to be avoided in most patients. There is evidence that the complete surgical excision of residual malignancy contributes to cure, and that relapse from deposits of fully differentiated tumors may be averted.

Surgery in this context forms a valuable

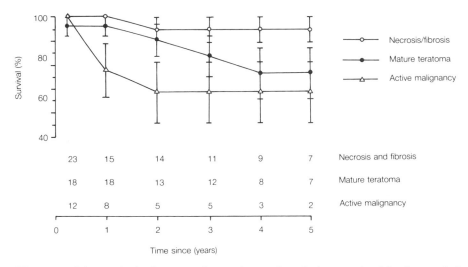

Fig. 27.8 The actuarial survival of our patients shown in relation to the histology of the resected deposits. The data are expressed ± the standard error of the mean. The number entering the analysis each year is shown above the horizontal axis.

adjunct to the multimodality treatment of disseminated malignancy.

ACKNOWLEDGEMENTS

The author wishes to acknowledge the support of the Cancer Research Campaign in funding the collection of these data, and to thank his oncological colleagues in the Royal Marsden Hospital and University College Hospital for their cooperation and support.

REFERENCES

Donohue, J.P. and Rowland, R.G. (1984) The role of surgery in advanced testicular cancer. *Cancer*, **54**, 2716–21.

Einhorn, L.H. and Donohue, J.P. (1977) Cis-diamminedichloroplatinum, vinblastine and bleomycin combination chemotherapy in disseminated testicular cancer. *Ann. Intern. Med.*, **87**, 293–8.

Einhorn, L.H., Williams, S.D., Mandelbaum, I. and Donohue J.P. (1981) Surgical resection in disseminated testicular cancer following chemotherapeutic cytoreduction. *Cancer*, **48**, 904–8.

Goldstraw, P. (1987) Surgical management of pulmonary metastases, in *Clinical Oncology –*

Management of Metastases (ed. M.L. Slevin), Baillière Tindall, London, pp. 601–22.

Gothard, J.W.W. and Macrae, D.J. (1987) Thoracic anaesthetic problems. in *Thoracic Anaesthesia* (ed. J.W.W. Gothard), Baillière Tindall, London, pp. 107–31.

Hendry, W.F., Goldstraw, P., Husband, J.E. *et al.* (1981) Elective delayed excision of bulky para-aortic lymph node metastases in advanced nonseminoma germ cell tumours of testis. *Br. J. Urol.*, **53**, 648–53.

Hendry, W.F., Goldstraw, P. and Peckham, M.J. (1987) The role of surgery in the combined management of metastases from testicular teratomas of testis. *Br. J. Urol.*, **59**, 358.

Javadpour, N., Ozols, R.F., Anderson, T. *et al.* (1982) A randomised trial of cytoreductive surgery followed by chemotherapy versus chemotherapy alone in bulky Stage III testicular cancer with poor prognostic features. *Cancer*, **48**, 2004–10.

Lehrman, F.G. (ed.) (1979) *Carcinoembryonic Proteins*, Elsevier, Amsterdam.

Logothetis, C.J., Samuels, M.L., Trindale, A. and Johnson, D.E. (1982) The growing teratoma syndrome. *Cancer*, **50**, 1629–35.

Peckham, M.J., Barrett, A., Liew, K.H. *et al.* (1983) The treatment of metastatic germ-cell testicular tumours by bleomycin, etoposide and cisplatin (BEP). *Br. J. Cancer*, **47**, 613–19.

Peckham, M.J., Hendry, W.F., McElwain, T.J. and Calman, F.M.B. (1977) The multimodality management of testicular teratoma, in *Adjunct Therapy of Cancer* (eds E.E. Salmon and S.E. Jones), North Holland Publishing Co, Amsterdam, pp. 305–20.

Pillai, R., Blauth, C., Peckham, M.J. *et al.* (1986) Intracardiac metastases from malignant teratoma of the testis. *J. Thorac. Cardiovasc. Surg.*, **92**, 118–20.

Pizzocaro, G. (1986) Primary, secondary and salvage surgery in the management of germinal testis cancer, in *Advances in the Biosciences – Germ Cell Tumours II* (eds W.G. Jones, A. Ward and C.K. Anderson), Pergamon Press, Oxford, pp. 395–402.

Pizzocaro, G. (1989) Cancer of the testis, in *Surgical Oncology – A European Handbook* (eds U. Veronesi, B. Arnesjo, I. Burn *et al.*), Springer-Verlag, Berlin, p. 758.

Schrafford Koops, H., Gelderman, W.A.H., Sleijfer, D.Th. *et al.* (1986) Adjuvant surgery after PVB chemotherapy for Stage II and Stage III non-seminomatous testicular tumours, in *Advances in the Biosciences – Germ Cell Tumours II* (eds W.G. Jones, A. Ward and C.K. Anderson), Pergamon Press, Oxford, pp. 403–7.

Smith, T.K., Stallone, R.J. and Yee, J.M. (1979) The thoracic surgeon and anterior spinal surgery. *J. Thorac. Cardiovasc. Surg.*, **77**, 925–8.

Tait, D., Peckham, M.J., Hendry, W.F. and Goldstraw, P. (1984) Post-chemotherapy surgery in advanced non-seminoma germ cell tumours: The significance of histology with particular reference to differentiated (mature) teratoma. *Br. J. Cancer*, **50**, 601–9.

Venn, G.E., Sarin, S. and Goldstraw, P. (1989) Survival following pulmonary metastasectomy. *Eur. J. Cardiothor. Surg.*, **3**, 105–10.

Vugrin, D., Whitmore, W.F. and Golbey, R.B. (1983) VAB-6 combination chemotherapy without maintenance in the treatment of disseminated cancer of the testis. *Cancer*, **51**, 211–15.

Vugrin, D., Whitmore, W.F., Sogani, P.C. *et al.* (1981) Combined chemotherapy and surgery in treatment of advanced germ cell tumours. *Cancer*, **47**, 2228–31.

MALIGNANT EXTRAGONADAL GERM CELL TUMORS IN ADULTS

D. Raghavan and M. Boyer

28.1 INTRODUCTION

Malignant germ cell tumors occur most commonly in the testicles, and represent the commonest cancer in men aged 18–35 years (see Chapter 1). Occasionally, tumors that are histologically identical arise in the ovaries or in extragonadal sites, including mediastinum, retroperitoneum, pineal gland and sacrococcygeal region. Rarely such tumors have been reported in the liver, prostate, bladder, esophagus and stomach, uterus, heart and many other extragonadal sites (Hyman and Leiter, 1943; Holt, Melcher and Conquhoun, 1965; Hart, 1975; Benson, Segura and Carney, 1978; Gonzalez-Crussi, 1982; Kikuchi et al., 1988). However, doubts have been raised regarding the stringency of criteria for the exclusion of a possible primary testicular neoplasm in some of these cases, and the certainty of germ cell histology has been questioned in others. In some instances, however, 'burnt out' primary foci of scar tissue or even occult primary tumors have been demonstrated in the testicles of patients with presumed extragonadal germ cell tumors (EGCT) (Azzopardi and Hoffbrand, 1965). Despite the uncertainty of origin in some cases, there have been many well-documented reports of such tumors in which the testes have been assessed carefully and have been found to be histologically normal (Utz and Buscemi, 1971; Johnson et al., 1973; Cox, 1975; Raghavan and Barrett, 1980).

It is clear that these tumors constitute very different entities from their gonadal counterparts, with respect to natural history, management and prognosis, and it is appropriate to review these issues in a separate section of this book. We have addressed specifically the malignant EGCT that occur in adults, in particular the mediastinum, the retroperitoneum and the pineal gland. Consistent with the theme of this text, we have not discussed pediatric malignancies, such as sacrococcygeal teratomas, in detail, although these have been reviewed elsewhere (Donnellan and Swenson, 1968; Miles and Stewart, 1974; Schey, Shkoinik and White, 1977; Gonzalez-Crussi, 1982). Malignant germ cell tumors occasionally occur in adults in the sacrococcygeum or other extragonadal sites, and the principles of management are similar to those for the more common presentations, as outlined below.

28.1.1 HISTOGENESIS

The origins of EGCT have been the subject of considerable debate. Several bizarre theories have been proposed, including their development from displaced germ cell layers during embryogenesis (Schlumberger, 1946) and the

Testicular Cancer: Investigation and management. Second edition. Edited by Professor A. Horwich. Published in 1996 by Chapman & Hall. ISBN 0 412 61210 0.

'included twin' hypothesis, as summarized by Gonzalez-Crussi (1982). However, it is now generally accepted that these tumors arise from primordial germ cells that have migrated from the yolk sac endoderm (Friedman, 1951). Witschi (1948) demonstrated the pathway of germ cell migration from endoderm to genital ridges. This passage occurs in the midline, and it is presumed that EGCT arise as a result of aberrant midline migration, with the germ cells lodging in the sites of common presentation. One feature that remains unexplained is the striking predominance of malignancy of these tumors in males, as distinct from an equal sex predominance of benign EGCT and a predominance of benign germ cell tumors in the ovaries (Kurman and Norris, 1977).

Bosl *et al.* (1989) have provided further support for a common origin of testicular and EGCT by demonstrating that tumors arising at each site share a chromosomal abnormality, isochromosome 12p, in which the long arm of chromosome 12 is lost and the short arm duplicated, with symmetry around the centromere. We have postulated that an event in the first trimester of pregnancy may give rise to the development of EGCT, based upon a case in which a mediastinal germ cell tumor occurred in a patient with congenital anomalies that probably arose during the first trimester (Raghavan and Barrett, 1980), as well as other associations between germ cell malignancy at various sites and the development of congenital anomalies with origins in the first trimester of development (Raghavan and Neville, 1982). There have also been other reported associations between EGCT and congenital and chromosomal anomalies, including Klinefelter's syndrome (Feun, Samson and Stephens, 1980; Logothetis *et al.*, 1985).

28.1.2 PATHOLOGY

Extragonadal germ cell tumors at each site are histologically identical to germ cell tumors that arise in the testicles (Friedman, 1951; Gonzalez-Crussi, 1982). Frequently the only means of identifying the site of presentation is by the assessment of the surrounding tissues (e.g. absence of testicular tubules, presence of lung, mediastinal structures, etc.).

Both seminoma (also termed 'dysgerminoma', or 'germinoma' in the pineal and suprasellar regions) and non-seminomatous germ cell tumor (NSGCT) may present in extragonadal sites, and are frequently found to coexist within the one deposit. In fact, we believe that this lends additional support to the concept of a common origin of seminoma and NSGCT in the testis and elsewhere (Raghavan and Neville, 1982). All subgroups of NSGCT have been reported in all extragonadal sites, including embryonal carcinoma, the spectrum of malignant teratoma (or teratocarcinoma), endodermal sinus tumor (yolk sac tumor) and choriocarcinoma (Borit, 1969; Dayan *et al.*, 1966; Raghavan and Barrett, 1980; Vogelzang *et al.*, 1982). Analogous to testicular tumors, the majority of advanced extragonadal NSGCT are associated with the production of the tumor markers, alphafetoprotein (AFP) and/or human chorionic gonadotrophin (HCG), as well as less specific markers such as lactic acid dehydrogenase (LDH) and carcinoembryonic antigen (CEA).

In patients with mediastinal EGCT, differentiation from thymoma and large cell lymphoma has often been difficult using conventional light morphological criteria (Lattes, 1962). However, with the introduction of immunohistochemical techniques (Heyderman and Neville, 1976, 1977), which allow the demonstration of AFP and HCG indicating germinal origin, or leukocyte common antigen (consistent with lymphoma within biopsied tumor tissue), this distinction has become somewhat more reliable. Furthermore, the electron microscope may sometimes resolve the issue through the demonstration of features consistent with germ cells, lymphocytes, mesenchymal or epithelial tissues. For example, germinal tumors are characterized by convoluted and complex nucleolar structures and, in the case of NSGCT, electron-dense extracellular material (Gonzalez-Crussi, 1982; Monaghan, Raghavan and Neville, 1982).

Precise histological classification is of particular importance in the retroperitoneum and mediastinum because of the presence of extensive lymph node tissue, and the consequent risk of misdiagnosis of metastases. In addition to the possibility of testicular germ cell tumors with nodal involvement, other differential diagnoses of importance in this age group include metastases from malignant melanoma, poorly differentiated renal adenocarcinoma (in the retroperitoneum in particular), large cell lymphoma, poorly differentiated carcinoma of unknown primary site (atypical teratoma syndrome), and the adult presentations of pediatric malignancies (Ewing's sarcoma, neuroblastoma, Wilm's tumor).

Dorothy Russell (1944) first reported the histological similarity of gonadal and primary intracranial germ cell tumors, drawing a clear distinction from the less common pineal parenchymal tumors. Further data have confirmed these morphological, ultrastructural and functional pathological similarities (Friedman, 1951; Dayan *et al.*, 1966; Beeley *et al.*, 1973; Gonzalez-Crussi, 1982).

The so-called 'atypical teratoma or germ cell syndrome', first described by Fox *et al.* (1979), has been the source of considerable clinical controversy (Greco, Vaughn and Hainsworth, 1986), as discussed below. This syndrome, which has been reported most often in young men, is characterized histologically by the presence of metastatic deposits of undifferentiated carcinoma cells, usually without the ultrastructural or functional (tumor marker) features of germinal malignancy (Logothetis *et al.*, 1985; Hainsworth *et al.*, 1987). It has been proposed that patients with this syndrome should be managed similarly to those with metastatic germ cell tumors (see below).

28.2 MALIGNANT GERM CELL TUMORS OF MEDIASTINUM

Primary mediastinal germ cell tumors account for only 2–6% of all mediastinal tumors (Cox, 1975). However, they do represent the most common site for EGCT (Kuhn and Weissbach, 1985) Although mediastinal germ cell tumors occur with equal frequency in both sexes, there is an excess of malignancy in males (Martini *et al.*, 1974; Cox, 1975; Polansky *et al.*, 1979). They usually occur between the ages of 17 and 35 years (Martini *et al.*, 1974; Polansky, Barwick and Ravin, 1979; Raghavan and Barrett, 1980), although cases have been reported in children (Canty and Siemens, 1978).

28.2.1 CLINICAL FEATURES

The presenting features of mediastinal malignant germ cell tumors are a function of: (i) the anatomical location of the tumor, (ii) local growth, with extrinsic compression of surrounding structures, (iii) invasion into adjacent tissues and (iv) metastatic deposits. The most common initial symptom is chest or upper back pain, although as many as 25% are detected at routine chest X-ray (Martini *et al.*, 1974; Cox, 1975; Lemarié *et al.*, 1992). In addition, patients present commonly with cough, hemoptysis, dyspnea, dysphagia and constitutional syndromes (including weight loss, fever and anorexia) (Schantz, Sewall and Castleman, 1972; Martini *et al.*, 1974; Raghavan and Barrett, 1980; Vogelzang *et al.*, 1982; Lemarié *et al.*, 1992; Childs *et al.*, 1993). Gynecomastia is sometimes associated with mediastinal choriocarcinoma (Fine, Smith and Pachter, 1962; British Medical Journal, 1969; Martini *et al.*, 1974). Headache may be due either to superior vena cava obstruction or to cerebral metastases. In fact, superior vena cava syndrome has been documented in as many as 25% of patients (Polansky, Barwick and Ravin, 1979; Vogelzang *et al.*, 1982).

These tumors characteristically are clinically silent early in the course of the disease, and thus are often locally extensive by the time of first representation (Vogelzang *et al.*, 1982; Jain *et al.*, 1984). Common sites of metastases include lung and pleura, liver, lymph nodes and bone (Martini *et al.*, 1974; Cox, 1975; Luna, 1975; Walden *et al.*, 1977; Raghavan and Barrett, 1980; Vogelzang *et al.*, 1982; Childs *et al.*, 1993). In less than 10% of cases, metastases are found in kidney, central nervous system, spleen, adrenals, soft tissues and pericardium (Luna, 1975; (Walden *et al.*, 1977; Polansky, Barwick and Ravin 1979; Raghavan and Barrett, 1980). The discrepancy between published clinical series and data from autopsies (in which there is a greater distribution and higher frequency of metastases) reflects the propensity of these tumors to metastasize widely, especially during periods of prolonged, but unsuccessful, treatment (Oberman and Libcke, 1964; Cox, 1975; Luna, 1975; Aliotta *et al.*, 1988). Furthermore, many of the sites of metastases may not manifest themselves clinically until the tumor is extensive.

28.2.2 INVESTIGATION

The investigation of the patient with an EGCT is similar to that for the patient with a testicular tumor, as discussed in Chapters 1 to 3. Important endpoints of investigations include the demonstration of the histological type of the tumor and the assessment of the extent or stage of disease. Routine biochemical and hematological assessment and the measurement of the tumor markers, AFP and HCG, are integral to initial staging. Plain radiography of the chest will usually provide a simple baseline for monitoring and follow-up after treatment. However, computed axial tomography (CAT) scanning of the chest and abdomen are essential to define the extent of solid versus cystic disease (Fig. 28.1), the potential for surgical resection, and the distribution of metastases. Of particular importance,

significant mediastinal lymphadenopathy may be masked by adjacent structures and thus may not be obvious on plain chest radiography.

To date, no clear role has been defined for nuclear magnetic resonance imaging in preference to CAT scanning in this context, although it may provide a clearer delineation of the local vasculature and differentiation between enlarged nodes and ectatic blood vessels. In the instance of a pure mediastinal seminoma, CAT scanning in the prone position is often necessary as an aid to the planning of radiotherapy, to ensure that the boundaries of the tumor are fully encompassed.

In the asymptomatic patient, the yield of routine radionuclide bone scanning is low and this technique is not routinely used in this context in our institutions, with the exception of the patient with predominant choriocarcinoma (with its frequent tendency to form osseous metastases).

During treatment of mediastinal NSGCT, especially with prolonged regimens of cytotoxic chemotherapy, routine monitoring of serum AFP and HCG, at least on a monthly schedule, is essential as a guide to the efficacy of treatment. More frequent sampling schedules should be used when more dose-intensive and frequently administered cytotoxic regimens are employed, for example, the POMB/ACE regimen, in which drugs are administered every 10 days (Newlands *et al.*, 1983; Rustin, *et al.*, 1986). A prolongation in tumor marker half-life will often be the first evidence of resistance to the cytotoxic regimen in use. As the outcome of cytotoxic chemotherapy for mediastinal NSGCT is less successful than for the testicular equivalent (see below), it is of crucial importance that these patients be monitored meticulously, to facilitate the early change of ineffective treatment. Conversely, the phenomenon of tumor marker release is commonly associated with successful chemotherapy (particularly in HCG-producing tumors), and frequent tumor mar-

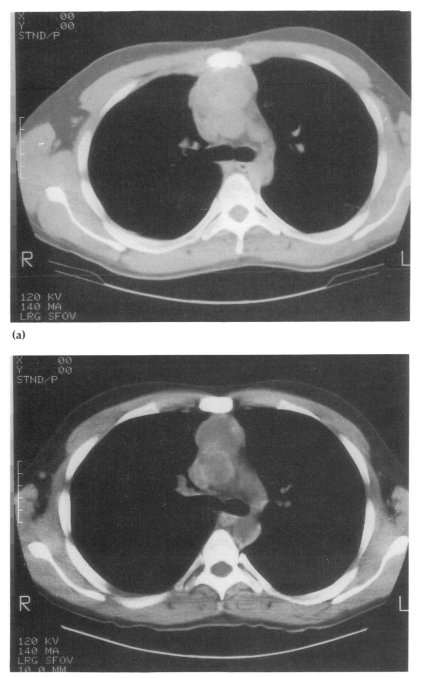

(a)

(b)

Fig. 28.1   Computed axial tomography scans of a mediastinal germ cell tumor. (a) Before treatment. (b) After treatment. Note diminution in size and variegation of tumor mass after two cycles of POMB/ACE; persistently raised tumor markers heralded locoregional relapse and the development of subcutaneous metastases.

ker sampling will allow the distinction between a prolonged marker clearance time, and an artefact created by an initial marker release into the circulation (due to tumor lysis), followed by normal clearance from a higher baseline value.

After the completion of treatment, the schedules of follow-up are similar to those employed for patients with testicular germ cell tumors. However, there is a greater propensity for late relapse, and thus a greater need for prolonged close follow-up. We routinely check serum markers and chest X-rays every 2–3 months for the first 3 years, then every 4 months until 5 years from presentation, and then follow the patients every 6–12 months indefinitely. There is no defined role for serial CAT scanning beyond the first 2–3 years, although we usually repeat the CAT scan of the chest and abdomen 5 years after presentation to document the disease-free status.

Of particular importance is the exclusion of a possible testicular primary tumor both at presentation and subsequently. Careful clinical examination can be supplemented by high resolution ultrasonography. In the presence of atrophic testicles, Skakkebaek has proposed fine needle biopsy as a means of screening for carcinoma *in situ* of the testicles (Chapter 29), although this issue remains controversial, especially in the presence of a completely normal ultrasound examination. For example, in a series of 48 patients with EGCT who underwent routine testicular biopsies, none of eight patients with mediastinal germ cell tumors were found to have carcinoma *in situ* (Daugaard *et al.*, 1992). By contrast, 16 of 39 cases of retroperitoneal GCT were associated with carcinoma *in situ* on testicular biopsy (implying that these cases were probably not true EGCT).

Finally, in the patient with mediastinal choriocarcinoma, the approach should be similar to that employed for the patient with metastatic testicular choriocarcinoma, as discussed in Chapters 1 and 19. Thus,

synchronous measurement of blood and cerebrospinal fluid levels of HCG should be carried out to determine whether there is local production of HCG by intracranial tumor deposits. In this situation, we routinely screen for intracerebral deposits by CAT scan before spinal tap is effected.

28.2.3 TREATMENT

28.2.3.1 Dysgerminoma/seminoma

Historically, the treatment of mediastinal dysgerminoma was based upon the use of radiotherapy, either alone or following surgery (Bagshaw, McLaughlin and Earle, 1969; Medini *et al.*, 1979; Polansky, Barwick and Ravin, 1979; Raghavan and Barrett, 1980; Bush, Martinez and Bagshaw, 1981). The results achieved with some of the more dated approaches to radiotherapy, antedating the use of current imaging techniques and the measurement of tumor markers, were unsatisfactory, with 5-year survival rates of less than 30%, and significant toxicity, especially to the lung. In some instances, inadequate field sizes or doses were employed. With the introduction of more modern techniques with CAT scan-guided treatment planning and the use of the shrinking-field technique (in which field sizes are progressively reduced as the size of the tumor shrinks) cure rates of greater than 60% have been achieved, accompanied by acceptable levels of toxicity. In general, a dose of 35–40 Gy, in 1.5 to 2 Gy fractions, has been used (Medini *et al.*, 1979; Economou *et al.*, 1982). With these approaches, deaths have occurred as a result of metastatic disease, but with the treatment proving effective in the control of the primary tumor. Our approach has been to use radiotherapy as the primary modality of treatment if: (i) the histology is pure seminoma; (ii) the maximum horizontal diameter of the tumor is less than 50% of the total transthoracic diameter; (iii) raised levels of AFP and HCG are not detected in the circulation; (iv) staging tests fail to reveal any evidence of metastatic disease. However, it is uncommon for mediastinal dysgerminomas to present with small volume disease, and we are increasingly using initial debulking cytotoxic chemotherapy (see below).

Since the introduction of cisplatin-containing chemotherapy regimens, a substantial change in approach has occurred in many centers. The demonstration that seminoma (dysgerminoma) is highly sensitive to the effects of cisplatin has led to the use of combination chemotherapy as one of the mainstays of treatment for mediastinal dysgerminoma (Jain *et al.*, 1984; Logothetis *et al.*, 1985; Motzer *et al.*, 1988).

During the evolution of our clinical approach, for large mediastinal dysgerminomas, or in the presence of metastases, we administered a conventional dosage of the PVB regimen, combining cisplatin/vinblastine/bleomycin (Levi *et al.*, 1988; Raghavan *et al.*, 1989) and then used radiotherapy to the site of the original primary tumor mass to consolidate the remission, especially in the presence of a residual tumor mass. This approach required particular care in the delivery of bleomycin, a potent pulmonary radiosensitizer. The demonstration that bleomycin does impact on cure rates in advanced germ cell tumors (Levi *et al.*, 1993) led us to maintain this agent in the combination, at least for the first one to two cycles of treatment. With the introduction of etoposide into clinical practice, we modified our approach to the use of the PEB regimen, incorporating cisplatin, etoposide and bleomycin (Williams *et al.*, 1987).

Others have merely relied upon the effects of chemotherapy alone (Newlands *et al.*, 1983). As yet, the true necessity for added radiotherapy in this context is unproven. Using chemotherapy as the primary modality of treatment, sometimes augmented by radiotherapy, cure rates of more than 80% have been achieved (Logothetis *et al.*, 1985, Motzer *et al.*, 1988). In some instances, surgical exploration will be effected for a residual mediastinal mass, although the surgery is technically difficult and demanding as the tumors tend to invade locally, and tissue planes for dissection have often been destroyed. Another option is to employ delayed gallium scanning, as there is a good correlation between residual gallium uptake and active remaining malignancy, once the acute post-chemotherapy inflammatory phase has resolved.

The demonstration of high response rates of advanced seminoma to carboplatin (Chapters 19, 20), with the associate substantial reduction of toxicity, appeared likely to change further the approaches to the management of this illness. The potential role of carboplatin as a radiosensitizer, as well as the modest profile of side-effects, might have facilitated combination regimens incorporating concurrent or sequential use of carboplatin and radiotherapy, with a view to the improvement of cure rates and the further reduction of toxicity. However, recent data that demonstrate a lower cure rate for metastatic NSGCT from carboplatin-containing regimens compared with more traditional cisplatin-based chemotherapy have retarded such research efforts.

28.2.3.2 Malignant non-seminomatous germ cell tumors

The results achieved in the treatment of malignant mediastinal NSGCT (as distinct from mediastinal seminomas or benign mediastinal teratomas) have been very disappointing (Table 28.1). Historically, the use of radiotherapy alone, or in combination with surgery, yielded cure rates of less than 20% (Oberman and Libcke, 1964; Johnson *et al.*, 1973; Martini *et al.*, 1974), analogous to the situation in the early management of metastatic testicular NSGCT. With the introduction of cisplatin, initial response rates as high as 60% were achieved (Feun, Samson and Stephens, 1980; Vogelzang *et al.*, 1982; Garnick, Canellos and Richie, 1983; Levi *et al.*, 1988; Tondini and Garnick, 1989; Nichols *et*

Table 28.1 Chemotherapy for mediastinal germ cell tumors

Number of patients	Regimen	Complete remission and disease-free survival*	Long-term survival (%) +	Reference
Seminoma				
8	PVB/EBAP	63	67**	Bukowski *et al.* (1993)
7	Carb±RT	86	100	Childs *et al.* (1993)
2	PV‡	0	0	Feun, Samson and Stephens (1980)
9	PVB±RT	67	67	Giaccone (1991)
9	various C-based	89	89	Goss *et al.* (1994)
2	C/P	100	100	Jain *et al.* (1984)
13	PVB/BEP/VAB-6	92	92	Lemarié *et al.* (1992)
4	CISCA2/CP	100	100	Logothetis *et al.* (1985)
17	VAB-6/EP	88	88	Motzer *et al.* (1988)
Non-seminomatous germ cell tumors				
16	PVB/EBAP	82	67**	Bukowski *et al.* (1993)
11	various C-based	82	73	Childs *et al.* (1993)
7	PV	0	0	Feun, Samson and Stephens (1980)
8	PVB	37	12	Garnick, Canellos and Richie (1983)
6	PVB/BEP	33	33	Giaccone (1991)
15	various C-based	53	47	Goss *et al.* (1994)
31	PVB±A	67	59¶	Hainsworth *et al.* (1982)
11	VAB-6	57	57	Israel *et al.* (1985)
12	PVB/BEP	50	42	Kay *et al.* (1987)
10	PVB±A	30	10¶	Kuzur *et al.* (1982)
64	various C-based	52	52#	Lemarié *et al.* (1992)
11	CISCA2/VB4	38	38	Logothetis *et al.* (1985)
7	VAB/VV	43	43	McLeod *et al.* (1988)
31	PVB/BEP	58	45	Nichols *et al.* (1990)
8	POMB/ACE	63	63	Parker *et al.* (1983)
7	PVB	41	41	Vogelzang *et al.* (1982)

* After resection.
** Kaplan Meier estimate, includes seminoma and non-seminoma.
+ Survival greater than 2 years in most series.
# Kaplan Meier estimate.
‡ Cisplatin dose of 75 mg m⁻².
¶ Split series from one group; separates endodermal sinus tumors; if combined 46% long-term survival. PVB, cisplatin/vinblastine/bleomycin. EP, etoposide/cisplatin. A, Adriamycin. BEP, bleomycin/etoposide/cisplatin. C/P, cyclophosphamide/cisplatin. CISCA2/VB4 cisplatin/cyclophosphamide/Adriamycin/vinblastine/bleomycin. VAB-6, vinblastine/actinomycin-D/bleomycin/cyclophosphamide/cisplatin. VV, etoposide/vincristine. POMB, cisplatin/vincristine/methotrexate/bleomycin. ACE, actinomycin-D/cyclophosphamide/etoposide; carb, carboplatin.

al., 1990; Lemarié *et al.*, 1992; Bukowski *et al.*, 1993; Childs *et al.*, 1993). However, standard regimens such as PVB or PEB have achieved cure rates that have been substantially lower, predominantly in the range 20–40% (Volgelzang *et al.*, 1982; Garnick, Canellos and Richie, 1983; Israel *et al.*, 1985; Logothetis *et al.*, 1985; Tondini and Garnick, 1989), in marked contrast to the results achieved for metastatic testicular germ cell tumors.

One of the difficulties in evaluating the true efficacy of chemotherapy for mediastinal NSGCT has been the bias in reporting. For example, the exclusion of patients with predominant endodermal sinus tumor and the inclusion of mediastinal dysgerminomas has, in each case, improved the apparent survival figures (Hainsworth *et al.*, 1982). Nevertheless, despite small numbers of patients having been reported, the recent introduction of more dose-intensive regimens, incorporating higher doses of cisplatin and more frequent dosing schedules, may be yielding higher response rates and more durable remissions (Israel *et al.*, 1985; Logothetis *et al.*, 1985; Raghavan *et al.*, 1989; Nichols *et al.*, 1990; Lemarié *et al.*, 1992; Bukowski *et al.*, 1993; Childs *et al.*, 1993;) (Table 28.1).

A postchemotherapy syndrome has been described in patients with mediastinal EGCT – the development of acute leukemia or other myelodysplastic phenomena during or soon after completion of chemotherapy (Feun, Samson and Stephens, 1980; Hainsworth *et al.*, 1982; Nichols *et al.*, 1990). The demonstration of an isochromosome of 12, *i*(12p), in the cytogenetic analysis of the bone marrow and in tumor tissue in such cases implies that both malignancies arise from a common progenitor cell (Landanyi *et al.*, 1990), or at least share a common mechanism of oncogenesis. It has also been postulated that chemotherapy may cause the hematological abnormalities. However, the short interval between treatment and the development of leukemia in these cases (median 6 months) contrasts with that usually observed in iatrogenic malignancies (Boyer and Raghavan, 1992).

Although the resection of residual masses after completion of chemotherapy is widely practiced in the management of metastatic testicular cancer (Chapters 26 and 27), this approach has not been proven to be of value in the management of EGCT, although it has been widely advocated (Vogelzang *et al.*, 1982; Parker *et al.*, 1983; Kay, Wells and Goldstraw, 1987; Nichols *et al.*, 1990; Wright *et al.*, 1990). Similarly, initial debulking surgery (prior to the use of chemotherapy) has not yet been evaluated in this context, although data from the management of metastatic testicular germ cell tumors would sug-

gest that this is unlikely to be a productive approach.

Despite these advances, the management of mediastinal NSGCT remains a difficult problem, and the results to date have been particularly disappointing in contrast to the successes achieved with metastatic testicular cancer. The reasons for this discrepancy are not clear. Paradoxically, the second Prognostic Factor Study of the British Medical Research Council suggested that the presence of a mediastinal primary *per se* is not an adverse prognostic factor (Mead *et al.*, 1992). Instead this report proposed that the adverse prognostic determinant in this context is locally advanced disease, rather than the site of origin itself.

28.3 MALIGNANT GERM CELL TUMORS OF THE RETROPERITONEUM

Traditionally it has been reported that the retroperitoneum is the second most common site of origin of EGCT, and that approximately 10% of primary retroperitoneal tumors are germinal in origin (Palumbo *et al.*, 1949). Seminomas and NSGCT (benign and malignant) have been reported in this site (Palumbo *et al.*, 1949; Arnheim, 1951; Abell, Fayos and Lampe, 1965; Pantoja, Llobet and Gonzalez-Flores, 1976; Gonzalez-Crussi, 1982). With the increasing sophistication of pathological diagnosis and of noninvasive staging techniques, it is likely that these estimates are inaccurate. Of particular importance is that many cases hitherto regarded as primary in the retroperitoneum are likely to have arisen from occult testicular neoplasms (Fig. 28.2)). Furthermore, many of the poorly differentiated neoplasms previously classified as teratomas or seminomas can be shown immunohistochemically to have other origins (e.g. lymphoma). There is a marked need for a detailed review of archival biopsy material from such tumors, with reprocessing for immunohistochemical staining and other techniques to define the true prevalence of

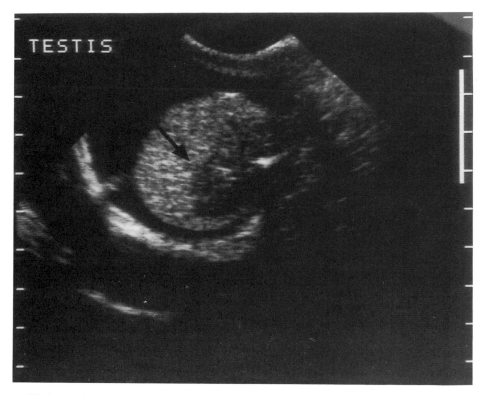

Fig. 28.2 High resolution ultrasound of a normal-sized testicle in a patient with a putative retroperitoneal germ cell tumor. Note the demonstration of an occult lesion.

primary retroperitoneal germ cell tumors. These tumors can be difficult to characterize morphologically, and all such cases should be referred for validation to a specialist tumor pathologist. We have previously demonstrated a significant change in histopathological diagnosis when specimens of germ cell tumors are reviewed in this fashion (Segelov *et al.*, 1993).

28.3.1   CLINICAL FEATURES

Notwithstanding the above concerns, the presentations of these tumors are quite well defined. Retroperitoneal NSGCT of childhood is most commonly a benign lesion, with only 10% showing malignant features (Palumbo *et al.*, 1949; Arnheim, 1951). There is a slight

female preponderance among patients with benign lesions. By contrast, retroperitoneal seminomas occur more commonly in older males, with mean ages at presentation ranging from 42 to 48 years (Abell, Fayos and Lampe, 1965; Medini *et al.*, 1979; Jain *et al.*, 1984).

The most common presenting symptoms include abdominal pain (80%), abdominal distension or an abdominal mass, back pain, weight loss, nausea and vomiting, or constipation (Arnheim, 1951; Abell, Fayos and Lampe, 1965; Pantoja, Llobet and Gonzalez-Flores, 1976). Occasionally urinary tract symptoms or the features of vascular obstruction may be noted. On examination, up to 75% of patients have a palpable abdominal mass. Other features include evidence of metastases, ascites or gynecomastia. We have previously reported the association of the syndrome of multiple atypical nevi with germ cell tumors (Raghavan *et al.*, 1994) and have observed this phenomenon in patients with retroperitoneal EGCT. Thus, in a patient with multiple atypical nevi and a large abdominal mass, greater consideration should be given to the diagnosis of EGCT or metastatic malignant melanoma.

28.3.2   INVESTIGATION

The most important diagnostic problem in the management of retroperitoneal EGCT is the exclusion of a testicular primary tumor. While this is pertinent in the management of mediastinal EGCT, the issue is more important in retroperitoneal tumors because of the pattern of spread of testicular neoplasia (Chapter 1). With more widespread use of high resolution testicular ultrasonography, an increasing proportion of patients with apparent retroperitoneal EGCT have been shown to have occult testicular primaries (Kirschling *et al.*, 1983; Bohle *et al.*, 1986; Saltzman, Pitts and Vaughan, 1986).

Thus careful clinical examination of the testes, supplemented by high resolution ultrasonography (Fig. 28.2) is integral to the staging of these tumors. In addition, the routine tests discussed above for mediastinal tumors should also be applied. In particular, meticulous histological assessment, with special stains for germ cell markers, leukocyte common antigen, etc., is mandatory. In the absence of elevated blood levels of AFP or HCG, negative fine needle aspiration cytology is usually inadequate to define the absence of malignancy in a retroperitoneal germ cell tumor because of the risk of sampling error, and accordingly we advocate a core biopsy or open surgical biopsy to ensure the acquisition of an adequate tissue sample.

28.3.3   TREATMENT

The management of retroperitoneal germ cell tumors depends upon the histology and the size of the lesion. If there is a high index of suspicion of an occult testicular neoplasm, we routinely perform exploration of the ipsilateral testis via an inguinal approach, and this is usually followed by an orchidectomy (depending somewhat upon the level of surgical suspicion of the presence of a primary testicular tumor). Even when it is anticipated that chemotherapy will be used, resection of a testicular primary is required as the testis constitutes a sanctuary site in up to one-third of cases. In the patient who refuses surgery, fine needle aspiration cytology of the testis may be helpful, notwithstanding concerns about sampling error.

28.3.3.1   Retroperitoneal dysgerminomas

It has been suggested that retroperitoneal seminomas (dysgerminomas) of less than 5 cm diameter should be managed by radiotherapy, with doses in the range 20–40 Gy (Abell, Fayos and Lampe, 1965; Medini *et al.*, 1979). However, because of the lack of symptoms associated with small retroperitoneal masses, this clinical situation is extremely uncommon. Analogous to metastatic testicular seminoma and large mediastinal dysgerminoma, we believe that the optimal approach is to treat these tumors with initial cisplatin-based combination chemotherapy. For patients with residual masses, depending upon the clinical context, we may elect to follow the patient closely but expectantly, to irradiate the residual mass or occasionally to attempt surgical resection. If surgery is contemplated, it should be undertaken only by an expert urological oncologist, as there is a substantial risk of tearing the vascular structures during the attempted dissection because of the lack of defined tissue planes.

Table 28.2   Treatment of retroperitoneal germ cell tumors

Number of patients	Regimen	Complete remission and disease-free survival* (%)	Long-term survival (%)	Reference
Seminoma				
2	PVB/EBAP	50	80#	Bukowski *et al.* (1993)
2	PVB‡	0	0	Feun, Samson and Stephens (1980)
2	various C-based	100	100	Goss *et al.* (1994)
3	VAB-6	100	100	Jain *et al.* (1984)
13	C/P	85	85	Logothetis *et al.* (1985)
Non-seminomatous germ cell tumors				
4	PVB/EBAP	70	80#	Bukowski *et al.* (1993)
4	PVB‡	25	25	Feun, Samson and Stephens (1980)
5	PVB	80	60	Garnick, Canellos and Richie (1983)
4	various C-based	?	50	Goss *et al.* (1994)
6	VB	?	33	Logothetis *et al.* (1985)
6	CISCA2/+VB4	66	66	Logothetis *et al.* (1985)
5	POMB/ACE	?	60	Newlands *et al.* (1983)

* After resection.
# Kaplan Meier estimates, includes seminoma and non-seminomatous germ cell tumors.
+ Survival greater than 2 years in most series.
‡ Cisplatin dose of 75 mg m^{-2}.
PVB, cisplatin/vinblastine/bleomycin. C/P, cyclophosphamide/cisplatin. CISCA1/VB4, cisplatin/cyclophosphamide/Adriamycin/vinblastine/bleomycin. VAB6, vinblastine/actinomycin-D/bleomycin/cyclophosphamide/cisplatin. VV, etoposide/vincristine. POMB, cisplatin/vincristine/metholoenate/bleomycin. ACE, actinomycin-D/cyclophosphamide/etoposide.

28.3.3.2   Retroperitoneal NSGCT

In the situation of an unequivocally benign retroperitoneal germ cell tumor, surgical resection is the treatment of choice. Further treatment is usually not required unless histological assessment reveals occult malignant elements (in which case the tumor is managed as outlined below).

Combination chemotherapy is the first line treatment of choice for malignant retroperitoneal NSGCT (Table 28.2), and it now appears that the cure rates are equivalent to those for metastatic testicular germ cell tumors of equivalent volume (McAleer, Nicholls and Horwich, 1992). Others have suggested a possible improvement of outcome if regimens of high dose intensity are employed (Garnick, Canellos and Richie, 1983; Logothetis *et al.*, 1985). Our view is that tumor volume and other conventional prognostic determinants, such as amplitude of tumor markers (Levi *et al.* 1988; Mead *et al.*, 1992), should

govern the selection of treatment, rather than the retroperitoneal extragonadal primary site *per se*. After chemotherapy for retroperitoneal NSGCT, it is our practice to resect residual masses whenever feasible to remove occult elements of residual malignancy or residual differentiated teratoma (Reddell *et al.*, 1983). Particular attention should be paid to the testicles as we have seen testicular relapse 10 years after the treatment of a retroperitoneal NSGCT with cisplatin, vinblastine and bleomycin (Boyer *et al.*, 1990). Furthermore, as noted previously, there has been clear documentation that residual cancer may remain viable in the testicle after systemic chemotherapy for metastatic disease (Greist *et al.*, 1984).

28.4   INTRACRANIAL GERM CELL TUMORS

In Western populations, primary germ cell tumors of the pineal gland and suprasellar region account for less than 5% of all primary intracranial tumors (Jellinger, 1973), and the figure is lower if childhood cases are excluded (Gonzalez-Crussi, 1982). By contrast, in the Far East, these tumors constitute up to 10% of intracranial malignancy, for reasons that are not known (Koide, Watanabe and Sato, 1980). They occur most commonly in the first two decades of life (Jenkin, Simpson and Keen, 1978; Jennings, Gelman and Hochberg, 1985; Edwards *et al.* 1988), although Jennings *et al.* (1985) have reported a case in a patient aged 69 years. Pineal germ cell tumors occur twice as frequently in males as in females (Jenkin, Simpson and Keen, 1978; Jennings, Gelman and Hochberg, 1985), although there is no sex difference in suprasellar germ cell tumors (Simson, Lampe and Abell, 1968; Jenkins, Simpson and Keen, 1978; Sung, Hariusiadis and Chang, 1978).

These tumors occur most commonly in pineal and suprasellar sites, although 5% of cases may be found in the third ventricle, basal ganglia, thalamus or other ventricles (Gonzalez-Crussi, 1982; Bloom, 1983; Jennings, Gelman and Hochberg, 1985). Germinomas (seminomas or dysgerminomas) are the most common tumors in pineal and suprasellar regions. However, when NSGCT does occur it is found more often in the pineal gland (Jennings, Gelman and Hochberg, 1985).

All histological types of germ cell tumors have been described in this context, including germinoma (dysgerminoma or seminoma), embryonal carcinoma, pure choriocarcinoma and pure yolk sac tumor, and different histological types may coexist (Dayan *et al.*, 1966; Bestle, 1968; Simson, Lampe and Abell, 1968; Borit, 1969; Beeley *et al.*, 1973; Ho and Rassekh, 1979; Gonzalez-Crussi, 1982).

Isochromosome 12p has been reported in one case of nongerminomatous pineal GCT, implying a common pathogenesis with other GCT and EGCT (deBruin *et al.*, 1994).

28.4.1 PRESENTATION

There is often a prolonged period of non-specific central nervous system symptoms antedating the diagnosis (Jennings, Gelman and Hochberg, 1985). The symptoms are usually related to the involved anatomical structures. Pineal tumors, which are located near the midbrain and aqueduct, usually present with headache (more than 80% of cases), nausea and vomiting, consistent with raised intracranial pressure and hydrocephalus. A range of nonspecific (and falsely localizing) symptoms may be associated, including memory disturbance, impaired concentration and lassitude (Bloom, 1983). Suprasellar tumors, which abut the optic chiasm, pituitary and hypothalamus, commonly present with visual disturbance, polyuria and polydypsia, lethargy and somnolence.

Physical examination of the patient with a pineal germ cell tumor frequently reveals papilledema (up to 65% of cases) and the features of Parinaud's syndrome, with paralysis of upward gaze, pupillary areflexia and paralysis of convergence (Simson, Lampe and Abell, 1968; Sung, Hariusiadis and Chang, 1978; Bloom, 1983; Jennings, Gelman and Hochberg, 1985; Legido *et al.*, 1989). Precocious puberty occurs in up to 40% of cases (Gonzalez-Crussi, 1982). By contrast, suprasellar tumors are more commonly associated with signs of hypopituitarism and visual field loss. It should, however, be noted that there is likely to be a reporting bias in favor of patients with neurological or endocrinological syndromes, and the prevalence figures reported may represent an overestimate.

The most common site of metastases is the spinal subarachnoid space. However, systemic metastases have been reported, sometimes in association with ventriculosystemic shunts (Giuffre and DiLorenzo, 1975; Jennings, Gelman and Hochberg, 1985). In most series, spinal metastases have been reported in 10–20% of cases (Jenkin, Simpson and Keen, 1978; Sung, Hariusiadis and Chang, 1978;

Chapman and Linggood, 1980; Watterson and Priest, 1988), and it has been proposed that biopsy of the primary tumor may be a pre-disposing feature (Jenkin, Simpson and Keen, 1978; Sung, Hariusiadis and Chang, 1978; Leibel and Sheline, 1987).

28.4.2　INVESTIGATION

The emphasis of investigation is somewhat different from the protocols used for mediastinal and retroperitoneal tumors. In the case of intracranial germ cell tumors, there is a much lower probability of an associated testicular primary in the absence of systemic metastases. In fact, only 4–6% of unselected cases of testicular cancer have associated cerebral metastases (Kaye *et al.*, 1979; Raghavan *et al.*, 1987). Thus careful clinical examination of the testes is probably sufficient to exclude a testicular primary. Routine assessment of serum biochemistry will define the presence of diabetes insipidus. The measurement of serum HCG and AFP levels is mandatory to screen for systemic involvement, and cerebrospinal fluid should also be assessed for HCG and AFP at the same time (Kida *et al.*, 1986; Watterson and Priest, 1988), although it has been reported that cerebrospinal fluid AFP is an unreliable index of the presence of an intracranial germ cell tumor (Kaye *et al.*, 1979). Because of the anatomical location of the tumor, a biopsy and histological diagnosis may not always be possible. In that situation, measurement of tumor markers is of particular importance in defining its nature. If a patient is first seen after a neurosurgical procedure with a ventriculosystemic shunt in place, caution must be exercised in the interpretation of the levels of serum tumor markers (which may be artefactually high, representing spillover from the cerebrospinal fluid).

The delineation of the primary tumor is of particular importance. Cerebral CAT scans, with closely spaced serial sections, sagittal and coronal views, may define the extent of disease, and are often helpful in monitoring the progress of treatment (Inoue *et al.*, 1979). Nuclear magnetic resonance imaging (Fig. 28.3) is particularly helpful in defining the intracranial anatomy and the extent of tumor involvement, occasionally demonstrating tumor tissue that has not been shown by CAT scanning (Edwards *et al.*, 1988). Where sophisticated imaging techniques are not initially available, assessment of the pituitary fossa and surrounds by plain radiography may be helpful. However, this is a complex and subtle area of clinical oncology, in which the potential for a life-threatening error of management is high, and we believe that, if such a diagnosis is suspected, the patient should be referred to a subspecialist or tertiary referral center, and considerations of lack of necessary equipment should not really apply. A CAT scan of the chest, abdomen and pelvis is a useful ancillary staging test to assess whether systemic metastases are present.

Serial measurement of blood and cerebrospinal fluid tumor marker levels and cerebral CAT scans are essential in the monitoring and follow-up of these patients. In patients with ventriculosystemic shunts in place, regular measurement of serum AFP and HCG will provide a simple and effective mechanism for follow-up. For example, we have previously diagnosed relapse in a patient with a pineal NSGCT in whom cerebrospinal fluid HCG was 2000 IU ml^{-1} with a concomitant serum level of 50 IU ml^{-1} (accompanied by a cerebral CAT scan with no demonstrable deposit of tumor).

28.4.3　TREATMENT

As noted above, because of the site of the tumor, it has traditionally been quite common for a biopsy-proven tissue diagnosis not to have been obtained (Schmidek, 1977). This has been one of the contributing factors to the controversy regarding the outcome of treatment and optimal management (i.e. because of the uncertainty regarding whether the

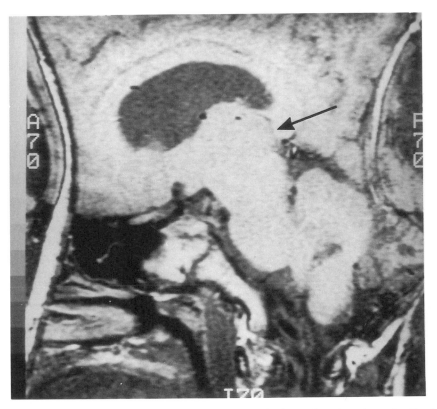

Fig. 28.3 Magnetic resonance imaging scan in a sagittal plane showing clear detail of normal brain structures and a pineal germ cell tumor abutting the third ventricle.

treated tumor is a germinoma or a NSGCT). The traditional approach to the management of intracranial germ cell tumors consisted of a shunting procedure to relieve hydrocephalus, followed by radiotherapy to the tumor (with or without craniospinal extension of fields) (Simson, Lampe and Abell, 1968; Jenkin, Simpson and Keen, 1978; Sung, Hariusiadis and Chang 1978; Abay *et al.*, 1981). More recently, with the evolution of microsurgical techniques and improved approaches to tumor imaging, a more aggressive surgical stance is being taken when there is uncertainty that the lesion is a pure dysgerminoma, with attempted definitive biopsy and/or resection, and adjuvant systemic chemotherapy with or without cerebral irradiation (Edwards *et al.*, 1988).

The techniques of radiotherapy vary, with a wide range of published fractionation sched-

ules and field sizes (Jenkin, Simpson and Keen, 1978; Sung, Hariusiadis and Chang, 1978; Rich *et al.*, 1985). Most commonly, a dose to the tumor volume of 50 Gy in 25 fractions has been used (Jenkin, Simpson and Keen, 1978; Rich *et al.*, 1985; Edwards *et al.*, 1988). Little agreement exists regarding the need for adjuvant craniospinal irradiation. Its proponents cite a cerebrospinal metastatic rate of more than 30% as justification for extended fields (Legido *et al.*, 1989). However, others emphasize that spinal metastasis is rare in the absence of an antecedent biopsy procedure, and that spinal prophylaxis is a morbid process (Salazar *et al.*, 1979; Leibel and Sheline, 1987), although this applies more to a pediatric population. In some centers, patients receive whole brain irradiation with a tumor boost, and in others the radiotherapy is targeted to the environs of the tumor alone (Bloom, 1983). In our institutions, radiotherapy remains the treatment of choice for adults with pure germinoma, patients usually receiving a tumor dose of 50 Gy in 25 fractions over 5 weeks, without routine spinal prophylaxis. The availability of the new localization techniques of radiosurgery has facilitated increased precision of treatment, and has allowed higher doses to be delivered directly to the tumor, while sparing the surrounding tissues. However, the increased precision of neurosurgical microsurgical techniques has also allowed a change in practice, with a more aggressive approach to these tumors. As yet, no comparative trial of modern surgical and radiotherapy techniques has been effected.

In general, the results achieved by these approaches have been quite satisfactory, at least for the management of pineal and suprasellar germinomas, with 5 year survival rates of 60–90% (Jenkin, Simpson and Keen, 1978; Sung, Hariusiadis and Chang, 1978; Rich *et al.*, 1985; Legido *et al.*, 1989). However, patients with intracranial NSGCT have a substantially worse prognosis (Bloom, 1983, Jennings, Gelman and Hochberg, 1985; Kida *et al.*, 1986; Watterson and Priest, 1988). In fact, the absence of histological confirmation probably explains the broad range of reported 5-year survival rates for patients treated for the presumptive diagnosis of germinoma (Table 28.3).

In patients with biopsy-proven NSGCT, the results of external beam irradiation have been poorer than those achieved for pure germinoma, even when combined with adjuvant chemotherapy. In the Royal Marsden Hospital experience, patients with NSGCT had an 18% 5-year survival, with most recurrences being found at the primary site (Dearnaley *et al.*, 1990). The lack of success of conventional treatment, in contrast to the moderately successful management of brain metastases from testicular NSGCT (Rustin *et al.*, 1986; Raghavan *et al.*, 1987) has prompted

the assessment of systemic chemotherapy as first line treatment (Rustin *et al.*, 1986; Allen, Kim and Packer, 1987; Edwards *et al.*, 1988). To date, we are unaware of any published large series of primary intracranial germ cell tumors treated by chemotherapy alone. Rustin *et al.* (1986) have reviewed their experience of primary intracranial and metastatic testicular NSGCT, reporting high objective response rates in a series that included only two primary intracranial germ cell tumors. Graziano *et al.* (1987) reported an apparent cure in a 15-year-old patient with a mixed pineal NSGCT treated with cisplatin, vinblastine and bleomycin after subtotal surgical resection and radiotherapy, and similar clinical anecdotes have been reported by others predominantly in the context of children and teenage patients (Edwards *et al.*, 1988; Watterson and Priest, 1988).

Ginsberg *et al.* (1987), in a detailed pharmacokinetic study of a single patient with intracranial germ cell tumor, demonstrated objective response after the administration of intravenous cisplatin, bleomycin and vinblastine. They reported the achievement of a peak cerebrospinal fluid level of bleomycin that was 40% of plasma level about 2 h after the administration of a bolus intravenous dose of 30 U. Clearance from the cerebrospinal fluid was substantially slower than from plasma, with an elimination half-life of 2 h. These workers also showed that peak levels of cisplatin in the cerebrospinal fluid were approximately 25% of those in plasma, and that the peak occurred about 30 min after a short intravenous infusion of 50 mg cisplatin. It is of interest to note that vinblastine was not detected in the cerebrospinal fluid, although it is possible that the drug was taken up directly by tumor tissue, which was not sampled in this study. Kobayashi *et al.* (1989) reported apparent *in vitro* antitumor synergy of cisplatin and etoposide, when tested against a germ cell tumor cell line, although the interpretation of their experimental data is open to question. Nevertheless, these workers also

Table 28.3   Treatment of intracranial germ cell tumors

Number of patients	Regimen	Complete remission and disease-free survival* (%)	Long-term survival (%)	Reference
Surgery/radiotherapy only				
Germinomas				
11	Radiotherapy	81	81	Edwards *et al.* (1988)
10	Radiotherapy	90	100	Legido *et al.* (1989)
4	Radiotherapy	75	75	Rich *et al.* (1985)
72	Radiotherapy	61	78	Sung, Hariusiadis and Chang (1978)
Non-seminomatous germ cell tumors				
45	Radiotherapy	?	3	Graziano *et al.* (1987)
7	Radiotherapy	1	0	Kida *et al.* (1986)
7	Radiotherapy	1	57	Rich *et al.* 1985)
No biopsy				
27	Radiotherapy	48	48	Abay *et al.* (1981)
31	Radiotherapy	55	55	Jenkin, Simpson and Keen (1978)
14	Radiotherapy	86	93	Rich *et al.* (1985)
Chemotherapy (± surgery/radiotherapy)				
Non-seminomatous germ cell tumors¶				
4	PVB/etc.	100	'50'	Allen, Kim and Packer (1987)
5	PVB+E	'80'	'60'	Edwards *et al.* (1988)‡
1	PVB	'100'	?	Ginsberg *et al.* (1987)
1	PVB	'100'	'100'	Graziano *et al.* (1987)
10	P±VB	50	20+	Kida *et al.* (1986)
3	E/P	'66'	'66'	Kobayashi *et al.* (1989)
2	POMB/ACE	'50'	'50'	Rustin *et al.* (1986)
2	POMB/ACE	'50'	'50'	Raghavan (unpublished)
1	PVBE	'100'	'100'	Watterson/Priest (1988)

* N.E.D.: No evidence of disease (after resection).
† Survival greater than 2 years in most series.
‡ Includes patients treated with 'adjuvant' chemotherapy.
¶ NB. Numbers in italics do not represent true percentages because of small numbers (case reports included because of scant available data); note bias in reporting of 'good outcome'.
PVB, cisplatin/vinblastine/bleomycin. E/P, etoposide/cisplatin. E. etoposide.

achieved a response rate of three complete and one partial remissions among four treated patients, without recurrence during follow-up of 9 to 22 months. A series of 17 patients with AFP-secreting intracranial germ cell tumor had previously been reported from the same institution (Kida *et al.*, 1986). Prior to the introduction of cisplatin-based chemotherapy all such patients had died, whereas four of ten patients treated with cisplatin (with or without bleomycin and vinblastine) achieved complete remission, and two of these had

remained clear beyond 2 years (Kida *et al.*, 1986).

In the clinical situation in which biopsy has not been obtained, but cerebrospinal fluid or serum AFP levels are definitely elevated, the tumor should be managed as a NSGCT (Rustin *et al.*, 1986). From the data available from the management of testicular germ cell tumors, it is clear that elevated AFP correlates with elements of NSGCT, even if pure seminoma or germinoma is seen on biopsy (Raghavan *et al.*, 1982). If there is evidence of a pineal or suprasellar germ cell tumor on CT scan with elevated HCG only (and no biopsy), the management decision is more difficult as synctiotrophoblastic giant cells, which are sometimes found in pure testicular seminoma, have been shown to secrete HCG (Heyderman and Neville, 1976). There is no proven cut-off level beyond which the level of cerebrospinal HCG denotes NSGCT, rather than germinoma with syncytiotrophoblastic giant cells. Thus it is our arbitrary policy to commence systemic platinum-based chemotherapy in this situation if the level of cerebrospinal fluid HCG is greater than 100 IU ml^{-1}, and to consolidate with radiotherapy as necessary. Rustin *et al.*, (1986) have adopted a similar approach, but do not routinely prescribe radiotherapy after completion of chemotherapy.

28.5   ATYPICAL TERATOMA SYNDROME

The clinical features of a putative syndrome occurring in young men with metastatic undifferentiated carcinoma were first reported by Fox *et al.* (1979) and confirmed by others (Richardson *et al.*, 1981; Greco, Vaughn and Hainsworth, 1986). It was initially proposed that these cases represented unrecognized EGCT, base upon the age of the patients, lack of differentiation histologically, sporadic production of low levels of HCG or AFP and occasional responsiveness to cytotoxic chemotherapy. Subsequent study has shown that only a small proportion of such cases truly represents germ cell malignancy (Logothetis *et al.*, 1985; Hainsworth *et al.*, 1987), and it seems likely that at least some of the 'chemoresponsive' cases represented the initial sensitivity to cisplatin-based regimens that is characteristic of bronchogenic carcinoma or esophageal cancer. The majority of such patients simply have metastatic undifferentiated malignancy of uncertain origin, and the evolution of electron microscopy and special immunohistochemical stains has done little to clarify the true histogenesis of these

tumors. It is important to remember that AFP and HCG are not specific to germ cell malignancy and can be associated with tumors that arise in lung, liver, ovary, gastrointestinal tract and even lymphoma, as reviewed by Lange and Raghavan (1983) and in Chapter 3. Thus, in the case of pulmonary or supraclavicular presentations, the emphasis of pathological assessment should be to exclude such treatable entities as EGCT, malignant lymphoma or thymoma. In smokers in their fourth or fifth decades, bronchogenic carcinoma should also be excluded.

The pattern of presentation varies with the site of tumor involvement, although most commonly such patients have cancer in lungs, supraclavicular nodes or elsewhere in a midline distribution. While the presenting symptoms usually reflect the sites of tumor involvement, nonspecific constitutional symptoms are also a common feature (Fox *et al.*, 1979; Richardson *et al.*, 1981).

Such tumors continue to present a difficult problem in management. For some years there was the illusion that the outcome of systemic chemotherapy was as successful as in the instance of metastatic testicular cancer. With increasing experience, it has become clear that only occasional patients respond dramatically to cisplatin-based chemotherapy regimens, and cure is an uncommon outcome (Logothetis *et al.*, 1985).

The recognition of *i*(12p) as a characteristic chromosomal abnormality in patients with germ cell tumors of both testicular and extragonadal origin has helped in the classification of these tumors. Cytogenetic analysis has been used to identify a subgroup of patients with the atypical teratoma syndrome that probably do, in fact, have germ cell malignancy (Motzer *et al.*, 1991). Similarly, the emerging recognition of the significance of multiple atypical nevi in association with germ cell tumors (Raghavan *et al.*, 1994) may also contribute to a greater precision of classification, although this association will not help to distinguish atypical presentations of metastatic malignant melanoma. Nevertheless, most such patients do not have the *i*(12p) abnormality, nor multiple atypical nevi, and the diagnosis with currently available techniques remains metastatic undifferentiated cancer.

In view of the youth of such patients, an active approach to management should be considered, incorporating systemic chemotherapy, surgical resection if appropriate and, sometimes, locoregional radiotherapy. However, it is important not to confuse this syndrome with metastatic testicular cancer, nor to set unreasonable expectations of outcome. Since the majority of such patients ultimately die of malignancy, the currently available cytotoxic regimens cannot be considered as an acceptable standard treatment for this condition.

28.6   CONCLUSIONS

Extragonadal germ cell tumors occur predominantly in the young. Although histologically similar to their testicular equivalents, the results of treatment are not universally as satisfactory, especially in the case of mediastinal non-seminomatous germ cell tumors. Unresolved issues include the reasons for the marked difference in outcome between seminoma and NSGCT in this context, the differences in gender prevalence of malignancy at extragonadal sites and the definition of optimal care of such patients. The issue has been complicated further by the inappropriate inclusion of patients with the atypical teratoma syndrome within this spectrum of disease. In order for real progress to be made in the care of these rare malignancies, patients should be investigated and treated according to stringent protocols in which the diagnosis and staging are carefully reviewed, treatment programs rationalized and outcomes of care can be evaluated objectively.

REFERENCES

Abay, E.O., Laws, E.R., Grado, G.L. *et al.* (1981) Pineal tumors in children and adolescents: Treatment by CSF shunting and radiotherapy. *J. Neurosurg.*, **55**, 889–95.

Abell, M.R., Fayos, J.V and Lampe, I. (1965). Retroperitoneal germinomas (seminomas without evidence of testicular involvement). *Cancer* **18**, 273–90.

Aliotta, P.J., Castillo, J., Englander, L.S. *et al.* (1988) Primary mediastinal germ cell tumors: histologic patterns of treatment failure at autopsy. *Cancer*, **62**, 982–4.

Allen, J.C., Kim, J.H. and Packer, R.J. (1987) Neoadjuvant chemotherapy for newly diagnosed germ-cell tumors of the central nervous system. *J. Neurosurg.*, **67**, 65–70.

Arnheim, E.E. (1951) Retroperitoneal teratomas in infancy and childhood. *Pediatrics* **8**: 309–27.

Azzopardi, J.G. and Hoffbrand, A.V. (1965). Retrogression in testicular seminoma with viable metastases. *J. Clin. Pathol.*, **18**, 135–41.

Bagshaw, M.A., McLaughlin, W.T. and Earle, J.D. (1969) Definitive radiotherapy of primary mediastinal seminoma. *Am. J. Roentgenol.* **105**, 86–94.

Beeley, J.M., Daly, J., Timperley, W.R. and Warner, J. (1973) Ectopic pinealoma: an unusual clinical presentation and a histochemical comparison with a seminoma of the testis. *J. Neurol. Neurosurg. Psych.*, **36**, 864–73.

Benson, R.C., Segura, J.W. and Carney, J.A. (1978) Primary yolk sac (endodermal sinus) tumours originating in the region of the pineal gland. *Acta. Pathol. Microbiol. Scand.*, **74**, 214–22.

Bestle, J. (1968) Extragonadal endodermal sinus tumours originating in the region of the pineal gland. *Acta. Pathol. Microbial. Scand.*, **74**, 214–222.

Bloom, H.C.G. (1983) Primary intracranial germ cell tumours. *Clin. Oncol.* **2**, 233–57.

Bohle, A., Studer, U.E., Sonntag, R.W. and Scheidegger, J.R. (1986) Primary or secondary extragonadal germ cell tumors? *J. Urol.*, **135**, 939–13.

Borit, A. (1969) Embryonal carcinoma of the pineal region. *J. Pathol.*, **97**, 165–8.

Bosl, G.J., Dmitrovsky, E., Reuter, V. *et al.* (1989) *i*(12p): A specific karyotypic abnormality in germ cell tumors (GCT). *Proc. Am. Soc. Clin. Oncol.*, **8**, 131.

Boyer, M. and Raghavan, D. (1992) Toxicity of treatment of germ cell tumors. *Semin. Oncol.*, **19**, 128–42.

Boyer, M., Raghavan, D., Harris, P.J. *et al.* (1990) Lack of late toxicity in patients treated with cisplatin-containing combination chemotherapy for metastatic testicular cancer. *J. Clin. Oncol.*, **8**, 21–6.

British Medical Journal (1969) Leading article. Primary mediastinal choriocarcinoma. *BMJ*, **ii**, 135–6.

Bukowski, R.M., Wolf, M., Kulander, B.G., Montie, J., Crawford, E.D. and Blumenstein, B. (1993) Alternating combination chemotherapy in patients with extragonadal germ cell tumors. *Cancer*, **71**, 2631–8.

Bush, S.E., Martinez, A. and Bagshaw, M.A. (1981) Primary mediastinal seminoma. *Cancer*, **48**, 1877–82.

Canty, T.G. and Siemens, R. (1978) Malignant mediastinal teratoma in a 15 year old girl. *Cancer*, **41**, 1623–6.

Chapman, P.H. and Linggood, R.M. (1980) The management of pineal area tumour: a recent reappraisal. *Cancer*, **46**, 1253–7.

Childs, W.J., Goldstraw, P., Nicholls, J.E., Dearnaley, D.P. and Horwich, A. (1993) Primary malignant mediastinal germ cell tumours: improved prognosis with platinum-based chemotherapy and surgery. *Br. J. Cancer*, **67**, 1098–101.

Cox, J.D. (1975) Primary malignant germinal tumors of the mediastinum: a study of 24 cases. *Cancer*, **36**, 1162–8.

Daugaard, G., Rørth, M., von der Maase, H. and Skakkebaek, N.E. (1992) Management of extragonadal germ-cell tumors and the significance of bilateral testicular biopsies. *Ann. Oncol.* **3**, 283–9.

Dayan, A.D., Marshall, A.H.E., Miller, A.A. *et al.* (1966) Atypical teratomas of the pineal and hypothalamus. *J. Pathol. Bact.*, **92**, 1–28.

Dearnaley, D.P., A'hearn, R.P., Whittaker, S. and Bloom. H.J.G. (1990) Pineal and CNS germ cell tumours: Royal Marsden Hospital experience 1962–1987. *Int. J. Radiat. Oncol. Biol. Phys.* **8**, 773–7.

deBruin T.W.A., Slater, R.M., Defferrari, R. *et al.* (1994). Isochromosome 12p-positive pineal germ cell tumor. *Cancer Res.*, **54**, 1542–6.

Donnellan, W.A. and Swenson, O. (1968) Benign and malignant sacrococcygeal teratoma. *Surgery*, **64**, 834–46.

Economou, J.S., Trump, D.L., Holmes, E.C. and Eggleston, J.E. (1982) Management of primary germ cell tumours of the mediastinum. *J. Thorac. Cardiovasc. Surg.* **83**, 643–9.

Edwards, M.S.B., Hudgins, R.J., Wilson, C.B. *et al.* (1988) Pineal region tumors in children. *J. Neurosurg.*, **68**, 689–97.

Feun, L.G., Samson, M.K. and Stephens, R.L. (1980) Vinblastine (VLB), bleomycin (BLEO), *cis*-diamminedichloroplatinum (DDP) in disseminated extragonadal germ cell tumors: a Southwest Oncology Group study. *Cancer*, **45**, 2543–9.

Fine, G., Smith, R.W. and Pachter, M.R. (1962) Primary extragenital choriocarcinoma in the male subject: Case report and review of literature. *Am. J. Med.*, **52**, 776–94.

Fox, R.M., Woods, R.L., Tattersall, M.H.N. and McGovern, V.J. (1979) Undifferentiated carcinoma in young men: the atypical teratoma syndrome. *Lancet*, **i**, 1316–18.

Friedman, N.B. (1951) The comparative morphogenesis of extragenital and gonadal teratoid tumors. *Cancer*, **4**, 265–76.

Garnick, M.B., Canellos, G. and Richie, J.P. (1983). Treatment and surgical staging of testicular and primary extragonadal germ cell cancer. *JAMA*, **250**, 1733–41.

Giaccone, G. (1991) Multimodality treatment of malignant germ cell tumours of the mediastinum. *Eur. J. Cancer*, **27**, 273–7.

Ginsberg, S., Kirshner, J., Reich, S. *et al.* (1987) Systemic chemotherapy for a primary germ cell tumor of the brain: a pharmacokinetic study. *Cancer Treat. Rep.*, **65**, 477–83.

Giuffre, R. and DiLorenzo, N. (1975) Evolution of a primary intrasellar germinomatous teratoma into a choriocarcinoma. *J. Neurosurg.*, **42**, 602–4.

Gonzalez-Crussi, F. (1982) *Extragonadal Teratomas*, Armed Forces Institute of Pathology, Washington, DC, pp. 9–25, 77–191.

Goss, P.E., Schwertfeger, L., Blackstein, M.E., Iscoe, N.A., Ginsberg, R.J., Simpson, W.J., Jones, D.P. and Shepherd, F.A. (1994) Extragonadal germ cell tumors: a 14 year Toronto experience. *Cancer*, **73**, 1971–9.

Graziano, S.L., Paollozzi, F.P., Rudolph, A.R. *et al.* (1987) Mixed germ-cell tumor of the pineal region: Case report. *J. Neurosurg.*, **66**, 300–4.

Greco, F.A., Vaughn, W.K. and Hainsworth, J.D. (1986) Advanced poorly differentiated carcinoma of unknown primary site: recognition of a treatable syndrome. *Ann. Intern. Med.*, **104**, 547–53.

Greist, A., Einhorn, L.H., Williams, S.D. *et al.* (1984) Pathologic findings at orchidectomy following chemotherapy for disseminated testicular cancer. *J. Clin. Oncol.*, **2**, 1025–7.

Hainsworth, J.D., Einhorn, L.H., Williams, S.D. *et al.* (1982) Advanced extragonadal germ cell tumors. Successful treatment with combination chemotherapy. *Ann. Intern. Med.*, **97**, 7–11.

Hainsworth, J.D. Wright, E.P., Gray, G.F. and Greco, F.A. (1987) Poorly differentiated carcinoma of unknown primary site: correlation of light microscopic findings with response to cisplatin-based combination chemotherapy. *J. Clin. Oncol.*, **5**, 1275–80.

Hart, W.R. (1975) Primary endodermal sinus (yolk sac) tumour of the liver: first reported case. *Cancer*, **35**, 1453–8.

Heyderman, E. and Neville, A.M. (1976) Syncytiotrophoblasts in malignant testicular tumours. *Lancet*, **ii**, 103.

Heyderman, E. and Neville, A.M. (1977) A shorter immunoperoxidase technique for the demonstration of carcinoembryonic antigen and other cell products. *J. Clin. Pathol.*, **8**, 551–63.

Ho, K.L. and Rassekh, Z.S. (1979) Endodermal sinus tumor of the pineal region: Case report and review of the literature. *Cancer*, **44**, 1081–6.

Holt, L.P., Melcher, D.H. and Conquhoun, J. (1965) Extragonadal choriocarcinoma in the male. *Postgrad. Med. J.*, **41**, 134–41.

Hyman, A. and Leiter, H.E. (1943) Extratesticular chorioepithelioma in male, probable primary in urinary bladder. *J. Mt. Sinai Hosp.*, **10**, 212–16.

Inoue, Y. Takeuchi, T., Tamaki, M. *et al.* (1979) Sequential CT observations of irradiated intracranial germinomas. *Am. J. Roentgenol.*, **132**, 361–5.

Israel, A., Bosl, G.J., Golbey, R.B. *et al.* (1985). The results of chemotherapy for extragonadal germ-cell tumors in the cisplatin era: the Memorial Sloan Kettering Cancer Center experience (1975–1982). *J. Clin. Oncol.*, **3**, 1073–8.

Jain, K.K., Bosl, G.J., Bains, M.S. *et al.* (1984) The treatment of extragonadal seminoma. *J. Clin. Oncol.*, **2**, 820–7.

Jellinger, K. (1973) Primary intracranial germ cell tumours. *Acta Neuropathol.*, **25**, 291–306.

Jenkin, R.D., Simpson, W.J.K. and Keen, C.W. (1978) Pineal and suprasellar germinomas; results of radiation treatment. *J. Neurosurg.*, **48**, 99–107.

Jennings, M.T., Gelman, R. and Hochberg, F. (1985). Intracranial germ-cell tumours: natural history and pathogenesis. *J. Neurosurg.*, **63**, 155–67.

Johnson, D.E., Laneri, J.P., Mountain, C.F. and Luna, M. (1973) Extragonadal germ cell tumors. *Surgery*, **73**, 85–90.

Kay, P.H., Wells, F.C. and Goldstraw, P. (1987)

A multidisciplinary approach to primary non-seminomatous germ cell tumours of the mediastinum. *Ann. Thorac. Surg.*, **44**, 578–82.

Kaye, S.B., Bagshawe, K.D., McElwain, T.J. and Peckham, M.J. (1979) Brain metastases in malignant teratoma: A review of four years' experience and an assessment of the role of tumour markers. *Br. J. Cancer*, **39**, 217–23.

Kida, Y., Kobayashi, T., Yoshida, J. *et al.* (1986) Chemotherapy with cisplatin for AFP-secreting germ-cell tumors of the central nervous system. *J. Neurosurg.*, **65**, 470–5.

Kikuchi, Y., Tsuneta, Y., Kawai, T. and Aizawa, M. (1988) Choriocarcinoma of the esophagus producing chorionic gonadotrophin. *Acta Pathol. Jpn.*, **38**, 489–99.

Kirschling, R.J., Kvols, L.K., Charboneau, J.W. *et al.* (1983) High-resolution ultrasonographic and pathologic abnormalities of germ cell tumors in patients with clinically normal testes. *Mayo Clin. Proc.*, **58**, 648–53.

Kobayashi, T., Yoshida, J., Ishiyama, J. *et al.* (1989) Combination chemotherapy with cisplatin and etoposide for malignant intracranial germ-cell tumors. An experimental and clinical study. *J. Neurosurg.*, **70**, 676–81.

Koide, O., Watanabe, Y. and Sato, K. (1980) A pathologic survey of intracranial germinoma and pinealoma in Japan. *Cancer*, **45**, 2119–30.

Kuhn, M.W. and Weissbach, L. (1985) Localization, incidence, diagnosis and treatment of extratesticular germ cell tumors. *Urol. Int.*, **40**, 166–72.

Kurman, R.M. and Norris, H.J. (1977) Malignant germ cell tumors of the ovary. *Human Pathol.*, **8**, 551–63.

Kuzur, M.E., Cobleight, M.A., Greco, F.A. *et al.* (1982) Endodermal sinus tumor of the mediastinum. *Cancer*, **50**, 766–74.

Landanyi, M., Samaniego, F., Reuter, V.E., Motzer, R.J., Jhanwar, S.C. and Bosl, G.J. (1990) Cytogenetic and immunohistochemical evidence for the germ cell origin of a subset of acute leukemias associated with mediastinal germ cell tumors. *J. Natl. Cancer Inst.*, **82**, 221–7.

Lange, P.H. and Raghavan, D. (1983) Clinical applications of tumor markers in testicular cancer, in *Testis Tumors* (ed. J.P. Donohue), Williams and Wilkins, Baltimore, pp. 112–30.

Lattes, R. (1962) Thymoma and other tumors of the thymus. *Cancer*, **15**, 1224–60.

Legido, A., Packer, R.J., Sutton, L.N. *et al.* (1989) Suprasellar germinomas in childhood: A reappraisal. *Cancer*, **63**, 340–4.

Leibel, S.A. and Sheline, G.E. (1987) Radiation therapy for brain tumors. *J. Neurosurg.*, **66**, 1–22.

Lemarié, E., Assouline, P.S., Diot, P., Regnard, J.F., Levasseur, P., Droz, J.P. and Ruffié, P. (1992) Primary mediastinal germ cell tumors: results of a French retrospective study. *Chest*, **102**, 1477–83.

Levi, J.A, Raghavan, D., Harvey, V. *et al.* (1993). The importance of bleomycin in combination chemotherapy for good prognosis germ cell carcinoma. *J. Clin. Oncol.*, 11, 1300–5.

Levi, J.A., Thomson, D., Sandeman, T. *et al.* (1988) A prospective study of cisplatin-based combination chemotherapy in advanced germ cell malignancy: Role of maintenance and long-term follow-up. *J. Clin. Oncol.* **6.**, 1154–60.

Logothetis, C.J., Samuels, M.L., Selig, D.E. *et al.* (1985) Chemotherapy of extragonadal germ cell tumors. *J. Clin. Oncol.* **3**, 316–25.

Luna, M.A. (1975) Extragonadal germ cell tumors, in *Testicular Tumors* (ed. D.E. Johnson), Medical Examination Publishing Company, New York, pp. 261–91.

Martini, N., Golbey, R.B., Hajdu, S.L. *et al.* (1974) Primary mediastinal germ cell tumors. *Cancer*, **33**, 763–9.

McAleer, J.J., Nicholls, J. and Horwich, A. (1992) Does extragonadal presentation impart a worse prognosis to abdominal germ cell tumors? *Eur. J. Cancer*, **28**, 825–8.

McLeod, D.G., Taylor, H.G., Skoog, S.J. *et al.* (1988) Extragonadal germ cell tumors clinico-pathologic findings and treatment experience in 12 patients. *Cancer*, **61**, 1187–91.

Mead, G.M., Stenning, S.P., Parkinson, M.P., Horwich, A., Fosså, S.D. Wilkinson, P.M., Kaye, S.B., Newlands, E.S. and Cook, P.A. (1992) The second Medical Research Council study of prognostic factors in nonseminomatous germ cell tumours. *J. Clin. Oncol.* **10**, 85–94.

Medini, E., Levitt, S.H., Jones, T.K. and Rao, Y. (1979) The management of extra testicular seminoma without gonadal involvement. *Cancer*, **44**, 2032–8.

Miles, R.M. and Stewart, G.S. (1974) Sacrococcygeal teratomas in adults. *Am. Sur.*, **179**, 676–83.

Monaghan, P., Raghavan, D. and Neville, A.M. (1982) Ultrastructural studies of xenografted human germ cell tumors. *Cancer*, **49**, 683–97.

Motzer, R.J., Bosl, G.J., Geller, N.L. *et al.* (1988) Advanced seminoma: the role of chemotherapy and adjunctive surgery. *Ann. Intern. Med.*, **108**, 513–18.

Motzer, R.J., Rodriguez, E., Reuter, V.E., Samaniego, F., Dmitrovsky, E., Bajorin, D.F., Pfister, D.G., Parsa, N.Z., Chaganti, R.S.K. and Bosl, G.J. (1991) Genetic analysis as an aid in diagnosis for patients with midline carcinomas of uncertain histologies. *J. Natl. Inst.* **83**, 341–6.

Newlands, E.S., Begent, R.H.J., Rustin, G.J.S. *et al.* (1983) Further advances in the management of malignant teratomas of the testis and other sites. *Lancet*, **i**, 948–51.

Nichols, C.R. Saxman, S., Williams, S.D., Loehrer, P.J., Miller, M.D., Wright, C. and Einhorn, L.H. (1990) Primary mediastinal non-seminomatous germ cell tumors: a modern single institution experience. *Cancer*, **65**, 1641–6.

Oberman, H.A. and Libcke, J.H. (1964) Malignant germinal neoplasms of the mediastinum. *Cancer*, **17**, 498–507.

Palumbo, L.T., Cross, K.R., Smith, A.N. and Baronas, A.A. (1949) Primary teratomas of the lateral retroperitoneal spaces. *Surgery*, **26**, 149–59.

Pantoja, E., Llobet, R. and Gonzalez-Flores, B. (1976) Retroperitoneal teratoma; historical review. *J. Urol*, **115**, 520–3.

Parker, D., Holford, C.P., Begent, R.H.J. *et al.* (1983) Effective treatment for malignant mediastinal teratoma. *Thorax*, **38**, 897–902.

Polansky, S.M., Barwick, K.W. and Ravin, C.E. (1979) Primary mediastinal seminoma. *Am. J. Roentgenol.*, **132**, 17–21.

Raghavan, D. and Barrett, A. (1980) Mediastinal seminomas. *Cancer*, **46**, 1187–91.

Raghavan, D., Levi, J., Thomson, D. *et al.* (1989) Chemotherapy of advanced germ cell tumors; Overview of Australasian Germ Cell Tumor Group studies, in *Systemic Therapy for Genito-urinary Cancers* (eds D.E. Johnson, C.J. Logothetis and A.C. von Eschenbach), Year Book Medical Publishers, Chicago, pp. 342–8.

Raghavan, D., MacKintosh, J.F., Fox, R.M. *et al.* (1987) Improved survival after brain metastases in non-seminomatous germ cell tumours with combined modality treatment. *Br. J. Urol.*, **60**, 364–7.

Raghavan, D. and Neville, A.M. (1982) The biology of testicular cancer, in the *Scientific Foundations of Urology*, 2nd edn (eds D. Innes Williams and C.D. Chisholm), William Heinemann, London, pp. 785–96.

Raghavan, D., Sullivan, A.L., Peckham, M.J. and Neville, A.M. (1982). Elevated serum alpha-fetoprotein and seminoma: Clinical evidence for a histologic continuum? *Cancer*, **50**, 982–9.

Raghavan, D., Zalcberg, J., Grygiel, J.J. *et al.* (1994) Multiple atypical nevi: A cutaneous marker of germ cell tumors. *J. Clin. Oncol.*, **12**, 2284–7.

Reddell, R.R., Thompson, J.F., Raghavan, D. *et al.* (1983) Surgery in patients with advanced germ cell malignancy following a clinical partial response to chemotherapy. *J. Surg. Oncol.*, **23**, 223–7.

Rich, T.A., Cassady, J.R., Strand, R.D. and Winston, K.R. (1985) Radiation therapy for pineal and suprasellar germ cell tumors. *Cancer*, **55**, 932–40.

Richardson, R.L., Schoumacher, R.A., Fer, M.F. *et al.* (1981) The unrecognized extragonadal germ cell cancer syndrome. *Ann. Intern. Med.*, **94**, 181–6.

Russell, D.S. (1944) The pinealoma; its relationship to teratoma. *J. Pathol. Bact.*, **56**, 145–50.

Rustin, G.J.S., Newlands, E.W., Bagshawe, K.D. *et al.* (1986) Successful management of metastatic and primary germ cell tumours in the brain. *Cancer*, **57**, 2108–13.

Salazar, O.M., Castro-Vita, H., Bakos, R.S. *et al* (1979) Radiation therapy for tumors of the pineal region. *Int. J. Radiat. Oncol. Biol. Phys.*, **5**, 491–9.

Saltzman, B., Pitts, W.R. and Vaughan, E.D. (1986) Extragonadal retroperitoneal germ cell tumors without apparent testicular involvement: A search for a source. *Urology*, **27**, 504–7.

Schantz, A., Sewall, W. and Castleman, B. (1972) Mediastinal germinoma: A study of 21 cases with an excellent prognosis. *Cancer*, **30**, 1189–94.

Schey, W.L., Shkoinik, A. and White, H. (1977) Clinical and radiographic considerations of sacrococcygeal teratomas: an analysis of 26 new cases and review of the literature. *Radiology*, **125**, 189–95.

Schlumberger, H.G. (1946) Teratoma of the anterior mediastinum in the group of military age: a study of sixteen cases and a review of theories of genesis. *Arch. Pathol.*, **41**, 398–444.

Schmidek, H.H. (1977) Surgical management of pineal region tumors, in *Pineal Tumors* (ed. H.H. Schmidek), Masson Publishing, New York.

Segelov, E., Cox, K.M., Raghavan, D. *et al.* (1993) The impact of histological review on clinical management of testicular cancer. *Br. J. Urol.*, **71**: 736–8.

Simson, L.R., Lampe, I. and Abell, M.R. (1968) Suprasellar germinomas. *Cancer*, **22**, 533–44.

Sung, D.I. Hariusiadis, L. and Chang, C.H. (1978) Midline pineal tumors and suprasellar germinomas: highly curable by irradiation. *Radiology*, **128**, 745–51.

Tondini, C. and Garnick, M.B. (1989) Chemotherapy for extragonadal and poor-prognosis germ cell cancers; The Dana-Farber Cancer Institute approach, in *Systemic Therapy for Genitourinary Cancers* (eds D.E. Johnson, C.J. Logothetis and A.C. Von Eschenbach), Year Book Medical Publishers, Chicago, pp. 370–9.

Utz, D.C. and Buscemi, M.K. (1971) Extragonadal testicular tumors. *J. Urol.*, **105**, 271–4.

Vogelzang, N.J., Raghavan, D., Anderson, R.W. *et al.* (1982) Mediastinal nonseminomatous germ cell tumors: the role of combined modality therapy. *Ann. Thorac. Surg.*, **33**, 333–9.

Walden, P.A.M., Woods, R.L., Fox, B. and Bagshawe, K.D. (1977) Primary mediastinal trophoblastic teratomas. *Thorax*, **32**, 752–8.

Watterson, J. and Priest, J.R. (1988) Control of extraneural metastasis of a primary intracranial nongerminomatous germ cell tumor. *J. Neurosurg.*, **71**, 601–4.

Williams, S.D. Birch, R., Einhorn, L.H., Irwin, L., Greco, F.A. and Loehrer, P. (1987) Treatment of disseminated germ-cell tumors with cisplatin, bleomycin, and either vinblastine or etoposide. *N. Engl. J. Med.*, **316**, 1435–40.

Wright, C.D., Kesler, K.A., Nichols, C.R., Mahomed, Y., Einhorn, L.H., Miller, M.E. and Brown, J.W. (1990) Primary mediastinal nonseminomatous germ cell tumors: results of a multimodality approach. *J. Thorac. Cardiovasc. Surg.*, **99**, 210–17.

Witschi, E. (1948) Migration of the germ cells of human embryos from the yolk sac to the primitive gonadal folds. *Contrib. Embryol.*, **209**, 67–80.

DIAGNOSIS AND MANAGEMENT OF CARCINOMA *IN SITU* OF THE TESTIS

29

H. von der Maase

29.1 INTRODUCTION

Carcinoma *in situ* (CIS) of the testis represents a characteristic pattern of intratubular atypical germ cells that was first associated with subsequent development of invasive growth by Skakkebæk (1972a, b). In the following years, this important observation was confirmed in numerous studies and it is now generally accepted that the CIS cells are precursors of malignant germ cell tumors. Carcinoma *in situ* may precede seminomatous as well as non-seminomatous tumors. Accordingly, CIS changes are present in the tissue adjacent to testicular germ cell tumors in more than 90% of patients (Skakkebæk, 1975; Jacobsen, Henriksen and von der Maase, 1981; Klein, Melamed and Whitemore, 1985). Until recently, no differences between CIS in relation to seminomatous and non-seminomatous tumors have been demonstrated. However, Oosterhuis *et al.* (1993) have shown that CIS adjacent to the two types of germ cell tumors is in fact different when looking at the chromosomal constitution. The spermatocytic seminoma (Muller, Skakkebæk and Parkinson, 1987) and the yolk sac tumor in children (Manivel *et al.*, 1988) are the only tumor types that have not been associated with CIS.

The risk for CIS to progress to invasive growth has been estimated to be about 50% within 5 years (Skakkebæk, Berthelsen and Müller, 1982; von der Maase *et al.*, 1986). Whether all cases of CIS would progress in time into invasive cancer is unknown and will probably remain unknown as detection of CIS today would provide an indication for some kind of treatment. However, spontaneous disappearance of CIS has never been documented.

Detection of CIS of the testis and subsequent treatment of this premalignant condition makes it possible to prevent development of invasive cancer. This may be done without the use of toxic treatment regimens and without significantly affecting androgen production. Thus, diagnosis and management of CIS of the testis are of obvious importance.

29.2 HISTOPATHOLOGY

Carcinoma *in situ* of the testis is defined as the presence of atypical germ cells in the seminiferous epithelium (Fig. 29.1). The abnormal intratubular germ cells are larger than normal spermatogonia with an abundant, light and vacuolized cytoplasm. The nuclei are large, irregular and hyperchromatic, containing one or more prominent nucleoli. The average diameter of the nuclei of the CIS cells is about 10 μm compared with 7 μm in the normal spermatogonia (Müller and Skakkebæk, 1981). Mitotic abnormal figures are

Testicular Cancer: Investigation and management. Second edition. Edited by Professor A. Horwich.
Published in 1996 by Chapman & Hall. ISBN 0 412 61210 0.

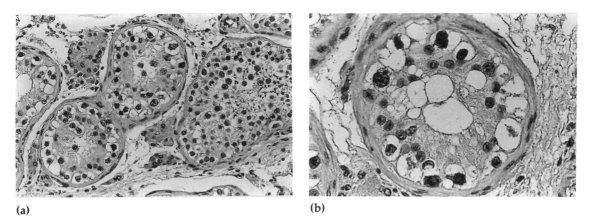

(a)   **(b)**

Fig. 29.1 Carcinoma *in situ* of the testis. (a) Biopsy sample showing seminiferous tubules with carcinoma *in situ* and single normal tubule (right). (b) Higher magnification of a single seminiferous tubule with characteristic carcinoma *in situ* changes.

often seen. The CIS cells are typically located in one layer close to the basement membrane of the seminiferous tubules and the tubular wall is generally thickened. Sertoli and Leydig cells are morphologically normal.

The atypical germ cells may also invade the interstitial tissue which is denoted as early invasive growth of undifferentiated tumor cells.

Carcinoma *in situ* may be difficult to diagnose following routine formalin fixation. Suitable fluids are Bouin's, Cleland's or Stieve's fixative. After fixation, the specimen is embedded in paraplast, sectioned and stained with hematoxylin and eosin. This routine staining is generally sufficient for easy recognition of the CIS changes. PAS staining can be used in doubtful cases to demonstrate the large amounts of glycogen in the cytoplasm of the CIS cells. Furthermore, a positive immunohistochemical reaction for placental-like alkaline phosphatase strongly supports the diagnosis of CIS testis. Thus, more than 90% of specimens containing CIS will stain for placental-like alkaline phosphatase whereas normal germ cells and Sertoli cells do not contain this isoenzyme (Jacobsen and Nørgaard-Pedersen, 1984; Hustin, Collette and Franchimont, 1987; Manivel *et al.*, 1987). CIS cells

can also be demonstrated by immunohistochemical staining with monoclonal antibodies (Giwercman, Cantell and Marks, 1991).

Detailed descriptions and excellent illustrations of the CIS pattern are given by Skakkebæk (1978), Skakkebæk, Berthelsen and Müller (1982) and Jacobsen and Talerman (1989).

29.3 DIAGNOSIS

At present, the only accurate method for diagnosing CIS of the testis is to perform a trans-scrotal surgical biopsy. The CIS changes are usually scattered throughout the testis and will, in nearly all cases, appear in a random biopsy (Berthelsen and Skakkebæk, 1981). The standard size of the biopsy specimen is about 3 mm. Larger biopsies are unnecessary and should be avoided. The testicular biopsy is associated with only a few, minor complications and can be carried out using local anesthesia as an outpatient procedured (Bruun *et al.*, 1987; Reinberg, Manivel and Fraley, 1989). Screening biopsies from the contralateral testis in patients with testicular cancer should be performed during orchidectomy for the primary tumor. Local spread of CIS cells caused by the biopsy procedure has never been reported. However, an open exploration of the testicle has to be performed instead of a trans-scrotal biopsy if there is any suspicion of a tumor.

Needle biopsies have also been used to detect CIS (Rajfer and Binder, 1989; Bracken-bury *et al.*, 1993; Heikkila *et al.*, 1993). However, the reliability of needle biopsies has not yet been sufficiently evaluated. We know that the predictive value of a negative surgical testicular biopsy for detection of CIS is very high. Thus, only few anecdotal cases of testicular cancer preceded by a negative biopsy have been demonstrated (von der Maase *et al.*, 1987; Dieckmann, Kaup and Loy, 1992).

In a prepubertal biopsy, CIS may be overlooked, as immature germinal cells may resemble CIS cells and because both cell types are located throughout the seminiferous tubules. The accuracy of a prepubertal biopsy is, thus, not clarified and it may be necessary to repeat the biopsy after puberty.

Establishment of noninvasive methods for the diagnosis of CIS of the testis would, obviously, be of great importance. Lenz *et al.* (1987) have shown that CIS changes may be associated with a very irregular echo pattern as seen by ultrasound. The sensitivity and specificity of this investigation is, however, far from clarified. CIS cells may also be detected by semen analysis (Giwercman, Clausen and Skakkebæk, 1988a; Giwercman, Marks and Skakkebæk, 1988b; Howard, Hargreave and McIntyre, 1989; Giwercman *et al.*, 1990). Unfortunately, the use of semen analysis in the detection of CIS cells has not yet proven to be a sufficiently reliable method. Further studies to elucidate the value of ultrasonography or semen analysis for the detection of CIS of the testis are ongoing.

29.4 INCIDENCE

The incidence of CIS of the testis in the general male population is unknown but probably very low. Thus, postmortem testicular biopsies from 399 men in the age range 18 to 50 years who suffered a sudden unexpected death revealed no CIS changes in any of the cases (Giwercman, Müller and Skakkebæk, 1991). For comparison, it can be noted that the lifetime risk for developing a testicular cancer in the Danish male population is 0.5% (Prener and Østerlind, 1985).

29.4.1 SUBFERTILE MEN

The frequency of CIS in subfertile men has been reported to be from 0.4 to 1.1% (Nüesch-Bachmann and Hedinger, 1977; Skakkebæk, 1978; Pryor *et al.*, 1983; Schütte, 1988). These data are the results of retrospective studies of biopsies from an inhomogenous group of men referred to testicular biopsies for different reasons and do not represent a systematic screening procedure. However, the very high number of cases (more than 6000 men) makes it probable that the frequency of 0.5–1% is representative for subfertile men in general. Systematic screening of this patient category is not indicated. On the other hand, it may be possible to identify subgroups among these men with a higher risk of CIS. Probable selection criteria could be men with severe oligozoospermia and an atrophic testis or a history of cryptorchidism.

29.4.2 MEN WITH A HISTORY OF CRYPTORCHIDISM

Carcinoma *in situ* of the testis has been demonstrated in patients with a current maldescended testicle as well as in men with a history of previously corrected cryptorchidism (Krabbe *et al.*, 1979; Ford, Parkinson and Pryor, 1985; Pedersen, Boiesen and Zetterlund, 1987; Giwercman *et al.* 1989). The high frequency of 8% in the study by Krabbe *et al.* (1979) may be due to some kind of selection as only 50 out of 180 men (28%) agreed to participate in the study. Ford, Parkinson and Pryor (1985) have also reported a high frequency (6.7%). However, in their study, testicular biopsies were performed at specific indications that probably selected patients with a higher frequency of CIS than in patients with cryptorchidism in general. The studies by Pedersen, Boiesen and Zetterlund (1987) and by Giwercman *et al.* (1989) were based on a systematic screening of 65 and 60% of the total study population, respectively. These two studies indicate a frequency of CIS in patients with a history of cryptorchidism of 2–3%.

Giwercman *et al.* (1989) have recommended that these men should be offered a testicular screening biopsy when they reach adulthood. This is a controversial statement and it may be pointed out that the incidence of 2–3% is too low to justify a systematic screening of the total patient population. A possibility would be to identify subgroups with a higher risk of CIS. However, Giwercman *et al.* (1989) found no clinical criteria indicating which patients should be selected for testicular biopsy. Noninvasive methods such as ultrasonography and semen analysis may be of value in the diagnosis of CIS and, thus, may aid in reducing the number of necessary biopsies in a screening program.

29.4.3 SOMATOSEXUAL AMBIGUITY

Individuals with somatosexual ambiguity and a Y chromosome in their karyotype have a very high risk of developing malignant germ cell tumors (Scully, 1981). Accordingly, CIS has been diagnosed in four out of four patients with gonadal dysgenesis (Müller *et al.*, 1985) and in three out of 12 with androgen insensitivity syndrome (Müller and Skakkebæk, 1984). These conditions are rare and it is not possible to indicate the actual risk of CIS in this group of individuals. The incidence is probably very high.

29.4.4 CONTRALATERAL TESTIS IN MEN WITH UNILATERAL TESTICULAR CANCER

The risk of bilateral tumors in patients with testicular germ cell cancer has been reported to be in the range 1–5% (Sokal, Peckham and Hindry, 1980; Scheiber, Ackermann and Studer, 1987; Thompson *et al.*, 1988; Fosså and Aass, 1989; Fordham *et al.* 1990; Østerlind *et al.*, 1991; Bokemeyer *et al.*, 1993; Dieckmann *et al.*, 1993). The true risk of developing a contralateral testicular tumor is probably 4–5%.

The first systematic screening for CIS of the contralateral testis in patients with unilateral testicular cancer was initiated in Denmark in 1972 and accelerated in 1978 (Berthelsen *et al.*, 1979). Carcinoma *in situ* has, consistently throughout the study, been found in about 5.5% of these patients (Berthelsen *et al.*, 1982; von der Maase *et al.*, 1986, 1987). The observed incidence of CIS of the contralateral testis has been confirmed in a German multicenter study. Thus, Loy and Dieckmann (1993) reported CIS of the contralateral testis in 4.5% of patients with unilateral testicular cancer. Altogether, the incidence of contralateral CIS seems to be about 5%, in accordance with the risk of developing a contralateral testicular tumor. In patients with contralateral CIS, the risk of developing a contralateral cancer has been estimated to be 40% within 3 years and 50% within 5 years (von der Maase *et al.*, 1986). Patients with testicular atrophy and/or a history of cryptorchidism have an increased risk of CIS (Berthelsen *et al.*, 1982; Harland *et al.*, 1993, Loy and Dieckmann, 1993). However, Loy and Dieckmann (1993) have demonstrated that reducing the screening population to patients with atrophy and a history of undescended testis may result in a situation where about half of the CIS-positive patients would be missed. A similar calculation has been made in relation to missing the second testicular cancer (Fordham *et al.*, 1990).

We recommend that all patients with unilateral testicular germ cell cancer should be offered a contralateral testicular biopsy concurrently with the orchidectomy for the primary tumor. The procedure is safe with only few and minor complications, and the investigation is of importance for all patients. If the biopsy specimen is without CIS, the patient can be assured that the risk of developing a contralateral cancer is negligible. If CIS is present, proper treatment can prevent development of a contralateral cancer without significantly affecting the testosterone production (von der Maase, Giwercman and Skakkebæk, 1986; von der Maase *et al.*, 1987).

29.4.5 EXTRAGONADAL GERM CELL CANCER

Böhle *et al.* (1986) have, in a retrospective study, showed CIS in three out of eight patients with extragonadal germ cell tumors. Two of these patients also had a microfocal tumor. As the histological examination in many of these patients was performed during or after chemotherapy, the frequency of CIS may have been underestimated. Daugaard *et al.* (1987, 1992) found CIS of the testis in 16 out of 38 patients with assumed extragonadal germ cell tumors in the retroperitoneum examined before chemotherapy was instituted. Four of these patients had also small areas of invasive tumor growth. In contrast, none out of eight patients with tumors in the mediastinum had CIS of the testis (Daugaard *et al.*, 1992). Carcinoma *in situ* or microfocal tumors in patients with assumed extragonadal germ cell tumor have also been reported by others (Saltzman, Pitts and Vaughan, 1986; Reinberg, Manivel and Fraley, 1989). These findings may indicate that a significant proportion of extragonadal germ cell tumors are disseminated testicular cancers and that CIS cells, thus, may have a metastatic potential. It seems, however, more probable that the extragonadal tumor and the CIS changes or the microfocal testicular tumor are independent lesions equivalent to what is seen in patients with a tumor in one testicle and CIS in the contralateral testis. This hypothesis will, of course, also implicate that some cases of assumed metastatic testicular cancer are in fact independently occurring testicular cancers and 'extragonadal' germ cell tumors.

Independently of these hypothetical considerations, it is obvious that the testis of all patients with assumed extragonadal germ cells tumors should be carefully examined, including ultrasound scanning and bilateral testicular biopsies.

The observed frequency and the presumed true incidence of CIS of the testis in the different risk populations are summarized in Table 29.1.

29.5 TREATMENT

The diagnosis of CIS suggests that a specific treatment should be instituted. However, if treatment, due to different reasons, is not instituted, patients should be followed by clinical examination of the testis including ultrasound scanning every 6 months and biopsy sampling every 1–2 years. The use of testicular follow-up biopsies allows progression to be detected at a stage of early invasive growth. When invasive cancer is diagnosed, orchidectomy has to be performed. The follow-up program seems to ensure that the tumor is diagnosed as a Stage I tumor and most patients can probably be cured by orchidectomy alone (von der Maase *et al.*, 1986). However, this does not change the fact that patients should be offered treatment in continuation of the diagnosis of CIS in order to prevent development of invasive cancer and, in patients with only one remaining testicle, to avoid a second orchidectomy.

The treatment strategy for patients with CIS of the testis depends on the patient category in question and whether CIS is present in one or both testes.

29.5.1 ORCHIDECTOMY

Subfertile men and those with a history of cryptorchidism with CIS in one testis should primarily have a biopsy on the other testis to

Table 29.1 Incidence of carcinoma *in situ* of the testis

Population	Reference	Reported cases of carcinoma in situ of the testis	Presumed incidence of carcinoma in situ of the testis
General male population	Giwercman *et al.* (1991)	0/399 (0%)	About 0.5%
Subfertile men	Nüesch-Bachmann and Hedinger (1977)	9/1635 (0.6%)	0.5–1%
	Skakkebæk (1978)	6/555 (1.1%)	
	Pryor *et al.* (1983)	8/2043 (0.4%)	
	Schütte (1988)	15/2047 (0.7%)	
Men with a history of cryptorchidism	Krabbe *et al.* (1979)	4/50 (8.0%)	2–3%
	Ford *et al.* (1985)	6/90 (6.7%)	
	Pedersen *et al.* (1987)	3/94 (3.2%)	
	Giwercman *et al.* (1989)	5/300 (1.7%)	
Androgen insensitivity syndrome	Müller and Skakkebæk (1984)	3/12 (25%)	High
Gonadal dysgenesis	Müller *et al.* (1985)	4/4 (100%)	
Contralateral testis of men with testicular cancer	von der Maase *et al.* (1987)	34/600 (5.7%)	5%
	Loy and Dieckmann (1993)	53/1188 (4.5%)	
Assumed retroperitoneal extragonadal germ cell tumors	Böhle *et al.* (1986)	3/8 (38%)	About 40%
	Daugaard *et al.* (1992)	16/38 (42%)	

ensure that the condition is truly unilateral. If so, orchidectomy is the choice of treatment, whereas localized irradiation is recommended in bilateral cases. It should, however, be noted that we have, as yet, no experience with radiation treatment of bilateral CIS testis. If CIS is diagnosed in a prepubertal boy, it seems sufficient to follow the patient with careful palpation and ultrasound scanning of the testis, confirm the diagnosis after puberty with a new biopsy at the age of 18–20 years and then perform an orchidectomy. This strategy is based on the observation by Giwercman *et al.* (1987b) that no testicular cancer had occurred among boys with a maldescended testis before the age of 20 years.

Treatment of patients with gonadal dysgenesis or androgen insensitivity syndrome is difficult and should be individualized. Gonadectomy is generally the treatment of choice because of the very high risk of developing a malignant germ cell tumor (Scully, 1981).

As discussed below, orchidectomy is also the treatment of choice in patients with extragonadal germ cell tumors who have unilateral CIS of the testis.

29.5.2 EFFECT OF CANCER CHEMOTHERAPY

We have previously reported that intensive chemotherapy, instituted because of dissemination of the initial testicular cancer, may eradicate CIS of the contralateral testis (von der Maase *et al.*, 1985, 1986, 1987). However, it has been demonstrated that CIS may persist or recur after chemotherapy (von der Maase, Meinecke and Skakkebæk, 1988; Bottomly *et al.*, 1990; Dieckmann and Loy, 1991). As previously discussed (von der Maase *et al.*, 1987), the possibility of relapse in these

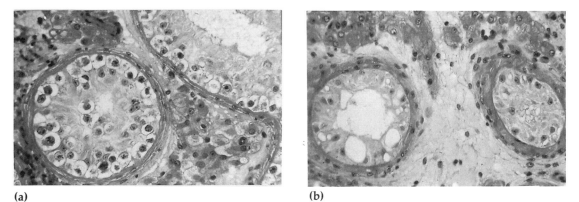

(a)   **(b)**

Fig. 29.2   (a) Before irradiation. Biopsy sample showing characteristic carcinoma *in situ* changes in all tubules. No invasive growth. (b) Three months after irradiation. Biopsy sample showing 'Sertoli-cell-only' pattern.

patients should, in fact, be expected. The testis may probably act as a sanctuary in agreement with the reports of residual germ cell cancers in orchidectomy specimens after cisplatin-based chemotherapy (Greist *et al.*, 1984; Böhle *et al.*, 1986; Chong *et al.*, 1986). Similarly, development of contralateral testicular cancer has been observed despite prior chemotherapy (Fowler *et al.*, 1979; Fosså and Aass, 1989). Our data seem, however, to indicate that chemotherapy postpones the occurrence of the second testicular cancer (von der Maase *et al.*, 1986). Thompson *et al.* (1988) have also observed prevention by chemotherapy, which, on the other hand, was not the case in the study by Fosså and Aass (1989). It is, thus, yet not clarified how to manage patients with CIS of the contralateral testis receiving chemotherapy for their initial testicular cancer. A possibility would be to offer these patients localized irradiation of the testis. If not, these patients should have close surveillance by use of ultrasonography and one should also consider the use of rebiopsies.

Patients with extragonadal germ cell tumors will generally receive intensive chemotherapy. Before starting the chemotherapy, bilateral testicular biopsies should be performed to ensure the presence or absence of CIS. As for patients with testicular cancer, CIS changes will apparently disappear, but the possibility of reappearance and development of invasive growth should be taken into consideration. Carcinoma *in situ* is most often found in only one of the testes and in such cases the patient should be offered an orchidectomy on the affected side or close surveillance as mentioned above. Localized irradiation of the testes is recommended in bilateral cases of CIS.

29.5.3   EFFECT OF LOCALIZED IRRADIATION

In 1985, we initiated a study of localized irradiation of CIS of the testis (von der Maase *et al.*, 1986, 1987; Giwercman *et al.*, 1991). The radiation treatment was given as 14–20 MeV to the scrotum placed in a cup of lead. The total dose was 20 Gy delivered in ten fractions of 2 Gy with five fractions per week. This radiation schedule was shown to eradicate the CIS changes as the postirradiation biopsy specimens revealed a 'Sertoli cells only' pattern in 20 out of 20 cases (Fig. 29.2). The follow-up time is now up to 10 years and none of the patients has developed a contralateral tumor. There have been no complaints of any change in libido or other sexual functions. However, an increase in the luteinizing hormone values and a decrease in the testosterone response to HCG have indicated an impairment of the Leydig cell function. Therefore, we are presently investigating the possibility of lowering the dose. Until now, we have treated 12 patients with total radiation doses from 18 to 14 Gy with 2 Gy per fraction. As with the 20 Gy radiation schedule, the postirradiation biopsy specimens have revealed a 'Sertoli cells only' pattern in all cases. The observation time is, however, yet too short to allow any valid conclusions concerning the effect of these radiation doses with respect to eradication of CIS cells as well as the influence on the Leydig cell function. The effect of doses in the range from 18 to 20 Gy has been confirmed by other centers (Mumperow *et al.*, 1992; Dieckmann, Besserer and Loy, 1993).

It has been reported that none of more than 1000 patients with unilateral testicular cancer receiving routine prophylactic radiotherapy to the remaining testicle has developed a contralateral testicular cancer (Read, 1987). This treatment strategy is now unconventional. The results, however, strongly support our conclusion that the localized radiation schedule effectively prevents development of a contralateral testicular cancer.

We recommend that patients with unilateral testicular cancer and CIS of the contralateral testis should be offered localized irradiation of the testis. It should be emphasized that this treatment will induce sterility. However, most patients with unilateral testicular cancer and CIS of the contralateral testis have, beforehand, azoospermia or a very poor semen quality (Giwercman *et al.*, 1993). This is in accordance with the observation that none of 38 men became fathers in a period from 0.5 to 14 years between the diagnosis of the first and second testicular cancer (Fordham *et al.*, 1990). Patients should, nevertheless, be carefully informed about this and offered a semen analysis and, if possible, storage of semen.

The ultimate goal for the management of CIS of the testis is to detect this condition at a premalignant stage and cure the patient without use of toxic treatment regimens and, if possible, without affecting the androgen production. The recommended screening and treatment strategy seems to meet that goal. In fact, application of this strategy may imply that future cases of bilateral testicular germ cell cancer can be prevented with the exception of the rare cases of synchronous bilateral tumors.

REFERENCES

Berthelsen, J.G. and Skakkebæk, N.E. (1981) Value of testicular biopsy in diagnosing carcinoma *in situ* testis. *Scand. J. Urol. Nephrol.*, **15**, 165–8.

Berthelsen, J.G., Skakkebæk, N.E., von der Maase, H. and Sørensen, B.L. (1982) Screening for carcinoma *in situ* of the contralateral testis in patients with germinal testicular cancer. *BMJ*, **285**, 1683–6.

Berthelsen, J.G., Skakkebæk, N.E., Mogensen, P. and Sørensen, B.L. (1979) Incidence of carcinoma *in situ* of germ cells in contralateral testis of men with testicular tumours. *BMJ*, **2**, 363–4.

Böhle, A., Studer, U.E., Sonntag, R.W. and Scheidegger, J.R. (1986) Primary or secondary extragonadal germ cell tumors? *J. Urol.*, **135**, 939–43.

Bokemeyer, C., Schmoll, H.J., Schoffski, P. *et al.* (1993) Bilateral testicular tumours: prevalence and clinical implications. *Eur. J. Cancer*, **29A**, 874–6.

Bottomley, D., Fischer, C., Hendry, W.F. and Horwich, A. (1990) Persistent carcinoma *in situ* of the testis after chemotherapy for advanced testicular germ cell tumours. *Br. J. Urol.*, **66**, 420–4.

Brackenbury, E.T., Hargreave, T.B., Howard, G.C. and McIntyre, M.A. (1993) Seminal fluid analysis and fine-needle aspiration cytology in the diagnosis of carcinoma *in situ* of the testis. *Eur. Urol.*, **23**, 123–8.

Bruun, E., Frimodt-Møller, C., Giwercman, A. *et al.* (1987) Testicular biopsy as an outpatient procedure in screening for carcinoma-*in-situ*: complications and the patient's acceptance. *Int. J. Androl.*, **10**, 199–202.

Chong, C., Logothetis, C.J., von Eschenbach, A. *et al.* (1986) Orchidectomy in advanced germ cell cancer following intensive chemotherapy: a comparison of systemic to testicular response. *J. Urol.*, **136**, 1221–3.

Daugaard, G., von der Maase, H., Olsen, J. *et al.* (1987) Carcinoma-*in-situ* testis in patients with assumed extragonadal germ-cell tumours. *Lancet*, ii, 528–9.

Daugaard, G., Rørth, M., von der Maase, H. and Skakkebæk, N.E. (1992) Management of extragonadal germ-cell tumors and the significance of bilateral testicular biopsies. *Ann. Oncol.*, **3**, 283–9.

Dieckmann, K.P., Besserer, A. and Loy, V. (1993) Low-dose radiation therapy for testicular intra-epithelial neoplasia. *J. Cancer Res. Clin. Oncol.*, **119**, 355–9.

Dieckmann, K.P., Kaup, F. and Loy, V. (1992) False-negative biopsy for testicular intraepithelial neoplasia. *J. Cancer Res. Clin. Oncol.*, **119**, 1–4.

Dieckmann, K.P. and Loy, V. (1991) Persistent testicular intraepithelial neoplasia after chemotherapy. *Eur. Urol.*, **20**, 258–60.

Dieckmann, K.P., Loy, V. and Büttner, P. (1993) Prevalence of bilateral testicular germ cell tumours and early detection based on contralateral testicular intra-epithelial neoplasia. *Br. J. Urol.*, **71**, 340–5.

Ford, T.F., Parkinson, M.C. and Pryor, J.P. (1985) The undescended testis in adult life. *Br. J. Urol.*, **57**, 181–4.

Fordham, M.V., Mason, M.D., Blackmore, C. *et al.* (1990) Management of the contralateral testis in patients with testicular germ cell cancer. *Br. J. Urol.*, **65**, 290–3.

Fosså, S.D. and Aass, N. (1989) Cisplatin-based chemotherapy does not eliminate the risk of a second testicular cancer. *Br. J. Urol.*, **63**, 531–4.

Fowler, J.E., Jr, Vugrin, D., Cvitkovic, E. and Whitmore, W.F., Jr. (1979) Sequential bilateral germ cell tumors of the testis despite interval chemotherapy. *J. Urol.*, **122**, 421–5.

Giwercman, A., Berthelsen, J.G., Müller, J. *et al.* (1987a) Screening for carcinoma-*in-situ* of the testis. *Int. J. Androl.*, **10**, 173–80.

Giwercman, A., Bruun, E., Frimodt-Møller, and Skakkebæk, N.E. (1989) Prevalence of carcinoma *in situ* and other histophathological abnormalities in testes of men with a history of cryptorchidism. *J. Urol.*, **142**, 998–1002.

Giwercman, A., Cantell, L. and Marks, A. (1991) Placental-like alkaline phosphatase as a marker of carcinoma-*in-situ* of the testis. Comparison with monoclonal antibodies M2A and 43-9F. *APMIS*, **99**, 586–94.

Giwercman, A., Clausen, O.P.F. and Skakkebæk N.E. (1988a) Carcinoma *in situ* of the testis: aneuploid cells in semen. *BMJ*, **296** 1762–4.

Giwercman, A., Grindsted, J., Hansen, B. *et al.* (1987b) Testicular cancer risk in boys with maldescended testis: a cohort study. *J. Urol.* **138**, 1214–16.

Giwercman, A., Hopman, A.H., Ramaekers, F.C. and Skakkebæk, N.E. (1990) Carcinoma *in situ* of the testis. Detection of malignant germ cells in seminal fluid by means of *in situ* hybridization. *Am. J. Pathol.*, **136**, 497–502.

Giwercman, A., Marks, A. and Skakkebæk, N.E. (1988b) Carcinoma-*in-situ* germ-cells exfoliated from seminiferous epithelium into seminal fluid. *Lancet*, i, 530.

Giwercman, A., von der Maase, H., Berthelsen, J.G. *et al.* (1991) Localized irradiation of testes with carcinoma *in situ*: Effects on Leydig cell function and eradication of malignant germ cells in 20 patients. *J. Clin. Endocrinol. Metab.*, **73**, 596–603.

Giwercman, A., von der Maase, H., Rørth, M. and Skakkebæk, N.E. (1993) Semen quality in testicular tumour and CIS in the contralateral testis. *Lancet*, **341**, 384–5.

Giwercman, A., Müller, J. and Skakkebæk, N.E. (1991) Prevalence of carcinoma *in situ* and other histopathological abnormalities in testes from 399 men who died suddenly and unexpectedly. *J. Urol.*, **145**, 77–80.

Greist, A., Einhorn, L.H., Williams, S.D. *et al.* (1984) Pathologic findings at orchidectomy following chemotherapy for disseminated testicular cancer. *J. Clin. Oncol.*, **2**, 1025–7.

Harland, S.J., Cook, P.A., Fosså, S.D. *et al.* (1993) Risk factors for carcinoma *in situ* of the contralateral testis in patients with testicular cancer. An interim report. *Eur. Urol.*, **23**, 115–19.

Heikkila, R., Heilo, A., Steinwig, A.E. and Fosså, S.D. (1993) Testicular ultrasonography and 18G biopty biopsy for clinically undetected cancer or carcinoma *in situ* in patients with germ cell tumours. *Br. J. Urol.*, **71**, 214–16.

Howard, G.D.W., Hargreave, T.B., McIntyre, M.A. (1989) Case report: Carcinoma-*in-situ* of the testis diagnosed on semen cytology. *Clin. Radiol.*, **40**, 323–4.

Hustin, J., Collette, J. and Franchimont, P. (1987) Immunohistochemical demonstration of placental alkaline phosphatase in various states of testicular development and in germ cell tumours. *Int. J. Androl.*, **10**, 29–35.

Jacobsen, G.K., Henriksen, O.B. and von der Maase, H. (1981) Carcinoma *in situ* of testicular tissue adjacent to malignant germ-cell tumors: a study of 105 cases. *Cancer*, **47**, 2660–2.

Jacobsen, G.K., and Nørgaard-Pedersen, B. (1984) Placental alkaline phosphatase in testicular germ cell tumours and in carcinoma-*in-situ* of the testis. *Acta Pathol. Microbiol. Immunol. Scand.*, **A, 92**, 323–9.

Jacobsen, G.K. and Talerman, A. (1989) Testicular Intratubular germ cell neoplasia (IGCN), in *Atlas of Germ Cell Tumours* (ed. G.K. Jacobsen and A. Talerman), Munksgaard, Copenhagen, pp. 194–204.

Klein, F.A., Melamed, M.R. and Whitmore, W.F., Jr (1985) Intratubular malignant germ cells (carcinoma *in situ*) accompanying invasive testicular germ cell tumors. *J. Urol.*, **133**, 413–15.

Krabbe, S., Skakkebæk, N.E., Berthelsen, J.G. *et al.* (1979) High incidence of undetected neoplasia in maldescended testes. *Lancet*, **i**, 999–1000.

Lenz, S., Giwercman, A., Skakkebæk, N.E. *et al.* (1987) Ultrasound in detection of early neoplasia of the testis. *Int. J. Androl.*, **10**, 187–90.

Loy, V. and Dieckmann, K.P. (1993) Prevalence of contralateral testicular intraepithelial neoplasia (carcinoma *in situ*) in patients with testicular germ cell tumour. Results of the German multicentre study. *Eur. Urol.*, **23**, 120–2.

von der Maase, H., Berthelsen, J.G., Jacobsen, G.K. *et al.* (1985) Carcinoma-*in-situ* of testis eradicated by chemotherapy, *Lancet*, **i**, 98.

von der Maase, H., Giwercman, A., Müller, J. and Skakkebæk, N.E. (1987) Management of carcinoma-*in-situ* of testis. *Int. J. Androl.*, **10**, 209–20.

von der Maase, H., Giwercman, A. and Skakkebæk, N.E. (1986) Radiation treatment of carcinoma-*in-situ* of testis. *Lancet*, **i**, 624–5.

von der Maase, H., Meinecke, B. and Skakkebæk, N.E. (1988) Residual carcinoma-*in-situ* of contralateral testis after chemotherapy. *Lancet*, **i**, 477–8.

von der Maase, H., Rørth, M., Walbom-Jørgensen, S. *et al.* (1986) Carcinoma *in situ* of contralateral testis in patients with testicular germ cell cancer: study of 27 cases in 500 patients. *BMJ*, **293**, 1398–401.

Manivel, J.C., Jessurun, J., Wick, M.R. and Dehner, L.P. (1987) Placental alkaline phosphatase immunoreactivity in testicular germ-cell neoplasms. *Am. J. Surg. Pathol.*, **11**, 21–9.

Manivel, J.C., Simonton, S., Wold, L.E. and Dehner, L.P. (1988) Absence of intratubular germ cell neoplasia in testicular yolk sac tumors in children. A histochemical and immunohistochemical study. *Arch. Pathol. Lab. Med.*, **112**, 641–5.

Müller, J. and Skakkebæk, N.E. (1981) Microspectrophotometric DNA measurements of carcinoma-*in-situ* germ cells in the testis. *Int. J. Androl.*, (Suppl. 4), 211–21.

Müller, J. and Skakkebæk, N.E. (1984) Testicular carcinoma *in situ* in children with the androgen insensitivity (testicular feminisation) syndrome. *BMJ*, **288**, 1419–20.

Müller, J., Skakkebæk, N.E. and Parkinson, M.C. (1987) The spermatocytic seminoma: views on pathogenesis. *Int. J. Androl.*, **10**, 147–56.

Müller, J. Skakkebæk, N.E., Ritzen, M. and Ploen L. (1985) Carcinoma *in situ* of the testis in children with 45, X/46, XY gonadal dysgenesis. *J. Pediatr.*, **106**, 431–6.

Mumperow, E., Lauke, H., Holstein, A.F. and Hartmann, M. (1992) Further practical experiences in the recognition and management of carcinoma *in situ* of the testis. *Urol. Int.*, **48**, 162–6.

Nüesch-Bachmann, I.H. and Hedinger, C. (1977), Atypische spermatogonien als präkanzerose. *Schweiz. Med. Wochenschr.*, **107**, 795–801.

Oosterhuis, J.W., Gillis, A.J.M., van Putten, W.J.L. *et al.* (1993) Interphase cytogenetics of carcinoma *in situ* of the testis. Numeric analysis of the Chromosomes 1, 12 and 15. *Eur. Urol.*, **23**, 16–22.

Østerlind, A., Berthelsen, J.G., Abildgaard, N., *et al.* (1991) Risk of bilateral testicular germ cell cancer in Denmark: 1960–84. *J. Natl. Cancer Inst.*, **83**, 1391–5.

Pedersen, K.V., Boiesen, P. and Zetterlund, C.G. (1987) Experience of screening for carcinoma-*in-situ* of the testis among young men with surgically corrected maldescended testes. *Int. J. Androl.*, **10**, 181–5.

Prener, A. and Østerlind, A. (1985) *Cancer in Denmark*, Danish Cancer Registry, Copenhagen.

Pryor, J.P., Cameron, K.M., Chilton, C.P. *et al.* (1983) Carcinoma *in situ* in testicular biopsies from men presenting with infertility. *Br. J. Urol.*, **55**, 780–4.

Rajfer, J. and Binder, S. (1989) Use of biopty gun

for transcutaneous testicular biopsy. *J. Urol.*, **142**, 1021–2.

Read, G. (1987) Carcinoma *in situ* of the contralateral testis. *BMJ*, **294**, 121.

Reinberg, Y., Manivel, J.C. and Fraley, E.E. (1989) Carcinoma *in situ* of the testis. *J. Urol.*, **142**, 243–7.

Saltzman, B., Pitts, W.R. and Vaughan, E.D. Jr (1986) Extragonadal retroperitoneal germ cell tumors without apparent testicular involvement. *Urology*, **27**, 504–7.

Scheiber, K., Ackermann, D. and Studer, U.E. (1987) Bilateral testicular germ cell tumors: a report of 20 cases. *J. Urol.*, **138**, 73–6.

Schütte, B. (1988) Early testicular cancer in severe oligozoospermia, in *Carl Schirren Symposium: Advances in Andrology* (eds A.F. Holstein, F. Leidenberger, K.H. Hölzer and G. Bettendorf), Diesbach Verlag, Berlin, pp. 188–90.

Scully, R.E. (1981) Neoplasia associated with anomalous sexual development and abnormal sex chromosomes. *Ped. Adolesc. Endocrinol.*, **8**, 203–17.

Skakkebæk, N.E. (1972a) Abnormal morphology of germ cells in two infertile men. *Acta Pathol. Microbiol. Scand.*, **A, 80**, 374–8.

Skakkebæk, N.E. (1972b) Possible carcinoma-in-situ of the testis. *Lancet*, **ii**, 516–17.

Skakkebæk, N.E. (1975) Atypical germ cell in the adjacent 'normal' tissue of testicular tumours. *Acta Pathol. Microbiol. Scand.*, **A, 83**, 127–30.

Skakkebæk N.E. (1978) Carcinoma *in situ* of the testis: frequency and relationship to invasive germ cell tumours in infertile men. *Histopathology*, **2**, 157–70.

Skakkebæk, N.E. Berthelsen, J.G. and Müller J. (1982) Carcinoma-in-situ of the undescended testis. *Urol. Clin. North Am.*, **9**, 377–85.

Sokal, M., Peckham, M.J. and Hendry, W.F. (1980) Bilateral germ cell tumours of the testis. *Br. J. Urol.*, **52**, 158–62.

Thompson, J., Williams, C.J., Whitehouse, J.M.A. and Mead, G.M. (1988) Bilateral testicular germ cell tumours: an increasing incidence and prevention by chemotherapy. *Br. J. Urol.*, **62**, 374–6.

N.J. Vogelzang

30.1 INTRODUCTION

The toxicities of chemotherapy have been recognized since Jacobson *et al.* (1946) first reported severe leukopenia, abrupt nausea and vomiting and sclerosing phlebitis following intravenous injection of nitrogen mustard. During the following years, over 50 different chemotherapeutic agents have reached the marketplace. Hundreds of other agents have been tested but have failed to pass Phase I, II or III trials.

Among the many chemotherapeutic agents available, only 14 have been widely used to treat patients with metastatic testis cancer (Table 30.1). These agents can be grouped by class of drug; the alkylating agents (cisplatin, carboplatin, cyclophosphamide, ifosfamide), the alkaloids (vincristine, vinblastine, etoposide, paclitaxel), the antibiotics (bleomycin, mithramycin, doxorubicin and actinomycin-D) and the antimetabolites (methotrexate, 5-fluorouracil). It is probable that other drugs within these classes are active against testis cancer, yet few reports on other drugs are available. The reason for this lack of data is quite simple; testis cancer is an uncommon cancer for which effective chemotherapy has been available since 1960 (Li *et al.*). Consequently the number of patients available for

Table 30.1 Single agents used to treat metastatic germ cell testicular malignancy

Drug	Class	Introduced	Reference
Cisplatin	Alkylator	1974	Higby *et al.* (1974)
Carboplatin	Alkylator	1987	Motzer *et al.* (1987)
Cyclophosphamide	Alkylator	1974	Buckner *et al.* (1974)
Ifosfamide	Alkylator	1986	Wheeler *et al.* (1986)
Vincristine	Alkaloid	1962	Costa, Hreshchyshyn and Holland (1962)
Vinblastine	Alkaloid	1970	Samuels and Howe (1970)
Etoposide	Epipodophyllotoxin	1980	Fitzharris *et al.* (1980)
Bleomycin	Antibiotic	1975	Samuels, Johnson and Holoye (1975)
Mithramycin	Antibiotic	1970	Kennedy (1970)
Doxorubicin	Antibiotic	1972	Monfardini *et al.* (1972)
Actinomycin-D	Antibiotic	1974	Merrin and Murphy (1974)
5-Fluorouracil	Antimetabolite	1959	Mendelson and Serpick (1970)
Methotrexate	Antimetabolite	1967	Wyatt and McAninch (1967)
Paclitaxel	Alkaloid	1994	Motzer *et al.* (1994)

Testicular Cancer: Investigation and management. Second edition. Edited by Professor A. Horwich.
Published in 1996 by Chapman & Hall. ISBN 0 412 61210 0.

formal Phase II studies has always been low and has declined even more with the increasing effectiveness of first line chemotherapy. Additionally, by the time patients are considered for a Phase II study they have frequently been heavily pretreated and subsequently may have decreased performance status, marrow reserve or renal function making them ineligible for study. New classes of antineoplastic agents (i.e. lymphokines/cytokines), should be tested in these patients, but, with rare exceptions (Roth *et al.*, 1985), such studies have also not been performed.

Thus this chapter will focus on the toxicities of the 14 agents alone and in combination. The acute and chronic toxicities are well known and published. Among these agents all, except carboplatin, paclitaxel and ifosfamide, were introduced into clinical practice prior to 1985. Thus reasonable amounts of data exist on the chronic toxicities of the agents singly and in combination. This chapter will detail the toxicities of the various chemotherapeutic agents using the outline summarized in Table 30.2.

30.2 TOXICITIES OF SINGLE AGENTS

30.2.1 CISPLATIN

Since cisplatin is the most active single agent and is widely used, both singly and in combination, its toxicities will be reviewed first. Numerous reports are available on the toxicity of cisplatin.

The bone marrow toxicity of cisplatin is modest and consists mostly of cumulative anemia and thrombocytopenia. The anemia of single agent cisplatin is generally felt to represent an erythropoietin-deficiency anemia and thus correlates modestly well with cisplatin nephrotoxicity and the total cumulative dose of cisplatin received (Ackland and Vogelzang, 1987). Clinical trials have documented the ability of recombinant erythropoietin to reverse the anemia (Miller *et al.*, 1992). The thrombocytopenia is felt to represent true toxicity to the megakaryocyte precur-

sors. Yet thrombocytopenia is rarely a clinical problem with the three to four courses of cisplatin given to most testicular cancer patients. Importantly, the lack of neutropenia following cisplatin therapy makes it an ideal agent to add to bone marrow suppressive agents. Also, after more than 15 years of clinical use, no case of secondary acute leukemia has been linked to cisplatin alone.

Severe nausea and vomiting has come to be inextricably linked with cisplatin, while other gastrointestinal toxicities (stomatitis, hepatic dysfunction and ileus) are extremely rare. The nausea and vomiting of cisplatin has been quantified precisely by Gralla *et al.* in an elegant series of trials with high dose metoclopramide (Gralla *et al.*, 1981; Kris *et al.*, 1985, 1989). Metoclopramide is superior to placebo or prochlorperazine in reducing by 90% the number of vomiting episodes in elderly patients receiving 120 mg m^{-2} of cisplatin. In young patients with testicular cancer a Parkinsonian-like state is commonly induced by the metoclopramide. Anticholinergics lead to rapid reversal. Such reactions require avoidance of further metoclopramide and have led to a search for more effective and less toxic antiemetics. Subsequent trials determined the need for diphenhydramine to control the extrapyramidal effects of metoclopramide, the additional value of an anxiety-lytic agent, lorazepam (Laszlo, 1985) and the further additional benefit of decadron (Markman *et al.*, 1984; Kris *et al.*, 1989). Other investigators using decadron and lorazepam without metoclopramide have achieved excellent control of cisplatin-induced emesis in testis cancer patients. Recently, the serotonin S$_3$ receptor antagonists granisetron (Addelmann *et al.*, 1990) and ondansetron have been able virtually to abrogate cisplatin-induced emesis (Einhorn *et al.*, 1990; Marty *et al.*, 1990). In the study by Marty *et al.* (1990) 75% of patients treated with ondansetron had two or less vomiting episodes compared with 42% of patients treated with metoclopramide. Einhorn *et al.* (1990) reported that 67% of patients

Table 30.2 Acute and chronic toxicity patterns of the single agents used to treat metastatic germ cell tumors of the testis

Toxicity	CDDP	Carbo	CTX	IFX	VCR	VLB	Etop	Bleo	Act-D	MTX	Dox	TAX
Anemia	+++	+++	+	+	−	−	+++	−	+	−	+	+
Leukopenia	+	+++	+++	+	+	++	+++	−	++	+	+++	+++
Thrombocytopenia	+++	+++	+	+	−	−	++	−	+	+	+	+
Secondary leukemia	−	−	+	+	−	−	++	−	−	−	−	−
Stomatitis	−	−	+	+	−	−	++	+++	+++	+++	++	++
Emesis/nausea	+++	+	+++	+++	−	−	+	+++	+++	+	++	+++
Ileus	+	−	−	−	++	++	−	−	−	−	−	+
Diarrhea	++	−	−	−	−	−	−	−	−	++	−	−
Hepatitis	−	−	−	−	+	+	+	−	+	++	+	−
Central nervous system	+	−	−	+	−	−	−	−	−	−	−	−
Peripheral nervous system	+++	−	−	−	+++	+	−	−	−	−	−	+++
Cranial nerves	+++	−	−	+	+	−	−	−	−	−	−	−
Pulmonary	−	−	−	−	−	−	−	+++	−	+	−	−
Hypertension	+	−	−	−	−	−	−	+	−	−	−	−
Cardiac muscle	−	−	+	+	−	−	−	+	−	−	++	+
Large vessels	−	−	−	−	+	+	−	+	−	−	−	−
Peripheral vessels	−	−	−	−	−	−	−	+	−	−	−	−
Nephrotoxiticy	+++	+	−	+++	−	−	−	−	−	+	−	−
Bladder	−	−	+	+++	−	−	−	AN	−	−	−	−
Endocrine	+	−	−	−	+	+	−	+	−	−	−	−
Hyperpigmentation	−	+	++	++	−	−	−	+++	+	++	+++	−
Alopecia	+	+	+++	+++	−	+	+++	+	++	+	+++	−
Azoospermia	+	+	+++	+++	−	−	+	−	−	+	−	−
Genetic damage	−	−	+	+	−	−	−	−	−	+	−	−
Orthopedic/muscular	−	−	−	−	+	+	−	+	−	−	−	−

AN, anecdotal.
−, not reported.
+, WHO Grade 1.
++, WHO Grade 2.
+++, WHO Grade 3.
++++, WHO Grade 4.
CDDP, cisplatin; Carbo, carboplatin; CTX, cyclophosphamide; IFX, ifosfamide; VCR, vincristine; VLB, vinblastine; Etop, etoposide; Bleo, bleomycin; Act-D, actinomycin-D; MTX, methotrexate; Dox, doxorubicin; TAX, paclitaxel.

treated with ondansetron had two or less vomiting episodes during 4–5-day cisplatin regiments. An appropriate dose and schedule of ondansetron appear to be an 8–12 mg dose each 8 hours. For patients receiving cisplatin, a reasonable regimen for antiemesis would be:

> Decadron 4 mg IV 0.5 h before cisplatin and repeated q. 6 h × 4 total doses. Oral administration is effective if the patient is not vomiting and is an outpatient.

> Lorazepam 1 mg IV 0.5 h before cisplatin and repeat q. 4–6 h. Reduce to 0.5 mg or 0.25 mg as necessary for excessive somnolence or hallucination.

> Ondansetron 8–12 mg IV q. 8h.

As the acute nausea and vomiting of cisplatin is controlled, the delayed nausea of cisplatin becomes more noticeable. Kris *et al.* (1985) described the value of oral metoclopramide in this setting. More recently, oral ondansetron 8 mg PO q. 8 h for 3–5 days after completion of the cisplatin appears to be highly effective in eliminating delayed nausea and vomiting.

A little recognized or investigated gastrointestinal effect of cisplatin is explosive diarrhea, which affects 10–20% of patients. Its etiology is unclear. Therapy is the use of standard antidiarrheal medications. The neuropathy of cisplatin has been long described and affects the large sensory fibers, leading to numbness, tingling and a decrease in vibratory sensation (Mollman, 1990). Ototoxicity, autonomic neuropathy, Lhermittes syndrome and, rarely, cortical blindness are also parts of the spectrum of cisplatin neuropathy. Pathologically, sural nerve biopsies reveal axonal dropout although some reports describe segmental demyelination. Anecdotally, phenytoin, amitriptyline and several other agents have provided symptomatic relief. Several recent reports (Mollman, 1990; van der Hoop *et al.*, 1990) have described the prevention of cisplatin neuropathy with a neurotrophic peptide Org 2766, an ACTH (4–9) analogue, but a trial in ovarian cancer patients failed to show prevention of cisplatin neurotoxicity. Recently, amifostine (WR-2721 Ethyol[R]) has been shown to protect against both the nephro- and the neurotoxicity of cisplatin (Alberts and Noel, 1995). The United States Food and Drug Administration approved amifostine on 7 June 1995. The value of this new agent in testicular cancer therapy remains speculative.

In surveys of testicular cancer patients cured with cisplatin-based chemotherapy, the incidence of symptomatic peripheral sensory neuropathy varies from 20 to 45%, and when detailed neurological studies are performed the incidence may be even higher (Hansen *et al.*, 1989; Aass *et al.*, 1990; Boyer, 1990; Gietema *et al.*, 1992; Gregg *et al.*, 1992). This incidence may decline as vinblastine use has declined.

The other major neuropathic effects of cisplatin include ototoxicity, retinal toxicity and seizures. Seizures appear to be related to severe hypomagnesemia (Schilsky, Barlock and Ozols, 1982). The ototoxicity (occurring in 10–20% of patients) is probably caused by cisplatin damage to the organ of Corti, and is manifest as high-frequency hearing loss and tinnitus. The retinal toxicity is probably direct toxicity to the rods and cones. It is manifested primarily as night blindness and loss of color discrimination. Neither toxicity is common with only four courses of cisplatin unless double-dose cisplatin 200 mg m^{-2} per course is used (Ozols *et al.*, 1985). Management of both toxicities demands permanent discontinuation of cisplatin.

Cardiovascular toxicity of single agent cisplatin is anecdotal and includes hypertension following intra-arterial cisplatin and case reports of myocardial infarction following cisplatin. This author is inclined to view such events as related to the stress of volume overload required for cisplatin and the vagal stimulation caused by cisplatin-induced nausea. The nephrotoxicity of cisplatin was recognized during early Phase I trials (Higby *et al.*, 1974; Hayes *et al.*, 1977). Hayes *et al.*

(1977) were the first to demonstrate that the renal toxicity of high dose bolus cisplatin (>100 mg m^{-2}) could be ameliorated by forced hydration and diuresis. Canine trials led to the initial clinical trials published in 1977, which in turn led directly to the vinblastine/cyclophosphamide/dactinomycin/bleomycin/cisplatin (VAB-2 to VAB-6) trials utilizing high dose bolus cisplatin (Reynolds *et al.*, 1981; Vugrin *et al.*, 1981). Meanwhile, Einhorn and Donohue (1977) added the cisplatin dose of Higby *et al.* (1974) (20 mg m^{-2} d^{-1} × 5) to a modification of the Samuels' regimen (Samuels, Johnson and Holoye, 1975) to develop the cisplatin/vinblastine/bleomycin (PVB) regimen. These two separate evolutionary paths of cisplatin utilization in germ cell tumor regimens were thus the direct outcome of two disparate methods of ameliorating cisplatin nephrotoxicity. Throughout the late 1970s and early 1980s it was believed that the two regimens were comparable in response rates and in toxicity parameters, although no direct comparative trials were performed.

Two recent studies have allowed a more direct comparison of the nephrotoxicity of a 'VAB-6-like' cisplatin regimen with a PVB-like cisplatin regimen. The first to be published was that of Bosl *et al.* (1988), in which 148 patients with good risk metastatic germ cell cancer were treated with either three cycles of VAB-6 or four cycles of etoposide/cisplatin (EP). The cisplatin dose of VAB-6 was 120 mg m^{-2} per course (single bolus) and of EP was 100 mg m^{-2} per course (20 mg m^{-2} d^{-1} × 5). Cumulative cisplatin doses of 360 mg m^{-2} and 400 mg m^{-2}, respectively, were achieved. The nephrotoxicity was virtually identical in both arms with the median serum creatinine of the VAB-6 patients being 1.3 mg dl^{-1} after completion of therapy, while those in the EP group had a median serum creatinine of 1.2 mg dl^{-1}. Another study compared the toxicity of two cycles of an adjuvant VAB regimen with two cycles of an adjuvant PVB regimen. Again no difference in renal toxicity could be ascertained (Williams *et al.*, 1987b).

In spite of the apparent equivalence in efficacy and toxicity of either standard cisplatin regimen there is prospective evidence that the peak serum free platinum is predictive of ultimate nephrotoxicity (Reece *et al.*, 1987). Thus, cisplatin bolus doses (≥100 mg m^{-2}) would be predicted to be more toxic than small daily doses (20 mg m^{-2} d^{-1} × 5). These data raise concerns about the chronic nephrotoxicity potential of double-dose cisplatin regimens and those regimens employing 120 mg m^{-2} of cisplatin on days 1 and 8. It must be emphasized that, in spite of the concern about nephrotoxicity, such concern must be tempered by a sober reality; doses of cisplatin at ≤75 mg m^{-2} at 3-week intervals result in inferior survival from metastatic germ cell cancer (Samson *et al.*, 1984). Thus oncologists must tread a careful path between underdosing and overdosing cisplatin.

The etiology of cisplatin nephrotoxicity has been the subject of many reports. Whether this is due to a direct toxic effect of filtered reactive platinum species on the proximal tubule cells, a toxic effect of secreted reactive platinum species on the proximal tubule cell or a toxic effect of reactive platinum species on the microvasculature of the kidney is unknown. What is clear is that the final common pathway for cisplatin nephrotoxicity is damage to the proximal tubular epithelial cell. This damage is most frequently clinically manifested as a magnesium-wasting nephropathy (Schilsky, Barlock and Ozols, 1982; Vogelzang, Torkelson and Kennedy, 1985; Boyer *et al.*, 1990). Yet with careful quantification of urinary electrolyte excretions, one can define defects in virtually all proximal tubular functions (Bitran *et al.*, 1982). These defects apparently are self-limiting or self-healing, as long-term follow-up studies rarely identify patients with chronic tubular abnormalities (Bosl *et al.*, 1986; Hansen *et al.*, 1988). Although minor elevation of the serum creatinine is common after four to six doses of cisplatin (≥100 mg m^{-2} per dose), there has been no evidence to date that these patients progress to chronic renal failure (Hamilton, Bliss and Horwich, 1989). Indeed, kidney biopsies done at various intervals after cisplatin administration commonly show interstitial fibrosis and tubular atrophy but little evidence of glomerular damage or drop-out (Dentino *et al.*, 1978). Some have postulated that these biopsy findings implicate cisplatin-induced vascular damage to individual nephrons (Meijer *et al.*, 1983). A corollary of such a hypothesis is that the rare cases of abrupt and permanent renal failure (acute cortical necrosis) secondary to cisplatin are vascular in origin.

In spite of the less than precisely understood pathophysiology of cisplatin nephropathy, clinical guidelines have evolved that can prevent or dramatically ameliorate the toxicity in all but the most unusual cases. These guidelines generally call for vigorous hydration with 2–3 l of normal saline per 24 h prior to and during cisplatin doses of 20–30 mg m^{-2} per day. At doses over 100 mg m^{-2} single bolus dose, fluid management is critical. Adequate prehydration with normal saline solution is essential in order to ensure urine output of over 100 ml h^{-1} and preferably 150–200 ml h^{-1} immediately prior to cisplatin. Although doses of $\geqslant$100 mg m^{-2} can be rapidly infused ($\leqslant$30 min) almost all investigators now infuse the cisplatin mixed with 25 g mannitol over 6 h while maintaining brisk urine flow with intravenous fluid at rates of 200 ml h^{-1} or greater, combined with diuresis induced by furosemide. Other precautions to be taken when administering cisplatin include the avoidance of other nephrotoxins, such as contrast dyes and aminoglycoside antibiotics. New agents that may provide even better kidney protection than forced diuresis include WR-2721, which may protect the renal tubular cells from cisplatin free-radical-induced damage. With these precautions, acute renal failure should occur in less than 1% of treated patients.

Other toxicities of cisplatin occur infrequently. Endocrine side-effects have not been reported except for transient syndrome of inappropriate antidiuretic hormone (SIADH) (Ginsberg, Comis and Miller, 1982). The resultant hyponatremia may be aggravated if hypotonic fluids are used for forced diuresis.

Dermatological effects have not been reported except for nail banding. Alopecia is usually partial.

Sperm counts after cisplatin are reproducibly suppressed, in some cases for up to 2 years after cisplatin (Stoter *et al.*, 1989). Since all tests have been done in patients who received PVB, it is possible that the vinblastine and bleomycin contributed to the azoospermia. Bleomycin and vinblastine, as single agents, have minimal gonadal toxicity; this implicated the alkylator cisplatin as the culprit.

No instances of genetic damage (i.e. fetal abnormalities) have been linked to single agent cisplatin.

Lastly, there have been no clear-cut examples of cisplatin-induced orthopedic problems, i.e. osteoporosis, rhabdomyolysis etc.

30.2.2 CARBOPLATIN

Carboplatin, a nonnephrotoxic analogue of cisplatin, entered clinical trials after preclinical and Phase I testing at the Royal Marsden Hospital (Calvert *et al.*, 1982; 1989). Although it was rapidly integrated into first line regimens for metastatic testis cancer (Horwich *et al.*, 1989; Motzer *et al.*, 1987), subsequent phase III trials documented reduced efficacy for carboplatin compared with cisplatin (Bajorin *et al.*, 1993; Kattan *et al.*, 1993; Tjulandin *et al.*, 1993; Horwich and Sleijfer, 1994). Bone marrow toxicity and nausea and vomiting are the major and virtually only important clinical toxicities.

Anemia occurs in 49% of patients treated with single agent carboplatin (400 mg m^{-2}), with about 30% of patients requiring transfusions (Vogelzang *et al.*, 1990). Myelosuppression is clinically insignificant with a single dose of 400 mg m^{-2} in chemotherapy-naive, high-performance patients but is dose limiting on all schedules. Nadir granulocytopenia occurs between days 21 and 28. Thrombocytopenia (50 000 mm^{-3}) will occur in 15–30% of patients at such doses and is somewhat more severe than the granulocytopenia. Nadirs occur at days 15–21, with recovery by day 35. Myelosuppression is greater in patients with impaired renal function (Christian, 1989). Secondary leukemia from carboplatin has not been reported.

Neurological toxicity of carboplatin has been remarkably rare, with only anecdotal cases of optic neuritis and ototoxicity being reported. As doses are escalated, neurological toxicity becomes more common.

No pulmonary, cardiovascular, endocrine, dermatological or orthopedic toxicity has been reported with carboplatin. Reproductive toxicity has not been systematically searched for. Rare reports of allergic reactions and hemolytic–uremic syndrome have occurred.

Renal toxicity of carboplatin is extremely rare and is essentially not seen in patients with normal renal function and no prior exposure to nephrotoxic agents. In those patients with renal dysfunction, dosage can be modified to achieve appropriate myelosuppression (Egorin *et al.*, 1984; Calvert *et al.*, 1982; 1989).

Since myelosuppression is the major toxicity of carboplatin, it has found a significant role in preparatory regimens for autologous bone marrow transplantation (see Chapter 25) (Shea *et al.*, 1989). It appears that at doses of 1600 mg m^{-2} myeloid reconstitution occurs by 14 days. At doses of 2000 and 2400 mg m^{-2} marrow support is required. At such doses in patients with prior cisplatin exposures, significant renal dysfunction is seen in over 50% of patients. When carboplatin doses are escalated as part of bone marrow transplant conditioning regimens, enterocolitis and hepatic dysfunction can also be dose-limiting toxicities.

30.2.3   CYCLOPHOSPHAMIDE AND IFOSFAMIDE

The role of cyclophosphamide (CTX) (one of the five drugs in the VAB-6 regimen) in germ cell tumor chemotherapy (Buckner *et al.*, 1974) has been greatly diminished by two recent studies; Bosl *et al.* (1988) demonstrated that VAB-6 was more toxic and no more effective than etoposide and cisplatin, while Loehrer, Einhorn and Williams (1986) and Wheeler *et al.* (1986) demonstrated a major role for ifosfamide (IFX) as salvage therapy. Since both CTX and IFX are classical alkylators with nearly identical chemical structures and with activity in germ cell cancer chemotherapy, this section will review the toxicities of both agents. Cyclophosphamide is profoundly myelosuppressive, with thrombocytopenia and anemia being much less of a clinical problem. The leukopenia is abrupt (nadir by day 10) with rapid recovery (usually by day 14 and full recovery by day 21) when doses of 600–1500 mg m^{-2} are used. With higher doses and in bone marrow ablative doses recovery is prolonged (Buckner *et al.*, 1974). Secondary leukemia has been reported following the VAB regimens, since earlier VAB regimens contained chlorambucil (a potent leukemogen) as part of the maintenance program (Redman *et al.*, 1984). Secondary leukemia following VAB-6, which contains the weak leukemogen CTX (600 mg m^{-2} IV at 4-week intervals × 3 cycles), is anecdotal. Ifosfamide is less myelosuppressive and secondary leukemia has not yet been reported.

Gastrointestinal toxicities of both CTX and IFX are limited to abrupt nausea and vomiting, which usually resolves 24 h post dosing. At very high doses CTX may cause hepatic veno-occlusive disease.

Neurological toxicities, including somnolence and confusion, and lethargy, can occur following IFX. The mechanism causing the toxicity is unknown. It appears to be related to delayed clearance of the drug or one of its metabolites (chloracetaldehyde) since prior cisplatin administration increases the risk of developing the complication. Treatment of the central nervous system toxicity is supportive as most patients' symptoms resolve within 3 days of onset (Goren *et al.*, 1988).

Cardiac toxicity appears to be restricted to high dose CTX. This hemorrhagic carditis is extremely rare and is usually rapidly fatal. If patients can be supported, recovery does occur and can be complete.

The renal toxicity of CTX is limited to hemorrhagic cystitis (Levine and Richie, 1989). Ifosfamide on the other hand may cause both a renal parenchymal lesion and hemorrhagic cystitis. The renal parenchymal lesion is identified by a rapidly rising serum creatinine level and oliguria. The etiology of the acute renal failure is presumably due to a tubular defect caused by a metabolite of IFX. Treatment is supportive with avoidance of future IFX (Zalupski and Baker, 1988).

Hemorrhagic cystitis is a major toxicity of both IFX and CTX. In initial studies, virtually 100% of patients treated with IFX developed the toxicity. Aggressive hydration and continuous infusion schedules of IFX obviated some of the toxicity. With the introduction of the sulfhydryl compounds (mesna and others) IFX could be safely given. These compounds scavenge or bind the acrolein derivatives that cause hemorrhagic cystitis. With mesna used in appropriate doses, hemorrhagic cystitis should occur in only 5–10% of patients receiving IFX (Zalupski and Baker, 1988). Hemorrhagic cystitis is rare in testicular cancer patients.

Once hemorrhagic cystitis occurs with either drug its management can be difficult (Levine and Richie, 1989). Bladder irrigation and instillation with formalin has been the usual management. Recently a prostaglandin E_2 analogue 'carboplast' instilled intravesically has shown considerable promise. Occasionally the bladder telangiectasias can be successfully fulgurated, but chronic intermittent hematuria can also result.

The feared long-term toxicity of both CTX and IFX on the bladder is the induction of bladder cancer. A recent report from Denmark suggested that chronic oral CTX (used to treat autoimmune disease) increased the risk of developing bladder cancer 20-fold (Pedersen-Bjergaard *et al.*, 1988). The increasing use of IFX in testis cancer patients may lead to a late risk of bladder cancer. Patients cured with IFX-containing regimens should be closely followed for this toxicity.

Endocrine side-effects of CTX and IFX appear to be rare. The syndrome of inappropriate antidiuretic hormone (SIADH) occurs following high dose CTX and is related to a circulating metabolite of CTX that causes impairment of free-water excretion (De Fronzo *et al.*, 1973).

Reproductive toxicity of CTX and IFX has been recently reviewed as well. The degree and reversibility of IFX gonadal toxicity (azoospermia) has not been determined. Cyclophosphamide gonadal toxicity appears to be irreversible.

30.2.4 VINCA ALKALOIDS; VINCRISTINE AND VINBLASTINE

Vincristine (VCR) and vinblastine (VLB) have substantial activity and continue to be a part of many second line treatment regimens. Vinblastine causes a brisk leukopenia (nadir by days 4–6, recovery by days 10–12) with an associated thrombocytosis. Anemia is minimal (Samuels and Howe, 1970). Vincristine has no marrow toxicity, which makes it an ideal agent in second or third line regimens. In patients with progressive disease and bone marrow fatigue or failure following previous chemotherapy, it may provide palliation.

Both drugs cause minimal nausea and vomiting except with high doses of VLB. Both are commonly associated with a paralytic ileus, presumably due to autonomic neuropathy (Costa, Hreshchyshyn and Holland, 1962; Samuels and Howe, 1970). The management of ileus induced by these drugs may

Table 30.3 Neuromuscular toxicity of cisplatin/vinblastine/bleomycin (percentage of patients)

Toxicity	None	Mild	Severe
Paresthesias	62%	27%	11%
Abdominal cramps	80%	12%	8%
Myalgias	81%	5%	14%

From Williams *et al.* (1987a).

require IV fluids and nasogastric suction for several days. Full recovery within 4–6 days is the rule.

Both drugs cause a dose-related peripheral sensory neuropathy of the 'stocking-glove' variety, presumably due to tubulin disruption in the axons. Vincristine is more potent than VLB in this regard. There is no effective treatment for the neurotoxicity, although the symptoms may slowly abate over several years. The frequency with which 'neuromuscular' toxicity occurs following PVB presumably due primarily to VLB has been documented by Williams *et al.* (1987a) and is shown in Table 30.3.

There are no known pulmonary or renal toxicities of the vinca alkaloids.

Cardiac toxicity of the vinca alkaloids is anecdotal, with scattered case reports describing myocardial infarctions during or within hours of administration of a dose (Subar and Muggia, 1986). There are no known valvular or myopathic toxicities.

Endocrine toxicities of the vinca alkaloids have been incompletely studied. Although reported to cause SIADH, the frequency of and the mechanism responsible for the toxicity are unclear, (Antony *et al.*, 1980). Ginsberg, Comis and Miller (1982) studied 12 patients receiving PVB prospectively for the occurrence of SIADH. All 12 had a fall in serum sodium or developed hypo-osmolality and four had symptoms attributable to hyponatremia. Whether the SIADH is attributable solely to VLB is unclear as all patients also received cisplatin. If one assumes a neurotoxic hypothalamic event leading to SIADH, other pituitary hormone changes should also

be present. Such changes have neither been looked for nor reported.

Vinblastine and vincristine are both vesicants that lead to blistering, pain, erythema and edema if extravasated. Neither agent, however, causes permanent skin necrosis or ulceration. They both cause partial to complete alopecia.

The gonadal toxicities of the vinca alkaloids are presumed to be minimal. Few direct experimental data are available to support that hypothesis however.

The 'orthopedic/muscular' toxicities of the vinca alkaloids are unique. Severe sensorimotor neuropathy with foot drop may, on rare occasions, progress to quadriparesis. Severe transient muscle pain may occur with high doses of either drug. Its etiology is not understood but is presumed to be a toxicity to the nerves innervating the muscles (i.e. jaw pain of vinblastine is clinically indistinguishable from trigeminal neuralgia).

The toxicities of the vinca alkaloids are highly dependent upon the dose and schedule of drug administration. For example, the dose-limiting toxicity of the long-term continuous infusion schedule is myelotoxicity for both drugs (Ratain and Vogelzang, 1986). At higher doses, or with shorter infusions, neurotoxicity and myelosuppression occur (Logothetis *et al.*, 1985). Krikorian *et al.* (1978) described a 70–80% probability of 'serious' toxicity when the vinblastine dose was escalated past $0.18 \, \text{mg kg}^{-1}$ daily for 2 days ($0.36 \, \text{mg kg}^{-1}$ as part of the PVB regimen). This threshold was lower for patients with a Karnofsky performance status ≤80. Einhorn and Williams (1980) confirmed those data by performing a three-armed randomized trial varying primarily in the total vinblastine dose; PVB ($0.4 \, \text{mg kg}^{-1}$), PVB ($0.3 \, \text{mg kg}^{-1}$) and PVB plus Adriamycin (doxorubicin hydrochloride) ($0.2 \, \text{mg kg}^{-1}$). Granulocytopenic fevers occurred in 35, 15 and 24% of patients and documented sepsis occurred in 12, 0 and 4% of patients, respectively. The $0.3 \, \text{mg kg}^{-1}$ dose was recommended as standard therapy since there was no difference in the complete response rate or 'free of disease' rate.

The chronic neuropathy that occurs after PVB has recently been the subject of four reports. Roth *et al.* (1988) reported a 43% incidence of paresthesia at a median follow-up of 7 years. Stoter *et al.* (1989) reported that 68% of long-term survivors by self-report had neuropathy. All patients, however, had received maintenance chemotherapy with vinblastine 0.2–0.3 mg kg^{-1} and cisplatin 50 mg m^{-2} at 3-week intervals for up to 2 years. Hansen *et al.* (1989) analyzed 30 patients cured with PVB, and found that 73% has sensory loss, 50% had paresthesia, and 80% had an increased vibration perception threshold. They attributed most of this chronic neuropathy to cisplatin, not vinblastine. The relative contribution of either agent is difficult to estimate. Boyer *et al.* (1990) performed nerve conduction studies on 30 long-term survivors treated with PVB and found that 50% had diminished sensory action potential amplitudes. Chronic neuropathy is a common late complication of PVB.

30.2.5   ETOPOSIDE (VP-16, VEPOSIDE^R)

This semisynthetic plant alkaloid is the second most active single agent in germ cell cancer (Fitzharris *et al.*, 1980; Vogelzang, Raghavan and Kennedy, 1982; Ozols *et al.*, 1985). Etoposide is virtually a purely myelo-suppressive agent given in the usual doses of 100 mg m^{-2} d^{-1} × 5 or 120–150 mg m^{-2} d^{-1} × 3. The nadir white blood cell and platelet counts occur on days 12–17. Anemia tends to be severe and progressive when etoposide is combined with cisplatin. This effect is much less apparent with single agent etoposide. With large cumulative doses after prolonged use and using an unusual weekly schedule rare cases of acute monocytic leukemia (M-5 FAB subtype) have been reported (Ratain *et al.*, 1987).

Secondary, or therapy-related malignancies, especially acute myelogenous leukemia (AML) are a dreaded toxicity of chemotherapy for testicular cancer. Acute leukemia was extremely rare following alkylating agent-containing (VAB1-6) chemotherapy (Redman *et al.*, 1984). With the introduction of etoposide-based salvage chemotherapy and the use of high dose etoposide in bone marrow transplant salvage chemotherapy regimens in the mid 1980s, sporadic reports began to appear of secondary AML in patients apparently cured with such salvage chemotherapy. Initially, the AML cases were thought to be related to either prior radiation use, prior alkylating agents, or a rare complication of mediastinal germ cell tumors which differentiated to leukemia (Downie, *et al.*, 1994). However, the cytogenetic analysis of the etoposide-related leukemias commonly showed a translocation at chromosome 11q23 (Ratain *et al.*, 1987). Furthermore, the clinical characteristics of the leukemias included a short latency of 2 to 3 years, the absence of a preleukemia myelo-dysplastic phase and a predominance of myelomonocytic or monocytic morphology. These leukemias appeared exclusively in germ cell tumor patients who had received high doses of etoposide, although other cases were reported following high dose doxo-rubicin, another topoisomerase-II-inhibiting drug (Pedersen-Bjergaard, 1995). The gene involved in this leukemia is called *MLL* (myeloid lymphoid leukemia) (Thirman *et al.*, 1993; Thirman and Larson, 1995) and is involved in all 11q23 leukemias. Its function remains unknown. There have now been at least five retrospective studies performed in germ cell tumor patients attempting to estimate the risk of etoposide-related leukemia (Table 30.4). There have been 19 cases in over 2267 patients analyzed (0.8%). This places these patients at a relative risk of 30–336 times the normal for the development of leukemia. The leukemia is characterized by an onset of 24 to 36 months postchemotherapy, usually of M-4 FAB subtype and abnormalities at 11q23 and t(8;21). According to Boshoff *et al.* (1995) five of six patients

Table 30.4 Risk of myelodysplasia and leukemia following etoposide/cisplatin-based chemotherapy for germ cell tumor

Reference	No. patients treated with VP-16	No. patients alive at risk (median surv)	No. patients with leukemia (%)	Relative risk (CI)
Pedersen-Bjergaard *et al.*, 1991	212*	Not stated	5 (67%)	336 (92–861)
Nichols *et al.*, 1993	538** (on clinical trials)	315 (4.9 years)	2 (0.6%)	66 (8–238)
Nichols *et al.*, 1993	Several hundred not on clinical trials	Unknown	3 (unknown)	Not stated
Bajorin *et al.*, 1993	503	343 (not stated)	2 (0.6%)	Not stated
Boshoff *et al.*, 1995	679	529 (5.7 years)	6 (0.8%)	150 (55–326)
Bokemeyer *et al.*, 1995	335	128 (4.5 years)	1 (0.8%)	30–35x
Total	2267+		19 (0.8%)	

* 82 received more than 2000 mg m^2 etoposide cumulative dose.
** All received less than 2000 mg m^2 etoposide cumulative dose.

responded to chemotherapy but four of five relapsed and died.

In summary, etoposide-related leukemia is a rare toxicity. A cumulative etoposide dose >2000 mg m^{-2} may be a risk factor but cases have occurred at low cumulative doses (720 mg m^{-2}). Lifelong follow-up of such patients is now suggested. The National Cancer Institute (USA) has in place a careful monitoring program of patients previously treated on clinical trials (Smith *et al.*, 1993).

No unusual types of gastrointestinal toxicity (other than nausea, vomiting and stomatitis) have been reported with etoposide. At high doses, veno-occlusive disease has been observed.

Other toxicities of etoposide are rare (Table 30.2) except for alopecia and oligospermia.

30.2.6 BLEOMYCIN

This high molecular weight polypeptide antineoplastic antibiotic has a unique mechanism of action and a unique spectrum of toxicity. The toxicities (cutaneous, pulmonary, vascular and allergic) are both idiopathic and dose related, occurring sporadically at low doses and with increasing frequency at cumulative doses over 360 U total dose. Thus, in germ cell tumor specific chemotherapy regimens,

cumulative bleomycin doses over 300–360 U are usually not allowed (see Chapter 20).

The chronic effect of bleomycin on pulmonary function in cured testis cancer patients has not been vigorously evaluated. Aass *et al.* (1990) reported that 17% of 72 cured patients reported 'pulmonary symptoms', while Stuart *et al.* (1990), using more sophisticated measures, reported that the majority of 27 patients had respiratory impairment related to the total dose of bleomycin.

The toxicity parameters of bleomycin may be schedule dependent. Bleomycin is given as a bolus (30 U IV q. week) in the bleomycin/etoposide/cisplatin (BEP), PVB and carboplatin/etoposide/bleomycin (CEB) regimens while it is given with a loading IV dose (30 mg) followed by an infusion (15 U d^{-1} × 3) in the VAB regimens. Preclinical data support a decreased pulmonary toxicity of the continuous infusion regimen (Comis *et al.*, 1979; van Barneveld *et al.*, 1985). A direct comparison of a VAB regimen with the PVB regimen was reported by the Testicular Cancer Intergroup Study (TCIS). These data suggest that the infusion schedule has less pulmonary and marrow toxicity while the bolus schedule is more myelosuppressive (Williams *et al.*, 1987b). Stomatitis was more frequent with the VAB regimen. Although other drugs may have contributed to the stomatitis, the data suggest a therapeutic advantage to the infusion schedule of bleomycin.

With these caveats about the toxicity parameters as a function of drug schedules, the toxicity patterns of bleomycin are rather predictable (see Table 30.2).

The bone marrow toxicity of bleomycin is minor, although occasionally severe thrombocytopenia occurs, possibly due to an autoimmune thrombocytopenia. Gastrointestinal toxicity is confined to stomatitis. The stomatitis is clinically similar to *Herpes simplex* virus (HSV) oral ulceration and thus HSV should be looked for and treated, if present, in patients with presumed bleomycin stomatitis. The stomatitis is more severe and longer lasting in patients with coexistent renal insufficiency, suggesting that delayed renal clearance leading to either higher peak levels, longer duration of drug or metabolite exposure or both is a predictor of the severity of bleomycin stomatitis.

The hyperpigmentation of bleomycin is not viewed by physicians as a major toxicity. However, patients who develop the diffuse yellowing followed by darkening of the skin can be significantly distressed, especially when the changes occur on the face. The classical 'flagellate striae' on the back and trunk may not disappear for years after completion of therapy. Similarly the darkened skin at the elbows, pressure points, finger tips and skin creases can be disfiguring and long lasting. The hyperpigmentation appears to be the end result of bleomycin-induced collagen cross-linking and an excessive accumulation of hydroxyproline in the skin. How this biochemical abnormality leads to hyperpigmentation is unclear.

Raynaud's phenomenon (RP) has occurred following single agent bolus doses of bleomycin (Von Gunten *et al.*, 1993). Likewise necrosis of the digits has anecdotally occurred in the setting of long-term maintenance bolus doses of bleomycin. Virtually all reports of Raynaud's phenomenon after testicular cancer chemotherapy have been in patients receiving BEP or PVB-type chemotherapy. Regimens of VAB and EP have virtually never been reported to induce Raynaud's phenomenon. This suggests (but does not prove) that bolus doses of bleomycin cause Raynaud's phenomenon in occasional patients.

Raynaud's phenomenon following vinblastine and bleomycin has been well documented since Teutsch, Lipton and Harvey (1977) reported a single case. Table 30.5 lists the reports that have described the phenomenon. On average, 19% of all patients will experience the toxicity; with bleomycin-containing regimens the incidence may be close to 50%. When both vinblastine and bleomycin are omitted and replaced by etoposide (Bosl *et al.*, 1988), Raynaud's phenomenon is not seen. Interestingly those series analyzing patients with ice-water immersion studies (Vogelzang *et al.*, 1981; Hansen *et al.*, 1988; Aass *et al.*, 1990) reported that 43–46% of patients had Raynaud's phenomenon following PVB. Series which report a lower incidence performed no provocative tests. The Raynaud's phenomenon appears to be relatively nonreversible, leading some patients to change jobs or places of residence. This toxicity has led to conjecture that other vessels could be affected by chemotherapy. Table 30.6 lists those reports. Several tentative conclusions can be drawn:

1. There appears to be both an acute and a chronic vascular toxicity of PVB. The acute toxicity usually involves coronary artery lesions and may be due to hypomagnesemia, fluid shifts or other intravascular changes. The chronic toxicity of Raynaud's phenomenon usually involves only digital arterial changes and is probably due to fibrosis of the small vessels. The variable frequency with which it is observed is

Table 30.5 Reports describing Raynaud's phenomenon following chemotherapy for germ cell tumors

Reference	Drug regimen	Number of cases/ number treated	Frequency (%)
Teutsch, Lipton and Harvey (1977)	VB	1	—
Rothberg (1978)	VB	1	—
Chernicoff, Bukowski and Young (1978)	VB	1	—
Vogelzang et al. (1981)	VB	3/14	21
Vogelzang et al. (1981)	PVB	19/46	41
Scheulen and Schmidt (1982)	VB/AP	8/271	3
Garnick et al. (1983)	PVB	7/54	13
Samson et al. (1984)	PVB	2/114	2
Vogelzang, Torkelson and Kennedy (1985)	PVB	13/30	43
Roth et al. (1988)	PVB	72/147	49†
Williams et al. (1987a)	BEP	15/224	7
Bosl et al. (1988)	EP	0/82	0
Boyer et al. (1990)*	PVB	8/30	27
Stefenelli et al. (1988)*	PVB	10/21	47.6
Hansen and Olsen (1989)*	PVB	14/32	44
Stoter et al. (1989)*	PVB	13/57	23
Bissett et al. (1990)*	Cisplatin-based	26/74	35
Aass et al. (1990)*	Cisplatin-based	33/72	46
Gietema et al. (1992)*	PVB/BEP	13/59	22
Total		256/1327	19

* Retrospective studies on long-term survivors.
† 'Digital cold sensitivity'.
V, vinblastine. B, bleomycin. P, cisplatin, E, etoposide. A, Adriamycin.

unexplained and may reflect investigator bias.

2. The toxicity is heterogeneous and is probably a continuum from micro- to macrovascular disease. Approximately 30–40% of patients treated with PVB will develop transient or chronic Raynaud's phenomenon. Approximately 20–25% of patients appear to develop hypertension (Stoter et al., 1989; Bissett et al., 1990; Boyer et al., 1990; Gietema et al., 1992). Such hypertension may be a manifestation of cisplatin-induced renal dysfunction, bleomycin-induced vascular disease, or a result of both.

Far fewer patients have yet developed large vessel disease, keeping in mind that the median follow-up of such patients is only 7 years (Gietema et al., 1992). In a long-term follow-up of patients receiving only two cycles of PVB or VAB, Nichols et al. (1992) found no significant vascular disease. Thus large vessel toxicity may be related to the cumulative doses of vinblastine and bleomycin.

3. The proximate cause for the toxicity remains conjectural. Vinca-induced vascular spasm, bleomycin-related endothelial cell damage, chemotherapy-induced coagulopathy and cisplatin-induced hypomagnesemia (leading to vascular hyperreactivity) are hypothetical causes. Recently Hansen et al. (1989) compared patients suffering PVB-induced Raynaud's phenomenon with normal control patients. Raynaud's phenomenon patients did not have structural intravascular obstruction but did have an increased vasoconstrictive response. They postulate hyperreactivity of the central sympathetic nervous system as the cause for vasospastic Raynaud's phenomenon. No specific cause for the

Table 30.6   Reports describing vascular toxicity (other than Raynaud's phenomenon) following chemotherapy for germ cell tumors of the testis

Reference	Drug regimens	Toxicity	Number of cases/ number treated
Edwards, Lane and Smith (1979)	PVB	CAD	2
Vogelzang, Frenning and Kennedy (1980)	VB+	CAD	2
Bodensteiner (1981)	PVB	AMI	1
Jackson *et al.* (1984)	PVB	Other	2
Roth *et al.* (1988)	PVB	CAD	6/147
Bosl *et al.* (1988)	VAB-6	Other	1
Stoter *et al.* (1989)	PVB	AMI	2/57
		Hypertension	10/56
Doll *et al.* (1986)	PVB	CAD	2
		CVA	2
Samuels, Vogelzang and Kennedy (1987)	PVB	AMI	3
		CVA	1
		Other	1
Stefenelli *et al.* (1988)	PVB	Angina	8/21
Nichols *et al.* (1992)	PVB or VAB	CVA, AMI	0/97
Boyer *et al.* (1990)	PVB	Hypertension	4/30
		AMI	0/30
Bissett *et al.* (1990)	Various	Hypertension	18/74
Gietema *et al.* (1992)	PVB or BEP	Hypertension	16/57
		AMI	1/57

CAD, Coronary artery disease. CVA, cerebrovascular accident. AMI, acute myocardial infarction. Other, peripheral arterial embolus, rectal infarction, thrombotic microangiopathy. PVB, cisplatin/vinblastine/bleomycin. VAB, vinblastine/cyclophosphamide/actinomycin-D/bleomycin/cisplatin. VB, vinblastine/bleomycin.

hyperreactivity of the sympathetic system was advanced.

4. Further clinical investigation of this intriguing toxicity has been hampered by its infrequency. The omission of bleomycin and vinblastine and the increased use of etoposide in germ cell tumor treatment regimens is apparently responsible for a declining incidence of such toxicity.

30.2.7   ACTINOMYCIN-D

This DNA-intercalating antibiotic has a consistent but low level of activity in germ cell cancers (Merrin and Murphy, 1974). It was an integral part of the VAB regimens and remains a part of the cisplatin/vincristine/methotrexate/bleomycin/etoposide/dactinomycin/cyclophosphamide (POMB/ACE) regimen. It is emetogenic and causes stomatitis (Table 30.2). It has few other major toxicities, and since its role in germ cell tumor chemotherapy is minimal, a detailed review of its toxicity will not be performed.

30.2.8   MITHRAMYCIN

This RNA-inhibiting antibiotic, although active as a single agent, has not been successfully integrated into combination chemotherapy. This is due in part to its unpredictable hepatic, renal and marrow toxicity (Brown and Kennedy, 1965; Kennedy, 1970). Since this drug has been rarely used to treat germ cell cancer in the 1980s and since anecdotal experience with using the drug suggests significant renal toxicity in cisplatin-exposed patients, a detailed review of its toxicity will not be performed.

30.2.9 DOXORUBICIN

This anthracycline antibiotic, although exhibiting single agent activity (Monfardini *et al.*, 1972), has not been successfully integrated into combination chemotherapy owing, in part, to the negative results from a randomized study (Einhorn and Williams, 1980). The major reports of its use in combination chemotherapy for germ cell cancer come from the M.D. Anderson Hospital. The regimen used at that institution, the cyclophosphamide/doxorubicin/cisplatin (CISCA)/VB-4, builds upon the Samuels *et al.* regimen of continuous infusion bleomycin and vinblastine using dose escalation of bleomycin and vinblastine (Logothetis *et al.*, 1985). To this 'base' regimen is added cisplatin and doxorubicin (50 mg m^{-2}). Although toxicity patterns can be difficult to attribute to specific drugs, doxorubicin causes a brisk neutropenia with mild anemia and thrombocytopenia. The only other clinically significant toxicities include stomatitis, alopecia, delayed cardiomyopathy (Lipshultz *et al.*, 1995) and skin necrosis at sites of extravasation. Numerous reviews on this important drug are available.

30.2.10 METHOTREXATE AND 5-FLUOROURACIL

These two antimetabolites are widely used in oncological medicine and yet are not integral parts of any standard regimen for germ cell cancer. 5-Fluorouracil (5-FU) was never studied in a systematic fashion as a single agent in germ cell tumors. It was used as part of the 'COMF' by several investigators (Mendelson and Serpick, 1970) without good rationale. Since 5-FU has no role in current management strategies, a detailed review will not be performed.

Methotrexate plays a significant role in the cure of gestational trophoblastic disease and metastatic choriocarcinoma (Wyatt and McAninch, 1967). It was an important drug in the curative 'triple therapy' regimens of Li *et al.* (1960) and has significant single agent activity. It has found little if any role in modern combination chemotherapy regimens for germ cell cancer, the exception being the POMB/ACE regimen used at the Charing Cross Hospital.

The Charing Cross Hospital regimen uses methotrexate at a dose of 300 mg m^{-2} IV infusion over 12 h on day 1 of treatment, followed by folinic acid rescue (Hitchins *et al.*, 1989). The contribution of methotrexate to the overall effectiveness of the regimen is unknown. Most physicians are reluctant to use methotrexate in cisplatin-treated patients owing to potential synergistic nephrotoxicity.

Recently Levi *et al.* (1990) designed a salvage regimen called EAM, etoposide (75 mg m^{-2} × 3), actinomycin-D (1 mg m^{-2} on day 1) and methotrexate (30 mg m^{-2} on day 1). This moderately toxic regimen induced a white blood cell count of less than 1000×10^9 l^{-1} in 2% of patients (one of 51), anemia in 28% of patients, severe nausea and vomiting in 79% of patients and stomatitis in 42% of patients. The nausea and vomiting were attributed to the actinomycin-D and the stomatitis to the methotrexate. Fifteen of 51 patients achieved a long-term disease-free state, with this well-tolerated regimen. The role of methotrexate in refractory germ cell tumors should be explored.

30.3 TOXICITIES OF COMBINATIONS

Table 30.7 lists the toxicities of the nine chemotherapy regimens in common use today. Most of the toxicities have been reviewed in the section on single agents, but several facts are worth repeating.

1. Since effectiveness could not be retained, the replacement of cisplatin by carboplatin will not lead to a major reduction in cisplatin-associated toxicity.
2. Omission of bleomycin (or restricting its use to nine doses; Loehrer *et al.*, 1995) will eliminate hyperpigmentation, pulmonary

Table 30.7 Toxicity patterns of the chemotherapy regimens used to treat metastatic germ cell tumors of the testis

Toxicity	PVB	VAB-6	CISCA/ VB-4	PEB	PE	POMB/ ACE	CEB	CE	VIP
Anemia	+++	+++	+++	+++	+++	+++	+++	+++	+++
Myelosuppression	+++	++	++++	+++	+++	++	+++	+++	+++
Thrombocytopenia	+	++	+++	+++	+++	+++	+++	+++	+++
Secondary leukemia	—	AN	AN	—	—	AN	—	—	—
Stomatitis	++	+	+++	++	+	++	++	+	+
Emesis	+++	+++	+++	+++	+++	+++	+	+	+++
Ileus	++	++	+++	—	—	—	—	—	—
Diarrhea	++	++	++	++	++	++	—	—	++
Hepatic	—	—	—	—	—	—	—	—	—
Central nerves	—	—	—	—	—	—	—	—	+
Peripheral nerves	++	++	++	—	—	++	—	—	—
Cranial nerves	AN	AN	AN	—	—	AN	—	—	—
Pulmonary	++	+	+	++	—	—	—	—	—
Hypertension	+/−	+/−	+/−	+/−	+/−	+/−	—	—	+/−
Cardiac muscle	—	—	—	—	—	—	—	—	—
Large vessel	+/−	+/−	+/−	+/−	—	—	+/−	—	?
Small vessel	++	++	++	++	—	—	++	—	?
Nephrotoxicity	++	++	++	++	++	++	—	—	++
Bladder toxicity	—	—	—	—	—	+	—	—	+
Endocrine	—	—	—	—	—	—	—	—	—
Hyperpigmentation	+++	+++	+++	+++	—	+++	+++	—	—
Alopecia	+++	+++	+++	+++	+++	+++	+++	+++	+++
Azoospermia	+++	+++	+++	+++	+++	+++	+	+	?
Genetic damage	AN	AN	AN	AN	AN	AN	?	?	?
Muscular	++	+	+++	—	—	+	—	—	—

AN, anecdotal.
—, not reported.
+, WHO Grade 1.
++, WHO Grade 2.
+++, WHO Grade 3.
++++, WHO Grade 4.
PVB cisplatin/vinblastine/bleomycin. VAB, vinblastine/actinomycin-D/bleomycin/cyclophosphamide/cisplatin. CISCA/ VB-4, cyclophosphamide/doxorubicin/cisplatin/vinblastine/bleomycin. PEB, cisplatin/etoposide/bleomycin. PE, cisplatin/ etoposide. POMB/ACE, cisplatin/vincristine/methotrexate/bleomycin/etoposide/actinomycin-D/cyclophosphamide. CEB, carboplatin/etoposide/bleomycin. CE, carboplatin/etoposide. VIP, etoposide/ifosfamide/cisplatin.

toxicity and probably Raynaud's phenomenon. Stomatitis should also be decreased. The Australian trial comparing PEB with EP will be critical in this regard.

3. Azoospermia and infertility are a result of most current regimens. Carboplatin-based regimens appear to be less damaging to fertility (Horwich *et al.*, 1995). Time to recovery of fertility and extent of return are a complex function of pretreatment sperm counts, age at diagnosis and amount and type of chemotherapy. The Indiana University group has reported on 30 patients treated with 24 cycles of BEP

24–78 months prior to a single semen analysis. The median sperm count was only 33.9 × 10^6, with only one patient having more than 50% of normal spermatozoa. Such chemotherapy causes persistent semen abnormalities (Stephenson *et al.*, 1995).

30.4 CONCLUSIONS

In conclusion, the toxicities of chemotherapy for germ cell tumors have been significantly decreasing over the past five years as etoposide has replaced bleomycin and vinblastine. Further toxicity reduction has occurred through improved antiemetics and through improved prevention of nephrotoxicity.

The future will bring even greater reductions in toxicity as recombinant erythropoietin and the colony-stimulating factors reduce bone marrow toxicities. The day may come when the most significant toxicity of the chemotherapy is the time and cost of administering it.

REFERENCES

Aass, N. *et al.* (1990) Long-term somatic side-effects and morbidity in testicular cancer patients. *Br. J. Cancer*, **61**, 151–5.

Ackland, S.P. and Vogelzang, N.J. (1987) Cisplatin, platinum analogues, and other heavy metal complexes, in *Cancer Chemotherapy by Infusion* (ed. J.J. Lokich), Precept Press Inc. Chicago, IL.

Addelmann, M. *et al.* (1990) Phase I/II trial of granisetron: A novel 5-hydroxytryptamine antagonist for the prevention of chemotherapy-induced nausea and vomiting. *J. Clin. Oncol.*, **8**, 337–41.

Alberts, D.S. and Noel, J.K. (1995) Cisplatin-associated neurotoxicity: can it be prevented? *Anti-Cancer Drugs*, **6**, 369–83.

Antony, A. *et al.* (1980) Inappropriate antidiuretic hormone secretion after high dose vinblastine. *J. Urol.*, **123**, 783–4.

Bajorin, D.F., Motzer, R.J., Rodriguez, E., Murphy, B. and Bosl, G.J. (1993) Acute nonlymphocytic leukemia in germ cell tumor patients treated with etoposide-containing chemotherapy. *J. Natl. Cancer Inst.*, **85**, 60–2.

Bissett, D., Kunkeler, L., Zwaneburg, L., Paul, J.

Gray, C., Swan, I.R. Kerr, D.J. and Kaye, S.B. (1990) Long-term sequelae of treatment for testicular germ cell tumours. *Br. J. Cancer*, **62** (4), Oct., 655–9.

Bitran, J.D. *et al.* (1982) Acute nephrotoxicity following *cis*-dichlorodi-ammine-platinum. *Cancer*, **49**, 1784–8.

Bodensteiner, D.C. (1981) Fatal coronary artery fibrosis after treatment with bleomycin, vinblastine, and *cis*-platinum. *Southern Med. J.*, **74**, 898–9.

Bokemeyer, C., Schmoll, H.-J., Kuczyk, M.A., Beyer, J. and Siegert, W. (1995) Risk of secondary leukemia following high cumulative doses of etoposide during chemotherapy for testicular cancer. *J. Natl. Cancer Inst.*, **87**, 58–60.

Boshoff, C., Begent, R.H., Oliver, R.T., *et al.* (1995) Secondary tumours following etoposide containing therapy for germ cell cancer. *Ann. Oncol.*, **6**; 35–40.

Bosl G.J. *et al.* (1988) A randomized trial of Etoposide + Cisplatin versus Vinblastine + Bleomycin + Cisplatin + Cyclophosphamide + Dactinomycin in patients with good prognosis germ cell tumors. *J. Clin. Oncol.*, **6**, 1231–8.

Bosl, G.J. *et al.* (1986) Increased plasma renin and aldosterone in patients treated with cisplatin-based chemotherapy for metastatic germ-cell tumors. *J. Clin. Oncol.*, **4**, 1684–9.

Boyer, M. *et al.* (1990) Lack of late toxicity in patients treated with cisplatin-containing combination chemotherapy for metastatic testicular cancer. *J. Clin. Oncol.*, **8**, 21–6.

Brown, J.H. and Kennedy, B.J. (1965) Mithramycin in the treatment of disseminated testicular neoplasms. *N. Engl. J. Med.*, **272**, 111–18.

Buckner, C.D. *et al.* (1974) High dose cyclophosphamide (NSC26271) for the treatment of metastatic testicular neoplasms. *Cancer Chemother. Rep.*, **58**, 709–14.

Calvert, A.H. *et al.* (1982) Early clinical studies with *cis*-diammine-1-1-cyclobutanedicarboxylate platinum II. *Cancer Chemother. Pharmacol.*, **9**, 40–7.

Calvert, A.H. *et al.* (1989) Carboplatin dosage: Prospective evaluation of a simple formula based on renal function. *J. Clin. Oncol.*, **7**, 1748–56.

Chernicoff, D.P., Bukowski, R.M. and Young, J.R. (1978) Raynaud's phenomenon after bleomycin treatment. *Cancer Treat. Rep.*, **62**, 570–1.

Christian, M.C. (1989) Carboplatin, in *Principles and Practice of Oncology Updates. 3(11)* (eds V.T.

DeVita Jr, S. Hellman and S.A. Rosenberg), J.B. Lippincott Co., Philadelphia PA, pp. 1–16.

Comis, R.L. *et al.* (1979) Role of single-breath carbon monoxide-diffusing capacity in monitoring the pulmonary effects of bleomycin in germ cell tumor patients. *Cancer Res.*, **39**, 5076–80.

Costa, G., Hreshchyshyn, M.M. and Holland, J.F. (1962) Initial clinical studies with Vincristine. *Cancer Chemother. Rep.*, **24**, 39–44.

De Fronzo, R.A. *et al.* (1973) Water intoxication in man after cyclophosphamide therapy: Time course and relation to drug activation. *Ann. Intern. Med.*, **78**, 861–9.

Dentino, M. *et al.* (1978) Long-term effect of cisdiamminedichloride platinum (DDP) on renal function and structure in man. *Cancer*, **41**, 1274–81.

Doll, D.C. *et al.* (1986) Acute vascular ischemic events after cisplatin-based combination chemotherapy for germ-cell tumors of the testis. *Ann. Intern. Med.*, **105**, 48–51.

Downie, P.A., Vogelzang, N.J., Moldwin, R.L., *et al.* (1994) Establishment of a leukemia cell line with $i(12p)$ from a patient with a mediastinal germ cell tumor and acute lymphoblastic leukemia. *Cancer Res*, **54**; 4999–5004.

Edwards, G.S., Lane, M. and, Smith, F.E. (1979) Long-term treatment with *cis*-dichlorodiammineplatinum (II)-vinblastine-bleomycin: possible association with severe coronary artery disease. *Cancer Treat. Rep.*, **63**, 551–2.

Egorin, M.J. *et al.* (1984) Pharmacokinetics and dosage reduction of *cis*-diammine (1, 1-cyclobutanedicarboxylate) platinum in patients with impaired renal function. *Cancer Res.*, **44**, 5432–8.

Einhorn, L.H. and Donohue, J. (1977) *Cis*-diamminedichloroplatinum, vinblastine, and bleomycin combination chemotherapy in disseminated testicular cancer. *Ann. Intern. Med.*, **87**, 293–8.

Einhorn, L.H. and Williams, S.D. (1980) Chemotherapy of disseminated testicular cancer: A random prospective study. *Cancer*, **46**, 1339–44.

Einhorn, L.H. *et al.* (1990) Ondansetron: A new antiemetic for patients receiving cisplatin chemotherapy. *J. Clin. Oncol.*, **8**, 731–5.

Fitzharris, B.M. *et al.* (1980) VP16–213 as a single agent in advanced testicular tumours. *Eur. J. Cancer*, **17**, 245–9.

Garnick, M.B. *et al.* (1983) Treatment and surgical staging of testicular and primary extragonadal germ cell cancer *JAMA*, **250**, 1733–41.

Gietema, J.A. *et al.* (1992) Long-term followup of cardiovascular risk factors in patients given chemotherapy for disseminated nonseminomatous testicular cancer. *Ann. Intern. Med.*, **116**, 709–15.

Ginsberg, O.J., Comis, R.L. and Miller, M. (1982) The development of hyponatremia following combination chemotherapy for metastatic germ cell tumors. *Med. Ped. Oncol.*, **10**, 7–14.

Goren, M.P. *et al.* (1988) Dechlorethylation of ifosfamide and neurotoxicity. *Lancet*, **ii**, 1219–20.

Gralla, R.J. *et al.* (1981) Antiemetic efficacy of high-dose metoclopramide: Randomized trials with placebo and prochlorperazine in patients with chemotherapy induced nausea and vomiting. *N. Engl. J. Med.*, **305**, 905–10.

Gregg, R.W. *et al.* (1992) Cisplatin neurotoxicity: the relationship between dosage time and platinum concentration in neurologic tissues and morphologic evidence of toxicity. *J. Clin. Oncol.* **10**, 795–803.

Hamilton, C.R., Bliss, J.M., and Horwich, A. (1989) The late effects of *cis*-platinum on renal function. *Eur. J. Cancer Clin. Oncol.*, **25**, 185–9.

Hansen, S.W. *et al.* (1988) Long-term effects on renal function and blood pressure of treatment with cisplatin, vinblastine and bleomycin in patients with germ cell cancer. *J. Clin. Oncol.*, **6**, 1728–31.

Hansen, S.W. *et al.* (1989) Long-term neurotoxicity in patients treated with cisplatin, vinblastine and bleomycin for metastatic germ cell cancer. *J. Clin. Oncol.*, **7**, 1457–61.

Hansen, S.W. and Olsen, N. (1989) Raynaud's phenomenon in patients treated with cisplatin, vinblastine and bleomycin for germ cell cancer: Measurement of vasoconstriction response to cold. *J. Clin. Oncol.*, **7**, 940–2.

Hayes, D.M. *et al.* (1977) High-dose *cis*-platinum diammine dichloride-amelioration of renal toxicity by mannitol diuresis, *Cancer*, **39**, 1372–81.

Higby, D.J. *et al.* (1974) Diamminodichloroplatinum II in the chemotherapy of testicular tumours. *J. Urol.*, **112**, 100–1.

Hitchins, R.N. *et al.* (1989) Long-term outcome in patients with germ cell tumours treated with POMB/ACE chemotherapy: Comparison of commonly used classification systems of good and poor prognosis. *Br. J. Cancer*, **59**, 236–42.

Horwich, A. *et al.* (1989) Simple nontoxic treatment of advanced metastatic seminoma with carboplatin. *J. Clin. Oncol.*, **7**, 1150–6.

Horwich, A. *et al.* (1995) Fertility after chemotherapy for metastatic germ cell tumors. *Proc. Am. Soc. Clin. Onc.*, **14**, 236.

Horwich, A. and Slejfer, D. (1994) Carboplatin-based chemotherapy in good prognosis metastatic non-seminoma of the testis (NSGCT): An interim report of an MRC/EORTC randomised trial. *Adv. Biosci.*, **91**, 221.

Jackson, A.M. *et al.* (1984) Thrombotic microangiopathy and renal failure associated with antineoplastic chemotherapy. *Ann. Intern. Med.*, **101**, 41–4.

Jacobson, L.O. *et al.* (1946) Nitrogen mustard therapy: Studies on the effect of methyl-*Bis* (Beta-chloroethyl) amine hydrochloride on neoplastic diseases and allied disorders of the hemopoietic system. *JAMA*, **132**, 263–71.

Kattan, J. *et al.* (1993) High failure rate of carboplatin–etoposide combination in good risk non-seminomatous germ cell tumours. *Eur. J. Cancer*, **29**A, 1504–9.

Kennedy, B.J. (1970) Mithramycin therapy in advanced testicular neoplasms. *Cancer*, **26**, 755–66.

Krikorian, J. *et al.* (1978) Variables for predicting serious toxicity (vinblastine dose, performance status, and prior therapeutic experience): Chemotherapy for metastatic testicular cancer with *cis* dichlorodiammine-platinum (II), vinblastine, and bleomycin. *Cancer Treat. Rep.*, **62**, 1455–63.

Kris, M.G. *et al.* (1985) Incidence, course, and severity of delayed nausea and vomiting following the administration of high-dose cisplatin. *J. Clin. Oncol.*, **3**, 1379–83.

Kris, M.G. *et al.* (1989) Double-blind, randomized trial comparing placebo, dexamethasone alone, and metoclopramide plus dexamethasone in patients receiving cisplatin. *J. Clin. Oncol.*, **7**, 108–11.

Laszlo, J. (1985) Lorazepam in cancer patients treated with cisplatin: A drug having antiemetic, amnesic and anxiolytic effect. *J. Clin. Oncol.*, **3**, 864–9.

Levi, J.A. *et al.* (1990) Effective salvage chemotherapy with etoposide, dactinomycin, and methotrexate in refractory germ cell cancer. *J. Clin. Oncol.*, **8**, 27–32.

Levine L.A. and Richie J.P. (1989) Urological complications of cyclophosphamide. *J. Urol.*, **141**, 1063–9.

Li, M.C. *et al.* (1960) Effects of combined drug therapy on metastatic cancer of the testis. *JAMA*, **174**, 145–53.

Lipschultz, S.E. *et al.* (1995) Female sex and higher drug dose as risk factors for late cardiotoxic effects of doxorubicin therapy for childhood cancer. *N. Engl. J. Med.*, **332**, 1738–43.

Loehrer, P.J. *et al.* (1995) Importance of bleomycin in favorable prognosis disseminated germ cell tumors: An Eastern Cooperative Oncology Group trial. *J. Clin. Oncol.*, **13**, 470.

Loehrer, P.J., Einhorn, L.J. and Williams, S.D. (1986) VP-16 + ifosfamide + cisplatin as salvage therapy in refractory germ cell cancer. *J. Clin. Oncol.*, **4**, 528–36.

Logothetis, C.J., Samuels, M.L., Selig, D.E. *et al.* (1985) Improved survival with cyclic chemotherapy for nonseminomatous germ cell tumors of the testis. *J. Clin. Oncol.*, **3**, 326–35.

Markman, M. *et al.* (1984) Antiemetic efficacy of dexamethasone: Randomized double-blind cross over study of prochlorperazine in patients receiving cancer chemotherapy. *N. Engl. J. Med.*, **311**, 549–65.

Marty, M. *et al.* (1990) Comparison of the 5-hydroxytryptamine$_3$ (serotonin) antagonist ondansetron (GR 38032F) with high-dose metoclopramide in the control of cisplatin-induced emesis. *N. Engl. J. Med.* **322**, 816–21.

Meijer, S. *et al.* (1983) Some effects of combination chemotherapy with *cis*-platinum on renal function in patients with nonseminomatous testicular carcinoma. *Cancer*, **51**, 2035–40.

Mendelson, D. and Serpick, A.A. (1970) Combination chemotherapy of testicular tumors. *J. Urol.*, **103**, 619–23.

Merrin, C.E. and Murphy, G.P. (1974) Metastatic testicular carcinoma: single-agent chemotherapy (actinomycin-D) in treatment. *NY State J. Med.*, April, 654–7.

Miller, C.B. Platanias, L.C., Ratain, M.J. *et al.* (1992) Phase I/II trial of erythropoietin in the treatment of cisplatin-associated anemia. *J. Natl. Cancer Inst.*, **84**, 98–103.

Mollman, J.E. (1990) Cisplatin neurotoxicity. *N. Engl. J. Med.*, **322**, 126–7.

Monfardini, S. *et al.* (1972) Clinical use of Adriamycin in advanced testicular cancer. *J. Urol*, **10**, 293–300.

Motzer, R.J. *et al.* (1987) Phase II trial of carboplatin in patients with advanced germ cell tumors refractory to cisplatin. *Cancer Treat. Rep.*, **71**, 187–8.

Motzer, R.J. *et al.* (1994) Phase II trial of paclitaxel shows antitumor activity in patients with previously treated germ cell tumors. *J. Clin. Oncol.*, **12**, 2277–83.

Nicols, C.R., Breeden, E.S., Loehrer, P.J. *et al.* (1993) Secondary leukemia associated with a conventional dose of etoposide: Review of serial germ cell tumor protocols. *J. Natl. Canc. Inst.*, **85**, 36–40.

Nichols, C., Roth, B., Williams, S. *et al.* (1992) No evidence of acute cardiovascular complications of chemotherapy for testicular cancer: an analysis of the testicular cancer intergroup study. *J. Clin. Oncol.*, **10**, 760–5.

Ozols, R.R. *et al.* (1985) High-dose cisplatin in hypertonic saline in refractory ovarian cancer. *J. Clin. Oncol.*, **3**, 1246–50.

Pedersen-Bjergaard, J. (1995) Editorial: Long-term complications of cancer chemotherapy. *J. Clin. Oncol.*, **13**, 1534–6.

Pedersen-Bjergaard, J. *et al.* (1988) Carcinoma of the urinary bladder after treatment with cyclophosphamide for non-Hodgkins lymphoma. *N. Engl. J. Med.*, **318**, 1028–88.

Pedersen-Bjergaard, J., Daugaard, G., Hansen, S.W. *et al.* (1991) Increased risk of myelodysplasia and leukaemia after etoposide, cisplatin and bleomycin for germ cell tumours. *Lancet*, Aug. 10, **338**, 359–63.

Ratain, M.J. *et al.* (1987) Acute non-lymphocytic leukemia following etoposide and cisplatin combination chemotherapy for advanced non-small-cell carcinoma of the lung. *Blood*, **70**, 1412–17.

Ratain, M.J. and Vogelzang, N.J. (1986) Phase I and pharmacologic study of vinblastine by prolonged continuous infusion. *Cancer Res.*, **46**, 4827–30.

Redman, J.R. *et al.* (1984) Leukemia following treatment of germ cell tumors in men. *J. Clin. Oncol.*, **2**, 1080–7.

Reece, P.A. *et al.* (1987) Creatinine clearance as a predictor of ultrafilterable platinum disposition in cancer patients treated with cisplatin: Relationship between peak ultrafilterable platinum plasma levels and nephrotoxicity. *J. Clin, Oncol.*, **5**, 304–9.

Reynolds, T.F. *et al.* (1981) VAB-3 combination chemotherapy of metastatic testicular cancer. *Cancer*, **48**, 888–98.

Roth, B.J. *et al.* (1985) Alpha-2 interferon (IFN) in the treatment of refractory malignant germ cell tumours. *Proc. Am. Soc. Clin. Oncol.*, **4**, 100 (Abstract).

Roth, B.J. *et al.* (1988) Cisplatin-based combination chemotherapy for disseminated germ cell-tumors: Long-term follow-up. *J. Clin. Oncol.*, **6**, 1239–47.

Rothberg, H. (1978) Raynaud's phenomenon after vinblastine, bleomycin chemotherapy. *Cancer Treat. Rep.*, **62**, 569–70.

Samson, M.K. *et al.* (1984) Dose-response and dose-survival advantage for high versus low-dose cisplatin combined with vinblastine and bleomycin in disseminated testicular cancer. A Southwest Oncology Group Study. *Cancer*, **53**, 1029–35.

Samuels, M.L. and Howe, C.D. (1970) Vinblastine in the management of testicular cancer. *Cancer*, **25**, 1009–21.

Samuels, M.L., Johnson, D.E. and Holoye, P.V. (1975) Continuous intravenous bleomycin (NSC-125066) therapy with vinblastine (NSC-49842) in stage III testicular neoplasia. *Cancer Chemother. Rep.*, **59**, 563–70.

Samuels, B.L., Vogelzang, N.J. and Kennedy, B.J. (1987) Severe vascular toxicity associated with vinblastine, bleomycin and cisplatin chemotherapy. *Cancer Chemother. Pharmacol.*, **19**, 253–6.

Scheulen, M.E. and Schmidt C.G. (1982) Raynaud's phenomenon and cancer chemotherapy. *Ann. Intern. Med.*, **96**, 256.

Schilsky, R.L., Barlock, A. and Ozols, R.F. (1982) Persistent hypomagnesemia following cisplatin chemotherapy for testicular cancer. *Cancer Treat. Rep.*, **66**, 1767–9.

Shea, T.C. *et al.* (1989) A phase I clinical and pharmacokinetic study of carboplatin and autologous bone marrow support. *J. Clin. Oncol.*, **7**, 651–61.

Smith, M., Rubinstein, L., Cazenave, L., *et al.* (1993) Report of the cancer therapy evaluation program monitoring plan for secondary acute myeloid leukemia following treatment with epipodophyllotoxins. *J. Natl. Cancer Inst.*, **85**, 554–8.

Stefenelli, T. *et al.* (1988) Acute vascular toxicity after combination chemotherapy with cisplatin, vinblastine, and bleomycin for testicular cancer. *Eur. Heart J.*, **9**, 552–6.

Stephenson, W.T., Poirier, S.M., Rubin, L. *et al.* (1995) Evaluation of reproductive capacity in germ cell tumor patients following treatment with cisplatin, etoposide and bleomycin. *J. Clin. Oncol.*, **13**, 2278–80.

Stoter, G. *et al.* (1989) Ten-year survival and late sequelae in testicular cancer patients treated with cisplatin, vinblastine, and bleomycin. *J. Clin. Oncol.*, **7**, 1099–104.

Stuart, N.S., Woodroffe, C.H., Grundy, R. and Cullen, M.H. (1990) Long-term toxicity of chemotherapy for testicular cancer – the cost of cure. *Br. J. Cancer*, **61**, 479–84.

Subar, M. and Muggia, F.M. (1986) Apparent myocardial ischemia associated with vinblastine administration. *Cancer Treat. Rep.*, **70**, 690–1.

Teutsch, C., Lipton, A. and Harvey, H.A. (1977) Raynaud's phenomenon as a side effect of chemotherapy with vinblastine and bleomycin for testicular carcinoma. *Cancer Treat. Rep.*, **61**, 925–6.

Thirman, M.J., Gill, H.J., Burnett, R.C., *et al.* (1993) Rearrangement of the *MLL* gene in acute lymphoblastic and acute myeloid leukemias with 11q23 chromosomal translocations. *N. Engl. J. Med.*, **329**, 909–14.

Thirman, M.J. and Larson, R.A. (1995) Therapy-related myeloid leukemia. *Sem. Hematol.*, (in press).

Tjulandin, S.A. *et al.* (1993) Cisplatin–etoposide and carboplatin–etoposide induction chemotherapy for good-risk patients with germ cell tumors. *Ann. Oncol.*, **4**, 663–8.

van Barneveld, P.W.C. *et al.* (1985) Changes in pulmonary function during and after bleomycin treatment in patients with testicular carcinoma. *Cancer Chemother. Pharmacol.*, **14**, 168–71.

van der Hoop, R.G. *et al.* (1990) Prevention of cisplatin neurotoxicity with an ACTH (4–9) analogue in patients with ovarian cancer. *N. Engl. J. Med.*, **322**, 89–94.

Von Gunten, X. *et al.* (1993) Raynaud's phenomenon in three patients with acquired immune deficiency syndrome related Kaposi sarcoma treated with bleomycin. *Cancer*, **72**, 2004–6.

Vogelzang, N.J., Frenning, D.H. and Kennedy, B.J. (1980) Coronary artery disease after bleomy-cin and vinblastine. *Cancer Treat. Rep.*, **64**, 1159–60.

Vogelzang, N.J. *et al.* (1981) Raynaud's phenomenon: A common toxicity after combination chemotherapy of testicular cancer. *Ann. Intern. Med.*, **95**, 288–92.

Vogelzang, N.J., Raghavan, D. and Kennedy, B.J. (1982) VP-16–213 (Etoposide): The mandrake root of Issyk-Kul. *Am. J. Med.*, **72**, 136–44.

Vogelzang, N.J., Torkelson, J.L. and Kennedy, B.J. (1985) Hypomagnesemia, renal dysfunction and Raynaud's phenomenon in patients treated with cisplatin, vinblastine and bleomycin. *Cancer*, **56**, 2765–71.

Vogelzang, N.J. *et al.* (1990) Carboplatin in malignant mesothelioma: A phase II study of the cancer and leukemia group B. *Cancer. Chem. Pharm.* **27**, 239–42.

Vugrin, D. *et al.* (1981) VAB-6 combination chemotherapy in disseminated cancer of the testis. *Ann. Intern. Med.*, **95**, 59–61.

Wheeler, B.M. *et al.* (1986) Ifosfamide in refractory male germ cell tumors. *J. Clin. Oncol.*, **4**, 28–34.

Williams, S.D. *et al.* (1987a) Treatment of disseminated germ cell tumors with cisplatin, bleomycin, and either vinblastine or etoposide. *N. Engl. J. Med.*, **316**, 1435–40.

Williams, S.D. *et al.* (1987b) Immediate adjuvant chemotherapy versus observation with treatment at relapse in pathological stage II testicular cancer. *N. Engl. J. Med.*, **317**, 1433–8.

Wyatt, J.K. and McAninch, L.N. (1967) A chemotherapeutic approach to advanced testicular carcinoma. *Can. J. Surg.*, **10**, 421–5.

Zalupski, M. and Baker, L.H. (1988) Ifosfamide. *J. Natl Cancer Inst.*, **80**, 556–66.

C. *Moynihan*

31.1 INTRODUCTION

The psychosocial aspects of cancer have become the focus of systematic attention in recent years, and many excellent reviews highlight important components of the current concern for the quality of a cancer patient's life (Cox and Mackay, 1982; Greer, 1983; de Haes and Knippenberg, 1987). New techniques and combinations of modalities of treatment have checked the course of rapidly fatal tumor types and, indeed, cure has been achieved in a large percentage of cases (Welch-McCaffrey *et al.*, 1989). The irony is that concomitant and associated with such medical triumphs are problems produced by these very successes. Anatomical and physiological defects result from aggressive treatment regimens, both in the short and long term (Devlin *et al.*, 1971; Dean *et al.*, 1983; Fobair *et al.*, 1986); psychological morbidity is known to exist at diagnosis (McIntosh, 1974), during treatment (Forester, Kornfeld and Fleiss, 1978; Maguire, Lee and Berington 1978; Silberfarb, 1980) and at follow-up (Schmale *et al.*, 1983).

Severe sexual difficulties have been reported in women who have undergone radical surgery for cancers of the cervix and vulva (Anderson, 1986) and studies of cancer patients in general indicate that 50% of those who were sexually active prior to their illness report a loss of sexual interest and frequency in performance. Problems arising from such changes were perceived as serious in 10–20% of patients (Hughes, 1987).

Relationships with family, friends and colleagues may be altered as a result of cancer (Maher, 1982). The need for interpersonal support of a familial kind, especially after the completion of treatment, has been found to be important but often unavailable (Maher, 1982). Although it is acknowledged that the family's role in the overall adjustment of the patient to diagnosis and treatment is important, little research has addressed the psychosocial dynamics of the family during treatment and survival from cancer (Greer, 1985).

Social dysfunction resulting from cancer may take the form of discrimination in the work place (Feldman *et al.*, 1982). Employers do not always realize that many cancer patients overcome their illness, that cancer is not contagious, and that cancer survivors have similar productivity rates to other workers (Welch-McCaffrey *et al.*, 1989). A number of longitudinal studies have convincingly demonstrated that mental health is affected by both anticipated loss of a job and becoming unemployed (Warr, 1984).

Testicular Cancer: Investigation and management. Second edition. Edited by Professor A. Horwich.
Published in 1996 by Chapman & Hall. ISBN 0 412 61210 0.

The need for formal counseling of cancer patients has been documented (Thomas, 1978; Watson, 1983). The form of intervention administered, is not always clear, however (Watson, 1983).

Research on the psychosocial implications of cancer is beset with methodological problems (Schipper and Clinch, 1988). The lack of definitional consensus of the quality of life and the use of heterogeneous subject pools provide diverse findings (de Haes and Knippenberg, 1987). The ongoing debate surrounding the scientific validity of objectivity versus subjectivity in the gathering of data has led to inconclusive evidence of the relevance of psychosocial parameters (de Haes and Knippenberg, 1987). Intuition alone is often used in the formation of indicators (Goldberg and Cullen, 1985; de Haes and Knippenberg, 1987) and little attention has been paid to the reliability and validity of instruments, or the theoretical underpinnings that would possibly explain the origin of certain psychosocial findings (de Haes and Knippenberg, 1987). Little research exists that provides baseline pretreatment measurement of psychosocial responses with which to compare longer-term findings (Greer, 1985). Many studies use little or no control for important intervening variables, such as age, sex, social class, the primary site of cancer, type of treatment, time since cancer diagnosis, end of treatment, and the relationship of disease to stage and psychological adjustment during treatment and survival time (de Haes and Knippenberg, 1987).

The design of the study and the importance of sensitive instruments become important imperatives if the dangers of falling into the trap of 'therapeutic nihilism' are to be avoided (Schipper and Clinch, 1988). For example, benefits of adjuvant chemotherapy may be compromised by a spurious focus on the quality of life by researchers. Patients may be given dangerous drug reductions because of the concern for toxic-free regimens, but the side-effects of chemotherapy may, in some cases, have less adverse effects on patients' quality of life than similar side-effects attributable to the disease.

Testicular cancer patients represent an ideal group for the study of psychosocial assessments and evaluation of a counseling intervention. Not only is the cure rate dramatic, reaching 93% for all combined stages, but the disease usually affects men between the ages of 19 and 34 years; a time when many are embarking on job and family responsibilities. Patients have, in the majority of cases, had to lose a sexual organ; strenuous treatment regimens have had to be endured and rigorous follow-up must be adhered to, especially by those patients who undergo a surveillance protocol. Thus, both short- and long-term physical, psychological and social outcomes and the interrelationship they have with one another may be investigated in a way that has hitherto been difficult, because of high mortality rates.

In this chapter, studies will be reviewed that have focused on the psychosocial aspects of patients with testicular tumors and suggestions will be made with regard to counseling interventions, which may help to alleviate specific problems experienced by this type of cancer patient and his relatives. These problems appear to center around psychological morbidity *per se* (and as it relates to other aspects of a man's experience), sexual adjustment, infertility distress and social dysfunction including work-related problems and social support.

In recent years studies have been undertaken which, in the main, are retrospective (Schover and von Eschenbach, 1984, 1985; Tross *et al.*, 1984; Rieker, Edbril and Garnick, 1985; Schover, Gonzaleo and von Eschenbach, 1986; Cassileth and Steinfeld, 1987; Herr, 1987; Moynihan, 1987; Schover, 1987; Blackmore, 1988; Gritz, Wellisch and Landsrerk, 1989a; Kaasa *et al.*, 1989; Rieker *et al.*, 1989; Stoter *et al.*, 1989). To date, four studies have investigated psychological morbidity prospectively (Malec, Romsaas and Trump,

1985; Trump *et al.*, 1985; Fosså, Aass and Kaalhus, 1988; Aass *et al.*, 1989) and a fifth is currently underway (Moynihan *et al.*, in press).

31.2 PSYCHOLOGICAL MORBIDITY

31.2.1 PYSCHOLOGICAL MORBIDITY AT DIAGNOSIS AND PRETREATMENT

A paucity of data makes it difficult to assess the true rate of psychological morbidity during diagnosis and the pretreatment period. Prospective data reveal low rates of morbid symptoms. One study reported 15% of the sample as 'often' feeling 'nervous' or 'anxious'; only 7% found it difficult to talk of their malignancy 'at diagnosis' (Fosså, Aass and Kaalhus, 1988). Results of a prospective study confirm this finding. The Hospital Anxiety and Depression Scale (HADS) (Zigmond and Snaith, 1983) reveals that men who have been told their diagnosis have low rates of severe psychological morbidity. At 1 month postdiagnosis and prior to treatment, 21% had levels of anxiety and 11% levels of depression that warranted an intervention (Moynihan *et al.*, in press).

Anecdotal evidence and retrospective data (with all its well-known limitations) (Morgan, 1983) indicate that the actual diagnosis is a time of fear of death and uncertainty (Moynihan, 1987). Subsequent uncertainty due to ongoing staging procedures and unresolved treatment decisions are recounted as times of concomitant fear and anxiety (Moynihan *et al.*, in press).

31.2.2 PSYCHOLOGICAL MORBIDITY DURING TREATMENT

Retrospective data reveal a vivid account of the horror of chemotherapy: 'it made me ill, not the cancer' (Moynihan, 1987). This sentiment is substantiated by data which suggest the heavy toll treatment places on patients' psychological state. Emotional problems were significantly more pronounced 6 months after treatment than they had been 'before diagnosis' (Gritz, Wellisch and Landsrerk, 1989). Prospective data do not always uphold these findings. Only 6% felt that they 'often' experienced 'nervousness', 'anxiety' or 'depression' (Fosså, Aass and Kaalhus, 1988). When patients were assessed 8 weeks after hospital admission, HADS scores showed that 17% and 9% were severely anxious and depressed respectively (Moynihan *et al.*, in press). These findings are contradicted by further prospective studies. A 20% rate of anxiety and a 40% rate of 'somatic concern' were experienced during treatment (Malec, Romsaas and Trump, 1985) and levels of 'anxiety', 'depression' and 'other psychological distress', were 'elevated' within 6 months of diagnosis (Trump *et al.*, 1985). These levels were significantly higher at this time than they were at 1 year following diagnosis.

Few studies have shown the effects of differing treatment regimens on psychological status during this time. Such evidence that does exist suggests that exhaustion was most pronounced in those who had undergone surgery and radiotherapy (Fosså, Aass and Kaalhus, 1988) and in those patients receiving vinblastine (Herr, 1987; Aass *et al.*, 1989). A prospective study reveals that men receiving chemotherapy were more likely to be anxious and depressed during treatment than those in a surveillance or radiotherapy group, although this finding was not statistically significant. In addition, mean differences of psychological morbidity between baseline, 8 weeks and 4 months postadmission showed no difference between treatment groups (Moynihan, in press).

31.2.3 PSYCHOLOGICAL MORBIDITY POST-TREATMENT

Studies report a consistent picture of psychological well-being in the majority of men (Tross *et al.*, 1984; Rieker, Edbril and Garnick, 1985; Trump *et al.*, 1985; Cassileth and Steinfeld, 1987; Moynihan, 1987; Schover, 1987;

Fosså, Aass and Kaalhus, 1988; Gritz, Wellisch and Landsrerk 1989; Kaasa *et al.*, 1989; Rieker *et al.*, 1989; Moynihan *et al.*, in prep). Indeed, in many cases, a more enhanced view of life is experienced, compared with prior conceptions (Rieker, Edbril and Garnick, 1985; Gritz, Wellisch and Landsrerk, 1989; Rieker, *et al.*, 1989) and control groups (Cassileth and Steinfeld, 1987; Gritz, Wellisch and Landsrerk 1989; Rieker, Edbril and Garnick, 1985; Rieker *et al.*, 1989). However, a significant minority suffer psychological symptoms, even years after treatment has ended (Schover and von Eschenbach, 1984, 1985; Tross *et al.*, 1984; Malec, Romsaas and Trump, 1985; Rieker, Edbril and Garnick, 1985; Trump *et al.*, 1985; Schover, Gonzaleo and von Eschenbach, 1986; Cassileth and Steinfeld, 1987; Moynihan, 1987; Schover, 1987; Fosså, Aass and Kaalhus, 1988; Gritz, Wellisch and Landsrerk, 1989; Kaasa *et al.*, 1989; Rieker *et al.*, 1989; Stoter *et al.*, 1989).

The rates of psychological symptoms vary between 10% (Fosså, Aass and Kaalhus, 1988) and 40% (Kaasa *et al.*, 1989), although the majority of studies show a 10–23% rate of moderate to severe psychological distress. While a few studies claim that patients manifest significantly more distress than controls (Tross *et al.*, 1984; Kaasa *et al.*, 1989), others show that patients are less prone to psychological morbidity than other groups (Malec, Romsaas and Trump, 1985; Rieker, Edbril and Garnick, 1985; 1989; Trump *et al.*, 1985; Cassileth and Steinfeld, 1987; Fosså, Aass and Kaalhus, 1988; Gritz, Wellisch and Landsrerk, 1989; Rieker *et al.*, 1989).

The lowest (Fosså, Aass and Kaalhus, 1988) and highest (Kaasa *et al.*, 1989) rates of morbidity were found where unvalidated subjective instruments were used. Elevated mood states were reported as 'negligible' 3 or more years post-treatment and were no higher than those in a comparison sample (Fosså, Aass and Kaalhus, 1988). Only 10% claimed 'anxious', 'nervous' or 'depressed' feelings 'much' or 'very much' during the past week. However, 72% reported feeling 'a little' or 'more' distressed during that time. A 40% rate of anxiety and depression was reported (Kaasa *et al.*, 1989) when patients were asked whether they 'often' or 'sometimes' experienced symptoms during the past 6 months. This finding conflicts with those studies that used a validated psychological measure: The Profile of Mood States (POMS) (Rieker, Edbril and Garnick, 1985, 1989; Trump *et al.*, 1985; Cassileth and Steinfeld, 1987; Gritz, Wellisch and Landsrerk, 1989), and the Hospital Anxiety and Depression Score (HADS) (Moynihan, in press). A rate of 14–18% morbidity was found 1–20 years post-treatment. Patients' mean scores of anxiety and depression in the previous month were lower than those of a self-selected but stratified group (Rieker, Edbril and Garnick, 1985; Cassileth and Steinfeld, 1987), college males (Rieker, Edbril and Garnick, 1985; Trump, *et al.*, 1985; Gritz, Wellisch and Landsrerk, 1989; Rieker *et al.*, 1989), psychiatric patients (Rieker, Edbril and Garnick, 1985; Gritz, Wellisch and Landsrerk, 1989; Rieker *et al.*, 1989) and other cancer groups (Rieker, Edbril and Garnick, 1985; Gritz, Wellisch and Landsrerk, 1989).

There are, however, inherent shortcomings in determining psychological health by comparing mean scores with those in comparison groups (Spinetta, 1982). Subsets of problems that testicular cancer patients may suffer are obscured. Moreover, by comparing patients with 'normal' men implies their 'abnormality' and little is learned about the patients themselves.

A previous psychiatric history (Rieker, Edbril and Garnick, 1985; Moynihan, 1987), age (Moynihan, 1987; Gritz, Wellisch and Landsrerk, 1989; Rieker, Edbril and Garnick, 1985; Rieker, *et al.*, 1989), time since diagnosis (Rieker, Edbril and Garnick, 1985; Moynihan, 1987; Rieker *et al.*, 1989), tumor types (Rieker, Edbril and Garnick, 1985; Moynihan, 1987; Gritz, Wellisch and Landsrerk, 1989; Rieker *et al.*, 1989), or marital status (Rieker, Edbril and

Garnick, 1985; Moynihan, 1987; Rieker *et al.*, 1989) were not significantly related to psychological morbidity. There was an indication that levels of distress decline between 6 months post-treatment and in the month previous to interview (Trump *et al.*, 1985; Gritz, Wellisch and Landsrerk, 1989). Men with sexual impairment (see below) reported more psychological symptoms and more areas of negative life functioning such as an inability to be active (Rieker, Edbril and Garnick, 1985; Rieker *et al.*, 1989). Men who had been unemployed (see below) and feared relapse were significantly more distressed than those who had retained their jobs or were not anxiously preoccupied about cancer returning (Moynihan, 1987).

Psychological distress was related to financial difficulties (Moynihan, 1987) and was more prevalent among lower-income groups (Rieker, Edbril and Garnick, 1985; Moynihan, 1987). When patients were asked to compare their current mental outlook with predisease states, 17% reported negative changes that were significantly related to high levels of psychological distress as measured by POMS (Rieker, Edbril and Garnick, 1985).

Neither treatment type nor stage of disease appeared to be related to long-term psychological morbidity (Rieker, Edbril and Garnick, 1985; Moynihan, 1987; Gritz, Wellisch and Landsrerk, 1989; Kaasa *et al.*, 1989; Rieker *et al.*, 1989). Those men in a surveillance policy suffered as much psychological morbidity as those who had undergone aggressive treatment regimens (Moynihan, 1987). However, men who had undergone retroperitoneal lymph node dissection (RPLND) had significantly higher infertility and sexual performance distress (see below) (Rieker, Edbril and Garnick, 1985).

Although psychological morbidity of a clinical kind will manifest itself in a minority of survivors, there are varying aspects of life that relate to negative outcomes. In the next section, the most important areas of dysfunction are detailed. They appear to center around sexual activity, infertility distress and social upheaval.

31.3 SEXUAL DYSFUNCTION AND INFERTILITY DISTRESS

It is now well established that reproductive and sexual function are often compromised as a result of treatment. Studies have shown that fertility after chemotherapy (Drasga *et al.*, 1983; Lange *et al.*, 1983) and/or radiation (Clark and Reswick, 1978) results in a period of sterility or subfertility that lasts from 12 months to 4 years (Lange *et al.*, 1983; Nijman *et al.*, 1987). Furthermore, permanent sterility or dry or retrograde ejaculation may result from RPLND (Kedia, Morkland and Frayley, 1977; Narayan, Lange and Frayley, 1982; Nijman *et al.*, 1987).

It is not surprising, therefore, that sexual dysfunction or dissatisfaction is reported among testicular cancer survivors at a rate of 10–50% in the populations investigated. These figures appear to vary according to specific types of dysfunction.

31.3.1 SEXUAL FUNCTION AT DIAGNOSIS AND PRETREATMENT

Little information exists on the sexual function of men prior to orchidectomy and diagnosis. Existing data corroborate anecdotal evidence: sexual dysfunction is minimal both prior and post diagnosis. (Moynihan, 1987, Fosså, Aass and Kaalhus, 1988, Gritz, Wellisch and Landsrerk, 1989, Aass *et al.*, 1993). When sexual function was assessed 1 month post orchidectomy and compared with the 30 days prior to surgery, 8% had an overall sexual dysfunction score that denoted a substantial deterioration (Moynihan *et al.*, in press). Increased age correlated with the incidence of sexual problems (Aass *et al.*, 1993). The main area of dysfunction was a decrease in sexual activity (Moynihan *et al.*, in press), which has been attributed to postsurgical discomfort (Gritz, Wellisch and Landsrerk,

1989). Dysfunction did not differ from a population control sample of age-matched men (Fosså, Aass and Kaalhus, 1988). At least 60% of patients felt it important that sexual function should be discussed before treatment (Aass *et al.*, 1993).

31.3.2 INFERTILITY DISTRESS AT DIAGNOSIS

Information is scant regarding what subjectively may be considered a major side-effect of testicular disease. Such data that exist are conflicting. One prospective study reported that 35% of men felt 'rather' or 'very afraid' of infertility at this time (Fosså, Aass and Kaalhus, 1988). When men were asked 1 month post diagnosis 'how much of a problem has infertility been in the past 4 weeks', 25 men (17%) said it had been the source of substantial worry (i.e. >50% of the time). Stage, histology, social class, marital status and educational levels were not related to levels of worry, although younger men (<40) and those who were childless were more likely to be distressed regarding this issue (Moynihan *et al.*, in press).

It is possible that patients are overwhelmed by the diagnosis of cancer at this time. This may overshadow all other considerations that may become areas of distress as treatment procedures progress.

31.3.3 SEXUAL FUNCTION AND INFERTILITY DISTRESS DURING TREATMENT

Few data exist that may shed light on sexual dysfunction and infertility distress during this time. A curtailment of sexual activity and a loss of sexual drive are reported, both prospectively (Trump, *et al.*, 1985; Fosså, Aass and Kaalkus 1988; Moynihan *et al.*, in prep.) and retrospectively (Gritz, Wellisch and Landsrerk, 1989). This type of dysfunction was more pronounced in radiotherapy and chemotherapy groups, but it was temporary (median duration 2.3 months). A

decrease in the quality of orgasm was reported by all treatment groups, but the highest rate was as a consequence of RPLND (median duration 3–4 months) (Fosså, Aass and Kaalkus, 1988). Side-effects of treatment procedures such as chemotherapy may have an effect on a man's self-esteem. This in turn may cause sexual anxiety and further sexual dysfunction (Schover, 1987).

An adverse impact on the spouse in terms of avoidance of sexual activity is reported (Gritz, Wellisch and Wang, 1989). Although of short duration, avoidance by partners was more frequent than patients realized.

31.3.4 SEXUAL FUNCTION POST-TREATMENT

Early studies of patients report little sexual dysfunction. This optimism may be caused by the lack of in-depth investigation on sexual function and the hesitancy of patients to disclose and physicians to seek information (Rieker *et al.*, 1989). However, a few studies looking specifically at sexual sequelae confirm this view: sexual function and activity are not unduly compromised in survivors (Trump *et al.*, 1985; Cassileth and Steinfield, 1987; Moynihan, 1987; Fosså, Aass and Kaalhus, 1988; Gritz, Wellisch and Wang, 1989) although there is evidence of sexual deterioration in as many as 30% of patients three years after treatment has ended (Aass *et al.*, 1993). Other studies conclude that testicular tumor patients report significantly more dysfunction than comparison groups (Tross *et al.*, 1984; Rieker Edbril and Garnick, 1985; Schover and von Eschenbach, 1985; Schover, 1987; Rieker *et al.*, 1989).

Studies investigating the **nature** of sexual dysfunction revealed consistent findings, although the overall incidence varied between 10 and 50%. Malfunction lay in the following areas: erectile dysfunction (6–29%) (Rieker, Edbril and Garnick 1985; Schover and von Eschenbach, 1985; Schover *et al.*, 1986; Moynihan, 1987; Nijman *et al.*, 1987;

Gritz, Wellisch and Wang, 1989b; Schover *et al.*, 1986; Aass *et al.*, 1993; Moynihan *et al.*, in prep.), difficulty in reaching orgasm (6–12%) (Rieker, Edbril and Garnick, 1985; Schover and von Eschenbach, 1985; Nijman *et al.*, 1987; Riecker *et al.*, 1989), a decrease in its intensity (6–38%) (Schover and von Eschenbach, 1985; Schover *et al.*, 1986; Moynihan, 1987), a moderate to severe reporting of sexual dissatisfaction (4–33%) (Rieker, Edbril and Garnick, 1985; Schover *et al.*, 1986; Moynihan, 1987; Gritz, Wellisch and Wang, 1989; Rieker *et al.*, 1989; Stoter *et al.*, 1989; Aass *et al.*, 1993; Moynihan *et al.*, in press), an inability to ejaculate (5–88%) (Rieker, Edbril and Garnick, 1985; Moynihan, 1987; Nijman *et al.*, 1987; Fosså, Aass and Kaalhus, 1988; Gritz, Wellisch and Wang, 1989; Rieker *et al.*, 1989; Stoter *et al.*, 1989; Aass *et al.*, 1993), a decline in semen volume (14–82%) (Schover and Eschenbach, 1985; Schover *et al.*, 1986; Gritz, Wellisch and Wang, 1989), a loss of libido (4–17%) (Rieker, Edbril and Garnick, 1985; Schover and von Eschenbach, 1985; Schover *et al.*, 1986; Moynihan, 1987; Fosså, Aass and Kaalhus, 1988; Gritz, Wellisch and Wang, 1989; Rieker *et al.*, 1989; Aass *et al.*, 1983; Moynihan *et al.*, in prep.) and a decrease in sexual frequency (10–35%) (Rieker, Edbril and Garnick, 1985; Schover and von Eschenbach, 1985; Schover *et al.*, 1986; Schover, 1987; Gritz, Wellisch and Wang, 1989b; Moynihan *et al.*, in prep.).

Differing treatment regimens are overtly responsible for the differences in the above rates of dysfunction. Although no differences were found to exist between histological groups *per se* (Rieker, Edbril and Garnick, 1985; Schover *et al.*, 1986; Moynihan, 1987; Rieker *et al.*, 1989; Gritz *et al.*, 1990; Aass *et al.*, 1993), non-seminoma patients with RPLND reported a greater decline in semen volume at ejaculation (Schover and von Eschenbach, 1984) when compared with those men who had seminoma and had been treated with radiotherapy alone (Schover, Gonzaleo and von Eschenbach, 1986). Within

a teratoma group, men who received RPLND and radiotherapy had significantly higher rates of erectile dysfunction (Schover and von Eschenbach, 1985; Nijman *et al.*, 1987), difficulty in reaching orgasm (Schover and von Eschenbach, 1984), reduced orgasmic intensity (Schover and von Eschenbach, 1984) and antigrade ejaculation (Nijman *et al.*, 1987) than those men who had RPLND or RPLND plus chemotherapy (Schover and von Eschenbach, 1985; Nijman *et al.*, 1987). In men with seminoma, a higher dosage of irradiation to the para-aortic field was predictive of erectile and/or orgasmic problems (Schover, Gonzaleo and von Eschenbach, 1986).

A composite variable 'sexual performance distress' (an inability to ejaculate, reach orgasm or keep an erection), revealed the radiotherapy-only group to have the lowest rates of dysfunction whilst the chemotherapy plus RPLND (Rieker, Edbril and Garnick, 1985) or chemotherapy plus radiotherapy (Gritz, Wellisch and Wang, 1989) reported the highest rates of distress.

Evidence strongly suggests that sexual dysfunction is related to the intensity of treatment regimens. It is especially evident in those men who have undergone RPLND (with concomitant ejaculatory dysfunction) plus or minus additional therapy (Rieker, Edbril and Garnick, 1985; Schover and von Eschenbach, 1985; Schover, Gonzaleo and von Eschenbach, 1986; Nijman *et al.*, 1987; Schover, 1987; Gritz, Wellisch and Wang, 1989; Rieker *et al.*, 1989; Aass *et al.*, 1993). This may account for low levels of sexual dysfunction in a UK group (Moynihan, 1987; Moynihan *et al.*, in press). Retroperitoneal lymph node dissection is not a routine procedure in that country.

Several authors have queried the practice of routine RPLND (Rieker, Edbril and Garnick 1985; Nijman *et al.*, 1987; Schover, 1987; Fosså, Aass and Kaalhus, 1988; Gritz, Wellisch and Wang, 1988), and indicate the advantages of a modified surgical intervention (Narayan *et al.*, 1982; Fosså, Aass and

Kaalhus, 1988) or a surveillance policy for Stage I non-seminomatous tumors (Rieker, Edbril and Garnick, 1985; Nijman *et al.*, 1987). Although 9% of these patients experienced some deterioration in their sexual function at 1 year (Moynihan *et al.* in prep.), fewer sexual problems were experienced by testicular cancer patients when compared with a group who had undergone orchidectomy for benign conditions and a group of 'normal men' (Blackmore, 1988).

Confounding variables, such as time since diagnosis and participation in sperm banking programs, do not affect sexual function post-treatment, or the distress it may cause (Rieker, Edbril and Garnick, 1985; Moynihan, 1987; Moynihan *et al.*, in prep.), although one prospective study did find a gradual reduction of sexual problems between diagnosis and 3 years post treatment (Aass *et al.*, 1993). However, age may be a contributing factor. Men in non-seminomatous and seminoma groups were found to have similar levels of sexual dysfunction (Schover and von Eschenbach, 1985; Schover, Gonzaleo and von Eschenbach, 1986). When the younger non-seminomatous group were compared with a well-matched control group, significantly higher rates in the former were recorded in the category of sexual inactivity only (Schover, Gonzaleo and von Eschenbach, 1986). However, when the older seminoma patients were compared with the same control group, they were found to have significantly **higher** rates of reduced sexual desire, erectile dysfunction and difficulty reaching orgasm (Schover, 1987). Differences may represent ageing effects rather than the effects of cancer treatment.

Sexual performance distress was more frequent in younger men and in those who concealed their emotions (making it more difficult to expose their problems) (Rieker, Edbril and Garnick, 1985). In turn, they were significantly more likely to come from lower income and educational groups and to suffer elevated moods states (Rieker, Edbril and

Garnick, 1985). Orgasmic difficulties and erectile dysfunction were found to be more common in men worried about sexuality (Schover and von Eschenbach, 1985). Men with sexual dysfunction (including infertility distress) reported a higher rate of negative mental outlook and were twice as likely to experience negative marital relationships (Rieker, Edbril and Garnick, 1985).

31.3.5 INFERTILITY DISTRESS POST-TREATMENT

Overall rates of distress due to infertility range from 7 (Schover, 1987) to 31% (Rieker, Edbril and Garnick, 1985; Moynihan *et al.*, in prep.). Differences appear to be related to differing treatment modalities, although scrutiny of data reveals additional associated factors. In the USA, the lowest rates of distress were found in seminoma patients treated with radiotherapy (Rieker, Edbril and Garnick, 1985; Schover and von Eschenbach, 1985) and the highest among those who had RPLND and chemotherapy (Rieker, Edbril and Garnick, 1985; Schover and von Eschenbach, 1985; Rieker, *et al.*, 1989).

Seminoma patients were, however, older than their non-seminoma counterparts and therefore more likely to have completed their families. This substantiates the overall consensus that younger, childless men were more likely to suffer infertility distress (Rieker, Edbril and Garnick, 1985; Schover and von Eschenbach, 1985; Rieker *et al.*, 1989; Gritz *et al.*, 1990), regardless of time elapsed since treatment (Rieker, Edbril and Garnick, 1985) or whether sperm was banked (Rieker, Edbril and Garnick, 1985), although childless men were more likely to have done the latter (Gritz *et al.*, 1990).

Age, however, was not a constant related factor. When tabulated separately within parental status groups, the univariate association between age and distress disappeared, suggesting that childlessness was the predominating factor of infertility distress (Rieker, Edbril and Garnick, 1985; Gritz *et al.*, 1990).

This finding was not confirmed in a UK study (Moynihan, 1987). Infertility perceived by the patient as a problem was not related to psychological distress, nor the latter to childlessness. Distress was more likely among those patients with children, especially if they had been affected by unemployment. In a later UK prospective study, infertility distress at 1 year was not associated with treatment, histology, number of children, age or educational levels. However, unskilled workers were significantly less likely to change in terms of the infertility distress experienced at diagnosis (Moynihan *et al.*, in prep.). In other studies, infertility distress was found to be significantly associated with low socio-economic and educational groups (Rieker, Edbril and Garnick, 1985), a conflicting marriage at an early stage of a man's cancer experience (Schover and von Eschenbach, 1985), negative changes in close interpersonal relationships (Rieker, Edbril and Garnick, 1985) and low self-esteem (Schover and von Eschenbach, 1985). A man's plight cannot be helped by concomitant psychological distress experienced by older childless spouses (≥31 years) (Moynihan, 1987).

It can be said with certainty that both sexual dysfunction and infertility distress cause profound difficulties for a minority of men.

31.4 SOCIAL ISSUES

31.4.1 MARITAL RELATIONSHIPS AND SOCIAL SUPPORT

Divorce rates were similar to those in the general population (Rieker, Edbril and Garnick, 1985; Moynihan, 1987; Rieker *et al.*, 1989). Indeed, marriages were, in the majority, perceived as strengthened by the cancer experience (Rieker, Edbril and Garnick, 1985; Cassileth and Steinfeld, 1987; Gritz, Wellisch and Wang, 1989b; Kaasa *et al.*, 1989; Rieker

et al., 1989; Gritz *et al.*, 1990), although lover relationships were more likely to become strained (Rieker *et al.*, 1989). Those men who reported strained relationships or had divorced, attributed this to sexual dysfunction and other cancer anxieties after treatment (Schover and von Eschenbach, 1985; Rieker *et al.*, 1989).

Reported rates of conflict differ. In one sample (Schover *et al.*, 1986) 8% of those who remained married reported interference due to cancer, compared with 39% who had divorced. Lower figures of conflict were reported in another study (Gritz *et al.*, 1990). Only 12% reported disharmony with high concordance between partners. However, the latter study did not include evaluations of those who had divorced or separated, thus lowering the prevalence of negative response.

The influence of the illness on marital relations, was independent of histological difference in a few studies (Rieker, Edbril and Garnick, 1985; Moynihan, 1987; Gritz *et al.*, 1990) and not in others (Schover and von Eschenbach, 1984, 1985; Schover, Gonzaleo and von Eschenbach, 1986). Short marriages among non-seminomatous patients were found to be more vulnerable and conflict was attributed mainly to infertility or sexual problems (Schover and von Eschenbach, 1984, 1985; Schover, Gonzaleo and von Eschenbach, 1986), although a loss of the expected role in a partnership was shown to cause strain (Schover and von Eschenbach, 1984, 1985). Unhappy relationships among seminoma patients were more prone to disruption, although the length of marriage was not a predictor of conflict (Schover, Gonzaleo and von Eschenbach, 1986).

Data on the psychological morbidity among partners and relatives are scarce. While it was reported to be at the rate of 22% in one study and significantly associated with childless wives (Moynihan, 1987), no undue distress was found in another study investigating dysfunction between partners (Gritz *et al.*,

1990). However, wives in the latter sample had completed their families.

While significant correlations between patient and spouse scores were seen for depression and anxiety (Gritz *et al.*, 1990), a high quality of communication between patients and spouses was reported and a special 'bonding' between patients and their partners was observed (Cassileth and Steinfeld, 1987; Gritz *et al.*, 1990). Data revealed a high beneficial level of relative partner and hospital support during and post treatment (Moynihan, 1987; Gritz *et al.*, 1990), although the partners' diligence was perceived by patients to diminish as time went by, despite the maintenance of its quality (Gritz *et al.*, 1990). Partners and relatives reported a need for inclusion, knowledge and general support throughout their ordeal (Moynihan, 1987).

31.4.2 EMPLOYMENT EXPERIENCE

A man's cancer experience does not appear to disrupt his career and work life seriously. Most men continued with educational plans and career goals (Rieker, Edbril and Garnick, 1985; Trump *et al.*, 1985; Moynihan, 1987; Reiker *et al.*, 1989; Stoter *et al.*, 1989; Edbril and Rieker, 1990), apparently without discrimination (Rieker, Edbril and Garnick, 1985; Edbril and Rieker, 1990).

A significant minority, however, experienced a negative impact in their work lives (Rieker, Edbril and Garnick, 1985; Moynihan, 1987; Edbril and Rieker, 1990). General dissatisfaction, a lack of confidence to handle strenuous work, the psychological stress of a job, an inability to work for long periods, apprehension about making further work plans, general worries about job maintenance (Moynihan, 1987; Edbril and Rieker, 1990) and worries about medical insurance and adequate medical benefits (Edbril and Rieker, 1990) helped to contribute to a negative impact in this area.

Whilst a prospective study has shown unemployment to be negligible among this group at 1 year post diagnosis and was not associated with psychological status (Moynihan *et al.*, in press), a retrospective study (Moynihan, 1987) reported a 26% rate of job loss over a 5-year period, and a 9% rate of current unemployment to be significantly associated with psychological symptoms and lower social status. While a man's psychological well-being was reinforced by employment status (Moynihan, 1987), (a factor substantiated by anecdotal evidence), data suggest that a simple return to work is not necessarily a useful indicator of patient well-being (Edbril and Rieker, 1990). Job dissatisfaction was evident and found to be significantly associated with anxiety, depression and fatigue, although satisfied workmen also exhibited psychological distress (Edbril and Rieker, 1990). The latter group were, however, unable to disclose emotions and were traditional in terms of masculine ideals, suggesting a need to overcompensate for physical and psychological loss through an overt expression of job satisfaction and security. Job satisfaction does not, however, preclude **the fear** of job loss or discrimination at work (Warr, 1984; Moynihan, 1987), which may account, in part, for the distress experienced by 'satisfied' workers.

Although it was not found to be a contributory factor in employment status (Moynihan, 1987), disclosure of cancer to employers was sometimes perceived as a jeopardizing strategy (Edbril and Rieker, 1990). Only 50% of unskilled labourers and 'the majority' of men in other occupational groups disclosed their cancer, implying fear or shame. Thus, the extent of discrimination as a result of cancer is difficult to assess.

Other less subtle aspects of employment include financial and social status. Those who had financial difficulties and were in low-income groups were more likely to be unemployed and suffer psychological distress, especially when there were children in the family (Moynihan, 1987).

Differences in results of unemployment and its ensuing distress may lie in political and cultural factors. Unemployment was high in the UK during the time of and preceding one study (Moynihan, 1987). This highlights the importance of considering the dynamics of change in all aspects of psychosocial research.

31.5 SUGGESTIONS FOR COUNSELING INTERVENTION

Counseling is advocated for the minority of men who suffer adverse psychosocial sequelae as a result of testicular cancer (Schover and von Eschenbach, 1984, 1985; Edbril and Rieker, 1985; Malec, Romsaas and Trump, 1985; Rieker, Edbril and Garnick, 1985; Schover, Gonzaleo and von Eschenbach, 1986; Moynihan, 1987; Fosså, Aass and Kaalhus, 1988; Gritz, Wellisch and Landsrerk, 1989; Gritz, Wellisch and Wang, 1989; Kaasa *et al.*, 1989; Rieker *et al.*, 1989). The literature depicts a diffuse profile of the patient in need of support. He is **likely** to be young, without social or marital support and of low income and educational groups. He may be unemployed, although employment *per se* may not necessarily be the sole indicator of a man's adjustment. He may be infertile or apprehend that state and he may suffer sexual dysfunction in varying degrees, especially if he has undergone aggressive treatments. However, the latter may not necessarily be the cause of distress. Those patients who have entered a 'watch and see' policy are just as likely to suffer psychological morbidity as others and may need help to surmount the 'Sword of Damacles' syndrome. However, many men will invariably be fearing that cancer will return, even years after treatment has ended. Anxieties may not be overt because of a propensity to conceal emotions.

It is recognized that men do not usually seek counseling services to deal with their distress (Edbril and Rieker, 1985). However, a prospective trial of a psychological therapy

with testicular cancer patients revealed that 40% ($n = 73$) agreed to be randomized (Moynihan *et al.*, in press). This did not necessarily depend on high levels of psychological morbidity. Moreover, patients who refused counseling were similar to those who took part with respect to age, marital status and social class. Patients with early stage disease, many of whom were in a surveillance program, were more likely to decline the intervention and had lower psychological and physical morbidity. Thus a blanket offer need not be instigated although it is important that clinicians and other interested parties initiate discussions (Rieker, Edbril and Garnick, 1985; Cassileth and Steinfeld, 1987; Moynihan, 1987), especially with young single men who may find it difficult to expose their feelings (Fosså, Aass and Kaalhus, 1988), particularly when sexuality may be an issue (Aass *et al.*, 1993). Although transient states may not warrant formal psychological intervention, and may even be healthy at initial diagnosis (Greer, 1985), clinicians can undertake a significant preventative service by giving accurate information about aspects of the patients' disease at a very early stage (Cassileth and Steinfeld, 1987; Moynihan *et al.*, in press). Justified reassurances greatly help to quell initial fears (Moynihan *et al.*, in press) and a reiteration of facts, post-treatment, will help to reinforce a status of well-being (Cassileth and Steinfeld, 1987; Moynihan *et al.*, in press).

Adequate information may also enhance follow-up compliance. This is particularly important for those in the surveillance group: strict adherence to regular checks is of paramount importance, but at the same time difficult to bear (Moynihan, 1987).

Infertility fears and problems may arise early and an intervention of counseling, prior to treatment, may help to alleviate future distress of a graver kind. Men of low socio-economic and educational groups may require additional help in this area (Rieker, Edbril and Garnick, 1985).

Some men may not be candidates for sperm

banking. While banking does not appear to enhance psychological well-being (Rieker, Edbril and Garnick, 1985; Moynihan, 1987), this finding may mask untapped anxieties only superseded by the cancer experience itself. Counseling should be given, especially to young and childless men and those undergoing aggressive treatment regimens (Schover and von Eschenbach, 1984).

Older (≥30) childless women (Moynihan, 1987) and couples who anticipate the normalcy of children (Schover, Gonzaleo and von Eschenbach, 1986) may be in particular need of support. Alternative options such as AID may wish to be explored when treatment is over (Schover, Gonzaleo and von Eschenbach, 1986). This important decision is often initially met with negative reactions by both men and their partners (Schover, Gonzaleo and von Eschenbach, 1986). Men may feel jealous: women guilty of manipulation and a sense of betrayal. Despite the potential of infertility, many patients and their partners require contraceptive counseling, especially up to 1 or 2 years posttreatment (Schover, Gonzaleo and von Eschenbach, 1986).

To-date, little research has focused on the well-being of children of parents with cancer. Attention to children's needs are particularly apposite in the population of testicular cancer patients, and, if possible, this most important area of potential disruption should be addressed in future research. Anecdotal evidence suggests that children benefit from open but sensitive discussions and accessibility to their sick father.

Although it has been found that the majority of men do not wish for a prosthesis (Moynihan, 1987), some men feel less attractive as a result of surgery (Gritz *et al.*, 1990) and this option should, if possible, be put forward as early as possible. Young men and those without sexual partners may feel particularly vulnerable about this aspect of their bodies.

Body image changes such as hair loss and scarring are sometimes perceived as stressful during and in some cases post-treatment, especially in patients who have undergone RPLND and chemotherapy (Gritz, Wellisch and Wang, 1989). Although partners are significantly less affected by such changes than the patients themselves, a certain amount of patient/partner concordance exists in areas of perceived unattractiveness, especially in those patients who have had chemotherapy (Gritz, Wellisch and Wang, 1989). Such patients and their partners may require counseling to help them with the effect these adverse responses may have on both short- and long-term marital and sexual relationships.

Sexual difficulties experienced at an early stage and during treatment may result in future dysfunction of a more serious kind. There is evidence that, if left untreated, resolution is not easy (Maguire, Lee and Bevington, 1978). If psychosexual difficulties arise, the techniques of sexual therapy, especially in the form of cognitive behavioral interventions, may be readily applied to, for example, loss of libido and orgasm problems experienced by testicular cancer patients (Schover and von Eschenbach, 1985).

Sexual counseling should, if possible, be extended to the special problems of the partners of men. The fear of venereal contagion is documented (Schover, Gonzaleo and von Eschenbach, 1986; Moynihan, 1987) and partners are reported to avoid sexual relationships (albeit for a short time) (Gritz, Wellisch and Wang, 1989). This may, in part, be due to fear. The unfounded idea of a causal link between sex and cancer can be explained, even to those couples in high social class and educational groups (Gritz, Wellisch and Wang, 1989).

Employment should not be the sole indicator of well-being (Edbril and Rieker, 1990). Employment status is, however, an important factor in the lives of these men, especially as unemployment or the fear of redundancy are linked with psychological distress (Warr, 1984; Moynihan, 1987). Those in lower social class groups, experiencing financial problems, with or without children to support, may be especially vulnerable and may need a counseling intervention for employment and related problems.

The importance of open communication to good adjustment is documented (Maguire *et al.*, 1983; Greer and Morrey, 1987). However, patients find it difficult to voice anxieties, both in clinical settings (Rieker, Edbril and Garnick, 1985; Moynihan, 1987; Fosså, Aass and Kaalhus, 1988; Riecker *et al.*, 1989) and within close family circles (Moynihan, 1987). Moreover, relatives have voiced their sense of helplessness but feel intrusive in their quest for knowledge (Moynihan, 1987). Thus, a psychological intervention should attempt to improve communication between all parties concerned.

Open discussions with clinicians and active participation by patients in their treatment decisions when possible, and if desired, will contribute towards a sense of reassurance and personal control (Cassileth and Steinfeld, 1987), and, at the same time, help to alleviate communication problems which may exist between patients and their partners or relatives over treatment and related decisions.

An individual psychological intervention at an early stage of the cancer experience was a preference made by a group of testicular cancer patients who had been 'cured' (Moynihan, 1987). Those patients who entered a randomized trial of Adjuvant Psychological Therapy (APT) – a cognitive behavioral approach (Morrey and Greer, 1989) and who had received their diagnosis 4 to 8 weeks previously were shown to benefit 8 weeks after counseling had started. This was a time when men were undergoing aggressive treatment regimens. Differences between the counseled group and controls had disappeared at 4 months and 1 year (Moynihan *et al.*, in press) following a median of three sessions. Indeed, at 1 year post-diagnosis, the control group displayed greater reductions of anxiety from baseline than did the counseled group, suggesting that either a protracted counsel-

ing intervention may have been necessary or that men who are not suffering from clinical psychological morbidity may benefit from a more 'client centered approach' where the focus is primarily on the expression of emotions (Schut, de Keijser and van den Bout, 1991). Although an early intervention appears to provide benefit, it should not be forgotten that some patients also feel bereft after treatment has ended (Moynihan, 1987; Moynihan, *et al* in press).

31.6 DISCUSSION

All the studies cited indicate that testicular cancer patients experience positive and, in a minority of cases, negative psychosocial sequelae. While there are varying degrees of psychosocial morbidity which may be due to factors such as age, socioeconomic status, unemployment and treatment regimens, especially as the latter relates to psychosexual functioning, differing methods used by researchers may also account for the wide differences found in the range and intensity of psychosocial morbidity. Moreover, there are wide discrepancies in study design. Caution should therefore be exercised when comparing results.

All long-term follow-up studies differ greatly in terms of time since treatment ended with ranges of '6 months or more' (Malec, Romsaas and Trump, 1985; Nijman *et al.*, 1987), to 20 years (Cassileth and Steinfeld, 1987). Although data indicate that time was making no difference to the rate of psychological morbidity (Rieker, Edbril and Garnick, 1985; Moynihan, 1987; Rieker *et al.*, 1989), other findings suggest that psychological sequelae were more evident immediately post-treatment than they were at interview (Clark and Reswick, 1978; Gritz, Wellisch and Landsrerk, 1989).

The time span prior to the evaluation of mood states may have an effect on results (Huisman *et al.*, 1987). For example, a time frame of 1 week (Fosså, Aass and Kaalhus,

1988) may produce very different responses when compared with results of a time span of 1 month (Rieker, Edbril and Garnick, 1985; Moynihan, 1987; Nijman *et al.*, 1987; Gritz, Wellisch and Wang, 1989) or 6 months (Kaasa *et al.*, 1989). Little reference is made to pre-morbid adjustment.

When morbidity is measured 'at diagnosis', patients' knowledge of their disease is seldom explicit (Trump *et al.*, 1985; Fosså, Aass and Kaalhus, 1988). Without defining what is meant by 'at diagnosis' and 'before treatment', the extent and severity of emotional states at this critical time may go unnoticed and therefore untreated.

Many studies have relied on small numbers (Tross *et al.*, 1984; Malec, Romsaas and Trump, 1985; Schover and von Eschenbach, 1985; Trump *et al.*, 1985; Cassileth and Steinfeld, 1987; Schover, 1987; Blackmore, 1988; Stoter *et al.*, 1989) and a univariate analysis (Malec, Romsaas and Trump, 1985; Schover and von Eschenbach, 1985; Cassileth and Steinfeld, 1987; Schover, 1987; Blackmore, 1988; Fosså, Aass and Kaalhus, 1988; Gritz, Wellisch and Landsrerk, 1989; Gritz, Wellisch and Wang, 1989; Stoter, Gonzaleo and von Eschenbach, 1989). Furthermore, important confounding variables have not been controlled for (Cassileth and Steinfeld, 1987; Kaasa *et al.*, 1989; Stoter *et al.*, 1989). While two studies have used objective psychological measures (Tross *et al.*, 1984; Moynihan, 1987) others rely on self-administered responses (Malec, Romsaas and Trump, 1985; Rieker, Edbril and Garnick, 1985; Trump *et al.*, 1985; Cassileth and Steinfeld, 1987; Fosså, Aass and Kaalhus, 1988; Gritz, Wellisch and Landsrerk, 1989; Kaasa *et al.*, 1989; Rieker, Edbril and Garnick, 1985). Unvalidated instruments are sometimes used to measure psychological (Fosså, Aass and Kaalhus, 1988; Kaasa *et al.*, 1989; Stoter *et al.*, 1989), sexual (Rieker, Edbril and Garnick, 1985; Cassileth and Steinfeld, 1987; Moynihan, 1987; Fosså, Aass and Kaalhus, 1988; Kaasa *et al.*, 1989; Rieker *et al.*, 1989), and social dysfunction (Rieker, Edbril and Garnick, 1985; Cassileth and Steinfeld, 1987; Moynihan, 1987; Kaasa *et al.*, 1989; Rieker *et al.*, 1989; Stoter *et al.*, 1989). One retrospective study relied on open-ended questioning as well as standardized measures to assess sexual and social function (Moynihan, 1987). When validated measures are used to measure psychological status, or sexual function, they are often recommended for psychiatric populations (Malec, Romsaas and Trump, 1985) or those with sexual problems (Trump *et al.*, 1985; Blackmore, 1988). Thus high scores are often a reflection of extreme concern over physical functioning and poor health.

When testicular cancer groups are compared with comparison groups, a picture of psychological well-being emerges. Such optimistic findings must be read with a certain amount of caution. When the POMS score has been used to compare testicular tumor patients with other cancer groups or psychiatric patients (Rieker, Edbril and Garnick, 1985; Cassileth and Steinfeld, 1987; Gritz, Wellisch and Landsrerk, 1989; Rieker *et al.*, 1989) the confirmed association between physical symptoms and this measure of morbidity must be recognized. It is difficult, therefore, to distinguish between physiological states and anxiety and depression over cancer itself. As one report (Rieker, Edbril and Garnick, 1985) points out, patients with testicular cancer experience little physical disability compared with other types of cancer (or indeed, psychiatric patients). This would, in part, explain the consistent well-being reported in studies using this measure. Furthermore, a comparison of cancer patients' scores with the scores of college students (Rieker, Edbril and Garnick, 1985; Cassileth and Steinfeld, 1987; Gritz, Wellisch and Landsrerk, 1989; Rieker *et al.*, 1989), the 'normal population' (Fosså, Aass and Kaalhus, 1988; Kaasa *et al.*, 1989) or self-selected groups (Rieker, Edbril and Garnick, 1985) are misleading because of obvious differences in circumstances.

These optimistic findings may also be due

to judgements based on an adaptation level influenced by the experience of having cancer (de Haes and Knippenberg, 1987). Cancer patients may have experienced more negative stimuli and their neutral point on a verbal rating scale may refer to a more negative objective situation. Thus, more positive judgements may be made by cancer patients compared with other populations.

Rigorous methodology must be applied if differing treatment modalities are to be assessed in their relation to psychological morbidity (or other psychosocial factors) (Schipper and Clinch, 1988). For example, differences between the times of evaluation of treatment groups may bias results. This issue is addressed by one study (Fosså, Aass and Kaalhus, 1988) in which the chemotherapy group was evaluated **before** the start of the fourth cycle. Acute toxicity and ensuing psychological morbidity may have been higher if the evaluation had been carried out immediately **after** it. Radiotherapy patients were evaluated during treatment and the surgery group during discharge.

Caution should be demonstrated. At the present time 'counseling' is presented as a panacea of good medical practice. However, systematic evaluation of its efficacy must be demonstrated as well as clear descriptions of the counseling intervention to be deployed. Validated and reliable measures that are sensitive to change and the very special needs of testicular cancer patients within their cultural contexts will provide an essential basis for psychological intervention and an evaluation of its implementation. The triumphs achieved by these men warrant our efforts to help them to attain a quality of life which would embrace self-esteem, sexual pleasure and family closeness.

REFERENCES

Aass, N., Fosså, S.D., Otto, F. *et al.* (1989) Acute subjective morbidity after cisplatin based combination chemotherapy in patients with testicular cancer: a prospective study. *Radiother. Oncol.,* **14**, 27–33.

Aass, N., Grunfeld, B., Kaalhus, O. and Fosså, S.D. (1993) Pre and post treatment sexual life in testicular cancer patients: a descriptive investigation. *Brit. J. Cancer,* **76**, 1113–17.

Anderson, B.L. (1986) Sexual difficulties for women following cancer treatment, in *Women with Cancer* (ed. B.L. Anderson), Springer, New York, pp. 233–56.

Blackmore, C. (1988) The impact of orchidectomy upon the sexuality of the man with testicular cancer. *Cancer Nursing,* **11**, 33–40.

Cassileth, B. and Steinfeld, A. (1987) Pyschological preparation of the patient and family. *Cancer,* **60**, 547–52.

Clark, S. and Reswick, M. (1978) Infertility following radiation and chemotherapy. *Urol. Clin. North Am.,* **5**, 531–5.

Cox, T. and Mackay, C. (1982) Pyschosocial factors and pyscho-physiological mechanisms in the aetiology and development of cancers. *Soc. Sci. Med.,* **16**, 381–96.

de Haes, J.C. and Knippenberg, F.C. (1987) Quality of life of cancer patients: review of the literature, in *The Quality of Life of Cancer Patients* (eds N.K. Aaronson and J. Beckman), Raven Press, New York, **17**, pp. 167–82.

Dean, C., Chetty, V., Forrest, A.M.P. *et al.* (1983) Effects of immediate breast reconstruction on pyschosocial morbidity after mastectomy. *Lancet,* **i**, 459–62.

Devlin, H.B., Plant, J.A., Griffin, N. *et al.* (1971) Aftermath of surgery for anorectal cancer. *BMJ,* **3**, 413–18.

Drasga, R.E., Einhorn, L.H., Williams, S.D. *et al.*, (1983) Fertility after chemotherapy for testicular cancer. *J. Clin. Oncol.,* **1**, 179–83.

Edbril, S. and Rieker, P. (1985) Fertility issues facing testis cancer survivors. Paper presented at the meeting of the American Psychological Association, Los Angeles.

Edbril, S. and Rieker, P. (1990) The impact of testicular cancer on the worklives of survivors. *J. Psychosoc. Oncol.,* **7**(3), 17–20.

Feldman, J.G., Saunders, M., Carter, A.C. *et al.* (1982) Work and cancer health histories, in *Psychosocial Aspects of Cancer* (eds J. Cohen, J.W. Cullen and L.R. Martin), Raven Press, New York, pp. 199–208.

Fobair, R., Hoppe, R., Bloom, J. *et al.* (1986) Psychosocial problems among survivors of Hodgkin's disease. *J. Clin. Oncol.,* **4**, 805–14.

Forester, B.M., Kornfeld, R.S. and Fleiss, J. (1978) Psychiatric aspects of radiotherapy, *Am. J. Pysch.*, **135**, 960–3.

Fosså, S., Aass, N., Kaalhus, O. (1988) Testicular cancer in young Norwegians. *J. Surg. Oncol.*, **39**, 43–63.

Goldberg, R. and Cullen, L.O. (1985) Factors important to psychosocial adjustment to cancer: A review of the evidence. *Soc. Sci. Med.*, **20**, 803–7.

Greer, S. (1983) Cancer and the mind. *Br. J. Psych.*, **143**, 535–43.

Greer, S. (1985) Cancer: psychiatric aspects, in *Recent Advances in Clinical Psychiatry* (ed. K. Granville-Crossman), Churchill Livingstone, Edinburgh, pp. 87–104.

Greer, S. and Morrey, S. (1987) Adjuvant psychological therapy for patients with cancer. *Eur. J. Surg. Oncol.*, **13**, 511–16.

Gritz, E.R., Wellisch, D.K. and Landsrerk, J.A. (1989) Psychosocial sequelae in long-term survivors of testicular cancer. *J. Psychosoc. Oncol.*, **6**, 41–63.

Gritz, E.R., Wellisch, D.K., Sian, J. and Wang, H.J. (1990) Long term effects of testicular cancer on marital relationships. *Psychosomatics*, **31**(3), 301–12.

Gritz, E.R., Wellisch, D.K. and Wang, H.J. (1989) Long term effects of testicular cancer on sexual functioning in married couples. *Cancer*, **64**, 1560–7.

Herr, H.W. (1987) Quality of life measurement in testicular cancer patients. *Cancer*, **60**, 1412–14.

Hughes, J. (1987) Psychological and social consequences of cancer. *Cancer Surveys*, **6**, 455–76.

Huisman, S., van Dam, F., Aaronson, N. *et al.*, (1987) On measuring complaints of cancer patients: some remarks on the time span of the question, in *The Quality of Life of Cancer Patients* (eds N. Aarons and J. Beckmann), Raven Press, New York, **17**, 101–10.

Kaasa, S., Aass, N., Mastekaasa, A. *et al.* (1989) Psychological well being in patients cured for testicular cancer. Paper given at the British Psychological Oncology Group and the European Society for Psychosocial Oncology Meeting, Royal College of Physicians, London.

Kedia, K.R., Morkland, C. and Frayley, E.E. (1977) Sexual function after high retroperitoneal lymphadenectomy. *Urol. Clin. North. Am.*, **4**, 523–7.

Lange, P.H., Narayan, P., Vogelzang, N.J. *et al.* (1983) Return of fertility after treatment for nonseminomatous testicular cancer: changing concepts. *J. Urol.*, **129**, 1131–5.

Maguire, P., Brooke, M., Tait, A. *et al.* (1983) The effect of counselling on physical disability and social recovery after mastectomy. *Clin. Oncol.*, **9**, 319–24.

Maguire, G.P., Lee, E.G., Bevington, D.J. (1978) Psychiatric problems in the first year after mastectomy. *BMJ*, **1**, 963–5.

Maher, E.L. (1982) Anomic aspects of recovery from cancer. *Social Science and Medicine*, **16**, 907–12.

Malec, J.F., Romsaas, M.S. and Trump, M.D. (1985) Psychological and personality disturbance among patients with testicular cancer. *J. Psychosoc. Oncol.*, **3**, 55–64.

McIntosh, J. (1974) Process of communication, information seeking and control associated with cancer. *Social Science and Medicine*, **8**, 167–87.

McNair, D.N., Lorr, M. and Droppleman, L.F. (1981) *Profile of Mood States* (2nd edn) Santiago Educational and Industrial Testing Service.

Morrey, S. and Greer, S. (1989) *Psychological Therapy for Patients with Cancer: a New Approach.* Heinemann Medical Books, Oxford.

Morgan, G. (ed.) (1983) *Beyond Method*, Sage, Beverley Hills.

Moynihan, C.M. (1987) Testicular cancer: the psychosocial problems of patients and their relatives. *Cancer Surveys*, **6**, 477–510.

Moynihan, C., Bliss, J. Davidson, J., Burchell, L. and Horwich, A. A prospective study on the psychosocial aspects of testicular cancer and an evaluation of a psychological intervention. *BMJ* (in preparation).

Narayan, P., Lange, P.H. and Frayley, E.E. (1982) Ejaculation and fertility after extended retroperitoneal lymph node dissection for testicular cancer. *J. Urol.*, **127**, 685–8.

Nijman, J.M., Schraffordt Koops, H., Oldhoff, J. *et al.* (1987) Sexual function after surgery and combination chemotherapy in men with disseminated non-seminomatous testicular cancer, in *Some Aspects of Sexual Gonadal Function in Patients with a Non-seminomatous Germ Cell Tumour of the Testis* (ed. J.M. Nijman), Drukkerij van Denderen B.V. Groningen, pp. 39–45.

Rieker, P., Edbril, S.D. and Garnick, M.B. (1985) Curative testis cancer therapy: psychosocial sequelae. *J. Clin. Oncol.*, **3**, 1117–26.

Rieker, P., Fitzgerald, E.M., Kalish, L.A. *et al.* (1989) Psychosocial factors, curative therapies and behavioural outcomes: a comparison of testis cancer survivors and a control group of healthy men. *Cancer*, **64**, 2399–407.

Schipper, H. and Clinch, J. (1988) Assessment of treatment in cancer, in *Measuring Health: A Practical Approach* (ed. G. Teeling Smith), John Wiley, Chichester, pp. 109–55.

Schmale, A.H., Morrow, G.P., Schmitt, M.H. *et al.* (1983) The well being of cancer survivors. *Psychosomatic Med.*, **45**, 163–9.

Schover, L.R. (1987) Sexuality and fertility in urologic cancer patients. *Cancer*, **60**, 553–8.

Schover, L.R. and von Eschenbach, A.C. (1984) Sexual and marital counselling with men treated for testicular cancer. *J. Sex. and Marital Ther.*, **10**, 29–40.

Schover, L. and von Eschenbach, A. (1985). Sexual and marital relationships after treatment for non-seminomatous testicular cancer. *Urology*, **45**, 251–5.

Schover, L., Gonzaleo, M. and von Eschenbach, A. (1986) Sexual and marital relations after radiotherapy for seminoma. *Urology*, **29**, 117–23.

Schut, H.A., de Keijser, J. and van den Bout, J. (1991) A controlled efficacy study into short term individual counselling. Client variables. Paper presented to the Third International Conference on Grief and Bereavement in Contemporary Society, Sydney, Australia. June 30–July 4 1992 and personal communication.

Silberfarb, P.M. (1980) Psychosocial aspects of neoplastic disease. Functional status of breast cancer patients during different treatment regimes. *Am. J. Psychiatry*, **137**, 450–5.

Spinetta, J.J. (1982) A guide to psychosocial field research in cancer, in *Psychosocial Aspects of Cancer* (eds. J.W. Cohen, J.W. Cullen and L.R. Martin), Raven Press, New York, pp. 249–54.

Stoter, G., Koopman, A., Cornelis, P.J. *et al.* (1989) Ten year survival and late sequelae in testicular cancer patients treated with cisplatin, vinblastine, bleomycin. *J. Clin. Oncol.*, **7**, 1099–104.

Thomas, S.G. (1978) Breast cancer: the psychosocial issues. *Cancer Nursing*, **1**, 53–60.

Tross, S., Holland, J.C., Bosl, G. *et al.* (1984) A controlled study of psychosocial sequelae in cured survivors of testicular neoplasms. *Proc. Am. Soc. Clin. Oncol.*, **3**, 74.

Trump, D.L., Romsaas, F., Cumings, K.C. *et al.* (1985) Assessment of psychologic and sexual dysfunction in patients following treatment of testis cancer. A prospective study. *Proc. Am. Soc. Clin. Oncol.*, **4**, 250.

Warr, P. (1984) Job loss, unemployment and psychological well being, in *Role Transitions* (eds V.L. Allen and E. van der Niert), Plenum Publishing, New York.

Watson, M. (1983) Psychosocial intervention with cancer patients: a review. *Psychol. Med.*, **13**, 839–46.

Welch-McCaffrey, D., Hoffman, B., Leigh, S. *et al.* (1989) Surviving adult cancer. Part 2: Psychosocial implications. *Ann. Intern. Med.*, **III**, 411–32.

Zigmond, A.S. and Snaith, R.P. (1983) The Hospital Anxiety and Depression Scale. *Acta Psychiatr. Scand.*, **67**, 361–70.

INDEX

Page numbers in **bold** refer to figures and page numbers in *italic* refer to tables.